Muscle Biopsy: A Clinico-Pathological Approach

Muscle Biopsy: A Clinico-Pathological Approach

Edited by Jenna Whitney

hayle medical

New York

Hayle Medical,
750 Third Avenue, 9th Floor,
New York, NY 10017, USA

Visit us on the World Wide Web at:
www.haylemedical.com

ISBN: 978-1-63241-728-2

The publisher's policy is to use permanent paper from mills that operate a sustainable forestry policy. Furthermore, the publisher ensures that the text paper and cover boards used have met acceptable environmental accreditation standards.

Printed in China.

Cataloging-in-Publication Data

Muscle biopsy : a clinico-pathological approach / edited by Jenna Whitney.
p. cm.
Includes bibliographical references and index.
ISBN 978-1-63241-728-2
1. Muscles--Biopsy. 2. Muscles--Diseases--Pathogenesis. 3. Muscles--Diseases--Diagnosis.
4. Muscles--Diseases--Treatment. I. Whitney, Jenna.
RC925.6 .M87 2019
616.74--dc23

Table of Contents

Preface

This book aims to highlight the current researches and provides a platform to further the scope of innovations in this area. This book is a product of the combined efforts of many researchers and scientists, after going through thorough studies and analysis from different parts of the world. The objective of this book is to provide the readers with the latest information of the field.

The procedure of removing a piece of muscle tissue from the body of an organism and examining it microscopically is known as muscle biopsy. The common issues discovered through a muscle biopsy include problems associated with the connective tissue, vascular system, nervous system and musculoskeletal system. Muscle biopsy is helpful in distinguishing between myopathies and neuropathies. Myopathy is a disease in which the muscle fibers do not function properly. Some of its examples include spasm, muscle cramps and stiffness in the body. In order to diagnose problems with the help of muscle biopsy, a biopsy needle is inserted into the muscle. This book elucidates the concepts and innovative models around prospective developments with respect to muscle biopsy. It strives to provide a fair idea about this discipline and to help develop a better understanding of the latest advances within this field. The extensive content of this book provides the readers with a thorough understanding of the subject.

I would like to express my sincere thanks to the authors for their dedicated efforts in the completion of this book. I acknowledge the efforts of the publisher for providing constant support. Lastly, I would like to thank my family for their support in all academic endeavors.

Editor

1

Fibre-Specific Responses to Endurance and Low Volume High Intensity Interval Training: Striking Similarities in Acute and Chronic Adaptation

Trisha D. Scribbans[1], Brittany A. Edgett[1], Kira Vorobej[2], Andrew S. Mitchell[2], Sophie D. Joanisse[3], Jennifer B. L. Matusiak[1], Gianni Parise[3], Joe Quadrilatero[2], Brendon J. Gurd[1]*

1 School of Kinesiology and Health Studies, Queen's University, Kingston, Ontario, Canada, **2** Department of Kinesiology, University of Waterloo, Waterloo, Ontario, Canada, **3** Department of Kinesiology, McMaster University, Hamilton, Ontario, Canada

Abstract

The current study involved the completion of two distinct experiments. Experiment 1 compared fibre specific and whole muscle responses to acute bouts of either low-volume high-intensity interval training (LV-HIT) or moderate-intensity continuous endurance exercise (END) in a randomized crossover design. Experiment 2 examined the impact of a six-week training intervention (END or LV-HIT; 4 days/week), on whole body and skeletal muscle fibre specific markers of aerobic and anaerobic capacity. Six recreationally active men (Age: 20.7±3.8 yrs; VO_2peak: 51.9±5.1 mL/kg/min) reported to the lab on two separate occasions for experiment 1. Following a muscle biopsy taken in a fasted state, participants completed an acute bout of each exercise protocol (LV-HIT: 8, 20-second intervals at ~170% of VO_2peak separated by 10 seconds of rest; END: 30 minutes at ~65% of VO_2peak), immediately followed by a muscle biopsy. Glycogen content of type I and IIA fibres was significantly ($p<0.05$) reduced, while p-ACC was significantly increased ($p<0.05$) following both protocols. Nineteen recreationally active males (n = 16) and females (n = 3) were VO_2peak-matched and assigned to either the LV-HIT (n = 10; 21±2 yrs) or END (n = 9; 20.7±3.8 yrs) group for experiment 2. After 6 weeks, both training protocols induced comparable increases in aerobic capacity (END: Pre: 48.3±6.0, Mid: 51.8±6.0, Post: 55.0±6.3 mL/kg/min LV-HIT: Pre: 47.9±8.1, Mid: 50.4±7.4, Post: 54.7±7.6 mL/kg/min), fibre-type specific oxidative and glycolytic capacity, glycogen and IMTG stores, and whole-muscle capillary density. Interestingly, only LV-HIT induced greater improvements in anaerobic performance and estimated whole-muscle glycolytic capacity. These results suggest that 30 minutes of END exercise at ~65% VO_2peak or 4 minutes of LV-HIT at ~170% VO_2peak induce comparable changes in the intra-myocellular environment (glycogen content and signaling activation); correspondingly, training-induced adaptations resulting for these protocols, and other HIT and END protocols are strikingly similar.

Editor: Stephen E. Alway, West Virginia University School of Medicine, United States of America

Funding: Funding was provided by the Natural Sciences and Engineering Research Council of Canada (NSERC) and the Canada Foundation for Innovation (CFI). The funders had no role in study design, data collection and analysis, decision to publish, or preparation of the manuscript.

* E-mail: gurdb@queensu.ca

Introduction

Endurance (END) training and interval training, consisting of either sprint interval training (SIT; repeated bouts of 'all out' exercise [e.g. Repeated Wingates]) or high-intensity interval training (HIT; repeated bouts of exercise below an all out intensity) result in comparable adaptations in both performance and skeletal muscle metabolism. These include: improvements in maximal oxygen uptake (VO_2peak) [1–7] and aerobic exercise performance [7–9], increases in markers of mitochondrial content, oxidative capacity [1–3,8,10], intramuscular glycogen [8] and triglyceride stores [3], capillary density [4,6,11], lipid oxidation [1,3,10], and reductions in substrate level (phosphocreatine and glycogen) phosphorylation [1]. Given the markedly reduced training dose (exercise energy expenditure and training time) associated with many high-intensity protocols, these data demonstrate the ability of high intensity exercise to induce physiological adaptations without the requirement for large training volumes.

The potency of HIT high-intensity exercise has recently been demonstrated by several studies employing a low volume- (LV) high-intensity interval training (HIT) protocol requiring a fraction of the training dose (total training time of ~4 min/day) necessary for END and many other HIT protocols. Similar to other larger dose HIT protocols, studies utilizing LV-HIT have demonstrated improvements in VO_2peak [9,12,13], anaerobic exercise capacity [12,13], and increased mitochondrial protein content (cytochrome *c* oxidase (COX) subunit I and COX IV)[13] that are equivalent to those induced by END [9,12]. While there is an abundance of literature demonstrating the efficacy of HIT at inducing adaptations, the mechanisms by which substantially lower doses of high intensity exercise induce adaptations typically associated with high dose END are not completely understood, specifically, similarities/differences in fibre-type specific adaptations induced by HIT and END have not been completely described.

Table 1. Experiment 1 participant characteristics (N = 6), mean (SD) unless otherwise indicated.

Age (yrs)	20.7(3.8)
Height (cm)	183.7(9.3)
Body mass (kg)	77.8(2.8)
Absolute VO_2 (mL/min)	4025(306)
Relative VO_2 (mL/kg/min)	51.9(5.1)
HRpeak (BPM)	196(7)
WRpeak (W)	264.1(41.6)
Mean power (W) LV-HIT (actual)	481.4(60.1)
Mean power (W) LV-HIT (prescribed)	448.0(70.5)
Mean power (W) endurance (actual)	173.7(29.8)
Mean power (W) endurance (prescribed)	172.0(27.1)

Note: LV-HIT mean power represents the average power output during the 8 intervals not including rest periods. BPM, beats per minute; cm, centimeters; kg, kilograms; min, minute; RER, respiratory exchange ratio; s, seconds; W, watts; yrs, years.

For example, several recent reports suggest that improvements in aerobic exercise capacity and performance following HIT result primarily from peripheral adaptations [14,15]. These adaptations, specifically the induction of mitochondrial biogenesis, result from the activation of signaling cascades which increase transcription of mitochondrial genes via the activation [16,17] and/or increased expression of peroxisome proliferator-activated receptor gamma co-activator 1 alpha (PGC-1α) [18]. Given that END and HIT result in similar increases in whole-muscle markers of mitochondrial content and oxidative capacity [1–3,8,10], it is not surprising that acute activation of signaling pathways, measured in whole-muscle homogenates, following a single bout of END and HIT are also comparable [19–21]. However, it is not clear if these whole-muscle measures reflect similar adaptations across distinct fibre populations within a trained muscle, or whether HIT induces adaptations in different populations of fibres. More specifically, whether the well characterized recruitment of type II fibres associated with higher intensities of exercise, including continuous supramaximal [22–24] and intermittent maximal [25] exercise result in different fibre recruitment patterns between LV-HIT and END is unknown. Further, whether variations in acute fibre recruitment result in distinctive fibre adaptations following chronic LV-HIT and END is also not known; however, it is possible that different recruitment patterns and fibre-type specific adaptations may partially explain the potency of high intensity exercise and more specifically, LV-HIT.

To examine these issues we performed 2 distinct experiments. The purpose of experiment 1 was to examine: 1) fibre recruitment patterns, as reflected by reductions in glycogen content of each fibre-type population, and 2) whole-muscle and fibre-type specific signalling pathway activation following an acute bout of LV-HIT and END exercise. The purpose of experiment 2 was to examine: 1) changes in aerobic and anaerobic exercise performance, and 2) fibre-type specific adaptations in oxidative and glycolytic capacities, substrate storage and whole-muscle capillary density resulting from 6 weeks of LV-HIT and END training. We hypothesized that an acute bout of LV-HIT would result in the activation of a greater number of type II muscle fibres than END exercise, and that resulting fibre-specific metabolic adaptations following training would reflect these differences in acute fibre recruitment.

Materials and Methods

Ethics Statement

All experimental procedures performed on human participants were approved by the Health Sciences Human Research Ethics Board at Queen's University and conformed to the Declaration of Helsinki. Verbal and written explanation of the experimental protocol and associated risks was provided to all participants prior to obtaining written informed consent.

Experimental Design

The current study involved the completion of two distinct experiments. Experiment 1 compared fibre specific and whole muscle responses to acute bouts of either low-volume high-intensity interval training (LV-HIT) or moderate-intensity continuous cycle exercise (END) in a randomized crossover design. Experiment 2 examined the impact of a six-week training intervention (END or LV-HIT 4 days/week), on whole body and skeletal muscle fibre specific markers of aerobic and anaerobic capacity. All physiological testing and training for both experiments was performed on a Monark Ergomedic 874 E stationary ergometer (Vansbro, Sweden). Participants were asked to refrain from alcohol and exercise 24 hours before, and caffeine 12 hours before all experimental days in experiment 1 and pre- and post-training testing days in experiment 2.

Experiment 1

Participants. Six recreationally active males volunteered to participate in the study (participant characteristics are presented in Table 1). No participants were involved in more than 3 hours of aerobic exercise (running, jogging, etc.) per week.

Physiological testing. On their first visit to the lab participants completed a VO_2peak incremental ramp test to exhaustion as described previously [26], and height and weight were recorded. Gas exchange was measured throughout the test with a metabolic cart (Moxus AEI Technologies, Pittsburgh, PA), with VO_2peak and heart rate (HR) peak calculated as the highest value of continuous 30 second averages for each measure during the protocol. Peak O_2 pulse was calculated by dividing absolute VO_2peak by HRpeak from the incremental ramp protocol. Work rate (WR) was collected continuously throughout the test and peak aerobic power (WRpeak) was calculated using the average WR from the last 30 seconds of the test.

Exercise interventions. Participants reported to the lab in the morning following an overnight fast (≥12 h) after consuming a standardized dinner the night before [Stouffer's Sauté Sensations Country Beef Pot Roast (540 kcal; 56 g carbohydrate (CHO), 20 g fat, 14 g protein) and 500 mL of 2% milk (260 kcal; 12 g CHO, 5 g fat, 9 g protein)]. A fasted, resting muscle biopsy (Rest) was taken from the vastus lateralis under superficial local anaesthesia (2% lidocaine, with epinephrine) using the Bergstrom needle biopsy technique [27] adapted with suction. An additional incision was made, and covered with sterile gauze, approximately 1 cm from the resting biopsy site to allow for immediate removal of the post-exercise muscle sample. Participants then rested in the lab for 30 minutes or 55 minutes before completing a bout of END or LV-HIT, respectively. Immediately following each exercise bout a second muscle biopsy was taken (Ex). The LV-HIT exercise protocol was performed as described previously [12,13]. Briefly, participants completed eight 20-second intervals at 170% of VO_2peak separated by 10 seconds of rest eight times, for a total of four-minutes. During rest periods participants cycled against no load at a cadence of their choice. The END exercise protocol consisted of 30 minutes of continuous cycling at 65% of VO_2peak. Each exercise bout was performed at the same time of day for all subjects and were performed one week apart (7 days).

Experiment 2

Participants. Nineteen recreationally active males (n = 16) and females (n = 3) volunteered to participate in this study (participant characteristics are presented in Table 1). No participants were involved in more than 3 hours of aerobic exercise (running, jogging, etc.) per week or involved in any structured training program within the past six months. Participants were VO_2peak-matched and assigned to either the LV-HIT (n = 10) or endurance (n = 9) group.

Training interventions. All participants completed training four days a week for six weeks (week 4 only had 3 training sessions due to the mid-training VO_2peak test for a total of 23 sessions). Both the LV-HIT and END training protocols were the same as those utilized in experiment 1 (see above for descriptions). Participants descended and ascended 4 flights of stairs as a warm-up prior to all training sessions. Revolutions per minute (RPM) data was collected for each training session in order to confirm training intensity.

Physiological testing. During baseline testing (Pre) participants reported to the lab in the morning following an overnight fast (≥8 h). Participants were fed a standardized breakfast [plain bagel (190 kcal; 1 g fat, 36 g CHO, 7 g protein) with 15 g of peanut butter (90 kcal; 8 g fat, 4 g CHO, 3 g protein) and 200 mL of apple juice (90 kcal; 0 g fat, 22 g CHO, 0 g protein)] and rested for 1 hour before a muscle biopsy was taken from their vastus lateralis under superficial local anaesthesia (2% lidocaine, with epinephrine) using the Bergstrom needle biopsy technique (1) adapted with suction.

Forty-eight hours following the muscle biopsy participants returned to the lab to complete a VO_2peak incremental ramp test to exhaustion as described previously [26]. Following completion of the VO_2peak test, participants rested for 30 minutes before completing a repeated Wingate protocol consisting of 2 minutes of load-less cycling followed by four 30 second Wingates (7.5% body weight), separated by 4.5 minutes of load-less cycling. RPM was collected continuously and peak (first 5 second average) and mean power (average for total 30 seconds) were determined for the first Wingate. Total work performed during all 4 Wingate bouts was also calculated. Twenty-four hours after the VO_2peak and Wingate tests, participants reported to the lab and completed a 500 kcal time to completion (TTC) trial at a self-selected cadence as quickly as possible as described previously [28,29].

A VO_2peak incremental ramp test to exhaustion was performed half way through training (Mid) on the first day of week 4 in order to adjust training loads. As a result participants only completed 3 training sessions in week 4. Post-training (Post) testing began 72 hours following the last training session of week 6 and was conducted in an identical manner as the baseline testing. (See above for details).

Immunofluorescent and Histochemical Analysis

Immunofluorescent analysis of myosin heavy chain isoforms was performed as previously described [30] using primary antibodies against myosin heavy chain (MHC) I (BA-F8), MHCIIa (SC-71), and MHCIIx (6H1) (Developmental Studies Hybridoma Bank, Iowa City, IA, USA), followed by isotype-specific fluorescent secondary antibodies. This allowed for the identification of type I (blue), type IIA (green), type IIX (red), as well as hybrid fibre types (IIAX). For all analyses type IIX and type IIAX fibres were analyzed together (type IIAX/IIX) given their relatively low percentage. Fibre type composition was determined by counting all fibres within a muscle cross-section.

Quantification of capillary density [31] and fibre-type specific phosphorylated-AMP-activated protein kinase alpha (p-AMPKα) [32] was adapted from previous work. Briefly, sections were fixed in 4% paraformaldehyde for 10 minutes, followed by permeabilization with 0.5% TritonX-100 for 30 minutes, and then blocked in 10% goat serum for 30 minutes. Sections were incubated overnight in 5% goat serum with the appropriate primary antibodies specific for the endothelium (PECAM) and sarcolemma (dystrophin) (Developmental Studies Hybridoma Bank, Iowa City, IA, USA) or p-AMPKα (Thr^{172}) (Cell Signaling Technology, Danvers, MA, USA). After 3×5 minute washes in PBS, sections were incubated for 1 hour in 5% goat serum with the appropriate fluorescent secondary antibodies (Life Technologies, Burlington, ON, CA).

For all immunofluorescent procedures, sections were mounted with Prolong Gold Antifade Reagent (Life Technologies, Burlington, ON, CA) and imaged the following day. All sections were visualized with an Axio Observer Z1 microscope (Carl Zeiss, Jena, TH, DE). Individual images were taken across the entire muscle cross-section and assembled into a composite panoramic image using AxioVision software (Carl Zeiss). Compiled images were matched to fibre-type images and ~30 of each fibre type were randomly selected and analyzed. Data were expressed relative to the values obtained in type I fibers, which were assigned a reference value of 1.0, and reported as mean optical density in arbitrary units (AU). This method was utilized for all immunofluorescent and histochemical analyses except for the determination of capillary density where 3 separate areas per sample were analyzed for number of capillaries. Fibre-specific p-AMPKα fluorescence was performed in ImageJ (National Institutes of Health, Bethesda, MD, USA) and was determined by subtracting the average fluorescence of the slide background (>5 per slide) from each individual fibre's fluorescence.

As a general indicator of oxidative and glycolytic potential, histochemical staining for succinate dehydrogenase (SDH) [33] and α-glycerophosphate dehydrogenase (GPD) [34] activity was performed [30]. Intramuscular triglyceride (IMTG) content was determined with Oil Red O (ORO) staining [35], whereas glycogen content was determined using the Periodic Acid Schiff (PAS) [36]. Images were acquired with a bright field Nikon microscope linked to a PixelLink digital camera. Individual images were taken across the entire muscle cross-section and assembled

Table 2. Quantitative RT-PCR primer sequences.

	Forward Primer	Reverse Primer
PGC-1α	Cacttacaagccaaaccaacaact	caatagtcttgttctcaaatgggga
SIRT1	Agaacatagacacgctggaaca	caagatgctgttgcaaaggaacc
GCN5	Aaggaccccgaccagctcta	gggaagcggatgacctcgta
RIP140	Gttccactcagcccagcagt	agaccctgcacagcccaagt
GAPDH	cctcctgcaccaccaactgctt	gaggggccatccacagtcttct

Note: GAPDH, glyceraldehyde 3-phosphate dehydrogenase; GCN5, general control non-derepressible 5; PGC-1α, peroxisome proliferator-activated receptor gamma coactivator 1 alpha; RIP140, receptor-interacting protein 140; SIRT1, silent mating type information regulation 2 homolog 1.

into a composite panoramic image using Microsoft Image Composite Editor (ICE) (Microsoft, Redmond, WA, USA). Image analysis was performed in ImageJ by converting color images to 8-bit, and calculated by subtracting background staining from the mean grey value of individual fibres. Estimated oxidative and glycolytic capacities were calculated by summing the calculated capacities of each fibre type together. Capacities for each fibre type were calculated by multiplying the mean SDH (oxidative) or GPD (glycolytic) activity for each fibre-type by the percent of that fibre present within each participant's sample.

Western Blotting

Samples were homogenized, total protein was determined, and sample loading, separation and transfer were performed as described previously [29]. All phosphorylated protein contents are expressed relative to total protein content at rest. Samples were run in duplicate and equal protein loading was confirmed with GAPDH analysis. For protein detection, commercially available antibodies were used for GAPDH (Millipore, Billerica, MA, USA), p-p38 MAPK (Thr^{180}/Tyr^{182}), p-38 MAPK, p-AMPKα (Thr^{172}), AMPKα, p-ACC (Ser^{79}), and ACC (Cell Signaling Technologies, Danvers, MA, USA). Membranes were blocked with 5% bovine serum albumin (BSA) in Tris-buffered saline with Tween-20 (TBS-T) (0.1%) and were immunoblotted with primary antibodies (1:1000). Proteins were visualized by chemiluminescence detection, according to the manufacturer's instructions (Millipore, Billerica, MA, USA). Blots were quantified using the Fluorochem HD2 System (Cell Biosciences, Santa Clara, CA, USA).

RNA Extraction

RNA was extracted using the TRIzol/RNeasy method (Qiagen Sciences, Valencia, CA, USA). Briefly, approximately 20 mg of frozen muscle was added to Lysing Matrix D tubes (MP Biomedicals, Solon, OH, USA), containing 1 mL of TRIzol Reagent (Life Technologies, Burlington, ON, Canada). Muscle samples were homogenized using the FastPrep-24 Tissue and Cell Homogenizer (MP Biomedicals, Solon, OH, USA) for 40 sec at a setting of 6 m/sec. 200 μl of chloroform reagent was added to homogenized samples (Sigma-Aldrich, Oakville, ON, CA), mixed for 15 sec, incubated at room temperature for 5 minutes and centrifuged for 10 minutes at 12000 g at 4°C. The aqueous phase was transferred to a new tube and equal amounts of 70% ethanol was added and mixed. The mixture was transferred into an RNeasy mini-spin column and RNA was purified following the commercially available E.Z.N.A. Total RNA Kit 1 (Omega Bio-Tek, Norcross, GA, USA) as per manufacturer's instructions. The RNA concentration and purity was quantified using the NanoDrop 1000 spectrophotometer (Thermo Fisher Scientific, Rockville, MD, USA). RNA integrity was assessed using a bioanalyzer (Agilent 2100 Bioanalyzer; Agilent Technologies). Average RNA Integrity Number (RIN) values were 6.4.

Quantitative Real-time PCR

Individual samples were reverse transcribed using the commercially available high capacity cDNA reverse transcription kit (Applied Biosystems, Foster City, CA, USA), according to the manufacturer's instructions, using an Eppendorf Mastercycler epgradient thermal cycler (Eppendorf, Mississauga, ON, CA). Reactions were run using RT^2 real-time SYBR Green qPCR master mix (SABioscience; Qiagen Sciences, Germantown, MD, USA), prepared using the epMotion 5075 Eppendorf automated pipetting system (Eppendorf, Mississauga, ON, CA) and carried out in duplicate with an Eppendorf $realplex^2$ Master Cycler epgradientS (Eppendorf, Mississauga, ON, CA). Primer sequences are shown in Table 2. Relative mRNA expression was calculated using the ΔCt method and fold changes from PRE was calculated using the ΔΔCt method [37]. Gene expression was normalized to the housekeeping gene GAPDH.

Statistical Analysis

For both experiments, a two-way, repeated measures ANOVA was used to compare the effect of condition (END and LV-HIT) and time (Rest/Ex and Pre/Post) for all muscle derived data and pre- to post-training physiological testing data from experiment 2. All fibre-type specific analyses were performed within a particular fibre-type. Differences in fibre-type specific expression of p-AMPKα were determined using paired students t-tests comparing mean fluorescence between fibre-types at that time point (Rest and Ex). For estimated glycolytic capacity, where no interaction effect or main effects of training were observed, paired student t-tests were utilized to examine within group changes. All statistical analysis was performed using GraphPad Prism v 5.01 (GraphPad Software Inc., La Jolla, CA, USA). Statistical significance was accepted at $p<0.05$ and all data are presented as means ± SD.

Results

Experiment 1

Exercise bout characteristics. All participants completed each exercise protocol at a work rate corresponding to 65.7±3.8% and 183.2±9.5% VO_2peak for the END and LV-HIT exercise bouts, respectively. Mean prescribed and actual WR for both protocols are presented in Table 1.

Immunofluorescent and histochemical analysis. Representative images are presented in Figure 1A. While no interaction effect was observed for either type I or type IIA fibres, a significant ($p<0.05$) main effect of exercise for muscle glycogen content was present for type I (END–42%, LV-HIT–55%; Fig. 1B) and IIA (END–72%,

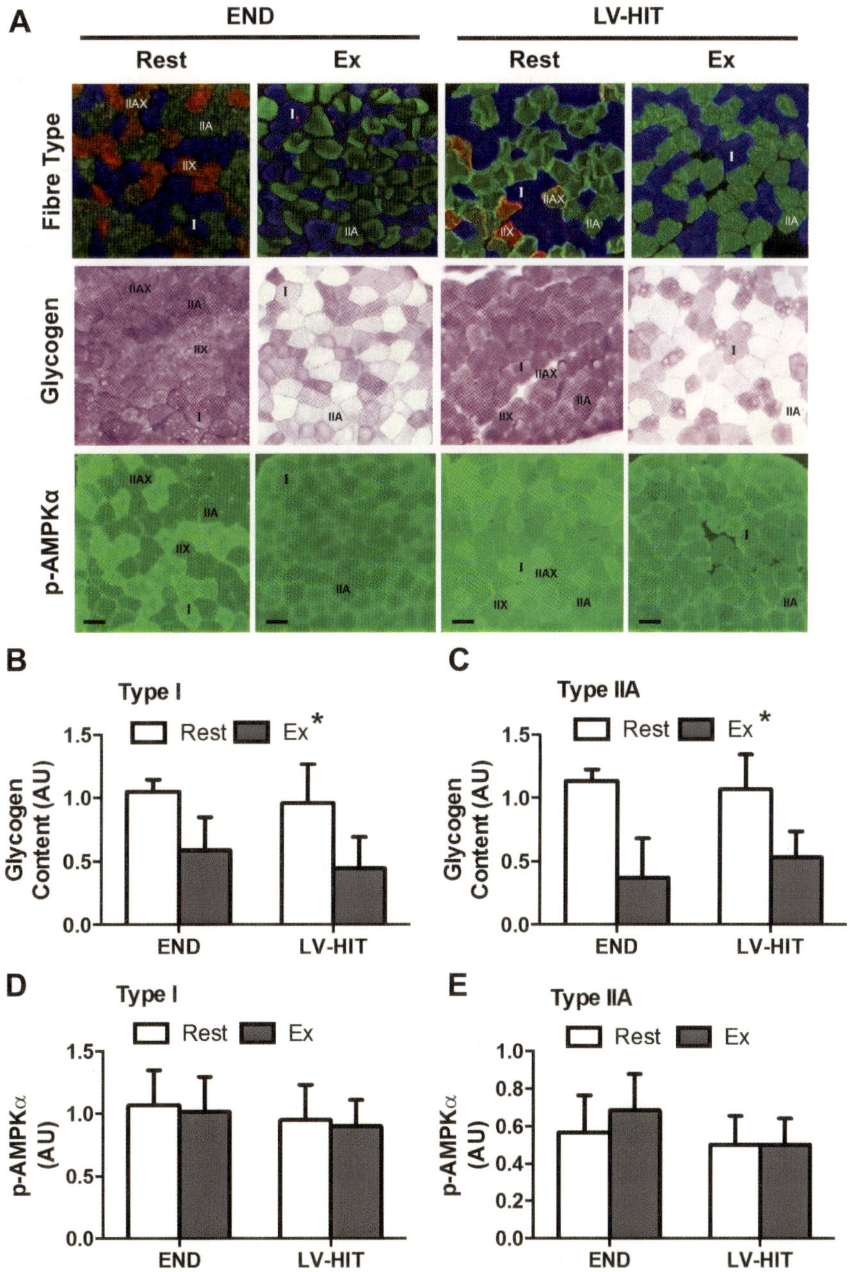

Figure 1. Effects of acute exercise on fibre-type specific glycogen depletion and phosphorylation of AMPKα. A: Representative slides of immunofluorescent fibre-type analysis (blue fibres are type I, green are type IIA, red/green are type IIAX/IIX) with serial sections of glycogen (periodic acid-Schiff staining) and p-AMPKα Thr^{172} content before (Rest) and immediately after (Ex) an acute bout of END or LV-HIT. B–C: Fold change in glycogen content from Rest and Ex in type I and IIA fibres. D–E: Fold change in p-AMPKα content from Rest and Ex in type I and IIA fibres. Bars represent 100 μm. AU, arbitrary units; μm, micrometre. *Significant ($p<0.05$) main effect of exercise.

LV-HIT–49%; Fig. 1C) fibres. As a result of type IIAX/IIX (END, n = 3; LV-HIT, n = 4) fibres not being present in all samples, they were excluded from analysis.

There was no interaction effect, or effect of exercise for p-AMPKα content in type I (Fig. 1D) or type IIA (Fig. 1E) fibres (see representative slides Fig. 1A). A similar lack of effect of exercise on p-AMPKα content was observed with whole muscle Western Blot analysis (see below). Type I fibres expressed significantly ($p<0.05$) greater levels of p-AMPKα than both type IIA and IIAX/IIX fibres at rest and post-exercise.

Western blotting. There was no effect (Fig. 2A and C) of exercise on p-AMPKα Thr^{172} or p-p38MAPK Thr^{180}/Tyr^{182} (see representative blots, Fig. 2D). However a main effect ($p<0.05$) of exercise was observed for p-ACC Ser^{79} (Fig. 2B).

Experiment 2

Aerobic exercise performance and oxidative capacity. A main effect of training ($p<0.05$) on relative VO_2peak (Fig. 3A) was observed at both Mid and Post testing (Percent change from pre: END: +15.5%, LV-HIT: +13.9%). A significant ($p<0.05$) main effect of training on absolute VO_2peak and peak HR was also

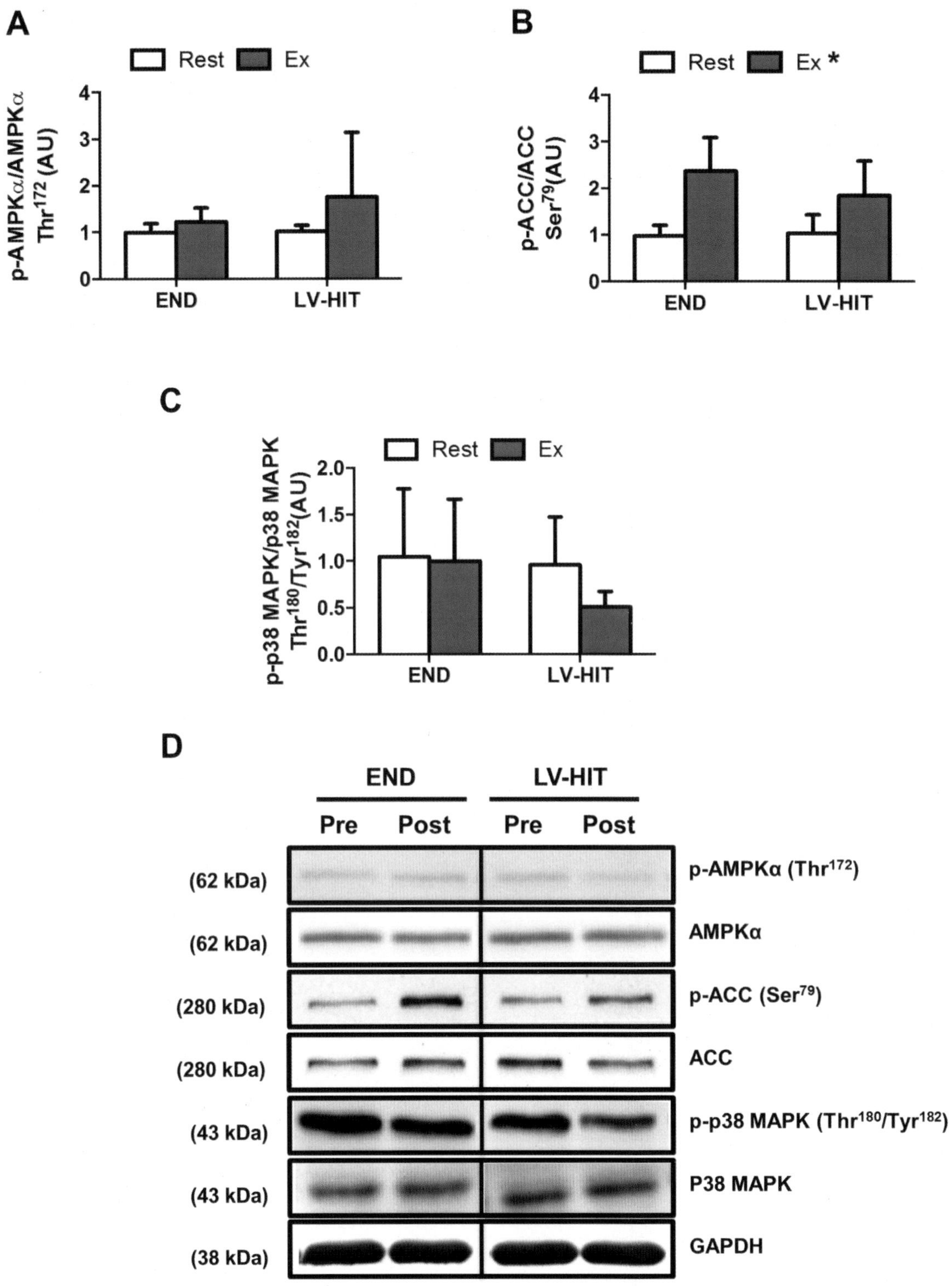

Figure 2. Effects of an acute bout of endurance (END) and low-volume high-intensity interval training (LV-HIT) on whole-muscle signaling. A–D: Fold change in p-AMPKα Thr^{172} (A), p-ACC Ser^{79} (B) and p38 MAPK Thr^{180}/Tyr^{182} (C) content from Rest and Ex. D: Representative western blots, including loading control are also shown. AU, arbitrary units. *Significant ($p<0.05$) main effect of exercise.

demonstrated, while no effect of training was observed for WRpeak (Table 3). A significant ($p<0.05$) main effect of training was also observed for the time to complete the 500 kcal test (Percent change from pre: END: +20.4%, LV-HIT: +15.3%; Fig. 3B).

A main effect of training ($p<0.05$) was demonstrated for fibre distribution of type I and type IIAX/IIX fibres, with the percentage of type I fibres increasing and type IIAX/IIX fibres decreasing following training (Fig. 3D). No effect of training was demonstrated for the percentage fibre distribution for type IIA

Table 3. Experiment 2 participant characteristics (N = 19) for low volume high-intensity interval (LV-HIT) training (n = 10) and endurance (END) training (n = 9) at baseline (pre), mid-training (mid) and following 6 weeks of training (post); mean (SD) unless otherwise indicated.

	END			LV- HIT		
	Pre	Mid	Post	Pre	Mid	Post
Age (yrs)	21(4)	-	-	21(2)	-	-
Height (cm)	180(7)	-	-	175(10)	-	-
Body mass (kg)	74(9)	74(8)	74(9)	71(17)	71(17)	71(17)
Absolute VO_2 (mL/min)*	3534(768)	3743(715)	4050(760)	3440(913)	3703(1007)	3910(1094)
Relative VO_2 (mL/kg/min)*	47.6(8.3)	50.6(7.4)	54.6(7.6)	48.3(6.1)	51.8(6.0)	54.9(6.2)
HRpeak (bpm)*	194(11)	190(9)	191(9)	195(7)	192(6)	193(3)
WRpeak (W)	255(62)	285(56)	281(58)	250(58)	262(53)	258(63)
Wingate peak power (W)*†	718(142)	-	704(147)	654(146)	-	718(184)
Wingate mean power (W)*†	570(119)	-	594(122)	498(141)	-	580(131)

Note: *Main effect of training, $p<0.05$; †significant interaction, $p<0.05$. BPM, beats per minute; cm, centimeters; kg, kilograms; min, minute; mL, milliliter; RER, respiratory exchange ratio; s, seconds; W, watts; yrs, years.

(Fig. 3D) fibres (see representative slides Fig. 3C). A main effect of training ($p<0.05$) was observed for fold change in SDH activity in type I (n = 9), type IIA (n = 9) and type IIAX/IIX (n = 6)(Fig. 3E, see representative slides Fig. 3C). A main effect of training ($p<0.05$) was also observed for estimated oxidative capacity (Fig. 3F).

Cardiovascular capacity and capillary density. A main effect of training ($p<0.05$) was observed for capillary density (Fig. 4B) (see representative slides Fig. 4A) and O_2 pulse (Fig. 4C).

Anaerobic exercise performance and glycolytic capacity. A significant interaction effect ($p<0.05$) and a main effect of training ($p<0.05$) were demonstrated for both peak and mean power in the first Wingate completed (Table 3), and for total work completed across all 4 Wingates (Fig. 5B). A main effect of training ($p<0.05$) was observed for fold change in GPD activity in type I fibres (see representative slides Fig. 5A). There was no effect of training observed for GPD activity in type IIA and IIAX/IIX fibres, while a significant ($p<0.05$) interaction was demonstrated for type IIA fibres (Fig. 5C). There was no main effect of training for estimated glycolytic capacity (Fig. 5D); however, paired students t-tests demonstrated a significant ($p<0.05$) increase in estimated glycolytic capacity post-training (Post) in the LV-HIT group only.

Intramuscular glycogen and triglyceride content. A main effect of training ($p<0.05$) was observed for glycogen content in type I fibres. There was no main effect of training for percent change of glycogen content in type IIA and IIAX/IIX fibres (Fig. 6B, see representative slides Fig. 6A). A main effect of training ($p<0.05$) was observed for IMTG content in type I, IIA and IIAX/IIX fibres (Fig. 6C, see representative slides Fig. 6A).

mRNA expression. Unpaired students t-tests demonstrated no difference in fold change of PGC-1α (END [n = 9]: 1.46±1.10 AU; HIT: 0.87±0.40 AU), general control non-derepressible (GCN) 5 (END [n = 9]: 1.04±0.74 AU; HIT: 0.81±0.45 AU) and receptor-interacting protein (RIP) 140 mRNA (END [n = 9]: 0.98±0.42 AU; HIT: 0.81±0.37 AU) expression between groups, and a significantly ($p<0.05$) higher fold change of silent mating type information regulation 2 homolog 1 (SIRT1) mRNA expression in the END group only (END [n = 9]: 1.19±0.57 AU; HIT: 0.74±0.23 AU) following training.

Discussion

The present study examined both fibre recruitment patterns in response to acute bouts of LV-HIT and END, and fibre-type specific adaptations following 6 weeks of either LV-HIT or END training. In experiment 1, we observed comparable changes in whole-muscle cellular signaling and glycogen depletion derived estimates of fibre recruitment following LV-HIT and END. Consistent with similar responses following the acute exercise bouts, results from experiment 2 demonstrate that 6 weeks of LV-HIT and END training induced comparable increases in aerobic capacity (VO_2peak) and exercise performance (TTC trial), changes in fibre-type distribution, fibre-type specific oxidative and glycolytic capacity, glycogen and IMTG storage, and whole-muscle capillary density. Interestingly, LV-HIT induced greater improvements in anaerobic exercise performance and estimated whole-muscle glycolytic capacity than END.

Experiment 1: Fibre Recruitment Patterns during LV-HIT and END

Whole-muscle measures of signaling pathway activation following acute exercise [19–21], and chronic increases in mitochondrial protein/oxidative capacity [1–3,8,10] are typically comparable following interval training and END. The current study was designed to investigate whether these similarities in whole-muscle measures are masking differences in fibre-type specific adaptations that may help explain the potency of high-intensity exercise and, more specifically, LV-HIT. Fibre recruitment, as indicated by fibre-type specific glycogen depletion, following steady state submaximal exercise is dependent on exercise intensity with type I fibres being preferentially recruited during low intensity exercise and type II fibres being progressively recruited with increasing exercise intensity [24,38,39]. Based on this relationship, we hypothesized that LV-HIT (~170% VO_2peak WR) would result in a greater number of recruited fibres (both type I and II) than END (~65% VO_2peak WR) which would recruit primarily type I fibres.

Contrary to our hypothesis, we observed equivalent reductions ($p<0.05$) in glycogen content in type I and IIA fibres following both protocols (Fig. 1B and C), suggesting that fibre recruitment during LV-HIT and END is comparable. While these data are

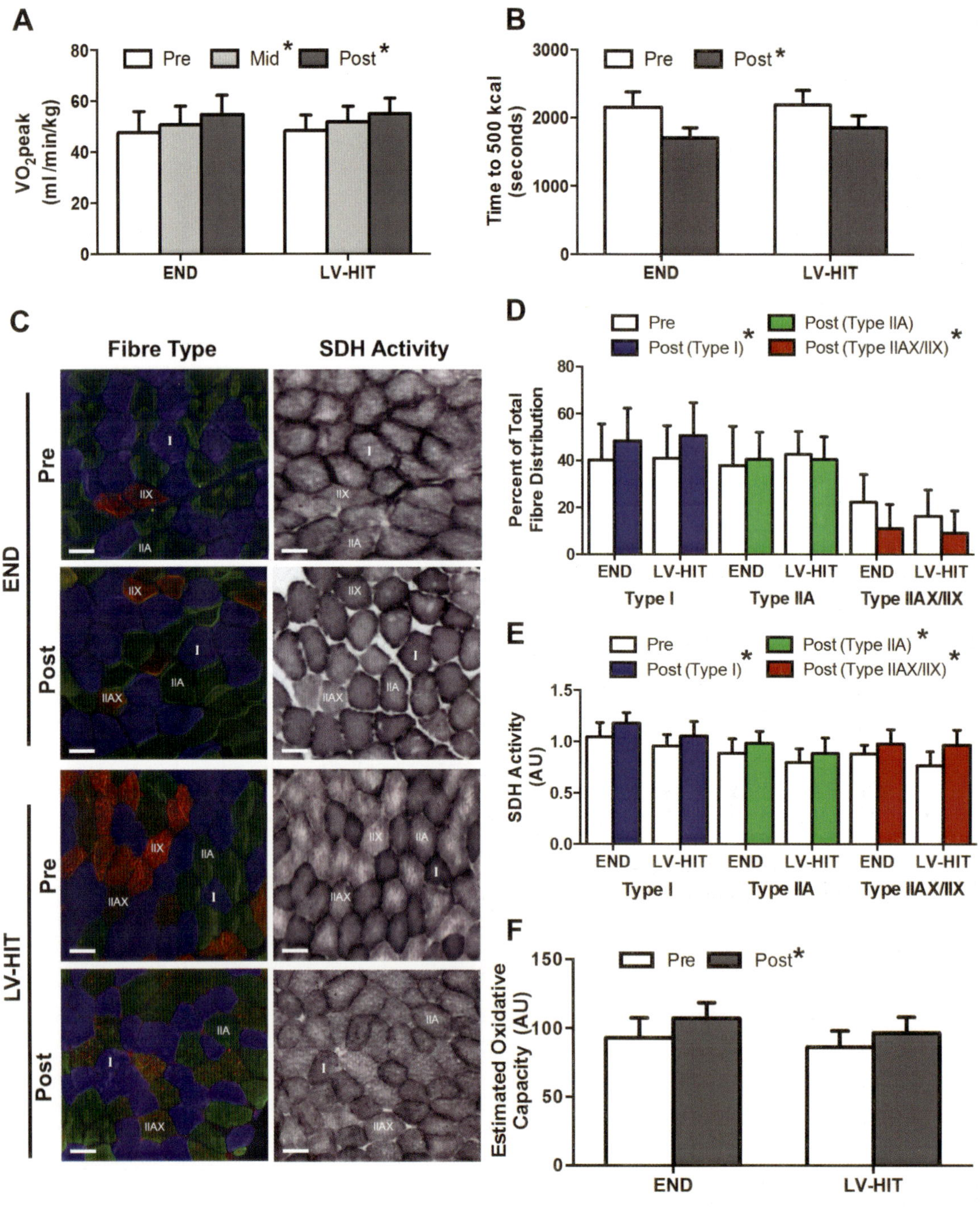

Figure 3. Effects of training (LV-HIT) on aerobic exercise performance, fibre-type distribution and fibre specific oxidative capacity. Relative VO_2peak (A) and time to 500 kcal (B) at Pre, Mid, and Post for both END and LV-HIT groups are shown. C: Representative slides of immunofluorescent fibre-type analysis (blue fibres are type I, green are type IIA, red/green are type IIAX/IIX) with serial sections of succinate dehydrogenase (SDH) activity Pre and Post END or LV-HIT. D: Percentage of total fibre distribution of type I, IIA and IIAX/IIX fibres Pre and Post END or LV-HIT. E: Fibre-type specific fold change in SDH activity post-training compared to pre-training in type I, IIA and IIAX/IIX fibres. F: Absolute change in estimated oxidative capacity. Bars represent 100 μm. AU, arbitrary units; μm, micrometre. *Significant ($p<0.05$) main effect of exercise.

consistent with both type I and IIA fibres being recruited during supramaximal exercise [22–25], the observed glycogen depletion in both fibre types following END is somewhat surprising [24,25,38]. Regardless, in combination with previous demonstrations of type IIA fibre glycogen depletion during submaximal exercise [38,39] our results suggest that there is a threshold intensity associated with the recruitment of a significant percentage of type IIA fibres and that this threshold is below ~65% of VO_2peak. Thus, it would appear that similarities in whole-muscle measures of signaling pathway activation between interval training and END observed previously [19–21], and between LV-HIT and END observed in the current study (Fig. 2), likely result from similar fibre recruitment patterns.

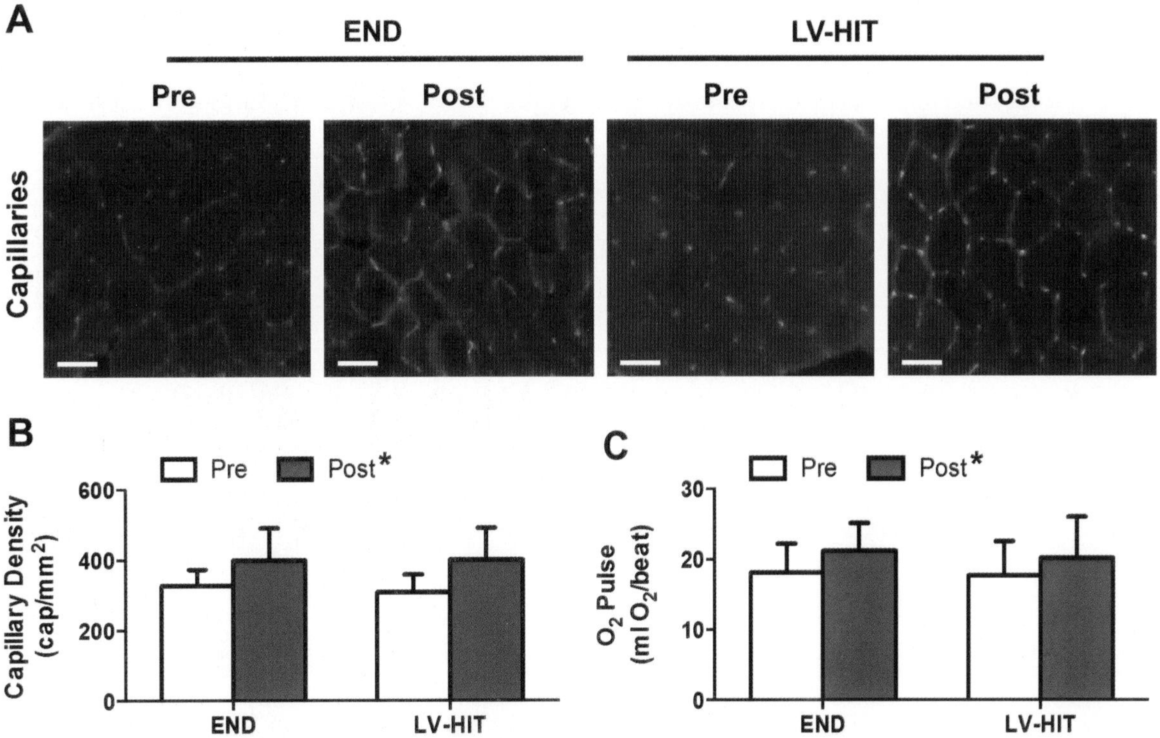

Figure 4. Effects of 6 weeks of endurance (END) and low-volume high-intensity interval training (LV-HIT) on cardiovascular capacity and capillary density. A: Representative slides of capillarisation Pre and Post training. B: Absolute change in capillary density (capillaries/mm^2). C: Change in O_2 pulse (mL O_2/beat). Bars represent 100 µm. mL, milliliter; mm, millimeter; O_2, oxygen; µm, micrometre. *Significant ($p<0.05$) main effect of exercise.

Given the equivalent fibre recruitment between LV-HIT and END, and the substantially greater power generation during LV-HIT, it seems reasonable to assume that a greater relative intensity of signal activation would be experienced within individual fibres during LV-HIT. It is therefore somewhat surprising that fibre-type specific phosphorylation of AMPK (Fig. 1D and E), whole-muscle phosphorylation of ACC (a downstream target of AMPK; Fig. 2) and p38 MAPK were not different between conditions. This finding is consistent with a previous report demonstrating similar activation of intramuscular signaling between END (~70% VO_2max) and submaximal (~90% VO_2max) HIT [19], but not with the recent observation that signaling events are intensity dependent when continuous submaximal exercise (~40 vs. ~80% VO_2peak) was compared [40]. Further, the finding that AMPK and p38 phosphorylation were not increased following LV-HIT is in contrast to observation made following SIT [18]. The reasons for this discrepancy in intramuscular signalling are unclear, however the brevity of the LV-HIT protocol utilized in the current study, compared to the longer duration of SIT protocols utilized previously, suggests that the duration of exercise may be an important factor underlying the activation of these pathways. Collectively, these results suggest that END exercise at an intensity >65% VO_2peak results in both similar fibre recruitment and activation of intramuscular signaling pathways as more intense, lower dose HIT. Additionally, it appears that the intensity/duration threshold required to activate intracellular signaling events associated with the induction of mitochondrial biogenesis within an individual muscle fibre is achieved by both LV-HIT and END exercise at intensities equal to, or greater than 65% VO_2peak and a duration of at least 30 minutes [19,40]. This assertion is supported by the presence of similar levels of PGC-1α mRNA and other genes related to mitochondrial biogenesis following 90 minutes of continuous submaximal (~65% VO_2peak) and supramaximal (~120% VO_2peak) interval exercise [20,21] in both type I and IIA fibres [21].

In summary, experiment 1 of the current study demonstrated that recruitment of muscle fibres (type I and IIA) during a single bout of LV-HIT or END are similar, as is activation of intracellular signaling pathways. Given that type I and IIA fibres represent ~90% of the total fibre population of the vastus lateralis (Fig. 3D) [30], the assumption that changes in both type I and type IIA fibres are accurately reflected in whole-muscle measures of intracellular signaling appears to be appropriate.

Experiment 2: Fibre Specific Adaptations to LV-HIT and END Training

Exercise training increases the maximal activity and content of mitochondrial enzymes involved in oxidative metabolism, capillary density, and intramuscular triglyceride and glycogen stores [1–4,6,8,10,11]. Collectively, these adaptations contribute to improved skeletal muscle oxidative potential, fatty acid oxidative capacity, and improve aerobic capacity and exercise performance (VO_2peak, time to fatigue trials, etc.). Based on the recent argument that improvements in aerobic capacity and performance following interval training are driven primarily by peripheral adaptations [14,15], and the previously discussed hypothesis that LV-HIT would recruit additional different muscle fibres than END, we examined fibre-type specific adaptations to both LV-HIT and END training.

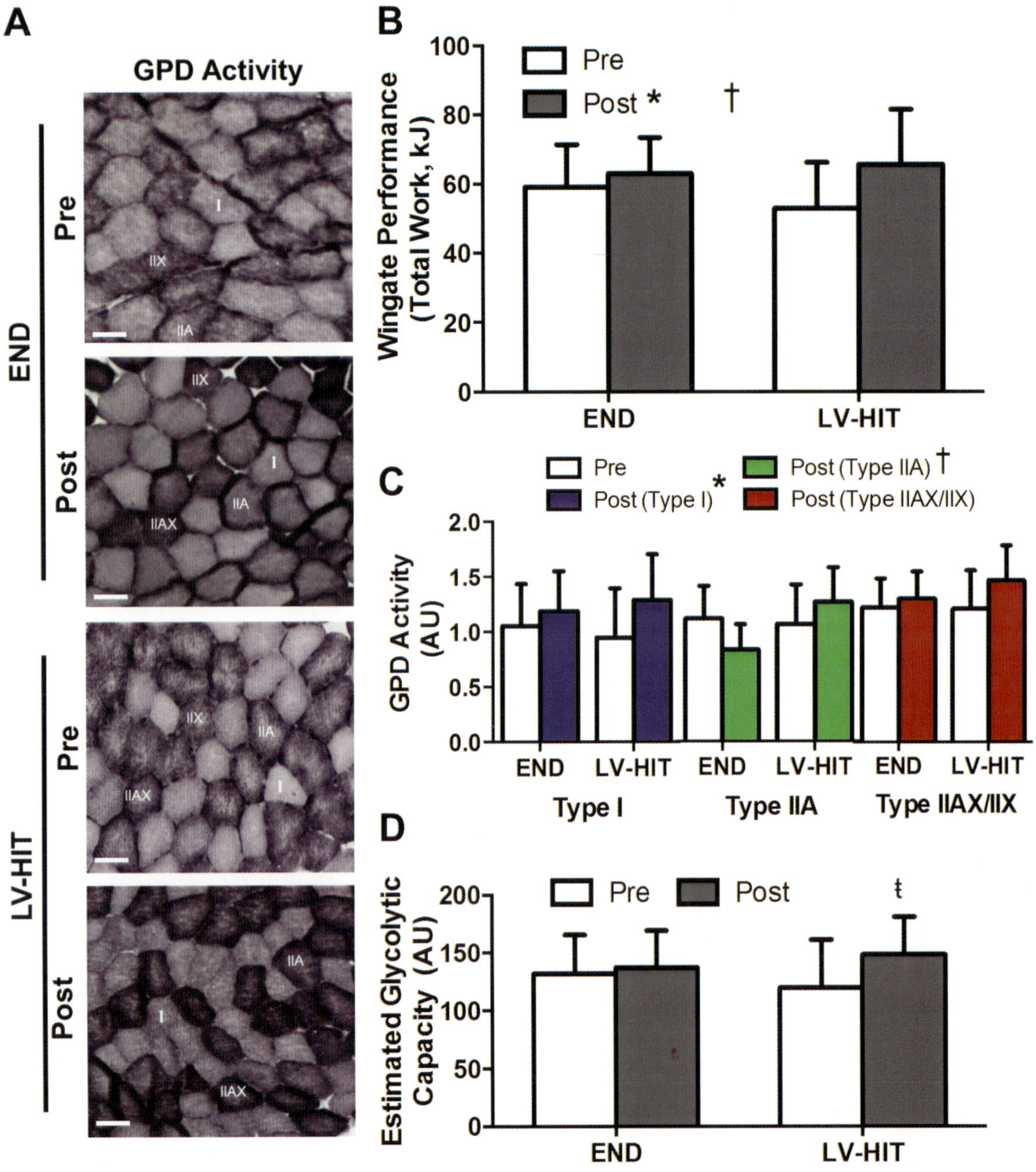

Figure 5. Effects of endurance (END) and low-volume high-intensity interval training (LV-HIT) on anaerobic exercise performance and glycolytic capacity. A: Representative slides of α-glycerophosphate dehydrogenase (GPD) activity Pre and Post training (see Fig. 3C for corresponding fibre-type slides). B: Total work performed during all 4 Wingate bouts. C: Fibre-type specific fold change in GPD activity post-training compared to pre-training in type I, IIA and IIAX/IIX fibres. D: Absolute change in estimated glycolytic capacity. Bars represent 100 μm. AU, arbitrary units; μm, micrometre. †Significant ($p<0.05$) group by time interaction, *Significant ($p<0.05$) main effect of exercise, ǂSignificant ($p<0.05$) within group difference (derived from paired t-test).

Aerobic Exercise Performance and Oxidative Capacity

As has been previously observed [9,12], we demonstrated similar improvements in VO_2peak and aerobic exercise performance (Fig. 3A and B) following 6 weeks of LV-HIT and END. Consistent with these whole body adaptations, comparable increases in SDH activity, a mitochondrial protein correlated with mitochondrial content [41], were observed across all fibre-types following both LV-HIT and END (Fig. 3E). Additionally, changes in whole muscle gene expression of proteins associated with mitochondrial biogenesis were similar following both training protocols. While others have reported comparable increases in fibre specific cytochorome c oxidase (COX) protein content following SIT and END [3], COX is not highly correlated with mitochondrial content ($r = 0.55$) [41]. Our results supports these assumptions but are derived from SDH activity, a protein which correlates much more highly with mitochondrial content ($r = 0.73$) [41]. These adaptations are also consistent with the muscle fibre activation patterns observed during a single bout of LV-HIT and END in experiment 1 suggesting that recruitment of fibres during repeated acute bouts of LV-HIT and END (i.e. training) results in

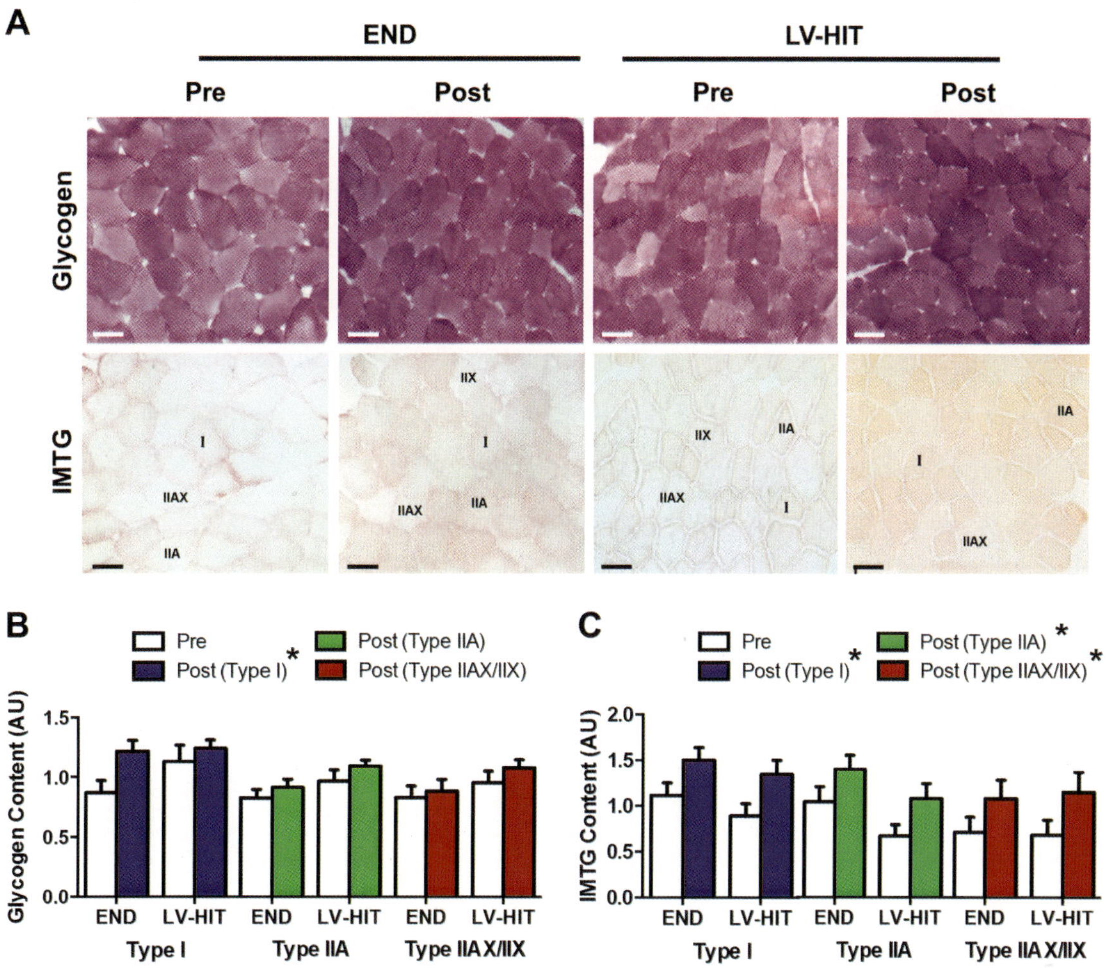

Figure 6. Effects of endurance (END) and low-volume high-intensity interval training (LV-HIT) on intramuscular glycogen and triglyceride storage. A: Representative slides of glycogen (periodic acid-Schiff reaction) and intramuscular triglyceride (IMTG) content (Oil red O staining) Pre and Post training (see Fig. 3C for corresponding fibre-type slides for IMTG stain only). B. Fibre-type specific fold changes in glycogen content in type I, IIA and IIAX/IIX fibres. C. Fibre-type specific fold changes in IMTG content in type I, IIA and IIAX/IIX fibres. Bars represent 100 μm. AU, arbitrary units; μm, micrometre. *Significant ($p<0.05$) main effect of exercise.

increases in oxidative capacity within those fibres. The results also further strengthen the assertion made above that the intensity/duration threshold required to induce increases in oxidative capacity within a given fibre are reached by both the LV-HIT and END protocols utilized in the present study.

Further, both groups demonstrated an increased proportion of type I fibres concomitant with a reduction in type IIAX/IIX fibres (Fig. 3D). While several studies have demonstrated myofiber transitions resulting in a greater percentage of oxidative fibres (type I) following HIT and END training [42,43], our results are not consistent with several reports demonstrating increases in type IIA fibres with concurrent reductions in type I fibres following several weeks of SIT [44–47]. While the exact mechanism(s) responsible for contraction-induced changes in myofiber composition remain to be completely described, contraction frequency has been demonstrated to influence fibre-type synthesis [48] with high-frequency activation inducing the synthesis of fast twitch myosin. Importantly, our END and LV-HIT protocols required participants to cycle at the same speed (80 RPM), while the load was changed in order to manipulate training intensity. This may explain why we observed increases in type I fibres and reductions in type IIAX/IIX fibres following 6 weeks of both LV-HIT and END, as opposed to those studies employing SIT, a training protocol typically demanding maximal pedaling frequency and contraction rates [44–47].

Combined, the increases in fibre-type specific SDH activity and the increase proportion of type I fibres resulted in an increase in estimated whole-muscle oxidative capacity (Fig. 3F) following both training protocols. These results support prior observations of comparable increases in whole-muscle markers of oxidative capacity and enzymes associated with oxidative metabolism [1,3,18,49,50] following HIT or SIT and END training. We also observed similar increases in capillary density (Fig. 4B), data which are consistent with previous studies reporting comparable increases in capillary density following SIT and END [4,6,11]. While these results are in agreement with improvements in aerobic capacity and performance following interval training being mediated by peripheral adaptations, the similar changes in estimated oxidative capacity, capillary density and O_2 pulse in both groups (Fig. 4C) are not consistent with suggestions that increases in VO_2peak are supported by different mechanisms following LV-HIT and END [14].

Anaerobic Exercise Performance and Glycolytic Capacity

Six weeks of LV-HIT and END resulted in improved anaerobic exercise performance (total work; Fig. 5B) and anaerobic capacity (peak and mean power; Table 3). Importantly, improvements for all indices of anaerobic performance/capacity were greater for LV-HIT than END. Consistent with these results, changes in GPD activity were similar in type I fibres (Fig. 5C) while a significant interaction effect was observed in type IIA fibres such that an increased GPD activity was only observed in this fibre population following LV-HIT. Additionally, our estimate of whole-muscle glycolytic capacity demonstrated a trend towards an increase following LV-HIT only (no main effect of training; paired t-test significant within LV-HIT only; Fig. 5D). These results are consistent with previous demonstrations that HIT and SIT improve anaerobic exercise performance [1,49], while changes in glycolytic enzyme activity have been observed following SIT but not END [5,50–52]. While the exact mechanisms responsible for our observed differences in anaerobic exercise capacity and performance between groups are unknown, it appears that they may be attributable to factors beyond the peripheral skeletal muscle adaptations examined in the present study. One such peripheral factor could be an improved skeletal muscle lactic acid buffering capacity, which has been observed following SIT [8], but not HIT [53]. Another potential mechanism may be differences in adaptations of central origin, such as rate of fibre recruitment, firing rate and motor unit synchronization. SIT in conjunction with END training results in increased motor unit recruitment and total work performed during a repeated Wingate test compared to END training alone [54], which suggests that improvements in neuromuscular characteristics may partially explain the greater improvements in Wingate performance and anaerobic capacity following LV-HIT.

Limitations and Future Directions

The sample size of experiment 1 ($n = 6$) was relatively small and it is therefore possible that a larger sample size may have yielded different results. However, while an increased sample size might have allowed for subtle differences between LV-HIT and END to be detected (for both glycogen depletion and intramuscular signalling), we do not believe that the limited statistical power associated with the small sample studies impaired our ability to conclude that both type I and IIA fibres are recruited during both of exercise protocols examined in the current study. Additionally, we have observed a dissociation between phosphorylation of AMPK and phosphorylation of ACC, an interesting result that reflects previously published results [18,40,55]. While we are unable to comment with certainty regarding why this dissociation exists, it is possible that differential phosphorylation of α1 and α2 AMPK sub-units [56,57] may impair the ability to estimate changes in AMPK activity based on changes in global AMPK phosphorytion. Thus, while we were unable to conduct this analysis on samples from the present study, the potential that phosphorylation of ACC is a more sensitive measure of AMPK activity than phosphorylation of AMPK itself raises the possibility the fibre specific differences in ACC phosphorylation may be present following exercise. This represents an important area for future research. It would also be of interest to investigate whether similar acute activation of intramuscular signalling pathways following LV-HIT and END result similar activation and expression of PGC-1α and other genes associated with the induction of mitochondrial biogenesis in the hours following exercise.

Perspectives/Conclusions

Numerous recent investigations have attempted to elucidate the mechanisms by which interval training and END training induce similar improvements in aerobic capacity and exercise performance (VO_2peak, time to fatigue trails, etc.) [18,19,40,55,58]. Collectively, these studies suggest that the intramuscular signaling required to elicit these adaptations are equivalently stimulated by both low intensity exercise of long duration and high-intensity exercise of short duration. While the minimum duration of low intensity exercise required to elicit adaptation remains unknown, very brief bouts of high-intensity exercise appear to be sufficient [9,12,13]. From an exercise prescription perspective, exercise resulting in the largest degree of intramuscular signaling activation in the greatest amount of muscle fibres would presumably result in the greatest degree of adaptation. What remains largely unknown, however, is whether differences in fibre recruitment and the magnitude of signal activation within individual fibre-types between interval training and END exercise are obscured by whole muscle analyses. Our results demonstrate that LV-HIT and END produce similar: a) glycogen depletion across fibre types (indicative of similar fibre recruitment), b) changes in intramuscular signaling, and c) fibre-type specific increases in oxidative capacity, intramuscular glycogen and triglyceride content, whole-muscle capillary density and O_2pulse. Remarkably, these results suggest that 30 minutes of END exercise at ~65% VO_2peak or 4 minutes of LV-HIT at ~170% VO_2peak induce comparable deviations of the intra-myocellular environment (glycogen content and signaling activation); correspondingly, training-induced adaptations resulting for these protocols, and other interval training and END protocols [1,8], appear comparable. The one exception to this equivocality is the capacity of LV-HIT to induce greater improvements in anaerobic adaptations than END. Thus, our results suggest that the mechanisms responsible for adaptation following chronic LV-HIT and END are the same, with the supramaximal exercise intensity inherent with LV-HIT permitting their manifestation in significantly less exercise time.

Collectively, results from this study suggest that the potency of high-intensity exercise resides is its ability to activate the mechanisms that trigger the induction of exercise-induced adaptation in a drastically reduced exercise time compared to traditional END training. However, while END exercise at intensities greater than ~65% VO_2peak are of adequate intensity to elicit "maximal" fibre recruitment (i.e. type I and IIA fibres) and the manifestation of chronic adaptations, at present the minimal duration of exercise at these relatively low intensities required for comparable adaptations is not known. Our results, and others [9], suggest that 30 minutes is adequate; however, given that our assumptions regarding the minimal dose of exercise required for adaptations having been recently challenged [59,60], the minimal duration of moderate intensity END required to induce adaptation is an interesting area for future research.

Acknowledgments

We would like to thank a very dedicated group of volunteers without whom this study would not have been possible.

Author Contributions

Conceived and designed the experiments: TDS BJG. Performed the experiments: TDS BAE KV ASM. Analyzed the data: TDS BAE KV ASM JBM SDJ GP JQ BJG. Contributed reagents/materials/analysis tools: GP JQ BJG. Wrote the paper: TDS BJG.

References

1. Burgomaster KA, Howarth KR, Phillips SM, Rakobowchuk M, MacDonald MJ, et al. (2008) Similar metabolic adaptations during exercise after low volume sprint interval and traditional endurance training in humans. J Physiol 586: 151–160. doi:10.1113/jphysiol.2007.142109.
2. Saltin B, Nazar K, Costill DL, Stein E, Jansson E, et al. (1976) The Nature of the Training Response; Peripheral and Central Adaptations to One-Legged Exercise. Acta Physiol Scand 96: 289–305.
3. Shepherd SO, Cocks M, Tipton KD, Ranasinghe AM, Barker TA, et al. (2013) Sprint interval and traditional endurance training increase net intramuscular triglyceride breakdown and expression of perilipin 2 and 5. J Physiol 591: 657–675. doi:10.1113/jphysiol.2012.240952.
4. Cocks M, Shaw CS, Shepherd SO, Fisher JP, Ranasinghe AM, et al. (2013) Sprint interval and endurance training are equally effective in increasing muscle microvascular density and eNOS content in sedentary males. J Physiol 591: 641–656. doi:10.1113/jphysiol.2012.239566.
5. Fournier M, Ricci J, Taylor AW, Ferguson RJ, Montpetit RR, et al. (1982) Skeletal muscle adaptation in adolescent boys: sprint and endurance training and detraining. Med Sci Sports Exerc 14: 453–456.
6. Daussin FN, Zoll J, Dufour SP, Ponsot E, Lonsdorfer-Wolf E, et al. (2008) Effect of interval versus continuous training on cardiorespiratory and mitochondrial functions: relationship to aerobic performance improvements in sedentary subjects. Am J Physiol Regul Integr Comp Physiol 295: R264–R272. doi:10.1152/ajpregu.00875.2007.
7. Eddy DO, Sparks KL, Adelizi DA (1977) The effects of continuous and interval training in women and men. Eur J Appl Physiol Occup Physiol 37: 83–92.
8. Gibala MJ, Little JP, van Essen M, Wilkin GP, Burgomaster KA, et al. (2006) Short-term sprint interval versus traditional endurance training: similar initial adaptations in human skeletal muscle and exercise performance. J Physiol 575: 901–911. doi:10.1113/jphysiol.2006.112094.
9. McRae G, Payne A, Zelt JGE, Scribbans TD, Jung ME, et al. (2012) Extremely low volume, whole-body aerobic-resistance training improves aerobic fitness and muscular endurance in females. Appl Physiol Nutr Metab. 37: 1124–1131. doi:10.1139/h2012-093.
10. Terada S, Tabata I, Higuchi M (2004) Effect of high-intensity intermittent swimming training on fatty acid oxidation enzyme activity in rat skeletal muscle. Jpn J Physiol 54: 47–52.
11. Vogiatzis I, Terzis G, Nanas S, Stratakos G, Simoes DCM, et al. (2005) Skeletal muscle adaptations to interval training in patients with advanced COPD. Chest 128: 3838–3845. doi:10.1378/chest.128.6.3838.
12. Tabata I, Nishimura K, Kouzaki M, Hirai Y, Ogita F, et al. (1996) Effects of moderate-intensity endurance and high-intensity intermittent training on anaerobic capacity and VO2max. Med Sci Sports Exerc 28: 1327–1330.
13. Ma JK, Scribbans TD, Edgett BA, Colin Boyd J, Simpson CA, et al. (2013) Extremely low-volume, high-intensity interval training improves exercise capacity and increases mitochondrial protein content in human skeletal muscle. OJMIP 03: 202–210. doi:10.4236/ojmip.2013.34027.
14. MacPherson REK, Hazell TJ, Olver TD, Paterson DH, Lemon PWR (2011) Run Sprint Interval Training Improves Aerobic Performance but Not Maximal Cardiac Output. Med Sci Sports Exerc 43: 115–122. doi:10.1249/MSS.0b013e3181e5eacd.
15. Jacobs RA, Lundby C (2013) Mitochondria express enhanced quality as well as quantity in association with aerobic fitness across recreationally active individuals up to elite athletes. J Appl Physiol 114: 344–350. doi:10.1152/japplphysiol.01081.2012.
16. Pilegaard H, Saltin B, Neufer PD (2003) Exercise induces transient transcriptional activation of the PGC-1 gene in human skeletal muscle. J Physiol 546: 851–858. doi:10.1113/jphysiol.2002.034850.
17. Wright DC, Han D-H, Garcia-Roves PM, Geiger PC, Jones TE, et al. (2007) Exercise-induced Mitochondrial Biogenesis Begins before the Increase in Muscle PGC-1 Expression. J Biol Chem 282: 194–199.
18. Gibala MJ, McGee SL, Garnham AP, Howlett KF, Snow RJ, et al. (2009) Brief intense interval exercise activates AMPK and p38 MAPK signaling and increases the expression of PGC-1 in human skeletal muscle. J Appl Physiol 106: 929–934. doi:10.1152/japplphysiol.90880.2008.
19. Bartlett JD, Hwa Joo C, Jeong TS, Louhelainen J, Cochran AJ, et al. (2012) Matched work high-intensity interval and continuous running induce similar increases in PGC-1 mRNA, AMPK, p38, and p53 phosphorylation in human skeletal muscle. J Appl Physiol 112: 1135–1143. doi:10.1152/japplphysiol.01040.2011.
20. Wang L, Psilander N, Tonkonogi M, Ding S, Sahlin K (2009) Similar Expression of Oxidative Genes after Interval and Continuous Exercise. Med Sci Sports Exerc 41: 2136–2144. doi:10.1249/MSS.0b013e3181abc1ec.
21. Wang L, Sahlin K (2011) The effect of continuous and interval exercise on PGC-1α and PDK4 mRNA in type I and type II fibres of human skeletal muscle. Acta Physiologica 204: 525–532. doi:10.1111/j.1748-1716.2011.02354.x.
22. Greenhaff PLP, Nevill MEM, Soderlund KK, Bodin KK, Boobis LHL, et al. (1994) The metabolic responses of human type I and II muscle fibres during maximal treadmill sprinting. J Physiol 478 (Pt 1): 149–155.
23. Vøllestad NK, Tabata I, Medbø JI (1992) Glycogen breakdown in different human muscle fibre types during exhaustive exercise of short duration. Acta Physiol Scand 144: 135–141.
24. Gollnick PD, Piehl K, Saltin B (1974) Selective glycogen depletion pattern in human muscle fibres after exercise of varying intensity and at varying pedalling rates. J Physiol 241: 45–57.
25. Essén B (1978) Glycogen depletion of different fibre types in human skeletal muscle during intermittent and continuous exercise. Acta Physiol Scand 103: 446–455. doi:10.1111/j.1748-1716.1978.tb06239.x.
26. Edgett BA, Foster WS, Hankinson PB, Simpson CA, Little JP, et al. (2013) Dissociation of Increases in PGC-1α and Its Regulators from Exercise Intensity and Muscle Activation Following Acute Exercise. PLoS One 8: e71623. doi:10.1371/journal.pone.0071623.t003.
27. Bergstrom J (1975) Percutaneous needle biopsy of skeletal muscle in physiological and clinical research. Scand J Clin Lab Invest 35: 609–616.
28. Jeukendrup A, Saris WH, Brouns F, Kester AD (1996) A new validated endurance performance test. Med Sci Sports Exerc 28: 266–270.
29. Boyd JC, Simpson CA, Jung ME, Gurd BJ (2013) Reducing the Intensity and Volume of Interval Training Diminishes Cardiovascular Adaptation but Not Mitochondrial Biogenesis in Overweight/Obese Men. PLoS One 8: e68091. doi:10.1371/journal.pone.0068091.t002.
30. Bloemberg D, Quadrilatero J (2012) Rapid Determination of Myosin Heavy Chain Expression in Rat, Mouse, and Human Skeletal Muscle Using Multicolor Immunofluorescence Analysis. PLoS One 7: e35273. doi:10.1371/journal.pone.0035273.t005.
31. Cebasek V, Kubínová L, Ribaric S, Erzen I (2004) A novel staining method for quantification and 3D visualisation of capillaries and muscle fibres. Eur J Histochem 48: 151–158.
32. Lee-Young RS, Canny BJ, Myers DE, McConell GK (2009) AMPK activation is fiber type specific in human skeletal muscle: effects of exercise and short-term exercise training. J Appl Physiol 107: 283–289. doi:10.1152/japplphysiol.91208.2008.
33. Blanco CE, Sieck GC, Edgerton VR (1988) Quantitative histochemical determination of succinic dehydrogenase activity in skeletal muscle fibres. Histochem J 20: 230–243.
34. Halkjaer-Kristensen JJ, Ingemann-Hansen TT (1979) Microphotometric analysis of NADH-tetrazolium reductase and alpha-glycerophosphate dehydrogenase in human quadriceps muscle. Histochem J 11: 127–136.
35. Koopman RR, Schaart GG, Hesselink MKM (2001) Optimisation of oil red O staining permits combination with immunofluorescence and automated quantification of lipids. Histochem Cell Biol 116: 63–68. doi:10.1007/s004180100297.
36. Quadrilatero J, Bombardier E, Norris SM, Talanian JL, Palmer MS, et al. (2010) Prolonged moderate-intensity aerobic exercise does not alter apoptotic signaling and DNA fragmentation in human skeletal muscle. Am J Physiol Endocrinol Metab 298: E534–E547. doi:10.1152/ajpendo.00678.2009.
37. Livak KJ, Schmittgen TD (2001) Analysis of relative gene expression data using real-time quantitative PCR and the 2(-Delta Delta C(T)) Method. Methods 25: 402–408. doi:10.1006/meth.2001.1262.
38. Vøllestad NKN, Blom PCP (1985) Effect of varying exercise intensity on glycogen depletion in human muscle fibres. Acta Physiol Scand 125: 395–405.
39. Vøllestad NK, Vaage O, Hermansen L (1984) Muscle glycogen depletion patterns in type I and subgroups of type II fibres during prolonged severe exercise in man. Acta Physiol Scand 122: 433–441. doi:10.1111/j.1748-1716.1984.tb07531.x.
40. Egan B, Carson BP, Garcia-Roves PM, Chibalin AV, Sarsfield FM, et al. (2010) Exercise intensity-dependent regulation of peroxisome proliferator-activated receptor γ coactivator-1α mRNA abundance is associated with differential activation of upstream signalling kinases in human skeletal muscle. J Physiol 588: 1779–1790. doi:10.1113/jphysiol.2010.188011.
41. Larsen S, Nielsen J, Hansen CN, Nielsen LB, Wibrand F, et al. (2012) Biomarkers of mitochondrial content in skeletal muscle of healthy young human subjects. J Physiol 590: 3349–3360. doi:10.1113/jphysiol.2012.230185.
42. Russell AP, Feilchenfeldt J, Schreiber S, Praz M, Crettenand A, et al. (2003) Endurance training in humans leads to fiber type-specific increases in levels of peroxisome proliferator-activated receptor-γ coactivator-1 and peroxisome proliferator-activated receptor-α in skeletal muscle. Diabetes 52: 2874–2881.
43. Simoneau JA, Lortie G, Boulay MR, Marcotte M, Thibault MC, et al. (1985) Human skeletal muscle fiber type alteration with high-intensity intermittent training. Eur J Appl Physiol Occup Physiol 54: 250–253.
44. Jansson E, Esbjörnsson M, Holm I, Jacobs I (1990) Increase in the proportion of fast-twitch muscle fibres by sprint training in males. Acta Physiol Scand 140: 359–363.
45. Allemeier CA, Fry AC, Johnson P, Hikida RS, Hagerman FC, et al. (1994) Effects of sprint cycle training on human skeletal muscle. J Appl Physiol 77: 2385–2390.
46. Esbjörnsson MM, Hellsten-Westing YY, Balsom PDP, Sjödin BB, Jansson EE (1993) Muscle fibre type changes with sprint training: effect of training pattern. Acta Physiol Scand 149: 245–246.
47. Dawson B, Fitzsimons M, Green S, Goodman C, Carey M, et al. (1998) Changes in performance, muscle metabolites, enzymes and fibre types after short sprint training. Eur J Appl Physiol Occup Physiol 78: 163–169.
48. Pette D, Vrbová G (1985) Invited review: neural control of phenotypic expression in mammalian muscle fibers. Muscle Nerve 8: 676–689.

49. Burgomaster KA, Hughes SC, Heigenhauser GJF, Bradwell SN, Gibala MJ (2005) Six sessions of sprint interval training increases muscle oxidative potential and cycle endurance capacity in humans. J Appl Physiol 98: 1985–1990. doi:10.1152/japplphysiol.01095.2004.
50. Rodas G, Ventura JL, Cadefau JA, Cussó R, Parra J (2000) A short training programme for the rapid improvement of both aerobic and anaerobic metabolism. Eur J Appl Physiol 82: 480–486. doi:10.1007/s004210000223.
51. MacDougall JD, Hicks AL, MacDonald JR, McKelvie RS, Green HJ, et al. (1998) Muscle performance and enzymatic adaptations to sprint interval training. J Appl Physiol 84: 2138–2142.
52. Phillips SM, Green HJ, Tarnopolsky MA, Heigenhauser GJ, Grant SM (1996) Progressive effect of endurance training on metabolic adaptations in working skeletal muscle. Am J Physiol 270: E265–E272.
53. Bishop D, Edge J, Thomas C, Mercier J (2008) Effects of high-intensity training on muscle lactate transporters and postexercise recovery of muscle lactate and hydrogen ions in women. Am J Physiol Regul Integr Comp Physiol 295: R1991–R1998. doi:10.1152/ajpregu.00863.2007.
54. Creer AR, Ricard MD, Conlee RK, Hoyt GL, Parcell AC (2004) Neural, metabolic, and performance adaptations to four weeks of high intensity sprint-interval training in trained cyclists. Int J Sports Med 25: 92–98. doi:10.1055/s-2004-819945.
55. Little JP, Safdar A, Cermak N, Tarnopolsky MA, Gibala MJ (2010) Acute endurance exercise increases the nuclear abundance of PGC-1 in trained human skeletal muscle. Am J Physiol Regul Integr Comp Physiol 298: R912–R917. doi:10.1152/ajpregu.00409.2009.
56. Treebak JT, Birk JB, Rose AJ, Kiens B, Richter EA, et al. (2007) AS160 phosphorylation is associated with activation of alpha2beta2gamma1- but not alpha2beta2gamma3-AMPK trimeric complex in skeletal muscle during exercise in humans. Am J Physiol Endocrinol Metab 292: E715–E722. doi:10.1152/ajpendo.00380.2006.
57. Birk JB, Wojtaszewski JFP (2006) Predominant α2/β2/3 AMPK activation during exercise in human skeletal muscle. J Physiol 577: 1021–1032. doi:10.1113/jphysiol.2006.120972.
58. Little JP, Safdar A, Bishop D, Tarnopolsky MA, Gibala MJ (2011) An acute bout of high-intensity interval training increases the nuclear abundance of PGC-1 and activates mitochondrial biogenesis in human skeletal muscle. Am J Physiol Regul Integr Comp Physiol 300: R1303–R1310. doi:10.1152/ajpregu.00538.2010.
59. Tjønna AE, Leinan IM, Bartnes AT, Jenssen BM, Gibala MJ, et al. (2013) Low- and High-Volume of Intensive Endurance Training Significantly Improves Maximal Oxygen Uptake after 10-Weeks of Training in Healthy Men. PLoS One 8: e65382. doi:10.1371/journal.pone.0065382.s002.
60. Hazell TJ, MacPherson REK, Gravelle BMR, Lemon PWR (2010) 10 or 30-s sprint interval training bouts enhance both aerobic and anaerobic performance. Eur J Appl Physiol 110: 153–160. doi:10.1007/s00421-010-1474-y.

2

Re-Evaluation of Sarcolemma Injury and Muscle Swelling in Human Skeletal Muscles after Eccentric Exercise

Ji-Guo Yu[1]*, Jing-Xia Liu[2], Lena Carlsson[2], Lars-Eric Thornell[2], Per S. Stål[2]

1 Department of Surgical and Perioperative Sciences, Sports Medicine Unit, Umeå University, Umeå, Sweden, 2 Department of Integrative Medical Biology, Section for Anatomy, Umeå University, Umeå, Sweden

Abstract

The results regarding the effects of unaccustomed eccentric exercise on muscle tissue are often conflicting and the aetiology of delayed onset muscle soreness (DOMS) induced by eccentric exercise is still unclear. This study aimed to re-evaluate the paradigm of muscular alterations with regard to muscle sarcolemma integrity and fibre swelling in human muscles after voluntary eccentric exercise leading to DOMS. Ten young males performed eccentric exercise by downstairs running. Biopsies from the soleus muscle were obtained from 6 non-exercising controls, 4 exercised subjects within 1 hour and 6 exercised subjects at 2–3 days and 7–8 days after the exercise. Muscle fibre sarcolemma integrity, infiltration of inflammatory cells and changes in fibre size and fibre phenotype composition as well as capillary supply were examined with specific antibodies using enzyme histochemistry and immunohistochemistry. Although all exercised subjects experienced DOMS which peaked between 1.5 to 2.5 days post exercise, no significant sarcolemma injury or inflammation was detected in any post exercise group. The results do not support the prevailing hypothesis that eccentric exercise causes an initial sarcolemma injury which leads to subsequent inflammation after eccentric exercise. The fibre size was 24% larger at 7–8 days than at 2–3 days post exercise ($p<0.05$). In contrast, the value of capillary number per fibre area tended to decrease from 2–3 days to 7–8 days post exercise (lower in 5 of the 6 subjects at 7–8 days than at 2–3 days; $p<0.05$). Thus, the increased fibre size at 7–8 days post exercise was interpreted to reflect fibre swelling. Because the fibre swelling did not appear at the time that DOMS peaked (between 1.5 to 2.5 days post exercise), we concluded that fibre swelling in the soleus muscle is not directly associated with the symptom of DOMS.

Editor: Nicole Beard, University of Canberra, Australia

Funding: This work was supported by grants from the Swedish National Centre for Research in Sports (139/07, 89/10, 105/11), the Swedish Research Council (12X-03934) and the Medical Faculty of Umeå University. The funders had no role in study design, data collection and analysis, decision to publish, or preparation of the manuscript. There is no actual or potential conflict of interest including financial, personal or other relationships with other people or organizations.

* E-mail: jiguo.yu@idrott.umu.se

Introduction

The aetiology of delayed onset muscle soreness (DOMS) induced by eccentric exercise (i.e., lengthening of a contracting muscle) is still unclear [1]. The prevailing hypothesis of the mechanisms of DOMS is that the excessive strain produced during eccentric muscular contraction induces extracellular or intracellular membrane disruption that may induce hydrolysis of structural proteins such as desmin intermediate filament network, leading to myofibrillar disorganization in the form of Z-band streaming or complete disruption [2,3]. This is followed by fibre necrosis and inflammatory cell infiltration that potentiate the nerve endings and perception of pain. Passive manipulation and active movement alter intramuscular pressure and stimulate mechanoreceptor nerve endings, contributing to the perception of soreness [4]. However, recent studies in humans provided evidence which did not support the hypothesis, e.g., voluntary eccentric exercise did not lead to desmin intermediate filament network hydrolysis [5,6], myofibrillar disruption [5,7] or muscle fibre inflammation and necrosis [5,6,8,9,10]. The Z-band streaming, classically proposed to be a hallmark of muscle damage after eccentric exercise [11,12] was also proved to represent myofibril remodelling [7,13,14,15,16].

As proposed in the prevailing hypothesis, sarcolemma damage has indeed been observed in animals soon after electrical stimulation-induced eccentric muscular contractions, and the damage was often amplified later [17,18,19]. In contrast, studies on humans after voluntary eccentric exercise revealed no [5,6,20,21,22,23] or only minor damage [10,24] in muscle fibre membrane. To our knowledge, no data is available in humans with regard to the initial reactions of muscle fibre membrane to acute voluntary eccentric exercise.

Eccentric exercise has been proposed to cause intracellular fibre swelling which is associated with the subsequent muscle soreness and stiffness [3,4,25,26]. Because of technique limitations in directly measuring intracellular fibre swelling, many studies measured muscle swelling using either sonography or circumference of the exercised extremity. Although many studies have reported muscle swelling in human muscles after voluntary eccentric exercise [27,28,29], none have shown a time course correlation between muscle swelling and DOMS. By measuring muscle fibre size and intracellular pressure, two studies observed fibre swelling after voluntary eccentric exercise [25,30]; however, the studies only analysed muscle biopsies taken 2 days after exercise and therefore there is no information on how fibre swelling develops in relation to the time course of DOMS after eccentric exercise.

In skeletal muscle the capillary network is very dynamic and general exercise can cause adaptive changes in capillary supply [31]. In human muscles a single bout of intensive exercise has been shown to up-regulate angiogenic factors [32], whereas in animals a few days of electrical stimulation induced increased capillarization [33]. Electrical stimulation-induced eccentric exercise and downhill running have been reported to cause morphological changes in capillary luminal area and microvascular dysfunction in rat skeletal muscle [34,35]. To date it is still unclear whether voluntary eccentric exercise in humans is also harmful to the microvascular system.

By analyzing muscle biopsies taken from human soleus muscle within 1 hour, at 2–3 days and 7–8 days after downstairs running, the present study aimed to reveal changes in 1) muscle fibre sarcolemma integrity; 2) muscle fibre swelling/fibre size; 3) microvascular system; and finally 4) to examine the time course of these changes (if any) in relation to the development of DOMS.

Materials and Methods

Ethics Statement

All participants were informed about the design of the study and were asked to refrain from unaccustomed exercise during the experimental period. Written informed consent was obtained from all participants. The study protocol was approved by the Ethics Committee, Medical Faculty, Umeå University.

Subjects

Sixteen healthy males (mean age 24 years, range 21–30) participated in the study. The subjects were young and healthy sedentary medical students, and none of them were accustomed to eccentric exercise or involved in any regular exercise regime. All the subjects were asked to refrain from any strenuous physical exercise before the experiment. Ten of the subjects were randomly assigned to exercise group and the rest served as controls.

Experimental Procedures

In brief, the subjects were asked to run downstairs from the 10th floor to the ground floor and then took the elevator back to the 10th floor, and to repeat the procedure 15 times. During the downstairs running, the subjects were asked to use the ball of the foot to touch the ground to support the body mass and then to the full foot. By doing so, the soleus muscle was subjected to eccentric contraction.

Muscle Soreness Evaluation and Muscle Biopsy

Evaluation of DOMS in the soleus muscle of all subjects was described in our previous work [14]. In brief, muscle soreness was self-evaluated over the middle of the soleus muscles with the muscle contracted (loaded) and relaxed (unloaded). The muscle soreness was rated by the subjects before and after the exercise twice daily for 8.5 days on a 0–10 subject rating scale (0 = no soreness and 10 = very, very sore).

Muscle biopsies were taken from the lateral border of the middle of the soleus muscle (accessible through contraction of the triceps surae). Biopsies from the soleus muscle were obtained under local anaesthesia from 6 controls, 4 exercised subjects within 1 hour (1 h group) and 6 exercised subjects at 2–3 days (2–3 day group) and 7–8 days (7–8 day group; the contralateral leg) after the exercise. The muscle biopsy was mounted in embedding medium (Tissue Tek®, O.C.T. Compound, Miles laboratories, Naperville, IL, USA), frozen in propane chilled with liquid N_2 (-160 °C) and stored at -80 °C until used.

Histochemistry and Immunohistochemistry (IHC)

Serial muscle cross-sections were cut at -25 °C by using a Reichert Jung cryostat (Leica, Nussloch, Germany). Eight μm thick sections were stained with haematoxylin-eosin and a modified Gomori trichrome staining for basic histopathology including detection of degenerative processes and inflammation [36].

Five μm thick sections were processed for IHC with different previously characterized antibodies. For fibre phenotype type classification, serial cross sections were stained with monoclonal antibodies (mAbs) against different adult and developmental myosin heavy chain (MyHC) isoforms [37]: A4.840 (strong affinity for MyHCI), A4.74 (strong affinity for MyHCIIa), N2.261 (strong affinity to MyHCIIa, weak affinity to MyHCI, no affinity to MyHCIIx), BF-35 (strong affinity for all MyHC isoforms except IIx), F1.652 (strong affinity to embryonic MyHC) and NCL-MHCn (strong affinity to fetal MyHC). All antibodies, except NCL-MHCn, were obtained from the Developmental Studies Hybridoma Bank, developed under the auspices of the NICHD and maintained by the University of Biological Sciences, Iowa City, Iowa, USA. NCL-MHCn was obtained from Novocastra Lab, Newcastle, UK.

A panel of antibodies was used for visualization of muscle fibre membrane integrity. Monoclonal Abs Dys1, Dys2, Dys3 (Novocastra laboratories, Newcastle upon Tyne, UK) and polyclonal antibody 5EM96 (gift from Dr. S. C. Watkins, CBI, Pittsburgh, PA, USA) stains muscle fibre plasma membrane protein dystrophin, and mAb 5H2 against laminin α2-chain (Novocastra Lab, Newcastle, UK) stains the basement membranes of muscle fibres. Muscle fibre membrane integrity was also evaluated through identification of cellular distribution of plasma proteins fibronectin and fibrinogen. Fibronectin has been previously used as an indicator for membrane injury in muscle fibre [18] and fibrinogen as a sensitive marker for membrane damage in cardiomyocytes after myocardial infarction [38]. Myocardial tissue samples obtained from experimental myocardial infarction in pigs were used as control for specificity of the staining reaction. MAb 52BF12 was used for plasma protein fibronectin [39]. Three different antibodies against plasma protein fibrinogen were used: mAb F 9902 (Sigma, Copenhagen, Denmark), polyclonal Ab A0080 (Dako, Carpinteria, USA) and polyclonal Ab Pc 056 (The Binding site Inc., San Diego, CA, USA).

Identification of capillaries was performed with mAb 4C7 against laminin α5-chain in the capillary basement membrane (Chemicon, Temecula, Calif., USA) [40] and Ulex europaeus agglutin 1 lectin (UEA-1, Dako, Glostrup, Denmark), an endothelial cell marker that previously has been shown to specifically recognize capillaries in skeletal muscle. The mAb 4C7 labels the basement membrane of capillaries strongly and the basement membrane of muscle fibre weakly [39]. To identify monocytes/macrophages, mAb F7135 (Dako, Glostrup, Denmark) against CD68 was used [41].

The IHC staining follows the same procedures as described previously [14]. Visualization of bound primary antibodies was performed by indirect fluorescence, using Alexa 488 (green) or Alexa 568 (red) conjugated secondary antibodies (Molecular Probes Inc., Eugene, USA) [14], or by indirect peroxidase-antiperoxidase (PAP) staining [37]. Control sections were treated as above, except that the primary antibody was exchanged with non-immune serum.

Sarcolemma Integrity

Analysis of the muscle sarcolemma integrity was performed on sections stained with antibodies against dystrophin, laminin α2-chain, fibronectin and fibrinogen. From each muscle sample randomly chosen areas covering a minimum of 300 fibres were scanned and photographed using a Nikon microscope (Eclipse, E800, Tokyo, Japan) equipped with a Spot RT camera (Diagnostic Instrument, Sterling Heights, USA). The sections stained with the antibodies against dystrophin and laminin α2-chain were examined for disruption or absence of staining from membrane, whereas the sections stained with antibodies against plasma proteins were examined for intracellular staining outlined by double labelling of dystrophin or laminin. The number of fibres with visible lack of staining on membrane or intracellular staining was counted separately and expressed as percentage of total fibres in the photographed area.

Morphometric Analysis

For estimation of muscle fibre size, fibre type classification and capillary network, four randomly chosen areas in each of the sections stained with antibodies against laminin α2-chain, UEA-I lectin and sections double stained for α5-chains and different MyHC isoforms were scanned and photographed with a MTI CCD 72 video camera (DAGE-MTI, Michigan City, USA) through a Zeiss microscope (Axiophot, Carl Zeiss, Oberkochen, Germany) equipped with an image analysis system (IBAS, Kontron Elektronik GMBH, Eching, Germany).

To estimate fibre size and capillary supply, the circumference of each fibre and capillary was traced on digital image along the periphery of the basement membrane revealed by staining for laminin α5-chain and UEA-I lectin. The IBAS program calculated the area of each individual muscle fibre in the muscle fibre cross-section. Fibre size variability as coefficient of variation (CV) was estimated according to the formula CV = (SD/mean fibre diameter) x 100%. Capillary density (CD) was calculated as the total number of capillary per mm^2 muscle cross-section and capillary per fibre (C/F) was expressed as the ratio CD/number of fibre per mm^2 cross-sectional tissue. For the analysis of the number of capillaries around each individual fibre (CAF), all capillaries within a distance of 5 μm from each muscle fibre were included. The variable of CAF related to the cross-sectional area of each individual fibre (CAFA) was calculated according to the formula: CAF/fibre cross-sectional area x 10^3. On average, 349 fibres per sample (totally 6821 fibres) were individually analysed for capillary supply, which is beyond the reported requirement (50 fibres/sample) for a reliable analysis of the capillary network in normal limb muscles [42].

Fibre type classification was based on the staining pattern of the fibres for the mAbs directed against different MyHC isoforms. According to a staining scheme of these antibodies (Fig. 1), the fibres were classified into fibre phenotypes containing solely slow MyHCI (type I), fast MyHCIIa (type IIA) or fast MyHCIIx (type IIX) or hybrid fibres co-expressing MyHCI+IIa (type I+IIA) or MyHCIIa+IIx (type IIAX).

The sections stained with antibodies F1.652 and NCL-MHCn were examined for detection of fibres containing developmental MyHCs. All positively stained fibres were counted and expressed as percentage of total fibres. For analysis of infiltration of inflammatory cells, the sections stained with mAb against CD68 were scanned thoroughly to identify positively stained monocytes/macrophages. The number of fibres with infiltration of monocytes/macrophages was counted and expressed as number of cells per mm^2 muscle cross-section. Necrotic muscle fibres containing monocytes/macrophages were not included in the counting.

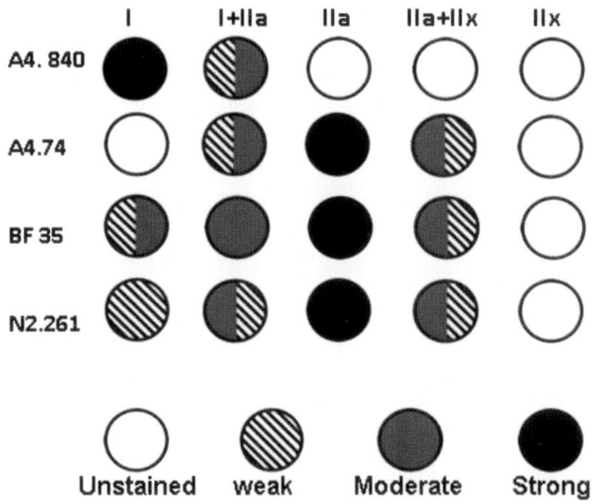

Figure 1. Scheme of fibre phenotype classification. The staining intensity of the four different antibodies in all fibres were briefly classified into "unstained", "weak", "Moderate" and "Strong". An individual fibre was classified into a specific fibre type according to its staining intensities with the four different antibodies against different MyHC isoforms.

Statistical Analysis

Statistical analyses were performed using the StatView program (SAS Company, Berkley, CA, USA). Data are presented as mean ± SD. Since no indication of non-normality was observed within each group, a *t*-test for unpaired data was used. Because the biopsies taken at 2–3 days and at 7–8 days were from the same group of subjects, data of the two groups was further analysed by using a paired sample *t*-test. Statistical significance was set at $p<0.05$.

Results

DOMS and Sarcolemma Injury

All exercised subjects experienced severe DOMS that reached peak values (7.8±1.4 for loaded and 7.7±1.7 for unloaded) between 1.5 to 2.5 days and returned to pre-exercise level by 6 days post-exercise. There was no significant difference in the mean values of DOMS between the loaded and unloaded soleus muscles at any time [14]. The dynamic changes of DOMS following the time course after the downstairs running have been published previously [14].

No visible lesions were observed in muscle fibre sarcolemma proteins revealed by staining for dystrophin and laminin (Fig. 2). Staining for plasma fibronectin was negative in all muscle samples, except for one biopsy from the 1 h group, where a few fibres contained some small and weakly stained subsarcolemmal dots (not shown). In the same fibres, where intracellular staining for fibronectin was observed, similar subsarcolemmal dots revealed by double staining for fibrinogen were present as well. However, intracellular staining for fibrinogen was more often observed in fibres where staining for fibronectin was negative. The intracellular staining for fibrinogen was usually seen as a rim adjacent to the plasmalemma close to capillaries and exhibited a diminishing gradient towards the centre of the fibres (Fig. 2). The intracellular staining for fibrinogen was observed in a low proportion of fibres (<5%) in both the controls and exercised groups. Statistical analysis of the number of fibres with intracellular staining for

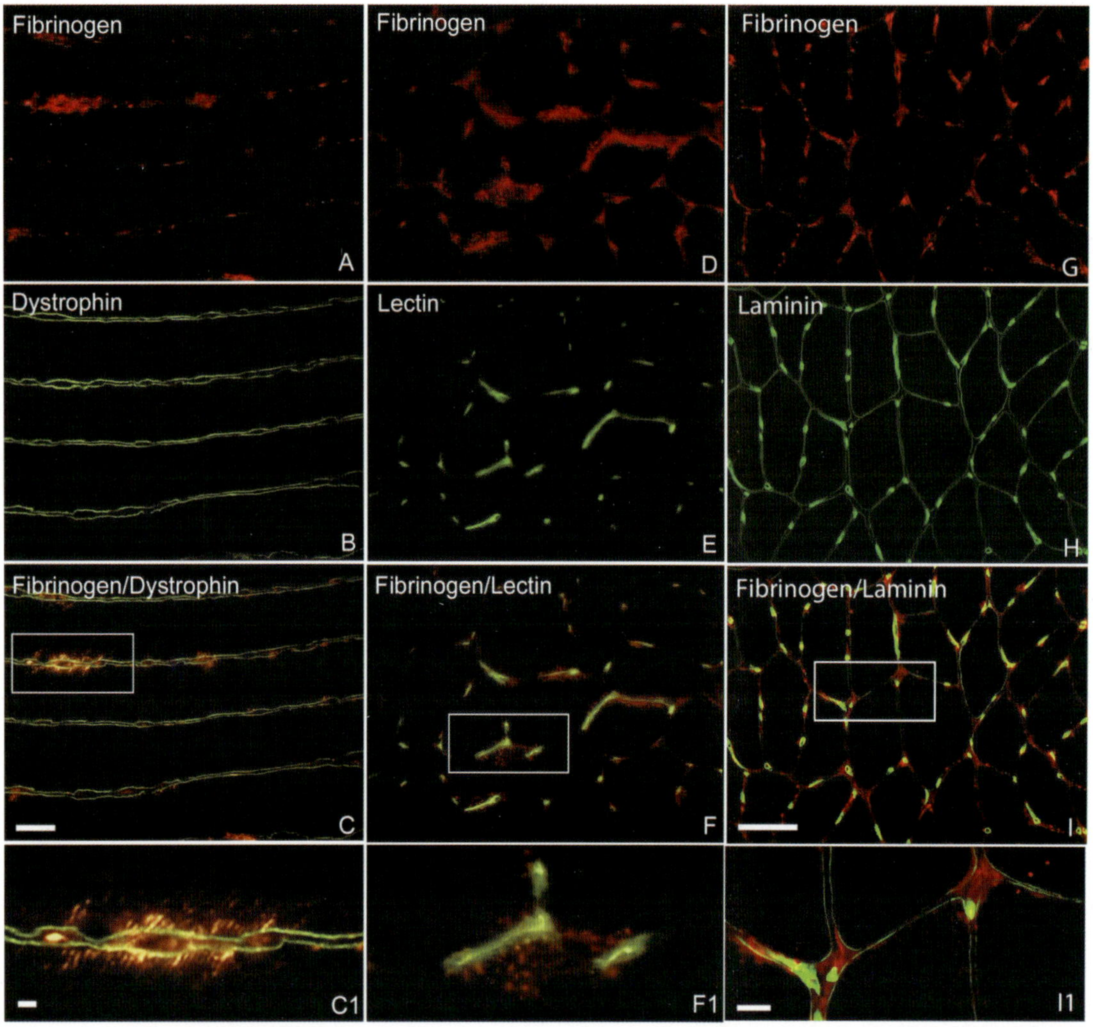

Figure 2. Immunofluorescence staining for visualization of muscle fibre sarcolemma integrity. A–C, one longitudinal section from a biopsy of 1 h group double stained for fibrinogen (**A**) and dystrophin (**B**). **C** is merged images of **A** and **B**, and **C1** is enlargement of boxed areas in **C**. Several sites of intracellular staining for fibrinogen outlined by dystrophin were seen along the length of a fibre, whereas staining for dystrophin did not reveal distinct disruption of plasma membrane. **D–F**, one transverse section from a biopsy of 1 h group double stained for fibrinogen (**D**) and lectin (**E**). F is merged images of **D** and **E**, and **F1** is enlargement of boxed areas in **F**. Intracellular staining for fibrinogen was seen close to capillaries revealed by lectin staining. **G–I**, one transverse section from a biopsy of control group double stained for fibrinogen (**G**) and laminin (**H**). **I** is merged images of **G** and **H**, and **I1** is enlargement of boxed areas in **I**. Several sites of distinct extracellular staining for fibrinogen outlined by laminin were seen. Bars 50 μm

fibrinogen did not reveal any significant difference between control and any post exercise groups.

In the samples of experimental myocardial infarction, all the three antibodies against fibrinogen showed distinct intracellular staining in necrotic cardiomyocytes as previously shown [38]. However, in the soleus muscle samples, positive staining for fibrinogen as small dots was seen in some areas in both muscle fibres and extracellular matrix (Fig. 2).

Necrotic Fibre and Infiltration of Inflammatory Cells

Routine histological staining showed that the fibres in both the controls and exercised samples had generally a polygonal shape and were tightly packed in well-ordered fascicles. A few monocytes/macrophages revealed by antibody against CD68 were seen in between fibres in both control and post exercise groups (Fig. 3). No significant difference was observed in the number of extracellular monocytes/macrophages per unit muscle cross-sectional area (CSA) between control (5.3 ± 3.3 per μm^2) and post exercise groups (1 h, 6.0 ± 1.7 per μm^2; 2–3 day, 11.9 ± 3.3 per μm^2; 7–8 day, 5.3 ± 3.5 per μm^2). Intracellular staining for CD68 was only observed in a few fibres that appeared to be necrotic (Fig. 3). Cells with intracellular staining for CD68 were not included in the data counting.

Developmental MyHCs

A few fibres expressing developmental MyHCs were observed in the 2–3 day and 7–8 day groups, but not in the control or 1 h group (Fig. 3). These fibres were generally extremely small in size in the 2–3 day group ($<100\ \mu m^2$) and somewhat larger ($<400\ \mu m^2$) in the 7–8 day group.

Muscle Fibre Phenotype Composition

The staining pattern for the different MyHC mAbs distinguished fibres containing MyHCI and MyHCIIa in all subjects

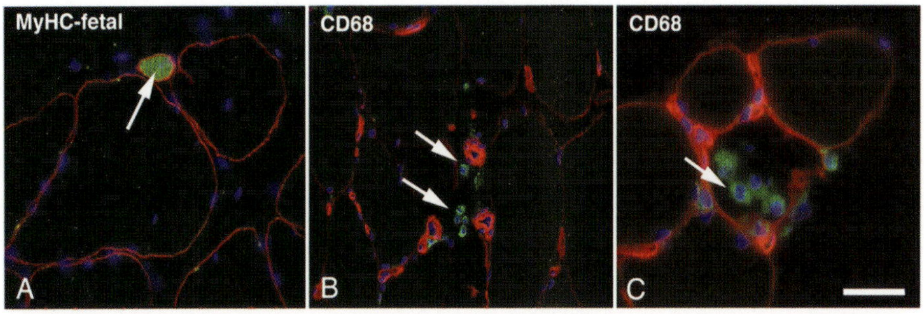

Figure 3. Immunofluorescence staining for visualization of developmental and inflammatory cells. A, one transverse sections from biopsy of 7–8 day group double stained with antibodies against MyHC-fetal (green) and dystrophin (red). One small neonatal fibre was seen between normal sized fibres (arrow). **B** and **C**, transvers sections from biopsies of 2–3 day group double stained with antibodies against CD68 (green) and laminin (red). Several extracellular monocytes/macrophages (arrows) were seen in **B** whereas in **C** monocytes/macrophages were seen inside a necrotic fiber. Nuclei (blue) were visualized in all sections by using mounting medium containing DAPI. Bar 100 μm

and nearly all samples contained a small proportion of hybrid fibres co-expressing MyHCI+IIa or MyHCIIa+IIx. The control soleus muscle was characterized by a very high proportion of fibres containing slow MyHCI (68%±9) and a population of fibres containing fast MyHCIIa (26%±8). No significant difference in proportion of the different fibre phenotypes was observed between any group, except that one subject contained a low proportion of fibres expressing MyHCIIx at 2–3 days (1%±4) and 7–8 days (2%±4).

Muscle Fibre Size

The mean fibre size was 5894 $\mu m^2 \pm 845$ for the control group and 4930 $\mu m^2 \pm 1418$ for the 1 h group, 4987 $\mu m^2 \pm 1367$ for the 2–3 day group and 6588 $\mu m^2 \pm 1551$ for the 7–8 day group. The fibre size at 7–8 days was significantly larger than that at 2–3 days ($p<0.05$; Fig. 4). Analysis of fibre size with respect to fibre phenotype revealed that type I and type IIa fibres in the 7–8 day group were significantly larger than in the 2–3 day group (Fig. 5). Variability in fibre size, expressed as CV, was approximately in the same range at 2–3 days and at 7–8 days (34% vs. 30%).

Capillary Supply

At the group level no significant difference in capillary parameters was observed between the control and the post-exercise groups, although a decreasing trend in capillary density (CD) was observed from 2–3 days to 7–8 days (330±6.1 vs. 289±71 cap/mm^2; $p = 0.07$). Paired analysis of the subjects in the 2–3 day and 7–8 day groups revealed a significant difference in CAF in 5 of the 6 subjects, where 3 subjects had higher values and 2 subjects had lower values at 7–8 days than at 2–3 days ($p<0.05$; Fig. 6). When CAF was further processed by fibre size (CAFA), paired comparison showed lower CAFA value in 5 of the 6 subjects at 7–8 days compared to 2–3 days ($p<0.05$; Fig. 6).

Discussion

The present study shows that the downstairs running leading to DOMS did not result in significant sarcolemma injury or serious inflammatory reactions in the soleus muscle. Thus, the hypothesis that eccentric exercise induces initial sarcolemma injury which triggers subsequent muscle fiber inflammation and necrosis seems not applicable for the human soleus muscle. The enlarged fiber size at 7–8 days post exercise was interpreted to represent fibre swelling due to edema. Since fiber swelling did not appear at the time of maximal DOMS (between 1.5 to 2.5 days post exercise), it seems not to be directly associated with the aetiology of DOMS.

Sarcolemma Injury

Previous studies have mainly used two different methods to evaluate sarcolemma integrity after eccentric exercise: direct visualization through examination of muscle biopsy and indirect evaluation by measuring serum levels of muscle enzymes such as creatine kinase (CK), lactate dehydrogenase (LDH) and glutamic

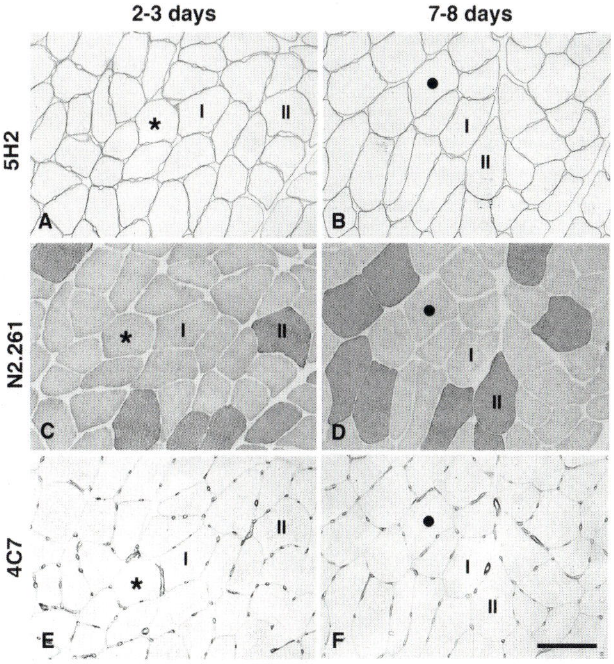

Figure 4. Immunohistochemical staining for visualization of muscle fibre size, fibre phenotype and capillary supply. Serial transverse sections from one biopsy in the 2–3 day group **(A, C, E)** and one from the 7–8 day group **(B, D, F)** stained with antibodies 5H2 for fibre profile **(A, B)**, N2.261 for fibre phenotypes **(C, D)** and 4C7 for capillaries **(E, F)**. Most fibres are larger in size in the 7–8 days group **(B)** compared to the 2–3 days group **(A)**. Type I and type II fibres are marked **(C, D)**. There was no distinct difference in number of capillaries around each fibre between the two groups **(E, F)** despite the fibre size was larger in the 7–8 day group **(F)**. Stars and black dots mark same fibre in series sections. Bar 100 μm

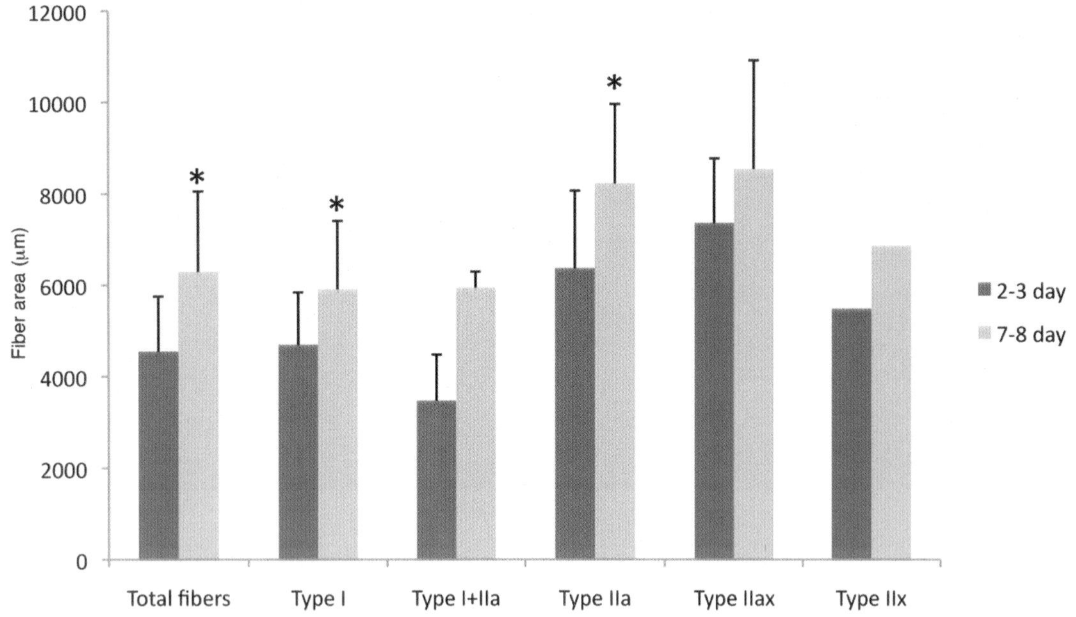

Figure 5. Comparison in fibre size between 2–3 day and 7–8 day groups. Fibre size in 7–8 day group was significantly larger than in 2–3 day group. Among the five different fibre phenotypes, only type I and type IIa fibres presented larger fibre size in 7–8 day group than in 2–3 day group (*p<0.05).

oxaloacetic transaminase (GOT), and of muscle proteins like slow myosin heavy chain (MyHC) fragments and myoglobin [1].

Many studies using animal models of eccentric muscular contraction have reported large proportions (around 10–30%) of muscle fibres with discontinuous or complete disruption of sarcolemma as evidenced by lack of staining for dystrophin, dystroglycans and sarcoglycans [43,44] and by intracellular staining for serum albumin, fibronectin and Evans blue [19,43,44,45]. In comparison, voluntary eccentric exercise of human muscles usually does not induce similar serious injury in sarcolemma integrity. In an early study on humans [10], ultra-marathon running (mainly downhill) induced very few fibres (in gastrocnemius muscle) with sarcolemma disruption. Using isolated high intensity eccentric exercise, two studies reported sarcolemma injury (in vastus lateralis muscle [46] and in biceps brachii muscle [47]), but the injury was only limited in a few of the subjects/biopsies (1 out of 8 subjects or 2 out of 24 biopsies [46], and 9 out of 61 biopsies [47]). Similarly, in a recent study, sarcolemma injury was only observed in 1 out of 18 biopsies (or 1 out of 9 subjects) from vastus lateralis muscle taken during (at 3 days) and after 6 days maximum voluntary eccentric exercise of knee joint [23]. The present study did not observe any significant lesion revealed by either sarcolemma proteins or by plasma proteins in any of the post exercise groups. The results of the study indicate that human soleus muscle sarcolemma was not as susceptible to the downstairs running as animal muscles to isolated eccentric exercise [18,19,43,44,45]. Importantly, the study did not observe sarcolemma damage at 1 hour after the downstairs running, indicating

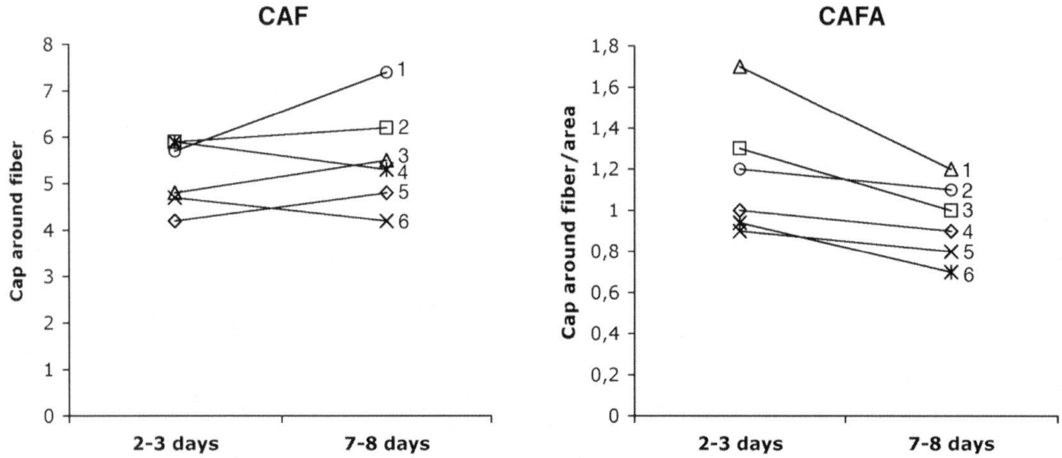

Figure 6. Comparison of individual values in CAF and CAFA from the same subjects in 2–3 day and 7–8 day groups. Compared to 2–3 day group, CAF was higher in three subjects (1, 3, 5) and lower in two subjects (4, 6), whereas CAFA was lower in five subjects (1, 3, 4, 5, 6) in 7–8 day group (p<0.05).

the previous hypothesis that early sarcolemma injury triggers subsequent deleterious reactions in muscles after eccentric exercise is not applicable to the human soleus muscles. The results of all these studies collectively indicate that sarcolemma disruption occurs in a minority of exercised subjects irrespective of how the voluntary eccentric exercise is performed.

Previous study has shown that disruptions of cell membranes are common in vivo and that the disrupted membranes can reseal within a minute even when a hole is up to 1 μm in diameter [48]. It is commonly believed that structural changes in muscles induced by eccentric exercise can be regarded as a continuum from mild changes to pathological-like changes [1]. We propose that the sarcolemma injuries in humans induced by voluntary eccentric exercise are mostly from mild to moderate in extent and therefore most injuries are temporary and reversible. The temporary injury in sarcolemma may allow the efflux of muscle enzymes such as CK, LDH and GOT, and even large molecular proteins like MyHC fragments and myoglobin into the plasma. Since such sarcolemma injuries are usually resealed very fast, no visible lesion in sarcolemma is available even if the level of muscle enzymes and muscle proteins are high in the serum. This might explain the poor correlation between serum CK level and changes in muscle histology [49].

In contrast, the electrical stimulation-induced eccentric muscular contractions might result in sarcolemma injuries too extensive in size to be resealed in animals (rabbit digitorum longus muscle [18] and rabbit and rat tibialis anterior muscle [18,19]) and in humans (vastus lateralis muscle [5]). This might lead to calcium influx and subsequent proteinase activation and hydrolysis of structural proteins like desmin and sarcolemma proteins, followed by complete sarcolemma disruption and fibre necrosis [5,18,19]. Of course, sarcolemma damage to such an extent will allow efflux of muscle enzymes and muscle proteins, and even influx of serum proteins such as fibronectin, albumin and tetranectin [1,5,18,19].

Sarcolemma injury in humans after voluntary eccentric exercise seems to be limited mainly in a few biopsies/subjects [10,23,46,47], which indicates individual variation in sensitivity of muscle fibre sarcolemma to the same mode of eccentric exercise. This is consistent with the observation that post-exercise plasma CK activity demonstrates large variation across individuals with high responders, median responders and low responders [49]. Interestingly, some studies (including the present study) have shown that sarcolemma injury [10,23,46,47] occurred often in the same biopsies/subjects where fibre necrosis were observed [5,10,46,50,51]. Currently, not much data is available about the relationship between sarcolemma injury and fibre necrosis after eccentric exercise; however, it seems plausible to speculate a close correlation between the two events, especially when sarcolemma injury is extensive.

The present study applied downstairs running to expose the soleus muscle to eccentric exercise. Compared with other studies using isolated maximal eccentric contraction on humans [5,46,47,50,51] and animals [17,18,19], the exercise mode used in the study might explain the lack of significant sarcolemma injury and inflammatory reaction.

Fibrinogen has been previously proved to be a good marker for cardiomyocyte damage after myocardial infarction [38]. However, in the present study, some small intracellular staining for fibrinogen existed not only in post exercise muscles ($<5\%$) but also in controls (around 3.7%). In addition, in some areas, positive staining for fibrinogen was also present in extracellular matrix. As a control for the antibodies, the samples of the experimental myocardial infarction were also tested in the study, and all the three different antibodies against fibrinogen revealed only distinct intracellular staining in the necrotic cardiomyocytes. On basis of the results, we concluded that plasma fibrinogen might be a good marker for necrotic fibres, but not for detection of mild membrane damage.

Necrotic Fibres and Infiltration of Inflammatory Cells

In the present study, very few necrotic fibres and a nearly negligible infiltration of monocytes/macrophages were observed in the exercised muscles. The findings were consistent with previous observations on humans after voluntary eccentric exercise [10,20,22,30,50,51]. Studies on lower body muscles (vastus lateralis) failed to present fibre necrosis after high intensity of knee eccentric activity (30 min eccentric cycling [20,22] and repetitive knee eccentric extension [30]). Even ultra-marathon footrace (160 km, mainly downhill) only resulted in very few necrotic fibres (1%) in gastrocnemius muscles [10]. Studies on upper body muscles (biceps brachii), however, indeed revealed fibre necrosis after maximal voluntary eccentric contractions of the elbow flexors, but it occurred only in a few of the exercise subjects/biopsies (3 out of 15 biopsies [50], and 8 out of 23 subjects [51]). These results seem in support of the observation that the upper body muscles are more prone to exercise-induced damage than lower body muscles [52].

In animal models of electrical stimulation-induced eccentric muscle contraction, massive muscular inflammation and necrotic fibres (over 30% necrotic fibres) were observed (in rabbit digitorum longus muscle [18] and in both rabbit and rat tibialis anterior muscle [18,19]). In this context, the study of Crameri et al (5) is of special interest and relevance. Massive fibre necrosis was observed in vastus laterlis muscles subjected to electrical stimulation-induced eccentric muscle contractions whereas in the same subjects, no fibre necrosis was observed in the muscle of the contralateral leg after maximal voluntary eccentric contractions. The authors suggested that the difference in the extent of muscle injury between the voluntary eccentric exercise and the electrical stimulation-induced eccentric muscle contraction may be due to the difference in motor unit recruitment pattern. This may also explain the difference in the extent of fibre necrosis and inflammation between animals and humans. Alternatively, the difference in exercise protocol may play an important role in the extent of muscle injury.

Developmental MyHCs

In the 2–3 day group, a few extremely small fibres expressed developmental MyHC. Such fibres were also observed in a very low number in the 7–8 day group, but these were relatively larger in size. In adult limb muscles, small fibres expressing developmental MyHC have been associated with newly formed/regenerated muscle fibres [53]. Satellite cells are considered to be involved in the process of repair and formation of new fibres after muscle damage [54]. Although we found no signs of serious muscle damage in the post exercise muscles, the findings of small fibres expressing developmental MyHCs in the post-exercise muscle biopsies may imply that the downstairs running induced a very restricted regenerative process in the soleus muscle.

Muscle Fibre Swelling

Muscle fibre swelling due to oedema has been associated with the mechanisms of DOMS induced by eccentric exercise [55]. Muscle fibre swelling evaluated by increased muscle fiber size and intramuscular pressure has been observed 2 days post exercise in human tibialis anterior muscle after 400 submaximal eccentric contractions [25] and vastus lateralis muscle after repetitive maximal eccentric exercise [30]. However, since the two studies did not examine serial biopsies following the time course of DOMS after the eccentric exercise, the association between muscle fibre swelling and DOMS was still inconclusive. In the present study, we observed a 24% greater increase in muscle fibre size at 7–8 days than at 2–3 days in the same group subjects. The increased fibre size was interpreted to reflect muscle fibre swelling. However, a single bout of eccentric exercise has been shown to stimulate net protein synthesis within 4–8 hours after exercise [56]. Thus, we could not exclude the possibility that increased protein synthesis is partly responsible for the dramatic enlargement in fibre size at 7–8 days after the exercise. Yet, the results of the relatively similar fibre size in different fibre phenotypes and the significant lower CAFA values in 5 out of the 6 subjects at 7–8 days compared to 2–3 days suggest that the larger fibre size was most likely due to fibre swelling. Since fibre swelling appeared at 7–8 days, not at 2–3 days when DOMS peaked, we conclude that fibre swelling is not associated with the aetiology of DOMS in human soleus muscle after the downstairs running.

Muscle Vascularization

In previous studies on rats, exhaustive eccentric exercise of spinotrapezius muscle [34] and 300 electrical stimulation-induced eccentric contractions of gastrocnemius muscles resulted in damage to microcirculation and thereby the delivery and exchange of O_2 and substrates [35]. The damage was exhibited more often in the capillary lumen rather than capillary collapse or capillary degeneration. In this study, we did not observe significant alterations in capillary network at the group level. However, a significant increase in the capillary network was observed 7–8 days post exercise in some individuals, whereas a regression of the capillary network was found in others. The different responses to the downstairs running might reflect individual variation in physical fitness or inherent genetic differences. Although it is not possible to make any reliable conclusions about the effect of eccentric exercise on the capillary network, the present results indicate that the same exercise could lead to completely different reactions in the microvascular system in different subjects.

Conclusions

The present study showed that the downstairs running did not induce early injury in sarcolemma or severe muscle fibre inflammation and necrosis. The result disproves the previous hypothesis that eccentric exercise leads to initial sarcolemma injury which triggers subsequent deleterious reactions such as muscle fibre inflammation and necrosis. The study revealed that the downstairs running indeed induced fibre swelling, but it appeared at 7–8 days, not at 2–3 days post exercise when DOMS peaked. The result also disproved previous hypothesis that muscle fibre swelling is directly associated with the symptom of DOMS. However, the study examined only the soleus muscles after downstairs running; thus, a definite conclusion cannot be made before evaluations of other muscles are performed in the same way. Furthermore, individual variation may confound the interpretation of the data since in the study only the 2–3 day group and the 7–8 day group are from the same subjects.

Acknowledgments

We thank M Enerstedt and A-K Olofsson for excellent technical assistance.

Author Contributions

Conceived and designed the experiments: JGY LET. Performed the experiments: JGY JXL LC. Analyzed the data: JGY JXL LC LET PSS. Wrote the paper: JGY PSS. Manuscript revision: JGY JXL LC LET PSS.

References

1. Paulsen G, Mikkelsen UR, Raastad T, Peake JM (2012) Leucocytes, cytokines and satellite cells: what role do they play in muscle damage and regeneration following eccentric exercise? Exerc Immunol Rev 18: 42–97.
2. Lieber RL, Friden J (2002) Morphologic and mechanical basis of delayed-onset muscle soreness. J Am Acad Orthop Surg 10: 67–73.
3. Clarkson PM, Hubal MJ (2002) Exercise-induced muscle damage in humans. Am J Phys Med Rehabil/Association of Academic Physiatrists 81: S52–69.
4. Lewis PB, Ruby D, Bush-Joseph CA (2012) Muscle soreness and delayed-onset muscle soreness. Clin Sports Med 31: 255–262.
5. Crameri RM, Aagaard P, Qvortrup K, Langberg H, Olesen J, et al. (2007) Myofibre damage in human skeletal muscle: effects of electrical stimulation versus voluntary contraction. J Physiol 583: 365–380.
6. Yu JG, Malm C, Thornell LE (2002) Eccentric contractions leading to DOMS do not cause loss of desmin nor fibre necrosis in human muscle. Histochem Cell Biol 118: 29–34.
7. Yu JG, Carlsson L, Thornell LE (2004) Evidence for myofibril remodeling as opposed to myofibril damage in human muscles with DOMS: an ultrastructural and immunoelectron microscopic study. Histochem Cell Biol 121: 219–227.
8. Malm C, Sjodin TL, Sjoberg B, Lenkei R, Renstrom P, et al. (2004) Leukocytes, cytokines, growth factors and hormones in human skeletal muscle and blood after uphill or downhill running. J Physiol 556: 983–1000.
9. Malm C, Yu JG (2012) Exercise-induced muscle damage and inflammation: re-evaluation by proteomics. Histochem Cell Biol 138: 89–99.
10. Crenshaw AG, Friden J, Hargens AR, Lang GH, Thornell LE (1993) Increased technetium uptake is not equivalent to muscle necrosis: scintigraphic, morphological and intramuscular pressure analyses of sore muscles after exercise. Acta Physiol Scand 148: 187–198.
11. Friden J, Sjostrom M, Ekblom B (1981) A morphological study of delayed muscle soreness. Experientia 37: 506–507.
12. Friden J, Lieber RL (1992) Structural and mechanical basis of exercise-induced muscle injury. Med Sci Sports Exerc 24: 521–530.
13. Yu JG, Furst DO, Thornell LE (2003) The mode of myofibril remodelling in human skeletal muscle affected by DOMS induced by eccentric contractions. Histochem Cell Biol 119: 383–393.
14. Yu JG, Thornell LE (2002) Desmin and actin alterations in human muscles affected by delayed onset muscle soreness: a high resolution immunocytochemical study. Histochem Cell Biol 118: 171–179.
15. Carlsson L, Yu JG, Moza M, Carpen O, Thornell LE (2007) Myotilin: a prominent marker of myofibrillar remodelling. Neuromuscul Disord 17: 61–68.
16. Carlsson L, Yu JG, Thornell LE (2008) New aspects of obscurin in human striated muscles. Histochem Cell Biol 130: 91–103.
17. Friden J, Lieber RL (2001) Eccentric exercise-induced injuries to contractile and cytoskeletal muscle fibre components. Acta Physiol Scand 171: 321–326.
18. Lieber RL, Thornell LE, Friden J (1996) Muscle cytoskeletal disruption occurs within the first 15 min of cyclic eccentric contraction. J Appl Physiol 80: 278–284.
19. Komulainen J, Takala TE, Kuipers H, Hesselink MK (1998) The disruption of myofibre structures in rat skeletal muscle after forced lengthening contractions. Pflugers Arch 436: 735–741.
20. Malm C, Nyberg P, Engstrom M, Sjodin B. Lenkei R, et al. (2000) Immunological changes in human skeletal muscle and blood after eccentric exercise and multiple biopsies. J Physiol 529 Pt 1: 243–262.
21. Newham DJ, McPhail G, Mills KR, Edwards RH (1983) Ultrastructural changes after concentric and eccentric contractions of human muscle. Neurol Sci 61: 109–122.
22. Friden J, Sjostrom M, Ekblom B (1983) Myofibrillar damage following intense eccentric exercise in man. Int J Sports Med 4: 170–176.
23. Costa A, Orosz Z, Apor P, Csaba N, Siamilis S, et al. (2009) Impact of repeated bouts of eccentric exercise on sarcolemma disruption in human skeletal muscle. Acta Physiol Hung 96: 189–202.
24. Stauber WT, Clarkson PM, Fritz VK, Evans WJ (1990) Extracellular matrix disruption and pain after eccentric muscle action. J Appl Physiol 69: 868–874.
25. Friden J, Sfakianos PN, Hargens AR, Akeson WH (1988) Residual muscular swelling after repetitive eccentric contractions. J Orthop Res 6: 493–498.
26. Proske U, Allen TJ (2005) Damage to skeletal muscle from eccentric exercise. Exerc Sport Sci Rev 33: 98–104.
27. Chleboun GS, Howell JN, Conatser RR, Giesey JJ (1998) Relationship between muscle swelling and stiffness after eccentric exercise. Med Sci Sports Exerc 30: 529–535.
28. Zainuddin Z, Newton M, Sacco P, Nosaka K (2005) Effects of massage on delayed-onset muscle soreness, swelling, and recovery of muscle function. J Athl Train 40: 174–180.
29. Jayaraman RC, Reid RW, Foley JM, Prior BM, Dudley GA, et al. (2004) MRI evaluation of topical heat and static stretching as therapeutic modalities for the

treatment of eccentric exercise-induced muscle damage. Eur J Appl Physiol 93: 30–38.
30. Crenshaw AG, Thornell LE, Friden J (1994) Intramuscular pressure, torque and swelling for the exercise-induced sore vastus lateralis muscle. Acta Physiol Scand 152: 265–277.
31. Laughlin MH, Roseguini B (2008) Mechanisms for exercise training-induced increases in skeletal muscle blood flow capacity: differences with interval sprint training versus aerobic endurance training. J Physiol Pharmacol 59 Suppl 7: 71–88.
32. Bloor CM (2005) Angiogenesis during exercise and training. Angiogenesis 8: 263–271.
33. Brown MD, Hudlicka O (2003) Modulation of physiological angiogenesis in skeletal muscle by mechanical forces: involvement of VEGF and metalloproteinases. Angiogenesis 6: 1–14.
34. Kano Y, Padilla DJ, Behnke BJ, Hageman KS, Musch TI, et al. (2005) Effects of eccentric exercise on microcirculation and microvascular oxygen pressures in rat spinotrapezius muscle. J Appl Physiol 99: 1516–1522.
35. Kano Y, Sampei K, Matsudo H (2004) Time course of capillary structure changes in rat skeletal muscle following strenuous eccentric exercise. Acta Physiol Scand 180: 291–299.
36. Dubowitz V, Sewry CA (2007) Muscle biopsy. A practical approach. Bailliere Tindall, City.
37. Liu JX, Eriksson PO, Thornell LE, Pedrosa-Domellof F (2002) Myosin heavy chain composition of muscle spindles in human biceps brachii. J Histochem Cytochem 50: 171–183.
38. Holmbom B, Lindstrom M, Naslund U, Thornell LE (1991) A method for enzyme- and immunohistochemical staining of large frozen specimens. Histochem 95: 441–447.
39. Vartio T, Laitinen L, Narvanen O, Cutolo M, Thornell LE, et al. (1987) Differential expression of the ED sequence-containing form of cellular fibronectin in embryonic and adult human tissues. J Cell Sci, 88: 419–430.
40. Stal PS, Lindman R (2000) Characterisation of human soft palate muscles with respect to fibre types, myosins and capillary supply. J Anat 197 (Pt 2): 275–290.
41. Micklem K, Rigney E, Cordell J, Simmons D, Stross P, et al. (1989) A human macrophage-associated antigen (CD68) detected by six different monoclonal antibodies. Br J Haematol 73: 6–11.
42. Porter MM, Koolage CW, Lexell J (2002) Biopsy sampling requirements for the estimation of muscle capillarization. Muscle Nerve 26: 546–548.
43. Lehti TM, Kalliokoski R, Komulainen J (2007) Repeated bout effect on the cytoskeletal proteins titin, desmin, and dystrophin in rat skeletal muscle. J Muscle Res Cell Motil 28: 39–47.
44. Lovering RM, De Deyne PG (2004) Contractile function, sarcolemma integrity, and the loss of dystrophin after skeletal muscle eccentric contraction-induced injury. Am J Physiol 286: C230–238.
45. McNeil PL, Khakee R (1992) Disruptions of muscle fiber plasma membranes. Role in exercise-induced damage. Am J Pathol 140: 1097–1109.
46. Crameri RM, Langberg H, Magnusson P, Jensen CH, Schroder HD, et al. (2004) Changes in satellite cells in human skeletal muscle after a single bout of high intensity exercise. J Physiol-London 558: 333–340.
47. Paulsen G, Egner I, Raastad T, Reinholt F, Owe S, et al. (2012) Inflammatory markers CD11b, CD16, CD66b, CD68, myeloperoxidase and neutrophil elastase in eccentric exercised human skeletal muscles. Histochem Cell Biol Dec 7.
48. McNeil PL, Steinhardt RA (1997) Loss, restoration, and maintenance of plasma membrane integrity. J Cell Biol 137, 1–4.
49. Clarkson PM, Nosaka K, Braun B (1992) Muscle function after exercise-induced muscle damage and rapid adaptation. Med Sci Sports Exerc 24: 512–20.
50. Lauritzen F, Paulsen G, Raastad T, Bergersen LH, Owe SG (2009) Gross ultrastructural changes and necrotic fiber segments in elbow flexor muscles after maximal voluntary eccentric action in humans. J Appl Physiol 107: 1923–1934.
51. Paulsen G, Egner IM, Drange M, Langberg H, Benestad HB, et al. (2010) A COX-2 inhibitor reduces muscle soreness, but does not influence recovery and adaptation after eccentric exercise. Scand J Med Sci Sports 20: e195–e207.
52. Jamurtas AZ, Theocharis V, Tofas T, Tsiokanos A, Yfanti C, et al. (2005) Comparison between leg and arm eccentric exercises of the same relative intensity on indices of muscle damage. Eur J Appl Physiol, 95: 179–85.
53. Schiaffino S, Gorza L, Dones I, Cornelio F, Sartore S (1986) Fetal myosin immunoreactivity in human dystrophic muscle. Muscle nerve 9: 51–58.
54. Kadi F, Eriksson A, Holmner S, Butler-Browne GS, Thornell LE (1999) Cellular adaptation of the trapezius muscle in strength-trained athletes. Histochem Cell Biol 111: 189–195.
55. Lieber RL, Friden J (1999) Mechanisms of muscle injury after eccentric contraction. J Sci Med Sport 2: 253–265.
56. Moore DR, Phillips SM, Babraj JA, Smith K, Rennie MJ (2005) Myofibrillar and collagen protein synthesis in human skeletal muscle in young men after maximal shortening and lengthening contractions. Am J Physiol Endocrinol Metab 288: E1153–E1159.

3

A Comparative Study of *N*-glycolylneuraminic Acid (Neu5Gc) and Cytotoxic T Cell (CT) Carbohydrate Expression in Normal and Dystrophin-Deficient Dog and Human Skeletal Muscle

Paul T. Martin[1,2,3]*, Bethannie Golden[1], Jonathan Okerblom[4], Marybeth Camboni[1], Kumaran Chandrasekharan[1], Rui Xu[1], Ajit Varki[4], Kevin M. Flanigan[1,2], Joe N. Kornegay[5]

1 Center for Gene Therapy, The Research Institute at Nationwide Children's Hospital, Columbus, Ohio, United States of America, **2** Department of Pediatrics, The Ohio State University College of Medicine, Columbus, Ohio, United States of America, **3** Department of Physiology and Cell Biology, The Ohio State University College of Medicine, Columbus, Ohio, United States of America, **4** Departments of Medicine and Cellular and Molecular Medicine, University of California, San Diego, La Jolla, California, United States of America, **5** Department of Veterinary Integrative Biosciences, Texas A&M University, College Station, Texas, United States of America

Abstract

The expression of *N*-glycolylneuraminic acid (Neu5Gc) and the cytotoxic T cell (CT) carbohydrate can impact the severity of muscular dystrophy arising from the loss of dystrophin in mdx mice. Here, we describe the expression of these two glycans in skeletal muscles of dogs and humans with or without dystrophin-deficiency. Neu5Gc expression was highly reduced (>95%) in muscle from normal golden retriever crosses (GR, n = 3) and from golden retriever with muscular dystrophy (GRMD, n = 5) dogs at multiple ages (3, 6 and 13 months) when compared to mouse muscle, however, overall sialic acid expression in GR and GRMD muscles remained high at all ages. Neu5Gc was expressed on only a minority of GRMD satellite cells, $CD8^+$ T lymphocytes and macrophages. Human muscle from normal (no evident disease, n = 3), Becker (BMD, n = 3) and Duchenne (DMD, n = 3) muscular dystrophy individuals had absent to very low Neu5Gc staining, but some punctate intracellular muscle staining was present in BMD and DMD muscles. The CT carbohydrate was localized to the neuromuscular junction in GR muscle, while GRMD muscles had increased expression on a subset of myofibers and macrophages. In humans, the CT carbohydrate was ectopically expressed on the sarcolemmal membrane of some BMD muscles, but not normal human or DMD muscles. These data are consistent with the notion that altered Neu5Gc and CT carbohydrate expression may modify disease severity resulting from dystrophin deficiency in dogs and humans.

Editor: Atsushi Asakura, University of Minnesota Medical School, United States of America

Funding: This work was funded by NIH grant R01 AR060949 to PTM. Support for dogs came from 1U24NS059696-01A1 (NINDS) Co-operative Program in Translational Research: Proposal for Establishment of the Center for Canine Models of Duchenne Muscular Dystrophy (NCDMD) to JNK and Muscular Dystrophy Association Infrastructure Grant to the Translational Research Advisory Committee (TRAC) to JNK. The funders had no role in study design, data collection and analysis, decision to publish, or preparation of the manuscript.

* E-mail: Paul.Martin@nationwidechildrens.org

Introduction

Duchenne muscular dystrophy (DMD) is a severe X-linked myopathy of childhood that arises from the loss of dystrophin protein expression in cardiac and skeletal muscles[1,2]. Becker muscular dystrophy (BMD) also results from mutations or deletions in the dystrophin gene, but BMD mutations allow for expression of partially functional dystrophin protein and are typically associated with phenotypically milder muscle disease than is seen in DMD. A number of animal models have been used to better define disease pathophysiology and treatments that might ameliorate DMD and BMD[3]. The model used to test most MD therapies is the mdx mouse, which lacks dystrophin in cardiac and skeletal muscles due to a nonsense point mutation in exon 23 of the dystrophin gene[4,5]. Spontaneous mutations and deletions in the dystrophin gene also occur in dogs[6–8] and cats[9–11]. The Golden Retriever Muscular Dystrophy (GRMD) dog is one such DMD model that has been bred for research purposes[6,12]. GRMD dogs harbor a single base pair change in the 3′ consensus splice site of intron 6, resulting in the skipping of exon 7 and an out-of-frame transcript with a stop codon immediately downstream[6,13]. GRMD dogs model a number of features of muscle pathophysiology found in DMD, including increased muscle membrane fragility, weakened muscle force, increased force decrement in response to eccentric contractions, altered pelvic and limb joint angles arising from combined muscle hypertrophy and atrophy, increased muscle inflammation, cardiomyopathy, loss of ambulation and premature death[6,12,14–20]. In addition, treatment of GRMD dogs with corticosteroids, which can prolong ambulation in DMD[21], yields improvement in muscle outcome measures[22]. Thus, while each animal model has its own advantages, GRMD dogs are generally thought to be a very good model of the more severe aspects of DMD pathophysiology and therefore potentially more appropriate for testing DMD therapies.

It is clear from a number of recent studies that glycosylation of the sarcolemmal membrane with particular carbohydrate structures can impact muscle membrane integrity and disease[23–27]. One such modifier of disease severity in the mdx mouse model is the *Cmah* gene[28]. *Cmah* encodes the CMP-Neu5Ac hydroxylase, the only enzyme known to hydroxylate the sugar nucleotide precursor for sialic acids at the 5-N-acyl position, converting CMP-Neu5Ac to CMP-Neu5Gc[29,30]. The twenty or so sialyltransferases in mammals utilize these substrates to add sialic acids to glycoproteins and glycolipids[31]. In all mammals studied to date, save humans, *Cmah* encodes an active enzyme that can result in Neu5Gc on glycoproteins and glycolipids. In mouse skeletal and cardiac muscle, Neu5Gc and Neu5Ac are the predominant sialic acid forms[28]. About 2–3 million years ago, after the divergence of humans from the great apes, a 92 base pair deletion in exon 6 of the human *CMAH* gene led to its inactivation from a resulting frame shift[32], and as a result all humans lack the biosynthetic ability to create Neu5Gc[33,34]. Deletion of mouse *Cmah* to reiterate this event in human evolution does not grossly impact muscle function, but loss of *Cmah* in mdx mice leads to more severe disease pathology, resulting in additional reductions in the strength of diaphragm and cardiac muscles as well as reduced lifespan[28]. While many other modifiers of disease severity occur in mdx mice, for example integrin α7[35], utrophin[36,37], MyoD[38], sarcospan[39,40] and telomerase[41], this is the first example of a disease modifier where the genetic change actually reiterates a human-specific genetic event.

As *Cmah*$^{-/-}$mdx mice show more severe disease severity than mdx animals, the question arises as to how Neu5Gc may impact disease in other animal models, such as dogs and cats. One comparative study of muscle glycolipids has shown that dog muscle has very low Neu5Gc levels, with Neu5Gc comprising 2% of total sialic acid as compared to much higher levels in the mouse, cow and monkey[42]. This raises the possibility that dog muscles are hypomorphic for Neu5Gc, even though they appear to express a functional canine *CMAH* gene.

Another carbohydrate structure that can modify muscular dystrophy is the Cytotoxic T cell (CT) carbohydrate (GalNAcβ1-4[Neu5Ac/Gcα2-3]Galβ1-4GlcNAc-)[43–45]. The CT carbohydrate is normally confined to the neuromuscular junction in adult mouse and human skeletal muscle, with additional expression in intramuscular capillaries[46,47]. The enzyme that defines the synaptic expression of the CT carbohydate is encoded by the *Galgt2* gene (also called *b4Galnt2*). *Galgt2* encodes a β1-4GalNAc glycosyltransferase that creates the terminal β1-4GalNAc linkage on the CT carbohydrate[48–50]. Overexpression of *Galgt2* in mouse skeletal myofibers stimulates the glycosylation of α dystroglycan with the CT carbohydrate and induces the ectopic overexpression of normally synaptic dystroglycan-binding proteins, including utrophin, laminin α4, laminin α5 and agrin[48,51–56]. Such overexpression of Galgt2 can ameliorate muscular dystrophy in three different mouse models of muscular dystrophy, the mdx model for DMD[55], the *Sgca*$^{-/-}$ model for LGMD2D[53] and the dy^{W} model for MDC1A[52]. *Galgt2* overexpression correlates with increased laminin and agrin binding to α dystroglycan[54] and with increased resistance of skeletal muscles to injury resulting from eccentric contractions[24].

Despite the demonstrated functional effects of these carbohydrates on muscle disease, there is no published information on CT carbohydrate expression and little to no information on Neu5Gc expression in BMD or DMD muscles or in golden retriever (GR) or GRMD muscles. As low levels of Neu5Gc and CT carbohydrate correlate with more severe disease in mice, we asked here whether a similar relative deficit might potentially contribute to worsened disease severity in dystrophin-deficient dog and human muscles.

Materials and Methods

Ethics Statement

mdx and wild type (both in a C57Bl/10 genetic background) mice were bred at Nationwide Children's Hospital in accordance with protocols approved by the Institutional Animal Care and Use Committee and specifically approved for use in this study (Permit AR07-00033). The full name of this committee is the "Institutional Animal Care and Use Committee at Nationwide Children's Hospital".

GR crosses and GRMD dogs were bred at University of North Carolina, Chapel Hill, in accordance with protocols approved by their Institutional Animal Care and Use Committee under a protocol that included the experiments described in this study (Permit 06-338). The full name of this committee is the "Institutional Animal Care and Use Committee at the University of North Carolina".

Blinded sections from human muscle biopsies were obtained from clinical specimens archived as part of the United Dystrophinopathy project in accordance with approval from the Institutional Review Board (IRB) at Nationwide Children's Hospital. The full name of this committee is the "Institutional Review Board at Nationwide Children's Hospital". All samples were obtained with patient's written informed consent. As part of the consent process approved by the IRB, we received written consent from guardians on behalf of children/minors. Dated and signed consent forms were archived.

Mice

mdx and wild type (both in a C57Bl/10 genetic background) mice were bred at Nationwide Children's Hospital in accordance with protocols approved by the Institutional Animal Care and Use Committee. mdx mice were originally obtained from Jackson Laboratory and *Cmah*$^{-/-}$ mice and *Cmah*$^{-/-}$mdx mice were generated previously[28,57]. Muscles from mdx mice treated with Adeno associated virus (AAV) vector to overexpress the human *GALGT2* gene (also termed *B4GALNT2*), using rAAV(rh.74).MCK.GALGT2, were utilized from a previous study[24].

Dogs

GR crosses and GRMD dogs were bred at University of North Carolina, Chapel Hill, in accordance with protocols approved by their Institutional Animal Care and Use Committee. Assessment of severity of muscle disease was measured by observation of gait and ambulation as well as measures of tibiotarsal joint (TTJ) angle and maximal tibiotarsal flexion and extension, per previous studies[14,16,19]. For sake of defining disease severity in these GRMD dogs, we characterized several phenotypic features. Ringo and Napoleon were characterized as "severe" based on TTJ extension tetanic force and TTG angles below 1 N/kg and 145°, respectively, while values above these levels were associated with a "mild" phenotype in Tico, Jane and Summer (Table S1). Biopsy or necropsy samples of cranial sartorius (CS) and vastus lateralis (VL) muscles were serially obtained at 3, 6 and 13 months of age. Methods to measure muscle physiology and other measures describing dystrophic changes have been described in previous studies[16,19].

Human muscle biopsies

Blinded sections from human muscle biopsies were obtained from clinical specimens archived as part of the United Dystrophinopathy project in accordance with approval from the Institutional Review Board. Normal human muscles were from a 55 year-old (yo) male, a 5yo male and a 6yo female; DMD muscles were taken from 6 and 5yo males and BMD muscles from 11yo, 35yo and 67yo males. Biopsies were taken from the quadriceps muscle in most instances. "Normal" human samples were defined as biopsies where no myopathy or evidence of inflammation was present. For all normal cases, dystrophin protein expression was verified as being positive, and for all DMD cases, dystrophin protein expression was verified as being negative. DMD cases arose from a duplication of exons 29–43, c.3603+2T>C splice site mutation, or a duplication of exons 3–6. The three BMD cases arose from an intron 11 c.1331+17770C>G pseudoexon mutation (leading to mutant RNA r.1331_1332ins1331+17691_1331+17769 (case BZ), with loss of ambulation at age 23, an exon 2 c.40_41delGA frameshift mutation, with ambulation until at least 36 (case KG), and an intron 25 c.3432+3730G>T pseudoexon mutation, leading to mutant RNA r.3432_3433ins3432+3663_3432+3728, with ambulation until at least 67 (case RS). None of the cases were treated with steroids prior to biopsy.

Immunostaining

Human muscle biopsies and mouse skeletal muscles were snap frozen in liquid nitrogen-cooled isopentane; dog muscle biopsies were frozen in liquid nitrogen-cooled SUVA34A (Freon analogue). 8 μm cross-sections of all skeletal muscles were cut on a cryostat. For staining with antibody to glycans bearing *N*-glycolylneuraminic acid (Neu5Gc, affinity purified chick IgY; Sialix) or non-immune chick IgY control (Sialix), sections were blocked in phosphobuffered saline (PBS) with 10% human serum that was confirmed to be Neu5Gc-free. Sections were incubated with anti-Neu5Gc or control antibody (1:500 or 1:1000) in blocking solution (10% human serum) overnight at 4°C, washed in PBS, incubated with donkey anti-chicken IgY secondary antibody conjugated to FITC (1:250; 703-485-155, Jackson Immunoresearch), washed again in PBS and mounted in glycerol with paraphenylenediamene to inhibit fluorescence quenching. For *Maackia amurensis* agglutinin (MAA) staining, sections were blocked in 5% bovine serum albumin (BSA) in PBS. Sections were incubated with FITC-conjugated MAA (10 μg/mL, EY laboratories, F-7801), washed in PBS and then mounted. All MAA staining could be blocked by addition of exogenous excess sialic acid to demonstrate lectin-binding specificity. Anti-Neu5Gc immunostaining could be blocked with either 10% chimpanzee serum, which has excess Neu5Gc, or by pre-treating sections with mild periodate to destroy the immunogenic side chain of Neu5Gc. None of these methods, or staining with non-immune chick IgY serum, differed from the control images shown. *Wisteria floribunda* agglutinin (WFA) linked to FITC was used to stain muscle at 2 μg/mL (EY Laboratories, F-3101), with 5% BSA in PBS used as a blocking agent. CT1 and CT2 staining was performed as previously described using antibody purified from hybridoma supernatant[58]. Staining for CT1, CT2 or control anti-mouse IgM(only) was blocked in 3%(v/v) BSA in PBS for one hour, followed by incubation with hybridoma supernatant (used straight or diluted 1:2) overnight. Sections were then washed in PBS and incubated in goat anti-mouse IgM(only) conjugated to Cy2 (115-225-020, Jackson ImmunoResearch).

For double immunostaining, sections were first stained overnight at 4°C with anti-Neu5Gc or control-specific chicken IgY after blocking in 10% (Neu5Gc-free) human serum, or with CT1 or CT2 after blocking in 5 mg/mL BSA, as described above. For Pax7 co-staining, sections were fixed in 2% paraformaldehyde. After blocking in 10% human serum, sections were then incubated overnight mouse-anti Pax7 (clone P3U1, Developmental Studies Hybridoma Bank), followed by species- and isotype-specific fluorophore-conjugated secondary antibodies for one hour. Pax7 antibody was a generous gift from Michael Rudnicki (Ottawa Health Research Institute). For all other anti-Neu5Gc or anti-CT co-stains, sections were incubated overnight with both primary antibodies without fixation, washed for one hour and incubated with the appropriate secondary antibodies as above. All sections were washed and placed in mounting medium containing with DAPI. Co-staining antibodies used in dog were mouse anti-chicken Pax7 (Developmental Studies Hybridoma Bank, clone P3U1), mouse anti-dog CD4 (AbD Serotec, MCA1998S), rat anti-dog CD8 (AbD Serotec, MCA1039GA), mouse anti-dog CD11b (AbD Serotec, MCA1777S), mouse anti-dog CD21 (AbD Serotec, MCA1781R), mouse anti-human β spectrin (Novus, NB300-574) or mouse anti-rat embryonic myosin (NovaCastra, NCL-MHCd). Co-staining antibodies used in human were mouse anti-chicken Pax7 (Developmental Studies Hybridoma Bank, clone P3U1), FITC-conjugated rabbit anti-human CD4 (BD Bioscience, 550628), FITC-conjugated mouse anti-human CD8 (AbD Serotec, MCA1039GA), rabbit anti-human CD11b (Abcam, ab52478), mouse anti-human β spectrin (Abcam, ab2808), mouse anti-rat embryonic myosin (eMyosin; NCL-MHCd, NovaCastra), rabbit anti-human calnexin (Sigma, C4731), rabbit anti-human clathrin (Cell Signaling, P1663), rabbit anti-human LAMP1 (Sigma, L1418) or mouse anti-human 58K Golgi protein (Novus, NB600-412). Other sections were co-stained with WFA-FITC and mouse anti-rat embryonic myosin (eMyosin; NCL-MHCd, NovaCastra). Appropriate fluorophore-conjugated species or species- and isotype-specific secondary antibodies were obtained from Jackson Immunoresearch. Imaging was done on a Zeiss Axiophot epifluorescence microscope using AxioVision LE 4.1 imaging software (Zeiss; Jena, Germany) with fluorescein-, DAPI-, or rhodamine-specific optics. AAV(rh.74).MCK.*GALGT2*(human)-treated mdx muscles were infected for 12 weeks, as previously described[24]. All images shown in a figure use time-matched exposures for comparison and were representative of commonly seen staining patterns. For quantification of cell staining, 5 random 10x images per muscle were taken and counted as previously described[59].

Western blotting

Western blots for Neu5Gc and glyceraldehyde 3-phosphate dehydrogenase (GAPDH) were done and quantified as previously described using 15 or 30 μg per lane of NP40-extracted skeletal muscle protein separated on by SDS-PAGE on a 4–12% gradient gel[60].

Quantification of sialic acids

Quantification of total sialic acid and sialic acid species (relative Neu5Gc and Neu5Ac levels) was performed with modification from previously described methods of DMB (1,2-diamino-4,5-methylenedioxybenzene dihydrochloride) derivatization[61]. Briefly, 20–60 mg muscle tissue was homogenized in 10% PBS, base treated with 100 mM NaOH at 37°C for 30 minutes, then neutralized with 100 mM HCl. Small aliquots were taken for protein concentration determination using a Bradford assay. Sialic acids were then hydrolyzed with 2 M acetic acid at 80°C

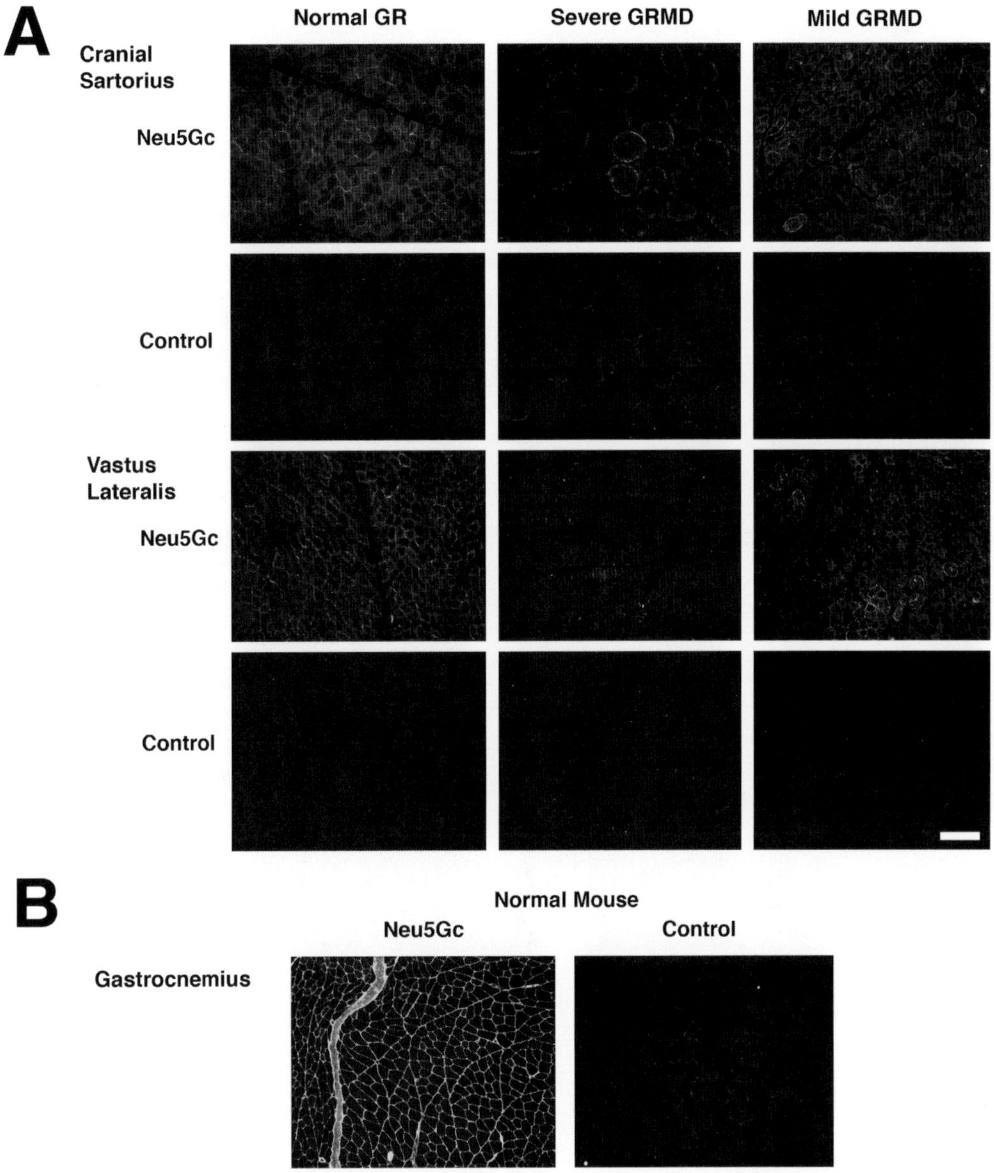

Figure 1. Neu5Gc expression in Golden Retriever cross (GR) and Golden Retriever Muscular Dystrophy (GRMD) dog skeletal muscle relative to mouse. (A) Neu5Gc-specific affinity-purified chicken IgY was used to stain skeletal muscles from 6 month-old normal Golden Retriever (GR) or Golden Retriever Muscular Dystrophy (GRMD) dogs. An example of staining from a severely affected and a mildly affected GRMD dog are shown. (B) Time-matched images in A were compared to normal mouse skeletal muscle immunostained with the same reagents. Non-immune chicken IgY was used as a control for background staining in A and B. Bar is 200 μm for all panels in A and B.

for 3 hours and passed through a 10 K molecular weight filter. Flow-through was concentrated and subjected to DMB derivatization at 50°C for 2.5 hours. Samples were then resolved using high performance liquid chromatography (HPLC) and Neu5Ac and Neu5Gc peaks quantified, as before[47].

Results

We chose to study two dog muscles, the vastus lateralis (VL) and the cranial sartorius (CS), because these muscles have been well documented to undergo differential changes relevant to muscular dystrophy in GRMD animals[17]. In particular, the CS shows more muscle necrosis during the neonatal period and subsequent hypertrophy by 6 months of age, while the VL has a more delayed pattern of muscle necrosis and regeneration that leads to atrophy (Figure S1). Muscle biopsies or necropsies from three GR and five GRMD dogs were used for this study. Of the five GRMD dogs, two (Ringo and Napoleon) showed severe muscular dystrophy by six months of age, as evidenced by decreased tibiotarsal joint angle and decreased force of tibiotarsal joint extension, two well-described measures of GRMD disease severity[16–18,62], while three others (Tico, Jane and Summer) were mildly affected, having measures for these parameters that neared or equaled wild type dogs despite having the same GRMD genetic defect (Table S1).

We first compared Neu5Gc staining in muscles from 6 month-old GR (Swiper), mildly affected GRMD (Tico) and severely affected GRMD (Ringo) dogs (Figure 1A). As expected from the previously documented low level of Neu5Gc in dog muscle gangliosides[42], we found very little Neu5Gc staining in GR or

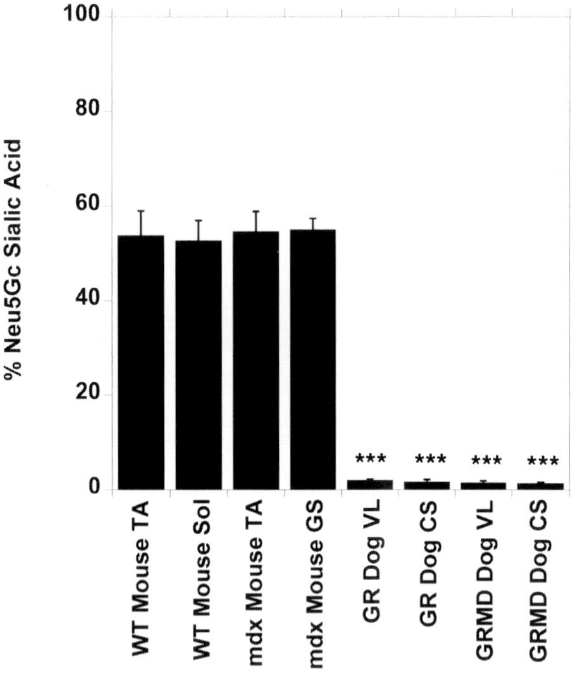

Figure 2. Quantification of Neu5Ac and Neu5Gc levels in normal and dystrophin-deficient mouse and dog muscles. Tibialis anterior (TA) and soleus (Sol) muscles were analyzed from 11 wild type (WT) mice, TA and gastrocnemius (GS) muscles were analyzed from 8 mdx mice, and vastus lateralis (VL) and cranial sartorius (CS) muscles were analyzed from 2 golden retriever (GR) and 5 golden retriever muscular dystrophy (GRMD) dogs. Average Neu5Gc as a percentage of total sialic acid is shown. Errors are standard deviation (SD). ***$P<0.001$, for all dog vs. mouse muscle comparisons.

GRMD muscle membranes. In addition, there was no Neu5Gc immunostaining of intramuscular connective tissue in any dog muscle (Figure 1A). There was some difference in fiber type between different GR and GRMD muscles, with CS showing a bias towards more slow fibers than the VL, as has been previously described[62]. Positively stained GR myofibers showed an uneven pattern of membrane staining, with some myofibers showing no staining, while GRMD muscles appeared to have even lower levels of staining than GR muscles (Figure 1A). While Neu5Gc staining of muscles from the severely affected GRMD dog appeared to be reduced relative to staining of the muscles from the mildly affected GRMD dog, this was not found to be significant when comparing all sections stained from all GRMD animals (not shown). By contrast, anti-Neu5Gc immunostaining of normal mouse gastrocnemius muscle showed very high and uniform staining of skeletal myofibers as well as intramuscular connective tissue (Figure 1B). Staining of muscles with pre-immune chicken IgY (Figure 1A and 1B, control) or secondary antibody alone (not shown) showed no background immunostaining. Thus, both GR and GRMD muscles showed very little Neu5Gc expression.

To investigate this further, we determined Neu5Gc levels, as a fraction of total sialic acids, in skeletal muscles from wild type and mdx mice and from GR and GRMD dogs (Figure 2). In addition, we compared Neu5Gc expression on GR and GRMD muscle glycoproteins to muscles from wild type (*Cmah*$^{+/+}$ and *Cmah*$^{-/-}$) mice (Figure S2). In both instances, both GR and GRMD muscles (CS and VL) expressed a fraction of the signal seen in mouse muscles (tibialis anterior, soleus and gastrocnemius). Neu5Gc levels did not exceed 2% of total sialic acids for any GR and GRMD muscle, while Neu5Gc levels in wild type and mdx mouse muscles averaged 52–55% (Figure 2). Thus, Neu5Gc levels in all GR and GRMD muscles were significantly reduced, by at least 95%, relative to mouse muscles ($P<0.001$, any dog muscle compared to any mouse muscle in Figure 2). Additionally, pooled GRMD muscles had a significant reduction in Neu5Gc relative to GR ($1.9\pm0.2\%$ of total sialic acid in GR vs. $1.4\pm0.1\%$ in GRMD, $P<0.05$). Total sialic acid content per mole protein, however, was not reduced in GRMD muscles compared to GR (not shown). Reduced Neu5Gc on glycoproteins was evident for both severely affected and mildly affected GRMD muscles (Figure S2). For example, Neu5Gc blot signals from all GRMD VL samples was $3\pm2\%$ of mouse *Cmah*$^{+/+}$ muscle signal and $16\pm6\%$ of GR VL signal. The low number of GRMD dogs precluded us from making definitive associations between muscle Neu5Gc levels and individual (severe versus mild) GRMD phenotypes.

To assess overall sialic acid expression, we also stained muscle sections from GR and GRMD animals with *Maackia amurensis* agglutinin (MAA), a sialic acid-binding lectin that recognizes sialic acid in a α2-3-linkage[63](Figure S3). GR and GRMD muscles, from both CS and VL, showed high levels of MAA staining along skeletal myofiber membranes and within intramuscular connective tissue. Increased fibrosis was evident from MAA staining of GRMD CS in a severely affected dog, as was the presence of hypertrophic skeletal myofibers. Thus, the low expression of Neu5Gc in GR and GRMD muscle was not due to a reduction in overall sialic acid levels.

We next performed a longitudinal study of anti-Neu5Gc staining for three different GRMD dogs, imaged at higher magnification, to assess expression at 3, 6 and 13 months of age (Figure 3). Muscles in all three GRMD dogs (GRMD1-3, Napoleon, Jane and Summer, respectively) showed higher Neu5Gc staining in mononuclear cells within the muscle than was seen on GRMD myofibers. There was faint Neu5Gc expression in some GRMD skeletal myofibers at 6 and 13 months of age compared to 3 months, however, this staining was not uniformly present. We stained the same GRMD dog muscles with MAA to assess relative total α2-3-linked sialic acid levels (Figure S4). MAA staining was high and relatively constant in both CS and VL muscles of GRMD dogs at 3, 6 and 13 months of age. MAA staining showed evidence of increased hypertrophic myofibers in the CS versus VL at 6 and 13 months, consistent with previous studies[17].

To further delineate which mononuclear cells expressed Neu5Gc in GRMD muscles, we triple stained muscle sections for Neu5Gc, DAPI (to stain nuclei) and markers for Pax7 (Figure 4A), to identify satellite cells, CD11b (Figure 4B), to identify macrophages, CD4 (Figure 4C), to identify helper T lymphocytes, or CD8 (Figure 4D), to identify cytotoxic T lymphocytes. We utilized mouse hybridoma clone P3U1 for Pax7 staining. A subset of cells that stained for Neu5Gc could be co-stained with each cell-specific marker used (except CD21, not shown, which did not stain muscle). Because each of these cell types co-expressed Neu5Gc, we quantified both the total number of each cell type per unit area (Figure 5A) as well as the percentage of each cell type that co-expressed Neu5Gc (Figure 5B). GRMD muscles showed higher numbers of Pax7−, CD4−, CD8− and CD11b−stained cells compared to GR muscles. Aside from CD4+ cells, however, all cell types showed a low percentage of co-expression with Neu5Gc in GRMD muscles, with only a quarter to half of Pax7+, CD8+ or CD11b+ cells co-expressing Neu5Gc (Figure 5B). For CD8 and Pax7, the percentage of cells expressing Neu5Gc in GRMD muscle was also significantly lower than it was in GR muscle (not shown).

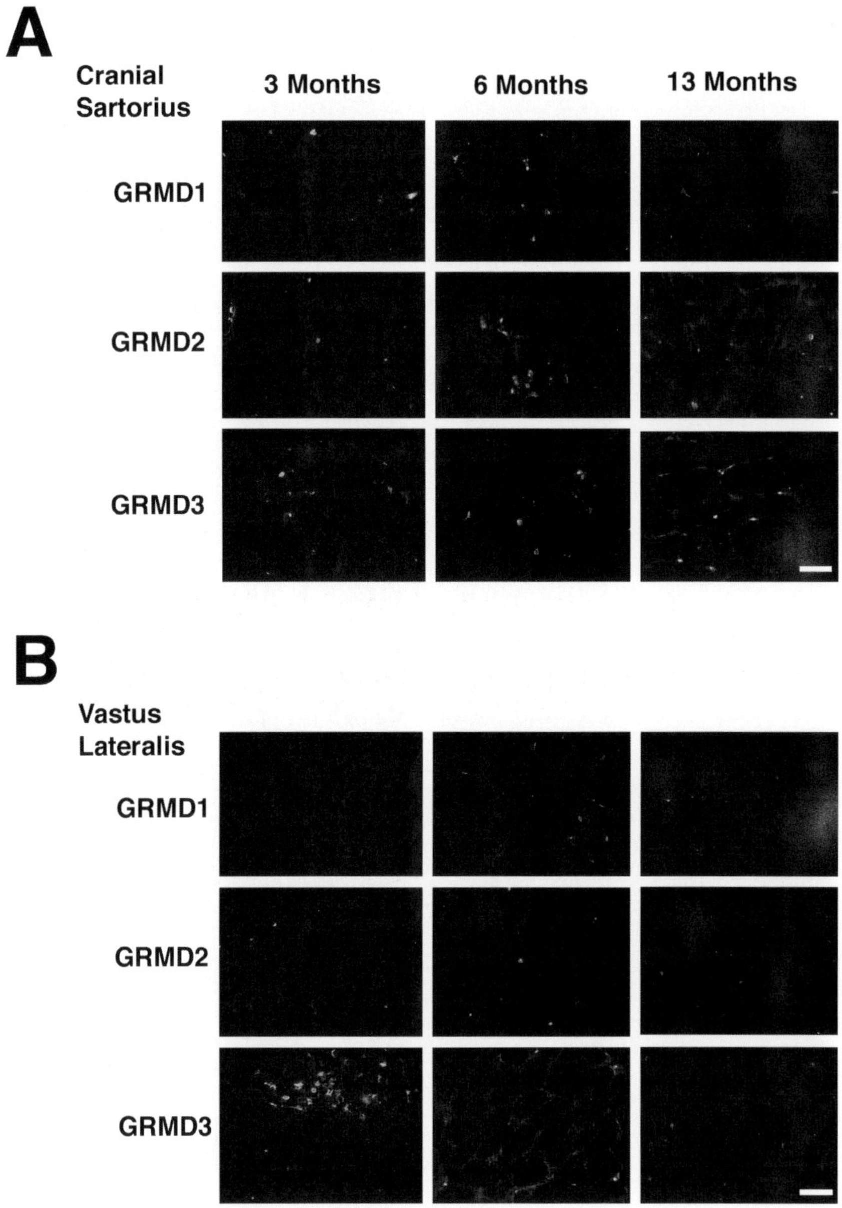

Figure 3. Neu5Gc expression in GRMD muscle at different ages. Three different GRMD cases (GRMD1, 2, and 3) were biopsied and muscles stained for Neu5Gc at 3, 6 and 13 months of age. Time-matched images of staining of the cranial sartorius (A) and vastus lateralis (B) muscles are shown. Bar is 50 μm for all panels in A and B.

We next analyzed Neu5Gc staining of muscle sections from biopsies of patients with Becker muscular dystrophy (BMD) or Duchenne muscular dystrophy (DMD) (Figure 6 Figure S5). These were compared to muscle sections from patients with an initial complaint that warranted muscle biopsy but where no muscle pathology could be identified (otherwise "normal" human muscle). We identified no Neu5Gc staining in normal human muscle, consistent with previous studies[28]. Unlike previously published Neu5Gc staining[28], however, we also identified some punctate intracellular Neu5Gc staining in BMD and DMD muscles. This was the case in all three DMD and all three BMD biopsies analyzed (Figure S5). Co-staining of Neu5Gc and β spectrin, a sarcolemmal membrane marker, showed that most Neu5Gc staining was localized within skeletal myofibers or near the sarcolemmal membrane, with greater concentrations being found within smaller myofibers (Figure 6A). By contrast, there was minimal to no co-staining of Neu5Gc with CD11b, CD8 or Pax7 in DMD muscle (Figure 6B). The intracellular aggregates of Neu5Gc within skeletal myofibers often co-stained with clathrin, a marker for endosomes (Figure 7A). In addition, some co-staining was evident with 58K Golgi protein, a marker for the Golgi apparatus (Figure 7B). There was minimal co-staining with LAMP1, a marker for lysosomes, or with calnexin, a marker for the endoplasmic reticulum (Figure 7B). Thus, the majority of Neu5Gc-stained puncta found within skeletal myofibers were co-stained with a marker for endosomes (Figure 7), suggesting that Neu5Gc is internalized by endocytosis into dystrophin-deficient human muscles and concentrated in distinct intramuscular and perimembranous regions of skeletal myofibers.

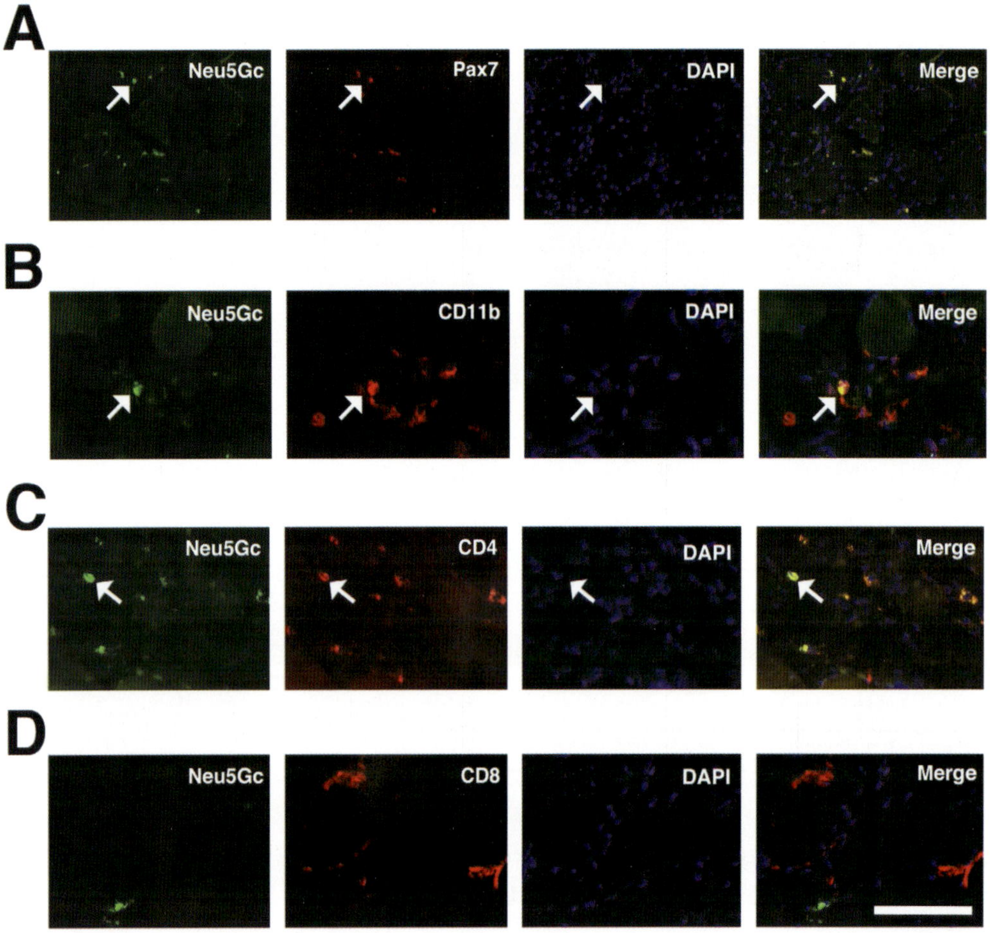

Figure 4. Neu5Gc immunostaining of satellite cells, T lymphocytes and macrophages in GRMD skeletal muscle. GRMD muscle (cranial sartorius) was triple stained for Neu5Gc (green), Pax7 (A), CD11b (B), CD4 (C), CD8 (D) (all red), and DAPI (blue). Arrows indicated co-staining of Neu5Gc and Pax7 (in A), CD11b (in B) or CD4 (in C). Bar is 100 μm (A) and 50 μm (B–D) for all panels.

We next surveyed CT carbohydrate and overall βGalNAc expression in GR and GRMD muscles, using the CT2 monoclonal antibody and *Wisteria floribunda* agglutinin (WFA), respectively (Figure 8 and Figure S6). In GR muscle, most WFA and CT2 staining was present at the neuromuscular junction (NMJ) (Figure S5). NMJs were identified by costaining with rhodamine-α-bungarotoxin, which labels nicotinic acetylcholine receptors (AChRs). In GRMD muscle, we also identified increased WFA staining on extrasynaptic regions of the muscle sarcolemmal membrane, as described previously in mdx mice[64]. WFA staining was not as abundant in eMyosin-positive myofibers as in eMyosin-negative myofibers (Figure 8C). In addition, we identified intense CT2 staining in mononuclear cell infiltrates in GRMD muscle. Here, CT2 co-stained with CD11b, suggesting that much of this CT expression was present on macrophages (Figure 8A). While CT2 co-stained large aggregates of macrophages in some muscle regions, an example with only a few macrophages present is shown here for clarity. CT2 co-stained with Pax7 far less frequently than with CD11b (Figure 8B). These data are similar to immunostaining results in mdx muscle[55] and show that CT carbohydrate expression can be increased in GRMD muscle relative to GR.

Last, we determined CT carbohydrate expression in DMD and BMD muscles, compared to normal human muscle (Figures 9, 10 and S7). We had previously demonstrated that CT2 shows a binding preference for the CT carbohydrate when Neu5Gc is the sialic acid present, while CT1 shows a binding preference for CT carbohydrates containing Neu5Ac[47]. We first compared CT1 and CT2 staining in DMD (Figure 9A) and normal human (Figure 9B) muscle to determine if CT1 would stain more strongly, as humans do not make Neu5Gc[32] (Figure 9). We also stained mdx muscles (Figure 9C) that had been infected with AAV(rh.74).MCK.*GALGT2*[24] to overexpress the CT carbohydrate. As expected, CT1 stained human muscle, but CT2 did not, while both antibodies stained AAV-*GALGT2*-infected mouse muscle (Figure 9). Normal human and DMD muscles did not show CT1 staining along the sarcolemmal membranes of myofibers, which were co-labeled with β spectrin, but some staining was evident in mononuclear cells (co-stained with DAPI) and also in peripheral nerve (Figure 10). All three BMD muscle biopsies, by contrast, showed increased CT1 staining along myofiber membranes (Figure 10, Figure S7). While it is impossible to generalize with only three cases, we observed at least some CT1-stained positive fibers in all three BMD cases used, and these cases ranged from relatively severe (loss of ambulation at 23) to relatively mild (ambulant at 67). In Figure S7, each BMD case is presented, respectively, with severity ranging from severe on the left to mild on the right.

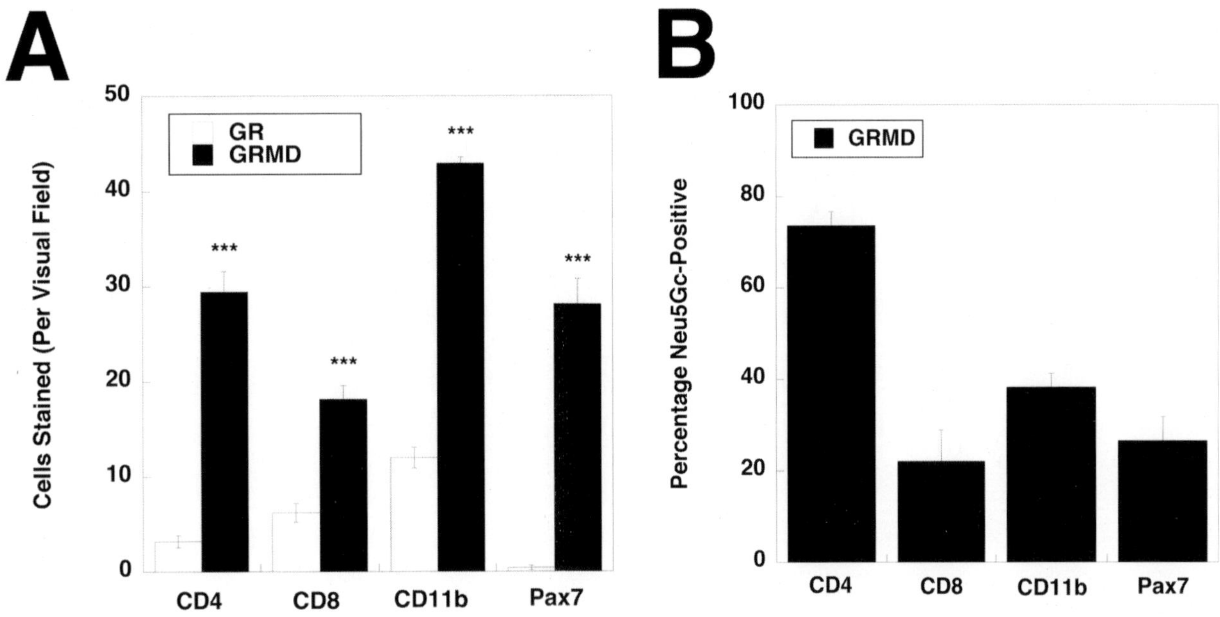

Figure 5. Quantification of CD4−, CD8−, CD11b− and Pax7−stained cells in GR and GRDM muscle and of Neu5Gc co-staining in GRMD muscle. (A) Cranial sartorius muscle sections from GR and GRMD dogs were stained with markers for satellite cells (Pax7), T lymphocytes (CD4 or CD8) or macrophages (CD11b) and quantified for numbers of cells stained per 40X visual field. (B) The percentage of cells co-stained for Neu5Gc and CD4, CD8, CD11b or Pax7 in GRMD muscles was quantified. Errors are SEM. ***$P<0.001$, for each GR vs. GRMD comparison in A.

Discussion

Both N-glycolylneuraminic acid (Neu5Gc), which requires the *Cmah* gene for its synthesis, and the Cytotoxic T cell (CT) carbohydrate, which requires the *Galgt2* gene for its synthesis, can, when altered, affect the severity of muscular dystrophy in mdx mice; Deletion of *Cmah*[28] or *Galgt2* (Xu et al., in preparation) increases severity of muscular dystrophy in the mdx mouse, decreasing lifespan and sometimes also muscle strength, while increasing *Galgt2* can ameliorate muscular dystrophy, increasing resistance of muscles to injury[24,55]. Here we have analyzed the expression of these two carbohydrates in patients with DMD and BMD and in GR and GRMD dogs. Both humans and dogs with dystrophin deficiency can show a range of disease severity, however, these phenotypes are generally more severe than those exhibited by the mdx mouse. All human cells lack a functional *CMAH* gene and therefore cannot synthesize Neu5Gc[32,65]. The data presented here demonstrate that Golden Retriever dog muscles also show little to no Neu5Gc expression (Figs. 1–3), despite lacking a human-like inactivating mutation in the canine *CMAH* gene. The low level of Neu5Gc found in skeletal muscle is consistent with a recent study showing little to no canine *CMAH* gene expression in cell lines made from Western dog breeds[66]. These data support the possibility that reduced Neu5Gc levels in GRMD dog muscles may contribute to their worsened disease severity relative to mdx mice. Similarly, we found very low levels of CT carbohydrate expression in both normal human and DMD muscles (Figure 9 and 10). Surprisingly, BMD muscles show increased membrane expression of CT carbohydrate (Figure 10). The fact that CT carbohydrate is not normally expressed in extrasynaptic membrane of normal, non-diseased, muscle gives an indication that CT carbohydrate may have a unique function in the setting of abnormal dystrophin expression. Because Galgt2 and CT carbohydrate expression are elevated in regenerating muscle, it is possible that elevated CT carbohydrate expression in BMD muscles may relate to some aspect of muscle regeneration. As increased CT carbohydrate can inhibit the development of muscular dystrophy in mdx mice[24,55], the elevated expression of the CT carbohydrate in BMD muscles, relative to DMD, suggests the potential for GALGT2 to contribute to lessened disease severity in BMD. The expression of a partially functional dystrophin protein, however, would be the primary effector of disease severity in BMD[67].

This study is also the first to describe the cellular and subcellular distribution of Neu5Gc in normal and dystrophin-deficient dog and human skeletal muscles (Figure 7). In addition to low to absent Neu5Gc expression on skeletal myofibers, GRMD muscles expressed Neu5Gc only on a minority of intramuscular satellite cells, CD8+ T lymphocytes and macrophages (Figure 4 and 5). Further, almost no such cells were stained for Neu5Gc in DMD muscles, consistent with loss of CMAH function in humans[32]. By contrast, we did identify intracellular accumulations of Neu5Gc in DMD and BMD skeletal myofibers (Figure 6). This presumably reflects the uptake of Neu5Gc by a salvage pathway from the diet[68,69]. Neu5Gc levels, for example, are particularly high in red meat[70], and Neu5Gc can be incorporated into cells from ingested glycoproteins in humans[70] and in *Cmah*-deficient mice[57,69]. Here we have shown that intracellular Neu5Gc co-stains with clathrin and Golgi 58K protein, and to a lesser extent with LAMP1 (Figure 7). This suggests a possible mechanism, much of which has been described previously[68], where internalization of Neu5Gc-containing glycoproteins via endosomes leads to their transport to the lysosome via the sialin transporter. There, Neu5Gc present on glycoproteins could be liberated by lysosomal sialidase. Such a mechanism would ultimately allow recycling of Neu5Gc into CMP-Neu5Gc, transport into the Golgi, and reintegration of Neu5Gc into proteins and lipids by sialyltransferases. The uptake and reincorporation of Neu5Gc into muscle cell proteins may affect muscle disease by altering muscle physiology or by increasing Neu5Gc-driven immune reactions. All humans possess serum antibodies that react with Neu5Gc-

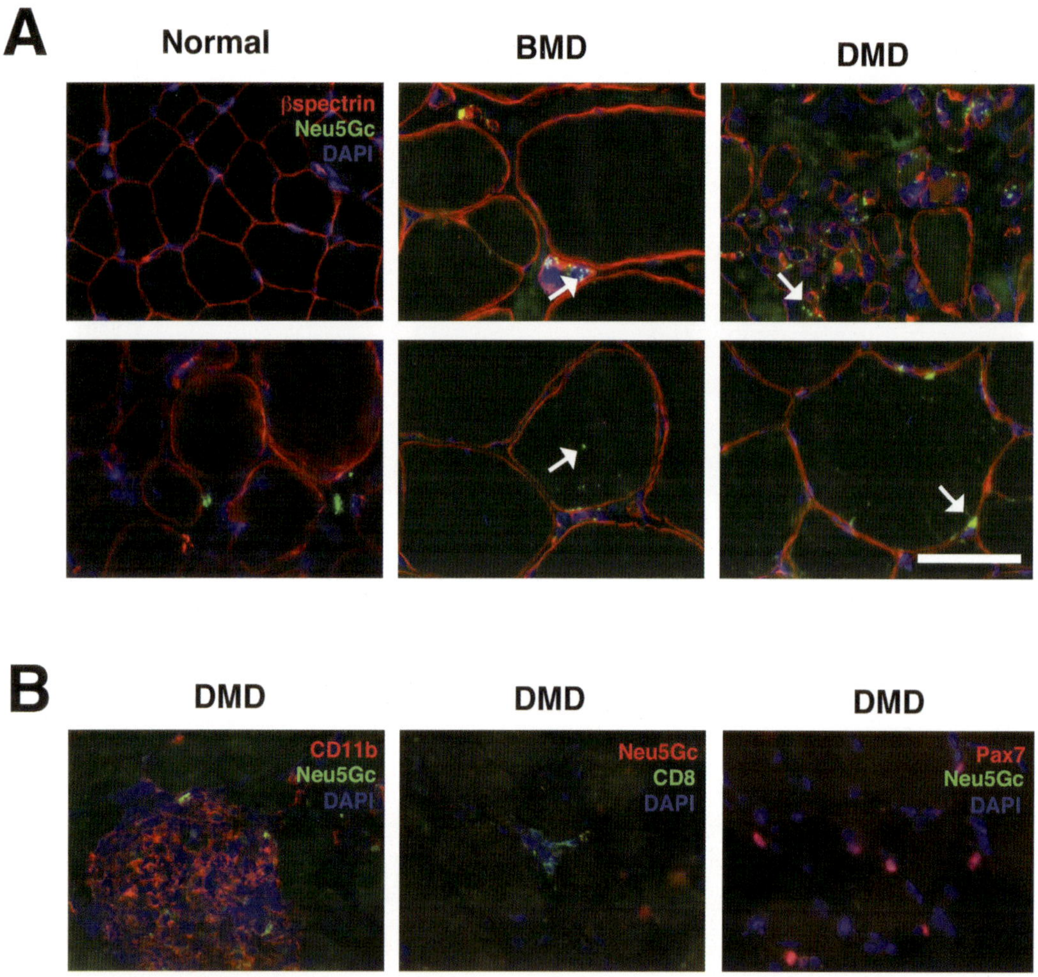

Figure 6. Neu5Gc co-staining with β spectrin, CD11b, CD8 or Pax7 in normal, BMD or DMD human muscle. (A) Otherwise normal, Becker muscular dystrophy (BMD) and Duchenne muscular dystrophy (DMD) muscle biopsy sections were stained for Neu5Gc (green), β spectrin (red) and DAPI (blue). Arrows indicate Neu5Gc puncta in cytoplasmic or perimembranous regions of BMD and DMD skeletal myofibers. (B) DMD muscle was co-stained for Neu5Gc and CD11b, CD8 or Pax7 (and DAPI). Bar is 50 μm for all panels in A and B.

containing glycans, and these antibodies could increase damage to Neu5Gc-containing muscle cells[33,71]. Future work will be required to delineate Neu5Gc's roles and the possible mechanisms controlling its functions.

Our findings in dog skeletal muscle suggest that reduced or absent Neu5Gc in dog muscles may be analogous to *Cmah*-deficient mdx mice, which, like GRMD dogs, have relatively severe muscle disease[28]. GRMD dogs should have no autoimmune response to Neu5Gc, as $Cmah^{-/-}$mdx mice [28]and humans can[33], but they may share the loss of function effects of lack of Neu5Gc expression found in $Cmah^{-/-}$mdx mice and in DMD patients. The percentage of sialic acid comprising Neu5Gc was reduced in both GR and GRMD muscles by at least 95% relative to mouse muscles (Figure 2). Only 1–2% of total sialic acid was Neu5Gc in any dog muscle studied. Further, Neu5Gc levels in GRMD muscles were reduced relative to GR. This was evident in Neu5Gc measurements of total muscle sialic acid (Figure 2), Neu5Gc immunoblots of muscle glycoproteins (Figure S2) and Neu5Gc immunostaining of muscle sections (Figure 1).

We also wished to determine if Neu5Gc expression plays a role in disease severity of individual dogs and the associated dramatic phenotypic variation. A range of phenotypic features have been used to allow a general definition of disease severity in GRMD dogs[62]. In particular, they have lower tibiotarsal joint (TTJ) tetanic force extension and a plantigrade posture exemplified by more acute tibiotarsal joint angles[16,19]. Paradoxically, some muscles (especially flexors) undergo early necrosis and then may recover or even hypertrophy. Accordingly, TTJ flexor tetanic force is typically increased in dogs with more severe postural abnormalities[62]. In keeping with this paradoxical functional muscle hypertrophy, the cranial sartorius muscle may become larger as disease progresses (represented by circumference [mm] divided by body weight [kg])[17]. While TTJ flexion does not involve the cranial sartorius muscle, force values tend to track with those of cranial sartorius hypertrophy. Interestingly, muscle membranes of hypertrophied muscle fibers appear to be partially protected against eccentric contraction-induced injury. As a result, the degree of decrement may actually be reduced in dogs with an otherwise severe phenotype (Kornegay JN, unpublished data). If Neu5Gc were playing a role in protecting dystrophic muscles, increased levels might therefore be expected in the VL of mildly affected dogs, which might prevent their subsequent atrophy, or the CS of dogs with a more severe phenotype, which might contribute to increased hypertrophy. With a small number of

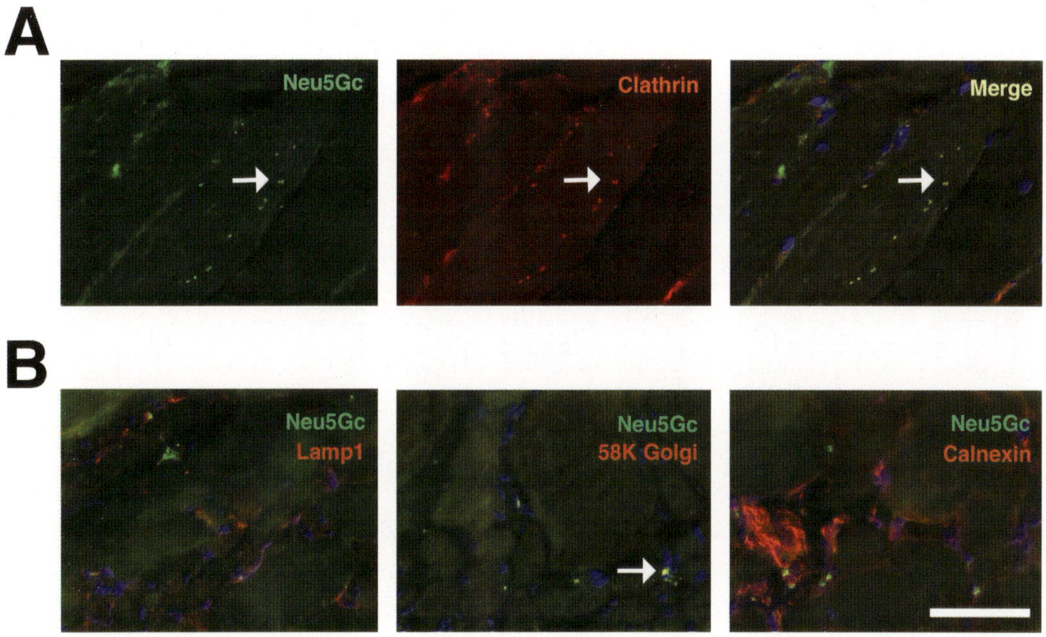

Figure 7. Co-localization of Neu5Gc staining with markers for endosomes and Golgi in BMD and DMD muscle. (A) BMD muscle co-stained for Neu5Gc (green) and clathrin (red), a marker of endosomes. Merged image on right shows overlap of Neu5Gc and clathrin expression in yellow. Arrow marks several examples of co-staining. (B) DMD muscle co-stained for Neu5Gc (green) with LAMP1, a lysosomal marker, 58K Golgi, a Golgi marker, or calnexin, and endoplasmic reticulum marker, all in red, and DAPI (blue). Arrow marks region of coincident staining (yellow) for Neu5Gc and 58K Golgi. Bar is 50 μm for all panels in A and B.

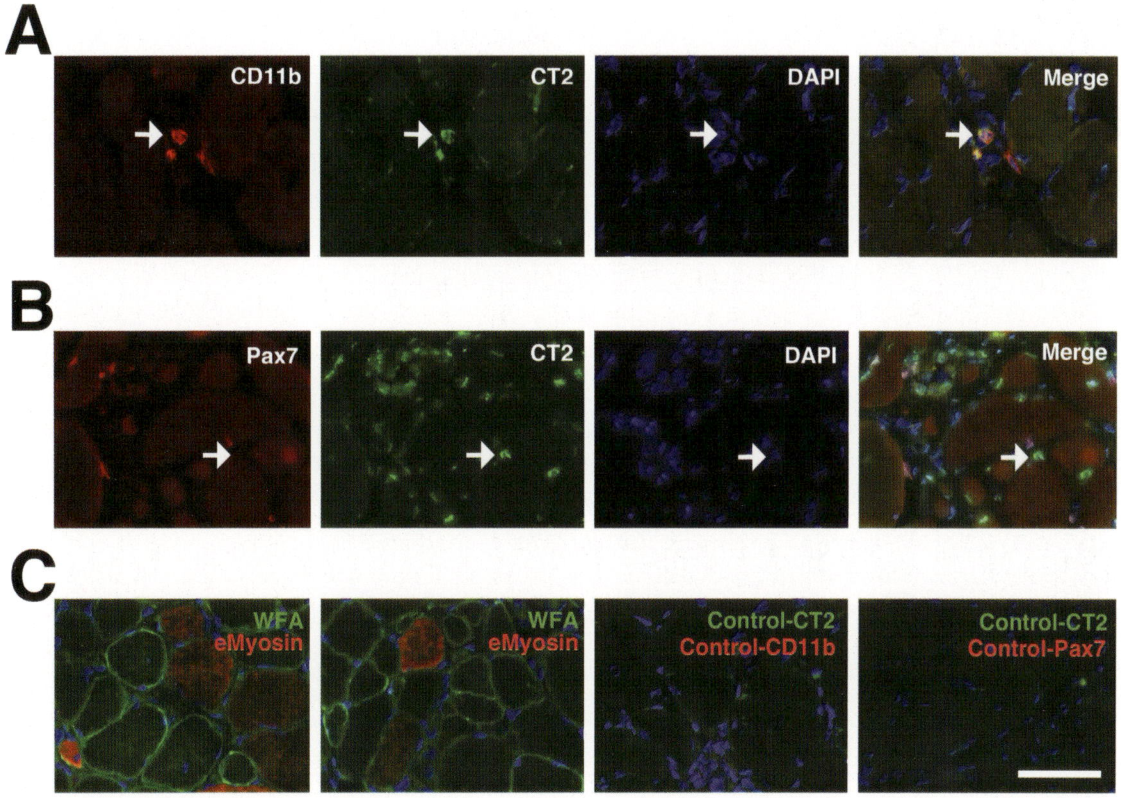

Figure 8. Co-staining of CT carbohydrate with macrophages in GRMD muscle. (A) Single and merged staining for CT2 (green) with CD11b (red, to mark macrophages) and DAPI (blue). Arrow shows co-incident staining for CT2 and CD11b. (B) Single and merged staining for CT2 (green) with Pax7 (red, to mark satellite cells) and DAPI (blue). Arrow shows lack of coincident staining for CT2 and Pax7. (C) Examples of WFA staining (green) with embryonic myosin (red) and DAPI (blue) (two left panels). Examples of control staining for staining shown in A and B using only secondary antibodies with DAPI (two right panels). Bar is 50 μm for all panels in A, B and C.

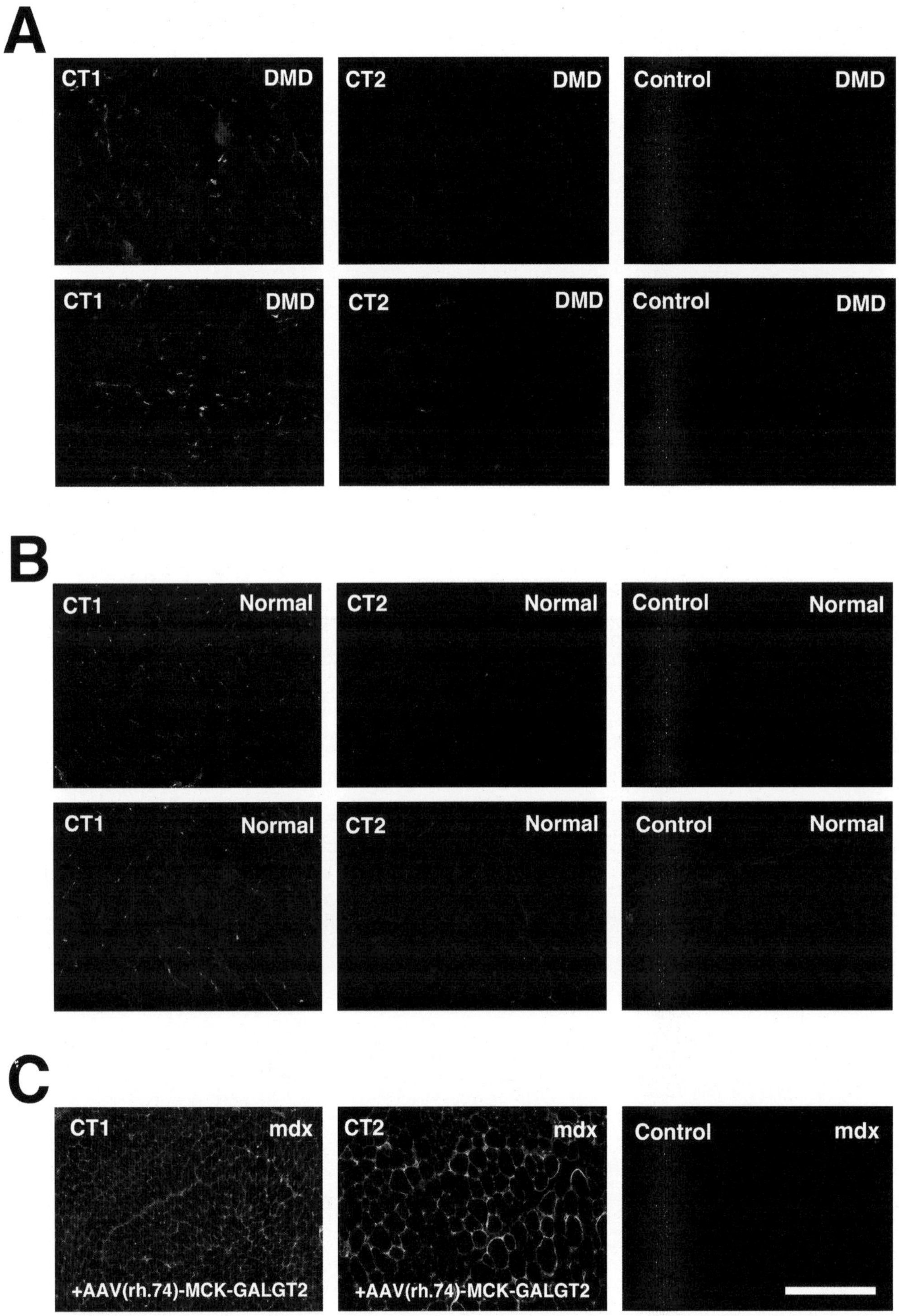

Figure 9. Comparison of CT1 and CT2 immunostaining in DMD and normal human muscle. CT1 and CT2 were used to immunostain two different DMD (A) and two different normal human (B) muscle biopsies, compared to secondary antibody control. These were compared to time-matched images taken from mdx muscles (C), diaphragm (left panel) or tibialis anterior (right panel), that had been infected with rAAV(rh.74).MCK.GALGT2 for 12 weeks. Bar is 200 μm for all panels in A, B and C.

GRMD dogs in this study, we were unable to draw definitive conclusions regarding the role of Neu5Gc expression in the individual phenotypes.

Similar to our Neu5Gc studies, we have shown that most DMD myofibers have very low to absent CT carbohydrate expression (Figure 9 and 10). By contrast, CT carbohydrate expression was increased in BMD muscles (Figure 10 and S7). Although these observations do not establish a causal relationship, they suggest an association between increased CT carbohydrate and BMD. CT carbohydrate was also increased in some myofibers and

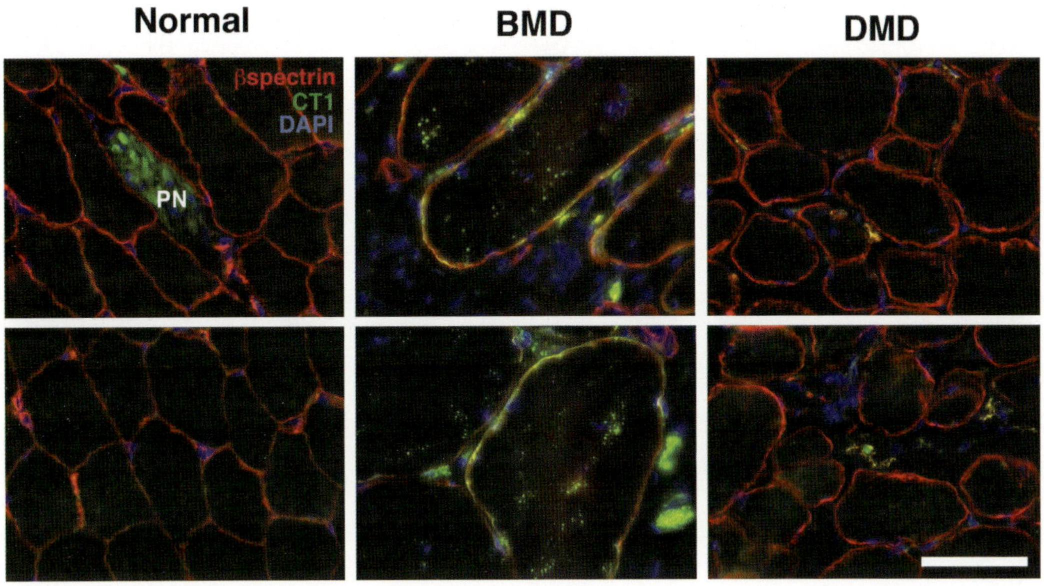

Figure 10. Co-staining of CT1 with βspectrin in BMD muscles. Sections from DMD, BMD and normal human muscle biopsies sections were co-stained with CT1 (green), β spectrin(red) and DAPI (blue). Merged sarcolemmal membrane staining for CT1 and β spectrin is orange-yellow. PN represents intramuscular peripheral nerve. Bar is 50 μm for all panels.

macrophages in GRMD muscles (Figure 8), where it may play additional roles. Further work will be required to understand if there is a direct relationship between CT carbohydrate expression and human or canine disease. However, the low expression of Neu5Gc and CT glycans in DMD and GRMD muscles suggests that they do not normally have the potential to ameliorate disease severity in dogs and humans lacking dystrophin protein.

Supporting Information

Table S1 GRMD Dog Functional Data (6 Mos). GRMD dogs have a range of phenotypic features that allow general definition of disease severity.[1] In particular, they have lower tibiotarsal joint (TTJ) tetanic extension force[2] and a plantigrade posture exemplified by more acute tibiotarsal joint angles.[3] Paradoxically, some muscles (especially flexors) undergo early necrosis and then may recover or even hypertrophy. Accordingly, TTJ flexor tetanic force may be increased in dogs with more severe postural abnormalities.[1] In keeping with this paradoxical functional muscle hypertrophy, the cranial sartorius muscle may be larger (represented by circumference [mm] divided by body weight [kg]).[4,5] While TTJ flexion does not involve the cranial sartorius muscle, force values tend to track with those of cranial sartorius hypertrophy. Interestingly, muscle membranes of hypertrophied muscle fibers appear to be partially protected against eccentric contraction injury. As a result, the degree of decrement may actually be reduced in dogs with an otherwise severe phenotype (Kornegay JN, unpublished data). For sake of defining disease severity in these GRMD dogs, we characterized several of these features. Ringo and Napoleon were characterized as "moderate/severe", while Tico, Summer, and Jane were "mild/moderate," based on TTJ extension tetanic force and TTJ angles below or above (1 N/kg) and (145°), respectively. 1. Kornegay JN, Bogan JR, Bogan DJ, Childers MK, Li J, Nghiem P, Detwiler DA, Larsen CA, Grange RW, Bhavaraju-Sanka RK, Tou S, Keene BP, Howard JF, Jr, Wang J, Fan Z, Schatzberg SJ, Styner MA, Flanigan KM, Xiao X, Hoffman EP: Canine models of Duchenne muscular dystrophy and their use in therapeutic strategies. Mamm Genome 23:85-108, 2012. 2. Kornegay JN, Bogan DJ, Bogan JR, Childers MK, Cundiff DD, Petroski GF, Schueler RO: Contraction torque generated by tarsal joint flexion and extension in dogs with golden retriever muscular dystrophy. J Neurol Sci 166:115–121, 1999. 3. Kornegay JN, Sharp NJH, Schueler RO, Betts CW: Tarsal joint contracture in dogs with golden retriever muscular dystrophy. Lab Anim Sci 44:331–333, 1994. 4. Kornegay JN, Cundiff DD, Bogan DJ, Bogan JR, Okamura CS: The cranial sartorius muscle undergoes true hypertrophy in dogs with golden retriever muscular dystrophy. Neuromuscul Disord 13:493–500, 2003. 5. Kornegay JN, Bogan JR, Bogan DJ, Childers MK, Grange RW: Golden retriever muscular dystrophy (GRMD): Developing and maintaining a colony and physiological functional measurements. In: Duan D (ed). Muscle Gene Therapy: Methods and Protocols. Methods in Molecular Biology, vol. 709, Humana Press, New York, 2011, 105–123.

Figure S1 Muscle damage in mild and severely affected GRMD muscles at 6 months of age. Hematoxylin and eosin staining of muscle cross-sections from GR and GRMD muscles. Cranial sartorius (A–C) and vastus lateralis (D–F) muscles from one normal dog (Heisenberg, A,D), one mildly affected GRMD dog (Summer, B, E) and one severely affected GRMD dog (Napoleon, C, F) are shown. Overall, histopathologic lesions in these GRMD dogs were in keeping with those we and others have described. There was small group muscle necrosis and regeneration in both the cranial sartorius and vastus lateralis. Each muscle had features of necrosis, including hyaline fibers and myophagocytosis (examples are circled). Myofiber mineralization was only seen in the cranial sartorius. Evidence of regeneration, with small basophilic myofibers and numerous central nuclei, was more pronounced in the vastus lateralis. The regenerative response was more mature in the cranial sartorius, with an increase in larger myofibers. Bar is 150 μm for all panels.

Figure S2 Neu5Gc expression on GR and GRMD glycoproteins relative to mouse. Western blots of NP-40 extracted muscle protein with anti-Neu5Gc antibody and anti-GAPDH control. Mouse *Cmah*$^{+/+}$ and *Cmah*$^{-/-}$ skeletal muscle lysates were compared to cranial sartorius (CS) and vastus lateralis (VL) muscles from GR and GRMD dogs that were either mildly or severely affected. Half the amount of mouse protein as dog protein is loaded per lane.

Figure S3 High expression of sialic acid in GR and GRMD muscle. *Maackia amurensis* agglutinin (MAA), a lectin that stains α2,3-linked sialic acid, both Neu5Ac and Neu5Gc, was used to stain skeletal muscles from 6 month-old Golden Retriever cross (GR) and Golden Retriever Muscular Dystrophy (GRMD) dogs. Time-matched images are shown. Bar is 200 μm for all panels.

Figure S4 High sialic acid expression in GRMD muscles at different ages. Three different GRMD cases (GRMD1, 2, and 3-Napoleon, Jane and Summer respectively) were biopsied and muscles stained for sialic acid using *Maackia amurensis* agglutinin (MAA) at 3, 6 and 13 months of age. Time-matched images of staining of the cranial sartorius and vastus lateralis muscles are shown. Bar is 50 μm for all panels.

Figure S5 Neu5Gc expression in DMD, BMD and normal human muscle. Muscle biopsies from Duchenne muscular dystrophy (DMD), Becker Muscular Dystrophy (BMD), or otherwise normal human muscle were immunostained with an antibody specific to *N*-glycolylneuraminic acid (Neu5Gc) or non-immune control sera. Each panel represents a different patient biopsy. Bar is 100 μm for all panels.

Figure S6 Neuromuscular junction staining of βGalNAc and the CT carbohydrate in GR muscle and elevated CT staining in GRMD muscle. GR muscle (6mo cranial sartorius) was co-stained with rhodamine-α-bungarotoxin, to label acetylcholine receptors (AChR) concentrated at the neuromuscular junction, and *Wisteria floribunda* agglutinin (WFA), which stains β-linked GalNAc, or CT2, which stains the CT carbohydrate. Below, GRMD muscle (cranial sartorius) was stained with WFA or CT2, compared to control secondary antibody alone. Bar is 100 μm for all panels.

Figure S7 CT1 immunostaining of DMD, BMD and normal human muscle. 3 DMD, 3 BMD, and 2 normal human biopsies were immunostained with CT1 and compared to secondary antibody control alone. BMD cases range in severity from severe (loss of ambulation at 23) to milder (ambulant at 36 and ambulant at 67), respectively, from left to right. Bar is 200 μm for all panels.

Acknowledgments

The authors would like to thank Daniel Bogan (UNC) for technical assistance and Michael Rudnicki (Ottawa Health Research Institute) for Pax7 antibody.

Author Contributions

Conceived and designed the experiments: PTM AV KMF JNK. Performed the experiments: PTM BG JO MC KC RX AV KMF JNK. Analyzed the data: PTM BG JO MC KC RX AV KMF JNK. Wrote the paper: PTM BG JO MC KC RX AV KMF JNK.

References

1. Hoffman EP, Brown RH Jr., Kunkel LM (1987) Dystrophin: the protein product of the Duchenne muscular dystrophy locus. Cell 51: 919–928.
2. Koenig M, Hoffman EP, Bertelson CJ, Monaco AP, Feener C, et al. (1987) Complete cloning of the Duchenne muscular dystrophy (DMD) cDNA and preliminary genomic organization of the DMD gene in normal and affected individuals. Cell 50: 509–517.
3. Willmann R, Possekel S, Dubach-Powell J, Meier T, Ruegg MA (2009) Mammalian animal models for Duchenne muscular dystrophy. Neuromuscul Disord.
4. Sicinski P, Geng Y, Ryder-Cook AS, Barnard EA, Darlison MG, et al. (1989) The molecular basis of muscular dystrophy in the mdx mouse: a point mutation. Science 244: 1578–1580.
5. Bulfield G, Siller WG, Wight PA, Moore KJ (1984) X chromosome-linked muscular dystrophy (mdx) in the mouse. Proc Natl Acad Sci U S A 81: 1189–1192.
6. Kornegay JN, Tuler SM, Miller DM, Levesque DC (1988) Muscular dystrophy in a litter of golden retriever dogs. Muscle & nerve 11: 1056–1064.
7. Cooper BJ, Winand NJ, Stedman H, Valentine BA, Hoffman EP, et al. (1988) The homologue of the Duchenne locus is defective in X-linked muscular dystrophy of dogs. Nature 334: 154–156.
8. Smith BF, Yue Y, Woods PR, Kornegay JN, Shin JH, et al. (2011) An intronic LINE-1 element insertion in the dystrophin gene aborts dystrophin expression and results in Duchenne-like muscular dystrophy in the corgi breed. Laboratory investigation; a journal of technical methods and pathology 91: 216–231.
9. Gaschen FP, Hoffman EP, Gorospe JR, Uhl EW, Senior DF, et al. (1992) Dystrophin deficiency causes lethal muscle hypertrophy in cats. J Neurol Sci 110: 149–159.
10. Winand NJ, Edwards M, Pradhan D, Berian CA, Cooper BJ (1994) Deletion of the dystrophin muscle promoter in feline muscular dystrophy. Neuromuscular disorders : NMD 4: 433–445.
11. Shelton GD, Engvall E (2005) Canine and feline models of human inherited muscle diseases. Neuromuscul Disord 15: 127–138.
12. Kornegay JN, Bogan JR, Bogan DJ, Childers MK, Li J, et al. (2012) Canine models of Duchenne muscular dystrophy and their use in therapeutic strategies. Mamm Genome 23: 85–108.
13. Sharp NJ, Kornegay JN, Van Camp SD, Herbstreith MH, Secore SL, et al. (1992) An error in dystrophin mRNA processing in golden retriever muscular dystrophy, an animal homologue of Duchenne muscular dystrophy. Genomics 13: 115–121.
14. Childers MK, Okamura CS, Bogan DJ, Bogan JR, Petroski GF, et al. (2002) Eccentric contraction injury in dystrophic canine muscle. Archives of physical medicine and rehabilitation 83: 1572–1578.
15. Childers MK, Okamura CS, Bogan DJ, Bogan JR, Sullivan MJ, et al. (2001) Myofiber injury and regeneration in a canine homologue of Duchenne muscular dystrophy. American journal of physical medicine & rehabilitation/Association of Academic Physiatrists 80: 175–181.
16. Kornegay JN, Bogan DJ, Bogan JR, Childers MK, Cundiff DD, et al. (1999) Contraction force generated by tarsal joint flexion and extension in dogs with golden retriever muscular dystrophy. Journal of the neurological sciences 166: 115–121.
17. Kornegay JN, Cundiff DD, Bogan DJ, Bogan JR, Okamura CS (2003) The cranial sartorius muscle undergoes true hypertrophy in dogs with golden retriever muscular dystrophy. Neuromuscular disorders : NMD 13: 493–500.
18. Kornegay JN, Sharp NJ, Bogan DJ, Van Camp SD, Metcalf JR, et al. (1994) Contraction tension and kinetics of the peroneus longus muscle in golden retriever muscular dystrophy. Journal of the neurological sciences 123: 100–107.
19. Kornegay JN, Sharp NJ, Schueler RO, Betts CW (1994) Tarsal joint contracture in dogs with golden retriever muscular dystrophy. Laboratory animal science 44: 331–333.
20. Valentine BA, Kornegay JN, Cooper BJ (1989) Clinical electromyographic studies of canine X-linked muscular dystrophy. American journal of veterinary research 50: 2145–2147.
21. Mendell JR, Moxley RT, Griggs RC, Brooke MH, Fenichel GM, et al. (1989) Randomized, double-blind six-month trial of prednisone in Duchenne's muscular dystrophy. N Engl J Med 320: 1592–1597.
22. Liu JM, Okamura CS, Bogan DJ, Bogan JR, Childers MK, et al. (2004) Effects of prednisone in canine muscular dystrophy. Muscle & nerve 30: 767–773.
23. Martin PT (2006) Mechanisms of Disease: congenital muscular dystrophies-glycosylation takes center stage. Nat Clin Pract Neurol 2: 222–230.
24. Martin PT, Xu R, Rodino-Klapac LR, Oglesbay E, Camboni M, et al. (2009) Overexpression of Galgt2 in skeletal muscle prevents injury resulting from eccentric contractions in both mdx and wild-type mice. Am J Physiol Cell Physiol 296: C476–488.

25. Barresi R, Michele DE, Kanagawa M, Harper HA, Dovico SA, et al. (2004) LARGE can functionally bypass alpha-dystroglycan glycosylation defects in distinct congenital muscular dystrophies. Nat Med 10: 696–703.
26. Godfrey C, Foley AR, Clement E, Muntoni F (2011) Dystroglycanopathies: coming into focus. Current opinion in genetics & development 21: 278–285.
27. Michele DE, Barresi R, Kanagawa M, Saito F, Cohn RD, et al. (2002) Post-translational disruption of dystroglycan-ligand interactions in congenital muscular dystrophies. Nature 418: 417–422.
28. Chandrasekharan K, Yoon JH, Xu Y, deVries S, Camboni M, et al. (2010) A human-specific deletion in mouse Cmah increases disease severity in the mdx model of Duchenne muscular dystrophy. Sci Transl Med 2: 42ra54.
29. Shaw L, Schneckenburger P, Carlsen J, Christiansen K, Schauer R (1992) Mouse liver cytidine-5'-monophosphate-N-acetylneuraminic acid hydroxylase. Catalytic function and regulation. Eur J Biochem 206: 269–277.
30. Kawano T, Koyama S, Takematsu H, Kozutsumi Y, Kawasaki H, et al. (1995) Molecular cloning of cytidine monophospho-N-acetylneuraminic acid hydroxylase. Regulation of species- and tissue-specific expression of N-glycolylneuraminic acid. J Biol Chem 270: 16458–16463.
31. Varki NM, Varki A (2007) Diversity in cell surface sialic acid presentations: implications for biology and disease. Lab Invest 87: 851–857.
32. Chou HH, Takematsu H, Diaz S, Iber J, Nickerson E, et al. (1998) A mutation in human CMP-sialic acid hydroxylase occurred after the Homo-Pan divergence. Proc Natl Acad Sci U S A 95: 11751–11756.
33. Padler-Karavani V, Yu H, Cao H, Chokhawala H, Karp F, et al. (2008) Diversity in specificity, abundance, and composition of anti-Neu5Gc antibodies in normal humans: potential implications for disease. Glycobiology 18: 818–830.
34. Varki A (2001) Loss of N-glycolylneuraminic acid in humans: Mechanisms, consequences, and implications for hominid evolution. Am J Phys Anthropol Suppl 33: 54–69.
35. Rooney JE, Welser JV, Dechert MA, Flintoff-Dye NL, Kaufman SJ, et al. (2006) Severe muscular dystrophy in mice that lack dystrophin and alpha7 integrin. J Cell Sci 119: 2185–2195.
36. Deconinck AE, Rafael JA, Skinner JA, Brown SC, Potter AC, et al. (1997) Utrophin-dystrophin-deficient mice as a model for Duchenne muscular dystrophy. Cell 90: 717–727.
37. Grady RM, Teng H, Nichol MC, Cunningham JC, Wilkinson RS, et al. (1997) Skeletal and cardiac myopathies in mice lacking utrophin and dystrophin: a model for Duchenne muscular dystrophy. Cell 90: 729–738.
38. Megeney LA, Kablar B, Perry RL, Ying C, May L, et al. (1999) Severe cardiomyopathy in mice lacking dystrophin and MyoD. Proc Natl Acad Sci U S A 96: 220–225.
39. Peter AK, Marshall JL, Crosbie RH (2008) Sarcospan reduces dystrophic pathology: stabilization of the utrophin-glycoprotein complex. J Cell Biol 183: 419–427.
40. Peter AK, Miller G, Crosbie RH (2007) Disrupted mechanical stability of the dystrophin-glycoprotein complex causes severe muscular dystrophy in sarcospan transgenic mice. J Cell Sci 120: 996–1008.
41. Sacco A, Mourkioti F, Tran R, Choi J, Llewellyn M, et al. (2010) Short telomeres and stem cell exhaustion model Duchenne muscular dystrophy in mdx/mTR mice. Cell 143: 1059–1071.
42. Nakamura K, Ariga T, Yahagi T, Miyatake T, Suzuki A, et al. (1983) Interspecies comparison of muscle gangliosides by two-dimensional thin-layer chromatography. J Biochem 94: 1359–1365.
43. Conzelmann A, Lefrancois L (1988) Monoclonal antibodies specific for T cell-associated carbohydrate determinants react with human blood group antigens CAD and SDA. J Exp Med 167: 119–131.
44. Lefrancois L, Bevan MJ (1985) Novel antigenic determinants of the T200 glycoprotein expressed preferentially by activated cytotoxic T lymphocytes. J Immunol 135: 374–383.
45. Lefrancois L, Bevan MJ (1985) Functional modifications of cytotoxic T-lymphocyte T200 glycoprotein recognized by monoclonal antibodies. Nature 314: 449–452.
46. Martin PT, Scott LJ, Porter BE, Sanes JR (1999) Distinct structures and functions of related pre- and postsynaptic carbohydrates at the mammalian neuromuscular junction. Mol Cell Neurosci 13: 105–118.
47. Hoyte K, Kang C, Martin PT (2002) Definition of pre- and postsynaptic forms of the CT carbohydrate antigen at the neuromuscular junction: ubiquitous expression of the CT antigens and the CT GalNAc transferase in mouse tissues. Brain Res Mol Brain Res 109: 146–160.
48. Xia B, Hoyte K, Kammesheidt A, Deerinck T, Ellisman M, et al. (2002) Overexpression of the CT GalNAc transferase in skeletal muscle alters myofiber growth, neuromuscular structure, and laminin expression. Dev Biol 242: 58–73.
49. Smith PL, Lowe JB (1994) Molecular cloning of a murine N-acetylgalactosamine transferase cDNA that determines expression of the T lymphocyte-specific CT oligosaccharide differentiation antigen. J Biol Chem 269: 15162–15171.
50. Singhal N, Martin PT (2011) Role of extracellular matrix proteins and their receptors in the development of the vertebrate neuromuscular junction. Developmental neurobiology 71: 982–1005.
51. Xu R, Camboni M, Martin PT (2007) Postnatal overexpression of the CT GalNAc transferase inhibits muscular dystrophy in mdx mice without altering muscle growth or neuromuscular development: evidence for a utrophin-independent mechanism. Neuromuscul Disord 17: 209–220.
52. Xu R, Chandrasekharan K, Yoon JH, Camboni M, Martin PT (2007) Overexpression of the cytotoxic T cell (CT) carbohydrate inhibits muscular dystrophy in the dyW mouse model of congenital muscular dystrophy 1A. Am J Pathol 171: 181–199.
53. Xu R, DeVries S, Camboni M, Martin PT (2009) Overexpression of Galgt2 reduces dystrophic pathology in the skeletal muscles of alpha sarcoglycan-deficient mice. Am J Pathol 175: 235–247.
54. Yoon JH, Chandrasekharan K, Xu R, Glass M, Singhal N, et al. (2009) The synaptic CT carbohydrate modulates binding and expression of extracellular matrix proteins in skeletal muscle: Partial dependence on utrophin. Mol Cell Neurosci 41: 448–463.
55. Nguyen HH, Jayasinha V, Xia B, Hoyte K, Martin PT (2002) Overexpression of the cytotoxic T cell GalNAc transferase in skeletal muscle inhibits muscular dystrophy in mdx mice. Proc Natl Acad Sci U S A 99: 5616–5621.
56. Singhal N, Xu R, Martin PT (2012) Distinct contributions of Galgt1 and Galgt2 to carbohydrate expression and function at the mouse neuromuscular junction. Mol Cell Neurosci.
57. Hedlund M, Tangvoranuntakul P, Takematsu H, Long JM, Housley GD, et al. (2007) N-glycolylneuraminic acid deficiency in mice: implications for human biology and evolution. Mol Cell Biol 27: 4340–4346.
58. Parkhomovskiy N, Kammesheidt A, Martin PT (2000) N-acetyllactosamine and the CT carbohydrate antigen mediate agrin-dependent activation of MuSK and acetylcholine receptor clustering in skeletal muscle. Mol Cell Neurosci 15: 380–397.
59. Wang CM, Devries S, Camboni M, Glass M, Martin PT (2010) Immunization with the SDPM1 peptide lowers amyloid plaque burden and improves cognitive function in the APPswePSEN1(A246E) transgenic mouse model of Alzheimer's disease. Neurobiol Dis 39: 409–422.
60. Martin PT, Camboni M, Xu R, Golden B, Chandrasekharan K, et al. (2013) N-Glycolylneuraminic acid deficiency worsens cardiac and skeletal muscle pathophysiology in alpha-sarcoglycan-deficient mice. Glycobiology 23: 833–843.
61. Spiro RG, Yasumoto Y, Bhoyroo V (1996) Characterization of a rat liver Golgi sulphotransferase responsible for the 6-O-sulphation of N-acetylglucosamine residues in beta-linkage to mannose: role in assembly of sialyl-galactosyl-N-acetylglucosamine 6-sulphate sequence of N-linked oligosaccharides. Biochem J 319 (Pt 1): 209–216.
62. Kornegay JN, Bogan JR, Bogan DJ, Childers MK, Li J, et al. (2012) Canine models of Duchenne muscular dystrophy and their use in therapeutic strategies. Mammalian genome : official journal of the International Mammalian Genome Society 23: 85–108.
63. Song X, Yu H, Chen X, Lasanajak Y, Tappert MM, et al. (2011) A sialylated glycan microarray reveals novel interactions of modified sialic acids with proteins and viruses. The Journal of biological chemistry 286: 31610–31622.
64. Marshall JL, Holmberg J, Chou E, Ocampo AC, Oh J, et al. (2012) Sarcospan-dependent Akt activation is required for utrophin expression and muscle regeneration. J Cell Biol 197: 1009–1027.
65. Varki A (2010) Colloquium paper: uniquely human evolution of sialic acid genetics and biology. Proc Natl Acad Sci U S A 107 Suppl 2: 8939–8946.
66. Lofling J, Michael Lyi S, Parrish CR, Varki A (2013) Canine and feline parvoviruses preferentially recognize the non-human cell surface sialic acid N-glycolylneuraminic acid. Virology 440: 89–96.
67. Chakkalakal JV, Thompson J, Parks RJ, Jasmin BJ (2005) Molecular, cellular, and pharmacological therapies for Duchenne/Becker muscular dystrophies. FASEB journal : official publication of the Federation of American Societies for Experimental Biology 19: 880–891.
68. Bardor M, Nguyen DH, Diaz S, Varki A (2005) Mechanism of uptake and incorporation of the non-human sialic acid N-glycolylneuraminic acid into human cells. J Biol Chem 280: 4228–4237.
69. Banda K, Gregg CJ, Chow R, Varki NM, Varki A (2012) Metabolism of vertebrate amino sugars with N-glycolyl groups: mechanisms underlying gastrointestinal incorporation of the non-human sialic acid xeno-autoantigen N-glycolylneuraminic acid. J Biol Chem 287: 28852–28864.
70. Tangvoranuntakul P, Gagneux P, Diaz S, Bardor M, Varki N, et al. (2003) Human uptake and incorporation of an immunogenic nonhuman dietary sialic acid. Proc Natl Acad Sci U S A 100: 12045–12050.
71. Taylor RE, Gregg CJ, Padler-Karavani V, Ghaderi D, Yu H, et al. (2010) Novel mechanism for the generation of human xeno-autoantibodies against the nonhuman sialic acid N-glycolylneuraminic acid. J Exp Med 207: 1637–1646.

4

Effect of 24 Sessions of High-Intensity Aerobic Interval Training Carried out at Either High or Moderate Frequency, a Randomized Trial

Håvard Hatle[1,2¶], Per Kristian Støbakk[1,2¶], Harald Edvard Mølmen[1,2], Eivind Brønstad[1,2,3], Arnt Erik Tjønna[1,2], Sigurd Steinshamn[1,2,3], Eirik Skogvoll[2], Ulrik Wisløff[1,2], Charlotte Björk Ingul[1,2], Øivind Rognmo[1,2]*

1 K.G. Jebsen Centre of Exercise in Medicine, Norwegian University of Science and Technology (NTNU), Trondheim, Norway, **2** Department of Circulation and Medical Imaging, NTNU, Trondheim, Norway, **3** Department of Pulmonary Medicine, St Olav University Hospital, Trondheim, Norway

Abstract

Purpose: The training response of an intensified period of high-intensity exercise is not clear. Therefore, we compared the cardiovascular adaptations of completing 24 high-intensity aerobic interval training sessions carried out for either three or eight weeks, respectively.

Methods: Twenty-one healthy subjects (23.0±2.1 years, 10 females) completed 24 high-intensity training sessions throughout a time-period of either eight weeks (moderate frequency, MF) or three weeks (high frequency, HF) followed by a detraining period of nine weeks without any training. In both groups, maximal oxygen uptake (VO_{2max}) was evaluated before training, at the 9th and 17th session and four days after the final 24th training session. In the detraining phase VO_{2max} was evaluated after 12 days and thereafter every second week for eight weeks. Left ventricular echocardiography, carbon monoxide lung diffusion transfer factor, brachial artery flow mediated dilatation and vastus lateralis citrate maximal synthase activity was tested before and after training.

Results: The cardiovascular adaptation after HF training was delayed compared to training with MF. Four days after ending training the HF group showed no improvement (+3.0%, $p = 0.126$), whereas the MF group reached their highest VO_{2max} with a 10.7% improvement ($p<0.001$: group difference $p = 0.035$). The HF group reached their highest VO_{2max} (6.1% increase, $p = 0.026$) twelve days into the detraining period, compared to a concomitant reduction to 7.9% of VO_{2max} ($p<0.001$) above baseline in the MF group (group difference $p = 0.609$).

Conclusion: Both HF and MF training of high-intensity aerobic exercise improves VO_{2max}. The cardiovascular adaptation following a HF programme of high-intensity exercise is however delayed compared to MF training.

Trial Registration: ClinicalTrials.gov NCT00733941.

Editor: Conrad P. Earnest, University of Bath, United Kingdom

Funding: The present study was supported by grants from the K.G. Jebsen Foundation, Norwegian Council of Cardiovascular Disease, The Norwegian Research Council, and Funds for Cardiovascular and Medical Research at St Olav's University Hospital, Trondheim. The funders had no role in study design, data collection and analysis, decision to publish, or preparation of the manuscript.

* E-mail: oivind.rognmo@ntnu.no

¶ These authors are joint first authors on this work

Introduction

Maximal oxygen uptake (VO_{2max}) is considered the best measure of aerobic capacity and an increase in VO_{2max} is the most common way of demonstrating an effect of aerobic exercise training [1]. The most efficient exercise intensity for improving VO_{2max} has been found to be close to maximal heart rate (HR_{max}) in both healthy subjects [2] as well as in different patient groups [3–5]. Interval training is an effective way of performing high-intensity aerobic exercise, and our research group have previously demonstrated that high-intensity interval exercise at 90–95% of HR_{max}, performed 2–3 times per week is superior to continuous moderate exercise at 60–70% of HR_{max} for improving VO_{2max} when total exercise volume is equalized [6].

The knowledge of how a short and intensified period of high-intensity exercise influences the progression of VO_{2max} is however less clear. Such block periodization could provide a highly time-efficient method for improving VO_{2max} within a very short time-period [7]. A recent study of Swiss alpine junior skiers found that 15 high-intensity exercise sessions at 90–95% of HR_{max} performed over 11 days improved VO_{2max} by 6% when measured seven days after completing training [8]. However, two earlier studies have reported a decrease in VO_{2max} and work performance after two weeks of highly intensified training in competitive cyclists [9,10]. This indicates that the assessment of VO_{2max} may be dependent of when the measurements are taking place after completing a highly intensified training period. Also the cardiovascular and pulmonary adaptations have shown to be depressed immediately after intensified exercise [11,12]. Therefore, the aim of the present study was to investigate the progression of aerobic adaptation in young, healthy individuals completing 24 interval training sessions carried out over either 3 weeks or 8 weeks, respectively. A secondary aim was to study the cardiovascular, pulmonary, endothelial and skeletal muscle adaptation induced by the two training programmes.

Methods

Participants

Twenty-one students (23.0±2.1 years, 10 females) were recruited from the Norwegian University of Science and Technology in Trondheim, Norway. Inclusion criteria were; healthy, non-smokers, BMI ≤27, age ≤30 years, not practising aerobic training more than twice per week and not exceeding a VO_{2max} of 50 and 60 ml · kg^{-1} · min^{-1} for women and men, respectively. The subjects were matched by gender and randomly assigned to a high frequency (HF) (n = 11; 6 females), or a moderate frequency (MF) (n = 10; 4 females) exercise group (Figure 1). The unit of Applied Clinical Research at the university carried out all randomization procedures to ensure complete blinded randomization. All participants signed written informed consent. The study protocol was approved by the regional committee for medical research ethics (REK midt 4.2008.1755) and registered by ClinicalTrials.gov (Identifier NCT00733941). The protocol for this trial and supporting CONSORT checklist are available as supporting information; see Checklist S1 and Protocol S1. The study was carried out from September 2008 to January 2009.

Exercise Protocol

The training period consisted of 24 training sessions carried out over a time span of either eight or three weeks for the MF group and the HF group, respectively. A subsequent detraining period consisted of nine weeks without aerobic training, except necessary daily activities. Both groups performed high-intensity aerobic training running uphill on a treadmill, with individually adjusted speed and inclination, supervised by a personal trainer. Each training session consisted of 10 minutes warm-up followed by 4×4-minute intervals at 90–95% of HR_{max}, alternating with 3-minute of active recovery at 70% of HR_{max}, ending with a 5-minute cool-down, giving a total exercise time of 40 minutes per session. Heart rate (HR) was monitored by HR recorders (Polar, Finland) to ensure that all training sessions was carried out at definitive intensities.

Maximal Oxygen Uptake Testing

Maximal oxygen uptake was tested using an individualized graded step incremental test on a treadmill (Woodway, PPS 55). After a 10 minutes warm-up, a facemask was placed on the subjects for metabolic measurements using a Metamax II (Cortex, Leipzig, Germany), where incline was constant at 10% and speed was increased by 1 km · h^{-1} every minute. Tests were terminated when candidates reached a VO_2 plateau that remained stable despite increased work load, i.e. VO_2 did not increase more than 2 mL · kg^{-1} · min^{-1} despite increased work load, and a respiratory exchange ratio (RER) >1.10. VO_{2max} was measured before study started (pre-test) and four days after the 24th and final training session (post-test). VO_{2max} was also tested during the training period, i.e. at the 9th and 17th training session, and after these tests the subjects performed 3×4-minute intervals. In the detraining phase the subjects were tested 12 days after the last training session and thereafter every second week until the end of the eight week detraining phase. Thus, a total of eight VO_{2max}-tests were conducted for both groups (Figure 2).

Echocardiographic Measurements

Echocardiography at rest was performed at baseline and repeated six days after the training period ended. Measurements were also repeated after the nine weeks of detraining. Complete echocardiographic examinations were performed using a Vivid 7 scanner (GE Vingmed Ultrasound, Horten, Norway) with a phased-array transducer (3MS probe). Three cine loops from the three standard apical planes (four-chamber, two-chamber and long-axis) as well as short-axis (basal, mid-papillary and apical) were recorded in gray scale harmonic mode and tissue Doppler mode. B-mode recordings were done with an average of 53 frames per second and tissue Doppler with 154 frames per second. Measurements and calculations obtained were in accordance to standard procedures recommended by the American Society of Echocardiography. LV volumes and ejection fraction (EF) were calculated from apical recordings by modified biplane Simpson's method. Inflow velocity of the left ventricle was measured by pulsed Doppler with the sample volume at the tips level of mitral valves. Measurements included early diastolic filling (E) and late diastolic filling (A). Stroke volume (SV) and cardiac output (CO) was calculated by Doppler flow measurement in the left ventricular outflow tract (LVOT). Tissue Doppler recordings of the mitral annulus were obtained from the septal and lateral points in four-chamber and in the anterior and inferior points in two-chamber views. Peak annulus velocity in systole (S'), early diastole (e') and late diastole (A') were measured as average of the four points.

Lung Function

Lung function testing was performed before and four days after the training period. Flow-volume spirometry [13] was performed with the Master Screen Pneumo Spirometer (Jaeger, GmbH & Co, KG). The spirometry was calibrated daily, and the highest of two measurements with <5% variation was recorded [14]. Transfer Factor of the Lung for Carbon Monoxide (TLCO) was measured by the "single breath"-method with gas mixture of 10% helium, 0.3% carbon monoxide, 21% oxygen and 68.7% nitrogen [13] with the Master Screen Diffusion (Jaeger, GmbH & Co, KG). All lung function tests were performed at sea level at room temperature (20–22°C).

Endothelial Function

Endothelial function was measured before and after the training phase. The measurements were done 1–3 weeks prior to study start and 10 days after the last training session for both groups. Endothelial function was measured as flow-mediated dilatation (FMD) with high-resolution vascular ultrasound using a 14 MHz echo Doppler probe (Vivid 7 System, GE Vingmed Ultrasound, Horten, Norway) according to guidelines [15]. The procedures for measuring FMD and blood pressure were recently published by our group [16]. All ultrasound images were analyzed in random order with EchoPACtm (GE Vingmed Ultrasound AS) by a blinded investigator.

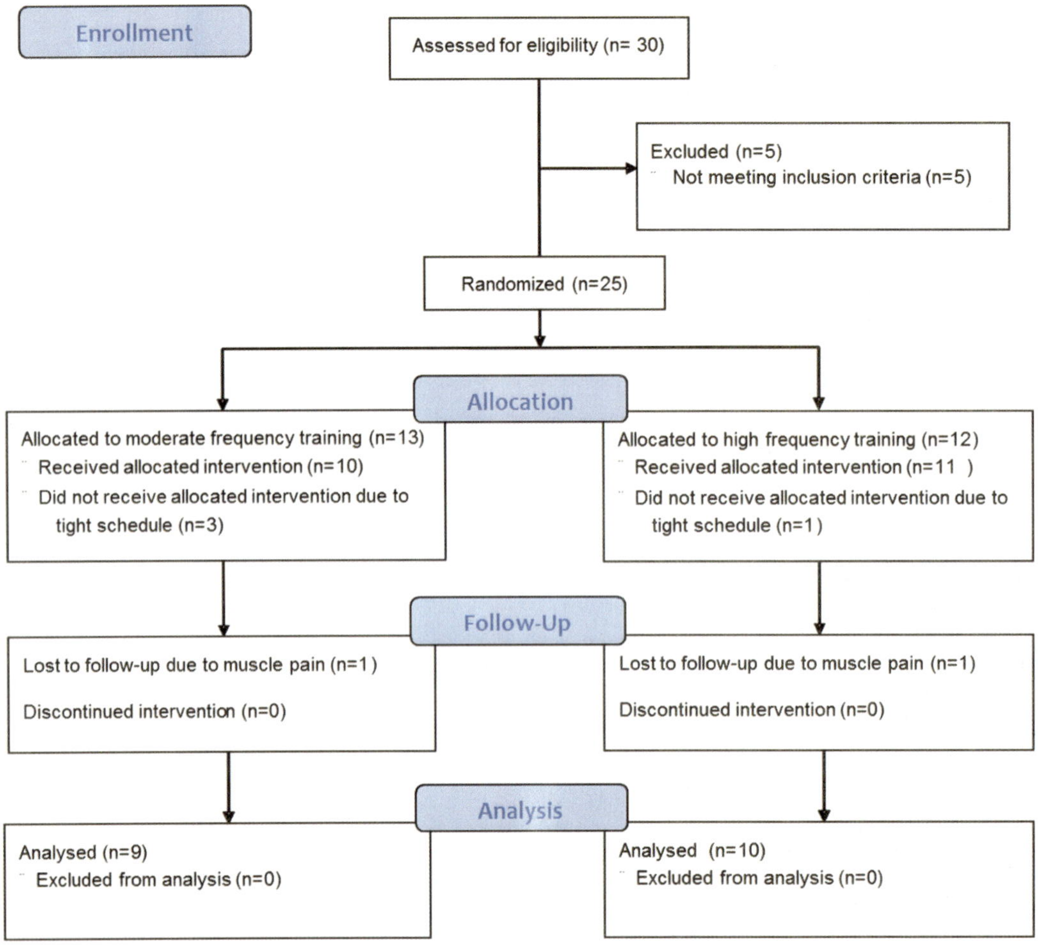

Figure 1. CONSORT flow diagram of the study design.

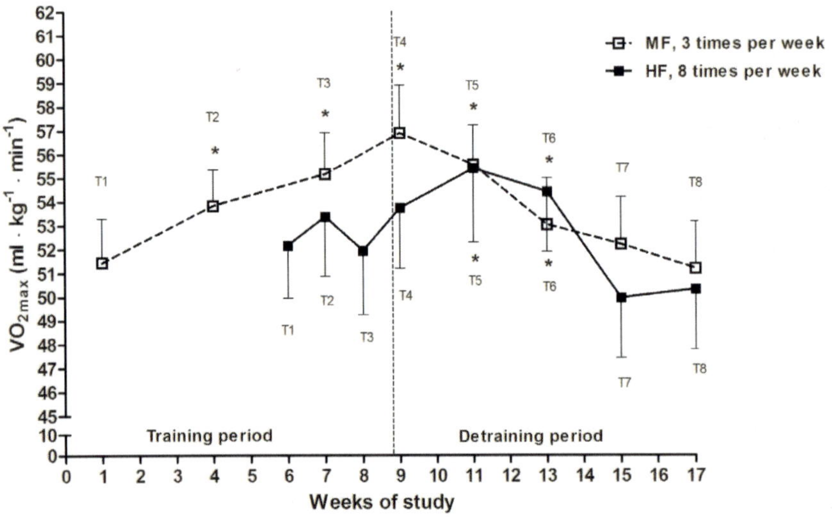

Figure 2. Mean values and standard error of the mean of VO_{2max} for the two groups during the training and the detraining period are shown. Vertical dotted line states the last day of training. Confer Table 2 for statistics and exact values at test points (T1–T8). * Indicates significant differences from baseline within groups.

Muscle Biopsies and Citrate Synthase Activity

Muscle biopsies were taken at baseline and five days after completing the training programme. The biopsies were obtained from the vastus lateralis with a sterile 5 mm diameter biopsy needle (Pelomi, Denmark) under local anaesthesia. All samples were snap-freezed in liquid nitrogen immediately after sampling. For citrate synthase (CS) maximal activity measurements, the muscle samples were homogenized in CelLytic buffer (Sigma-Aldrich, USA) at 6000 shakes/min for 2×8 seconds in a Precellys24 tissue homogenizer (Bertin, France). The homogenate was then centrifugated at 10000 g for 10 min at 4°C and supernatant tested for CS activity. The CS maximal activity was determined by the use of citrate synthase Assay Kit (CS 0720, Sigma-Aldrich). Absorbance at 412 nm was measured on a Fluostar Omega spectrometer (BMG Labtech, Germany). Specific activity was calculated by dividing measured activity on the muscle extract protein concentration. Protein concentrations were determined by the method of Bradford [17].

Statistical Analysis

Samples size was estimated for VO_{2max} as primary outcome measure using IBM SPSS SamplePower. The principal outcome variable VO_{2max} were analysed between groups using a linear model with correction for baseline value (ANCOVA) [18], and within groups comparisons were done using paired samples T-test. Values are expressed as mean and standard deviation (SD). A two-tailed significance-level of $p<0.05$ was acknowledged as statistical significant. All analyses were done by PASW 17.0 (SPSS Inc, Chicago). At five occasions a subject was unavailable for testing. Because of the Gaussian behaviour of the data and the low number of missing values, these time points were estimated by an imputed value using Missing Value Analysis (PASW 17.0) to complete the dataset [19].

Results

Subject Characteristics

There were no differences between the groups with respect to age, body weight, height and body mass index (BMI) at baseline (Table 1). One person in each group withdrew from the study reporting tight calf muscles, and a total of 19 subjects completed the training- and detraining phases and were included in the analysis (Figure 1). All subjects that completed the study fulfilled > 95% compliance to the prescribed training programme.

Adaptation of VO_{2max}

There was no baseline difference in VO_{2max} between the groups before the study started (Table 2). The MF group improved VO_{2max} by 4.6% ($p=0.036$) already after eight training sessions, whereas no significant improvement was seen in the HF group at the same time point (+2.3%, $p=0.128$; between group difference $p=0.449$). After finishing 16 of the 24 sessions, we found an improvement in VO_{2max} of 7.1% ($p=0.002$) in the MF group compared no improvement (−0.5% vs. baseline, $p<0.128$) in the HF group (between group difference $p=0.036$) (Figure 2 and Table 2). At post-test, i.e. four days after ending training, the MF group reached their highest achieved VO_{2max} by 10.7% ($p<0.001$) above baseline, whereas no improvement (+3.0%, $p=0.126$) was seen in the HF group (between group difference, $p=0.035$). Twelve days into the detraining period (week 11 of the study) the HF group reached their highest VO_{2max} with a value of 6.1% ($p=0.026$) above baseline, compared to a VO_{2max} of 7.9% ($p<0.001$) above baseline in the MF group at the same time point (group difference $p=0.609$) (Figure 2). When considering the individual subjects' highest VO_{2max} (Highest-VO_{2max}), irrespective of which VO_{2max}-test it was reached, the MF and HF groups improved their VO_{2max} with 12.1% ($p<0{,}001$) and 7.5% ($p=0.010$), respectively (between group difference, $p=0.319$) (Table 2).

After 4 weeks of detraining (week 13 into the study, Figure 2 and Table 2) the VO_{2max} in the MF group was still elevated compared to baseline (+2.9%, $p=0.029$), but was reduced compared to their highest achieved time point (i.e. 4 day post exercise: $p=0.003$). The VO_{2max} in the HF group was after 4 weeks of detraining 4.2% above baseline ($p=0.018$) and not reduced relative to the group's highest measurement (i.e. 12 d post exercise: $p=0.343$) (Figure 2 and Table 2). After 6 weeks of detraining (week 15 into the study) VO_{2max} was back to baseline level in both groups, i.e. +1.5% compared to baseline in the MF group, ($p=0.339$) and −4.2% in the HF group ($p=0.064$).

Left Ventricular Adaptations

Stroke volume increased by 14.5% after the training period in the MF group ($p=0.028$), while no change was observed in the HF group ($p=0.369$) (Table 3). Left ventricular ejection fraction (EF) increased in the MF group (12.1%, $p=0.050$), whereas it decreased by 11% ($p<0.001$) after HF training, but it is notable

Table 1. Group Characteristics.

	MF group (n = 9)	HF group (n = 10)	p-value
Age (yrs)	23.1±2.3	23.7±2.1	= 0.560
Weight (kg)	70.2±16.8	67.7±8.9	= 0.684
Height (cm)	175.0±11.3	173.0±8.7	= 0.709
BMI (kg/m^2)	22.7±3.1	22.6±2.3	= 0.938

Table 2. Values of VO_{2max} expressed as means ± SD for both groups during the training and detraining periods.

	MF group		HF group		Between gr.
Test points	**VO_{2max}**	**p-value**	**VO_{2max}**	**p-value**	**p-value**
1 (pre-test)	51.5±5.5	-	52.2±7.0	-	= 0.290
2 (after 8 sessions)	**53.8±4.6**	**= 0.036**	53.4±7.9	= 0.128	= 0.449
3 (after 16 sessions)	**55.2±5.3**	**= 0.002**	51.9±8.5	= 0.829	**= 0.036**
4 (post-test, 24 sessions)	**56.9±6.1**	**<0.001**	53.7±8.0	= 0.126	**= 0.035**
5 (12 d post exercise)	**55.6±5.0**	**<0.001**	**55.4±9.8**	**= 0.026**	= 0.609
6 (4 wk post exercise)	**53.0±5.9**	**= 0.029**	**54.4±7.9**	**= 0.018**	= 0.798
7 (6 wk post exercise)	52.2±5.9	= 0.339	50.0±8.1	= 0.064	= 0.115
8 (post-detraining)	51.2±5.9	= 0.758	50.3±8.1	= 0.118	= 0.493
Highest-VO_{2max}	**57.5±5.2**	**<0.001**	**56.0±9.7**	**= 0.010**	= 0.319

Post-test refers to values at the first test after training, which was four days after last exercise session. Highest-VO_{2max} refers to collected highest measured value of subjects within each group, independent of at which test point after training it occurred. VO_{2max} is presented as ml · kg^{-1} · min^{-1}. Significant differences from baseline within groups and differences between groups are typed in bold. Between group differences are post-test values.

that EF was 15% higher in the HF group compared to MF group at baseline (between group difference, $p = 0.050$). End diastolic volume (EDV) increased only in the HF group, by 10.1% ($p = 0.050$). S' tended to increase in the MF group (7.8%, $p = 0.056$), but no change was observed in the HF group (between group differences: $p = 0.490$). E, A and e' did not change in any group after the training period.

During the detraining period SV and EF returned to baseline values in the MF group. In the HF group SV increased by 10.0% ($p = 0.031$) during the detraining, and EF and S' returned to baseline values.

Lung Function

Flow volume spirometry values did not change at any point of measurement in either group. TLCO was reduced by 11.3% ($p = 0.004$) in the HF group after the training period, while the MF group increased diffusion capacity by 6.0% ($p = 0.041$) (Table 4). Haemoglobin levels did not differ during the study period, and thus TLCO was not corrected for haemoglobin levels.

Endothelial Function

Flow mediated dilation was unchanged from before to after training both within the MF group (7.4±3.6 vs. 7.5±2.5% ($p = 0.952$) and within the HF group (7.5±2.0 vs. 7.6±2.8% ($p = 0.910$) (between group difference $p = 0.943$) (Table 4).

Citrate Synthase Activity

The vastus lateralis citrate synthase maximal activity relative to the muscle extract protein concentration was increased by 39% in the MF group (from 0.38±0.10 to 0.52±0.10 $\mu mol \cdot ml^{-1} \cdot min^{-1} \cdot mg^{-1}$ protein, $p < 0.001$) (Table 4). We also found a 25% increase in activity in the HF group (from 0.30±0.12 to 0.37±0.11 $\mu mol \cdot ml^{-1} \cdot min^{-1} \cdot mg^{-1}$ protein), but this improvement did not reach statistical significance ($p = 0.185$; between group difference $p = 0.009$).

Discussion

The main finding of this study was that both HF and MF training of high-intensity aerobic exercise improves VO_{2max}. We found however no improvements in VO_{2max} immediately after ending the HF training programme. In addition, we found a reduction in lung diffusion capacity and indications of a reduction in cardiac function in HF immediately after training. This indicates a possibility of fatigue when exposed to such a high exercise dose. However, during the detraining period there was a delayed increase in VO_{2max} in the HF group demonstrating the necessity of sufficient rest to adapt from such a heavy exercise training programme. The MF training programme, in contrast, had a positive effect for improving the aerobic capacity in a progressive manner throughout the training period.

Maximal Oxygen Uptake

Previous studies have demonstrated that VO_{2max} improves after HF aerobic training [20,21], suggesting a possibility to improve VO_{2max} in reduced time compared to more moderate training regimes. In line with this, a recent study by Breil et al. [8] involving Swiss alpine skiers, showed that it is possible to boost the aerobic capacity by means of a 6% increase of VO_{2max} using a high-intensity interval training "shock" of 15 sessions in 11 days. In our study we found a quite different progression of the adaptation between MF- and HF-training, and the highest VO_{2max}-values occurred at different time points. In the MF group the adaptation to physical training progressed in a regular manner. VO_{2max} increased progressively in the MF group during the training period, and reached highest value at post-test, four days after ending training period (+10.7%, $p < 0.001$). Contrary, in the HF group there was no change in VO_{2max} during the training period. In fact, we measured a small, but not significant reduction at the VO_{2max}-test performed at the 16th training session, 14 days into the training regime. Furthermore, the HF group showed no improvements four days after ending 24 sessions of training (+ 2.9%, $p = 0.126$), and improved their VO_{2max} first after another week of detraining (+6.1%, $p = 0.026$), i.e. 12 days after finishing training. Interestingly, despite training for only 3 weeks the HF group still required 5 weeks to reach their highest measured VO_{2max} (+6.1% from baseline) whereas the MF group reached an improvement of 7.1% immediately after completing their 6 weeks of moderate training.

Our results show that the highly intensified training load experienced by the HF group was too severe to progressively adapt compared to the MF training programme. It is assumed that

Table 3. Parameters of heart function for both groups before and after training and after detraining.

	MF group					HF group				
	Pre-test	Post-test	p-value	Detraining	p-value	Pre-test	Post-test	p-value	Detraining	p-value
HR_{rest}, b/min	58±6	58±9	=0.997	59±9	=0.901	65±9	57±8	=0.034	66±12	=0.954
BP_{sys}, mmHg	117.0±10.0	118.0±11.0	=0.943	108.0±9.0	=0.025	118.5±10.5	123.0±9.0	=0.343	121.5±16	=0.561
BP_{dia}, mmHg	74.0±6.0	74.0±7.0	=0.992	68.0±3.0	=0.074	74.0±8.5	74.0±5.0	=0.784	71.0±9.5	=0.454
EDV, ml	120.0±28.0	129.0±40.0	=0.176	118.6±23.0	=0.408	119.5±20.0	131.5±25.0	=0.034	131.0±20.0	=0.024
SV, ml	77.0±21.0	88.0±18.0	=0.028	87.0±21.0	=0.192	85.0±14.1	89.0±18.5	=0.369	93.5±11.0	=0.031
S', cm/s	8.95±8.1	9.65±7.5	=0.056	9.05±10.5	=0.096	9.50±16.1	9.60±14.3	=0.813	9.70±14.6	=0.507
EF, %	58.0±5.8	65.0±4.3	=0.050*	63.5±5.9	=0.380	66.5±5.1	59.0±2.7	<0.001	66.0±5.2	=0.805
E/A	2.4±0.7	2.7±0.9	=0.239	2.4±0.7	=0.819	2.3±0.8	2.8±0.6	=0.070	2.3±0.7	=0.790
e'	15.9±2.2	16.1±2.4	=0.741	16.0±1.8	=0.524	15.6±2.6	15.7±1.9	=0.862	15.7±2.1	=0.734

Values are expressed as means ± SD. HR_{rest}; resting heart rate, BP_{sys}; systolic blood pressure, BP_{dia}; diastolic blood pressure, EDV; end diastolic volume, SV; stroke volume, S'; peak annulus velocity in systole, e'; early diastole, and A'; late diastole were measured as average of the four measures. EF; ejection fraction. P-values are within-groups differences from pre- to post-test, and between group differences for post-test values.
* Significant differences between groups ($p < 0.05$).

Table 4. Physiological variables for both groups before and after the training period.

	MF group			HF group			Between gr. p-value
	Pre-test	Post-test	p-value	Pre-test	Post-test	p-value	
FMD, %	7.4±3.6	7.5±2.5	=0.952	7.5±2.0	7.6±2.8	=0.910	=0.948
TLCO, conductance units	9.36±1.16	9.92±1.48	=0.041	10.61±2.14	9.40±1.79	=0.004	=0.094
CS, μmole/ml/min/mg protein	0.38±0.10	0.52±0.09	<0.001	0.30±0.12	0.37±0.12	=0.185	=0.009

Values are expressed as means ± SD. FMD; Brachial artery flow mediated dilatation, CS; citrate synthase activity, TLCO; transfer factor of the lung for carbon monoxide. Between group differences are post-test values. P-values are within-groups differences from pre- to post-test, and between group differences for post-test values.

recovery processes continue through homoeostatic restoration of the body after training until a compensation effect may occur [22]. The most common way to adapt and improve physical fitness after training is to recover sufficiently and then perform the next exercise session at the peak of the compensation phase [23]. However, It has been described that athletes may experience acute feelings of fatigue and decrease in performance following periods of intensified training [24]. Intensified training can thus result in a temporarily decline in performance, but when sufficient periods of recovery are provided, a supercompensation may occur with enhanced performance compared to baseline levels [24]. As it is possible to recover within a 2-week period [25], it may be argued that this is a relatively normal condition and thus a normal part of a strenuous training process. The lack of improvement of VO_{2max} in the HF group during the training period, along with the compensation effect in the detraining phase, suggests that too severe training load was induced, as opposed to the progressive improvement of VO_{2max} in the MF group suggesting sufficient rest between the exercise sessions. However, it is still possible that more well-trained athletes could have acquired greater adaptation to HF training compared with our moderately trained students. There was however only one drop-out in each group, despite the higher physical demands in the HF group. The high compliance rate might be due to the young healthy population and a strong will to complete the training programme.

After 6 weeks of detraining, that started after the last exercise session, VO_{2max} returned to baseline values both in the MF and HF group. Mujika and Padilla [26] found that recently trained subjects most often reverse their gained VO_{2max} when detraining extends 4 weeks [27], whereas Pedersen et al. [28] found that the inactivity period simply reverses the training effect in the same manner as it emerged. Coyle et al. found that the decline in VO_{2max} stabilized after 8 weeks of detraining [29]. Although VO_{2max} in both groups in our study were still elevated compared to baseline VO_{2max} at 4 weeks into the de-training period, our findings suggest an earlier reduction of VO_{2max} relative to highest measured value in the MF group, i.e. after 4 weeks compared to 6 weeks in the HF group. The reason for this may simply correspond to the latency of their highest VO_{2max} value in the HF group, which occurred 2 weeks after training cessation. The gained aerobic capacity in both groups thus declined in a similar pattern from the highest reached value, being back at baseline 4 weeks after their highest measurement.

Cardiovascular Response

We observed that stroke volume increased significantly in the MF group in response to the interval training in line with other studies [2,5,30]. In the HF group we found an increased end diastolic volume. In the HF group EF was reduced, suggesting a depressed left ventricular adaptation after the training period. The reduction in the systolic function is in concordance with another study that revealed a negative myocardial effect immediately after a strenuous exercise programme [12]. It should be emphasized that heart rate was reduced in the HF group after the exercise period, which may have affected the cardiac measurements. The cardiac measurements were secondary endpoints and the study is thus too small to draw firm conclusion. As expected, the diastolic measurements at rest did not improve, confirming existing literature that young healthy sedentary subjects on beforehand have a normal and optimal diastolic function [31].

During detraining in the MF group we observed that the stroke volume and the EF returned to baseline values. This indicates loss of the training induced adaptations caused by inactivity. The groups however differed in their adaptations during detraining. Stroke volume increased during detraining amongst the HF group and this was attributable to the increased end diastolic volume. EF was subsequently normalized. This indicates that recovery is crucial to achieve cardiac improvements after a strenuous physical activity programme. However, although the HF group increased stroke volume during detraining, the inactivity period returned VO_{2max} to baseline values.

It has previously been suggested that intense exercise may induce stress that impairs the systemic endothelial function [32]. We found however no signs of endothelial dysfunction as both groups showed the same FMD of the brachial artery both before and after training.

Lung Function

The MF group increased pulmonary diffusion capacity after the training period. Diffusion capacity may have increased in relation to the increased stroke volume seen in the MF group.

Peripheral Adaptations

The mitochondrial citrate synthase maximal activity improved more in the MF group compared to the HF group after the training programmes. Our results are in accordance with previous high-intensity exercise training studies showing that maximal activity of the citrate synthase is normally upregulated by 15–35% after strenuous training [33]. In line with our results, a recent study concluded that in skeletal muscle of trained individuals, the maximal activity of citrate synthase were enhanced to a greater extent by having a day of rest between the exercise sessions compared with training daily for 3 weeks [34].

Study Strengths and Limitations

This study is small with few subjects in each group. However, the high number of test points throughout the study with a steady incline and decline of VO_{2max} in the MF group, is indicating that changes not just being measurement variations. Also, the VO_{2max}-tests consistently showed plateaus of the O_2-curve and high RER-values above 1.10, suggesting maximal effort during all tests. As it is difficult to predict when each subject achieves their highest VO_{2max} value after a training programme, an even more frequent test programme could have revealed even higher maximum values. More frequent testing could on the other hand elicit an unwanted training effect in the detraining period. Another aspect would have been to elucidate which mechanisms were causing the signs of fatigue during and after HF training. However, this study was not designed to examine these underlying mechanisms. The study was originally designed also to investigate retraining after the detraining period, but due to the strain of the participants, this part of the study was not implemented.

Conclusions

It has previously been shown that it is possible to boost VO_{2max} by a short and intensified high-intensity interval training period. In our study we found a different progression of the adaptation between MF- and HF-training, and the highest VO_{2max}-values occurred at different time points. The adaptation following a HF programme of high-intensity exercise was delayed compared to training with MF. The HF programme may induce an initially fatigue which may limit the cardiopulmonary function whereas the latter programme follows a more progressive adaptation.

Acknowledgments

We would like to thank Cecilie Horvei for conducting the lung function measurements.

Author Contributions

Conceived and designed the experiments: HH PKS HEM EB AET SS ES UW CBI ØR. Performed the experiments: HH PKS HEM EB AET CBV ØR. Analyzed the data: HH PKS HEM EB SS ES UW CBV ØR. Contributed reagents/materials/analysis tools: HH PKS HEM EB CBV ØR. Wrote the paper: HH PKS HEM UW ØR.

References

1. Bassett DR Jr., Howley ET (2000) Limiting factors for maximum oxygen uptake and determinants of endurance performance. Med Sci Sports Exerc 32: 70–84.
2. Helgerud J, Hoydal K, Wang E, Karlsen T, Berg P, et al. (2007) Aerobic high-intensity intervals improve VO2max more than moderate training. Med Sci Sports Exerc 39: 665–671.
3. Rognmo O, Hetland E, Helgerud J, Hoff J, Slordahl SA (2004) High intensity aerobic interval exercise is superior to moderate intensity exercise for increasing aerobic capacity in patients with coronary artery disease. Eur J Cardiovasc Prev Rehabil 11: 216–222.
4. Tjonna AE, Lee SJ, Rognmo O, Stolen TO, Bye A, et al. (2008) Aerobic interval training versus continuous moderate exercise as a treatment for the metabolic syndrome: a pilot study. Circulation 118: 346–354.
5. Wisloff U, Stoylen A, Loennechen JP, Bruvold M, Rognmo O, et al. (2007) Superior cardiovascular effect of aerobic interval training versus moderate continuous training in heart failure patients: a randomized study. Circulation 115: 3086–3094.
6. Kemi OJ, Wisloff U (2010) High-intensity aerobic exercise training improves the heart in health and disease. J Cardiopulm Rehabil Prev 30: 2–11.
7. Laursen PB, Jenkins DG (2002) The scientific basis for high-intensity interval training: optimising training programmes and maximising performance in highly trained endurance athletes. Sports Med 32: 53–73.
8. Breil FA, Weber SN, Koller S, Hoppeler H, Vogt M (2010) Block training periodization in alpine skiing: effects of 11-day HIT on VO(2max) and performance. Eur J Appl Physiol.
9. Jeukendrup AE, Hesselink MK, Snyder AC, Kuipers H, Keizer HA (1992) Physiological changes in male competitive cyclists after two weeks of intensified training. Int J Sports Med 13: 534–541.
10. Snyder AC, Kuipers H, Cheng B, Servais R, Fransen E (1995) Overtraining following intensified training with normal muscle glycogen. Med Sci Sports Exerc 27: 1063–1070.
11. McKenzie DC, O'Hare TJ, Mayo J (2005) The effect of sustained heavy exercise on the development of pulmonary edema in trained male cyclists. Respiratory Physiology & Neurobiology 145: 209–218.
12. Aslani A, Babaee Bigi MA, Moaref AR (2009) Effect of extreme exercise on myocardial function as assessed by tissue Doppler imaging. Echocardiography 26: 1036–1040.
13. Macintyre N, Crapo RO, Viegi G, Johnson DC, van der Grinten CP, et al. (2005) Standardisation of the single-breath determination of carbon monoxide uptake in the lung. Eur Respir J 26: 720–735.
14. Miller MR, Hankinson J, Brusasco V, Burgos F, Casaburi R, et al. (2005) Standardisation of spirometry. Eur Respir J 26: 319–338.
15. Pyke KE, Tschakovsky ME (2005) The relationship between shear stress and flow-mediated dilatation: implications for the assessment of endothelial function. J Physiol 568: 357–369.
16. Tyldum GA, Schjerve IE, Tjonna AE, Kirkeby-Garstad I, Stolen TO, et al. (2009) Endothelial dysfunction induced by post-prandial lipemia: complete protection afforded by high-intensity aerobic interval exercise. J Am Coll Cardiol 53: 200–206.
17. Bradford MM (1976) A rapid and sensitive method for the quantitation of microgram quantities of protein utilizing the principle of protein-dye binding. Anal Biochem 72: 248–254.
18. Vickers AJ, Altman DG (2001) Statistics notes: Analysing controlled trials with baseline and follow up measurements. BMJ 323: 1123–1124.
19. Sterne JA, White IR, Carlin JB, Spratt M, Royston P, et al. (2009) Multiple imputation for missing data in epidemiological and clinical research: potential and pitfalls. BMJ 338: b2393.
20. Pollock ML, Miller HS, Linnerud AC, Cooper KH (1975) Frequency of training as a determinant for improvement in cardiovascular function and body composition of middle-aged men. Arch Phys Med Rehabil 56: 141–145.
21. Gettman LR, Pollock ML, Durstine JL, Ward A, Ayres J, et al. (1976) Physiological responses of men to 1, 3, and 5 day per week training programs. Res Q 47: 638–646.
22. Viru A (1994) Molecular cellular mechanisms of training effects. J Sports Med Phys Fitness 34: 309–322.
23. Kuipers H (1998) Training and overtraining: an introduction. Med Sci Sports Exerc 30: 1137–1139.
24. Halson SL, Jeukendrup AE (2004) Does overtraining exist? An analysis of overreaching and overtraining research. Sports Med 34: 967–981.
25. Halson SL, Bridge MW, Meeusen R, Busschaert B, Gleeson M, et al. (2002) Time course of performance changes and fatigue markers during intensified training in trained cyclists. J Appl Physiol 93: 947–956.
26. Mujika I, Padilla S (2000) Detraining: loss of training-induced physiological and performance adaptations. Part I: short term insufficient training stimulus. Sports Med 30: 79–87.
27. Mujika I, Padilla S (2001) Cardiorespiratory and metabolic characteristics of detraining in humans. Med Sci Sports Exerc 33: 413–421.
28. Pedersen PK, Jorgensen K (1978) Maximal oxygen uptake in young women with training, inactivity, and retraining. Med Sci Sports 10: 233–237.
29. Coyle EF, Martin WH, 3rd, Sinacore DR, Joyner MJ, Hagberg JM, et al. (1984) Time course of loss of adaptations after stopping prolonged intense endurance training. J Appl Physiol 57: 1857–1864.
30. Amundsen BH, Rognmo O, Hatlen-Rebhan G, Slordahl SA (2008) High-intensity aerobic exercise improves diastolic function in coronary artery disease. Scand Cardiovasc J 42: 110–117.
31. George KP, Naylor LH, Whyte GP, Shave RE, Oxborough D, et al. (2009) Diastolic function in healthy humans: non-invasive assessment and the impact of acute and chronic exercise. Eur J Appl Physiol.
32. Goto C, Higashi Y, Kimura M, Noma K, Hara K, et al. (2003) Effect of different intensities of exercise on endothelium-dependent vasodilation in humans: role of endothelium-dependent nitric oxide and oxidative stress. Circulation 108: 530–535.
33. Gibala MJ, McGee SL (2008) Metabolic adaptations to short-term high-intensity interval training: a little pain for a lot of gain? Exerc Sport Sci Rev 36: 58–63.
34. Yeo WK, Paton CD, Garnham AP, Burke LM, Carey AL, et al. (2008) Skeletal muscle adaptation and performance responses to once a day versus twice every second day endurance training regimens. J Appl Physiol 105: 1462–1470.

5

Alcohol Ingestion Impairs Maximal Post-Exercise Rates of Myofibrillar Protein Synthesis following a Single Bout of Concurrent Training

Evelyn B. Parr[1], Donny M. Camera[1], José L. Areta[1], Louise M. Burke[2], Stuart M. Phillips[3], John A. Hawley[4,5]*, Vernon G. Coffey[6]

1 Exercise and Nutrition Research Group, School of Medical Sciences, RMIT University, Bundoora, Victoria, Australia, **2** Department of Sports Nutrition, Australian Institute of Sport, Canberra, ACT, Australia, **3** Exercise Metabolism Research Group, Department of Kinesiology, McMaster University, Hamilton, Ontario, Canada, **4** Exercise and Nutrition Research Group, School of Exercise Science, Australian Catholic University, Fitzroy, Victoria, Australia, **5** Research Institute for Sport and Exercise Sciences, Liverpool John Moores University, Liverpool, United Kingdom, **6** School of Exercise and Nutrition Sciences and Institute of Health and Biomedical Innovation, Queensland University of Technology, Kelvin Grove, Queensland, Australia

Abstract

Introduction: The culture in many team sports involves consumption of large amounts of alcohol after training/competition. The effect of such a practice on recovery processes underlying protein turnover in human skeletal muscle are unknown. We determined the effect of alcohol intake on rates of myofibrillar protein synthesis (MPS) following strenuous exercise with carbohydrate (CHO) or protein ingestion.

Methods: In a randomized cross-over design, 8 physically active males completed three experimental trials comprising resistance exercise (8×5 reps leg extension, 80% 1 repetition maximum) followed by continuous (30 min, 63% peak power output (PPO)) and high intensity interval (10×30 s, 110% PPO) cycling. Immediately, and 4 h post-exercise, subjects consumed either 500 mL of whey protein (25 g; PRO), alcohol (1.5 g·kg body mass^{-1}, 12±2 standard drinks) co-ingested with protein (ALC-PRO), or an energy-matched quantity of carbohydrate also with alcohol (25 g maltodextrin; ALC-CHO). Subjects also consumed a CHO meal (1.5 g CHO·kg body mass^{-1}) 2 h post-exercise. Muscle biopsies were taken at rest, 2 and 8 h post-exercise.

Results: Blood alcohol concentration was elevated above baseline with ALC-CHO and ALC-PRO throughout recovery ($P<0.05$). Phosphorylation of mTOR^{Ser2448} 2 h after exercise was higher with PRO compared to ALC-PRO and ALC-CHO ($P<0.05$), while p70S6K phosphorylation was higher 2 h post-exercise with ALC-PRO and PRO compared to ALC-CHO ($P<0.05$). Rates of MPS increased above rest for all conditions (~29–109%, $P<0.05$). However, compared to PRO, there was a hierarchical reduction in MPS with ALC-PRO (24%, $P<0.05$) and with ALC-CHO (37%, $P<0.05$).

Conclusion: We provide novel data demonstrating that alcohol consumption reduces rates of MPS following a bout of concurrent exercise, even when co-ingested with protein. We conclude that alcohol ingestion suppresses the anabolic response in skeletal muscle and may therefore impair recovery and adaptation to training and/or subsequent performance.

Editor: Stephen E. Alway, West Virginia University School of Medicine, United States of America

Funding: This study was, in part, funded by a grant from the Australian Sports Commission to LMB. The funders had no role in study design, data collection and analysis, decision to publish or preparation of the manuscript. No additional external funding was received for this study.

* E-mail: john.hawley@acu.edu.au

Introduction

The focus of the early post-exercise period (i.e., 1–8 h) is to enhance physiological processes that are critical for reversing the exercise-induced disturbances to homeostasis and physiological function and for promoting adaptations to training [1]. Recommended nutritional strategies to maximize recovery in skeletal muscle include protein for enhancing rates of protein synthesis and carbohydrate for replenishing glycogen stores [2,3]. Muscle contraction and the intake of leucine-rich protein sources activate independent but complimentary signaling responses that converge at the mechanistic target of rapamycin (mTOR) to stimulate protein translation enhancing rates of muscle protein synthesis [4–6]. The ingestion of ~20–25 g of high quality protein soon after exercise [7], repeated every 4 h [8] has been shown to maximise the anabolic response in skeletal muscle.

The cultural environment surrounding some sports often involves the intake of large amounts of alcohol after training and competition, with athletes in several team sports being particularly at risk of "binge drinking" practices [9–11]. Indeed, a number of studies have reported that athletes are more likely than the general population to drink alcohol to excess, with a large proportion (~50–65%) consuming intakes above the threshold classified as hazardous drinking [12,13]. The outcomes of binge drinking after exercise are likely to include the direct effect of alcohol on physiological processes as well as the indirect effect on the athlete's recovery due to not eating or resting adequately as a result of intoxication. Although the concurrent consumption of carbohydrate can partially offset the deleterious effects of alcohol intake on post-exercise glycogen resynthesis [14], the effect of alcohol consumption on muscle protein synthesis is unknown.

Studies by Barnes and colleagues (2010, 2011) have investigated the effects of post-exercise alcohol consumption on human muscle function and performance [15,16]. However, data on the effects of alcohol intake on skeletal muscle protein synthesis is limited to work in rodents. These studies show that both acute and chronic alcohol ingestion can have a detrimental effect on cell signaling and protein synthesis in skeletal muscle [17–21]. The aim of the current study was to determine the effect of alcohol intake on anabolic cell signaling and rates of myofibrillar protein synthesis (MPS) in humans during recovery from a bout of strenuous exercise approximating stresses an athlete may experience in training and performance for various team sports such as various football and rugby codes, and court sports. We hypothesized that compared to post-exercise protein intake, co-ingestion of alcohol would down-regulate translation initiation signaling and decrease rates of MPS.

Methods

Subjects

Eight healthy physically active male subjects (age 21.4±4.8 yr, body mass (BM) 79.3±11.9 kg, peak oxygen uptake (VO_{2peak}) 48.1±4.8 $mL\cdot kg^{-1}\cdot min^{-1}$, leg extension one repetition maximum (1RM) 104±20 kg; values are mean ± SD) who had been participating in regular exercise (3 times wk^{-1} for >6 months) volunteered for this study. The experimental procedures and possible risks associated with the study were explained to each subject, who each gave written informed consent before participation.

Ethics statement

All subjects were informed of the purpose of the study, the experimental procedures involved and all the potential risks involved before giving written consent. No minors were involved in this study as subjects were required to be 18 years of age at the time of participation due to the legal age for alcohol consumption in Australia. All subjects were deemed healthy based on their response to a routine medical screening questionnaire. The study was approved by the Human Research Ethics Committee of RMIT University (43/11) and was carried out according to the NHMRC National Statement on Ethical Conduct in Human Research (2007) and the Australian Code for the Responsible Conduct of Research (2007).

Study Design

The study employed a randomized counter-balanced, cross-over design in which each subject completed bouts of consecutive resistance, continuous and intermittent high-intensity exercise with either post-exercise ingestion of alcohol-carbohydrate (ALC-CHO), alcohol-protein (ALC-PRO) or protein only (PRO) beverages on three separate occasions. Each experimental trial was separated by a two week recovery period, during which time subjects maintained their habitual physical activity pattern. Given the data showing little/no effect of carbohydrate ingestion on myofibrillar protein synthesis, the ALC-CHO treatment was used as an iso-energetic control. The decision not to use parallel groups was based on a within subject crossover design adding strength to the interpretation and conclusions of the study but limited the total number of treatments such that an exercise only trial was not undertaken. Finally, we based our exercise protocol incorporating the different metabolic stresses approximating those experienced in team sports due to published reports of the increased incidence of excessive alcohol consumption following performance in team/group sport [13].

Preliminary Testing

VO_2peak. VO_{2peak} and peak power output (PPO) were determined during an incremental test to volitional fatigue on a Lode cycle ergometer (Groningen, The Netherlands). The protocol has been described in detail previously [22].

Maximal strength. Quadriceps strength was determined on a plate-loaded leg extension machine until the 1RM load was established. Repetitions were separated by a 3-min recovery and were used to establish the maximum load/weight that could be moved through the full range of motion once, but not a second time.

Diet/exercise control

For the 48 h prior to an experimental trial subjects were instructed to refrain from strenuous exercise/training. Subjects were provided pre-packaged food and drinks (~6000 kJ; 3.1 g $CHO\cdot kg^{-1}$ BM, 0.5 g $fat\cdot kg^{-1}$ BM, 0.4 g $protein\cdot kg^{-1}$ BM) to be consumed for the last meal prior to an experiment. A food diary to record dietary intake was used to ensure adherence to the final meal and overall daily intake for the 24 h prior to an experiment day.

Experimental Procedure

The study employed a randomized cross-over design in which each subject completed three experimental trials. Each trial was separated by 14 d, during which subjects maintained their habitual level of physical activity and their normal diet. The three trials compared post-exercise protein synthesis with three different treatments: a post-exercise feeding regimen providing protein intake for optimal muscle protein synthesis [8] (2 feedings of 25 g high quality protein at 0 and 4 h of recovery: PRO), a trial in which the subjects consumed 1.5 $g\cdot kg^{-1}$ BM ethanol plus an energy match for recommended protein feedings in the form of carbohydrate (ALC-CHO), and ALC-PRO in which the same amount of alcohol was consumed in addition to protein intake in PRO also ingested at 0 and 4 h post-exercise (see Figure 1). All trials involved a further standardised carbohydrate-rich meal (1.5 g $CHO\cdot kg^{-1}$ BM) at 2 h post-exercise as post-event fuelling/eating.

On the morning of an experimental trial, subjects reported to the laboratory after a ~10-h overnight fast. After resting in a supine position for ~15 min, catheters were inserted into the antecubital vein of each arm and a baseline blood sample (~4 mL) was taken from one arm. A primed constant intravenous infusion (prime: 2 $\mu mol\cdot kg^{-1}$; infusion 0.05 $\mu mol\cdot kg^{-1}$ min^{-1}) of L-[*ring*-$^{13}C_6$] phenylalanine (Cambridge Isotopes Laboratories, Woburn, MA, USA) was then administered to the contralateral arm for the duration of the experiment. Under local anaesthesia (1% Xylocaine) a resting biopsy from the *vastus lateralis* of one leg was obtained 3 h after commencement of the tracer infusion using a 5-mm Bergstrom needle modified with suction, during the first trial only. This procedure was undertaken once during subjects first experimental trial to obtain resting fractional synthetic rates using the previously validated single biopsy method [23]. During subsequent trials tracer infusion commenced 1 h prior to the

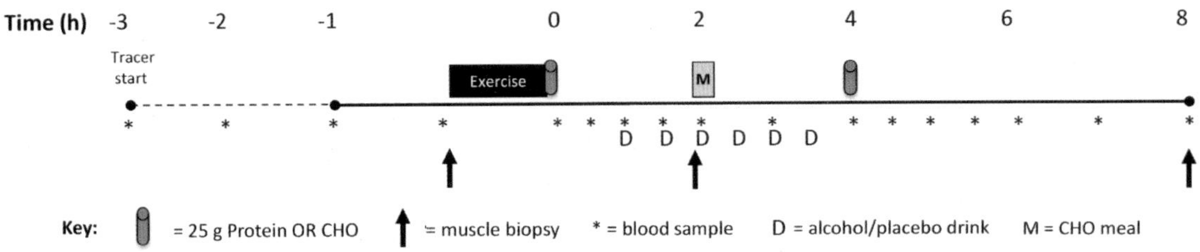

Figure 1. Schematic representation of the experimental trial. Subjects reported to the laboratory after an overnight fast where a constant infusion of L-[ring-$^{13}C_6$] phenylalanine was commenced (3 h in first trial; 1 h in trial 2/3), and subjects completed the concurrent exercise (8×5 repetitions at 80% one repetition maximum (1RM), 5 min rest, 30 min cycling at ~63% peak power output (PPO), 2 min rest, 10×30 s high intensity intervals at ~110% PPO). Immediately after exercise completion, and 4 h later, subjects consumed 500-mL of protein (25 g whey) or carbohydrate (25 g maltodextrin).

exercise protocol. The exercise bout incorporated the concurrent stimuli of resistance, continuous and intermittent high-intensity exercise to represent the key features of team sport activities. The specific protocol involved a standardized warm-up (5 repetitions at 50% and 5 repetitions at 60% 1RM) on a leg extension machine before the resistance exercise protocol was commenced. Resistance exercise consisted of eight sets of five repetitions at ~80% of 1RM. Each set was separated by a 3-min recovery period during which the subject remained seated. After completion of the final set, subjects rested for 5 min before commencing 30 min of continuous cycling at ~63% PPO (~70% VO_{2peak}). Upon completion, subjects rested on the bike for 2 min before undertaking 10×30 s high intensity intervals at ~110% of PPO, with 30 s active recovery (~50% PPO) between each work bout.

Immediately following exercise and after 4 h recovery, subjects ingested a 500 mL solution of either protein (PRO, 25 g whey protein powder; ISO8, Musashi, Melbourne, VIC Australia) or an energy-match in the form of CHO (25 g maltodextrin, International Health Investments, Helensvale, QLD Australia). Furthermore, a CHO-based meal (1.5 g·kg^{-1} BM) was consumed ~2 h post-exercise, immediately after the muscle biopsy, according to recommendations for post-exercise glycogen recovery [24]. Protein beverages included L-(*ring*-$^{13}C_6$] phenylalanine at 4% to prevent marked disturbance in isotopic enrichment and to maintain steady state enrichment. Blood (~4 mL) was collected immediately post-exercise and at regular intervals (30–60 min) throughout an 8 h recovery period, with additional muscle biopsies from separate incisions taken at 2 and 8 h post-exercise. Samples were stored at −80°C until analysis. The 8 h time frame represents an important phase of post-exercise recovery [1] as well as the period during which blood alcohol concentrations are likely to be elevated by a post-event drinking binge [14]. The alcohol dose in the present study represented the mean intake of alcohol reported by team athletes during a drinking binge [9,10] and an amount previously investigated in relation to post-exercise refuelling [14]. The alcohol ingestion protocol (1.5 g·kg^{-1} BM; 12±2 standard drinks) began 1 h post-exercise and was consumed in 6 equal volumes of 1 part vodka (~60 mL) to four parts orange juice (~240 mL, 1.8 g CHO·kg^{-1} BM) during a 3 h period. For the PRO condition, orange juice was consumed with a matched volume of water in place of the alcohol. Subjects ingested the beverages within 5 min every 30 min.

Analytical Procedures

Blood glucose and plasma ethanol concentrations. Whole blood samples (~25 µL) were immediately analysed for glucose concentrations using an automated analyser (YSI 2300, Yellow Springs, OH, USA). Blood samples were then centrifuged at 3,000 *g* at 4°C for 10 min, with aliquots of plasma frozen and stored at −80°C. On a separate occasion, plasma samples (~25 µL) were thawed and analysed for ethanol concentration using an automated analyser (YSI 2900, Yellow Springs, OH, USA).

Plasma amino acids and enrichment. Plasma amino acid concentrations and enrichments were analyzed by gas chromatography-isotope ratio mass spectrometry (MAT252; Finnigan, Breman, Germany) using EZ:faast kit (Phenomenex, CA, USA).

Rates of Myofibrillar Protein Synthesis. A single pre-infusion plasma sample, extracted by acetonitrile, was utilized as the baseline enrichment in tracer naïve subjects [23]. For the one non-tracer naïve subject a pre-infusion muscle biopsy was used for baseline enrichment. Muscle tissue was processed as previously described [7].

Calculations. The fractional synthetic rate (FSR) of myofibrillar protein synthesis was calculated using the standard precursor–product method:

$$FSR(\%{\cdot}h^{-1}) = [(E2_b - E1_b)/(E_{IC} \times t)] \times 100$$

Where $E2_b$ - $E1_b$ represents the change in the bound protein enrichment between two biopsy samples; E_{IC} is the average enrichment of intracellular phenylalanine between the two biopsy samples; and *t* is the time between two sequential biopsies. The inclusion of 'tracer-naive' subjects permitted use of the pre-infusion blood sample (i.e. single biopsy method) as the baseline enrichment ($E1_b$) for the calculation of resting MPS.

Western Blots. Intracellular signaling proteins were extracted, isolated and quantified as previously described [25]. The amount of protein loaded in each well was 50 µg. Polyclonal anti-phospho mechanistic target of rapamycin (mTOR) Ser2448 (no. 2971), elongation factor 2 (eEF2) Thr56 (no. 2331), 4E-BP1 Thr37/46 (no. 2855), monoclonal anti- 5′ adenosine monophosphate-activated protein kinase (AMPK) α Thr172 (no. 2535) and p70S6K Thr389 (no. 9234) were from Cell Signalling Technology (Danvers, USA). Data represent the volume and intensity quantified via densitometry and phosphorylation data and are expressed relative to α-tubulin reference protein expression at the equivalent time point on the same membrane (no. 3873, Cell Signalling Technology, Danvers, USA) in arbitrary units. All samples for each subject were run on the same gel.

Real Time PCR. Skeletal muscle (~20 mg) tissue RNA extraction, reverse transcription and real-time polymerase chain reaction (RT-PCR) was performed as previously described [25]. TaqMan-FAM labeled primer/probes (Applied Biosystems, Carlsbad, CA, USA) for muscle ring finger 1 (MuRF-1) (Cat

No. Hs00261590) and Atrogin (Cat No. Hs01041408) were used in a final reaction volume of 20 µL. Glyceraldehyde- 3-phosphate dehydrogenase (GAPDH, HS9999- 9905_m1) was used as the housekeeping gene. The relative amounts of mRNAs were calculated using the relative quantification (ΔΔCT) method [26].

Statistical Analysis

Blood, cell signaling and mRNA data were analyzed by two-way ANOVA (two factor: time × treatment) with repeated measures and myofibrillar protein synthesis was analyzed by one-way ANOVA with repeated measures. All data underwent Student-Newman-Keuls post hoc analysis when $P<0.05$ (Sigma-Plot for Windows; Version 12.5). All data are expressed as mean ± SD and the level of statistical significance was set at $P<0.05$.

Results

Blood Alcohol and Glucose Concentration

There were main effects for time and treatment for blood alcohol concentration ($P<0.05$; Figure 2). Blood alcohol concentration peaked 4 h post-exercise (ALC-CHO 0.059± 0.017 g·100 mL^{-1}; ALC-PRO 0.056±0.019 g·100 mL^{-1}) and remained elevated above rest throughout the 8 h recovery period (ALC-CHO: 0.023–0.059 g·100 mL^{-1}; ALC-PRO: 0.029–0.056 g·100 mL^{-1}; $P<0.05$). Blood alcohol concentration was higher ($P<0.05$) with ALC-CHO compared with ALC-PRO at 6 h (ALC-CHO: 0.055 g·100 mL^{-1}; ALC-PRO: 0.047 g·100 mL^{-1}) and 8 h (ALC-CHO: 0.043 g·100 mL^{-1}; ALC-PRO: 0.033 g·100 mL^{-1}) post-exercise. Blood glucose concentration increased above all time-points at 0.5 h (~17–41%) and 4.5 h (~16–40%) in the ALC-CHO treatment ($P<0.05$; Figure 3) but was not different from resting in ALC-PRO and PRO treatments. The blood glucose concentration measured in the ALC-CHO treatment was also different from ALC-PRO (~27–41%) and PRO (~26–42%) at 0.5, 1, 4.5 and 5 h post-exercise ($P<0.05$).

Plasma Amino Acids Concentration

There were main effects for time and treatment for plasma EAA, BCAA and leucine concentrations ($P<0.05$; Figure 4). Protein intake increased AA concentration at 1 h post-exercise: AA concentrations for ALC-PRO (EAA ~109%, BCAA ~118%, leucine ~203%) and PRO (EAA ~151%; BCAA ~170%; leucine

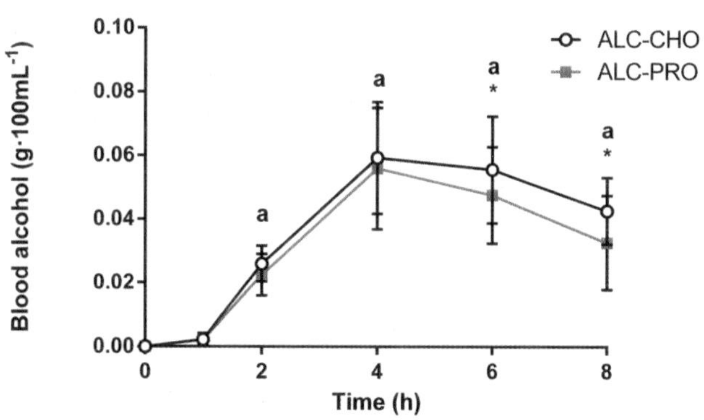

Figure 2. Blood alcohol levels after alcohol intake during recovery following a single bout of concurrent training. Data were analysed using a 2-way ANOVA with repeated measures and Student-Newman-Keuls post hoc analysis. Values are mean ± SD. Significant effect of treatment ($P=0.02$), time ($P<0.01$) with no interaction ($P=0.20$). Significantly different ($P<0.05$) vs. (a) rest, and (*) between treatments (ALC-CHO vs. ALC-PRO).

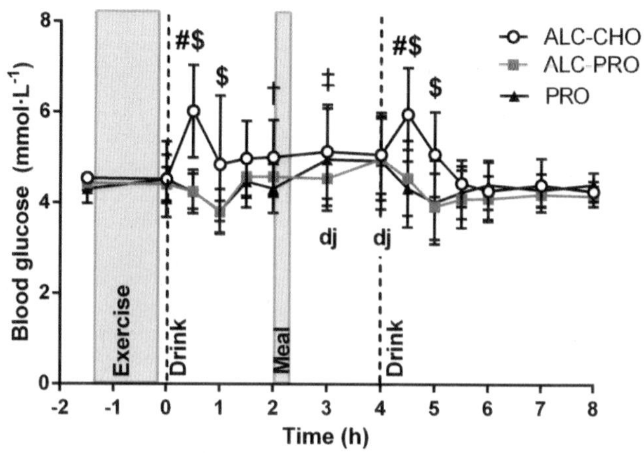

Figure 3. Blood glucose concentrations before and duringrecovery following a single bout of concurrent training. Drink = 25 g of whey protein (PRO and ALC-PRO) or 25 g maltodextrin (ALC-CHO); Meal = 1.5 g·kg^{-1} BM. Data were analysed using a 2-way ANOVA with repeated measures and Student-Newman-Keuls post hoc analysis. Values are mean ± SD. Significant effect of treatment, time and interaction (all $P<0.01$). Significantly different ($P<0.05$) (d) from 1 h within treatment, (j) from 5 h within treatment, ($) between treatments (ALC-CHO vs. ALC-PRO, PRO). (†) between treatments (ALC-CHO vs. PRO), (‡) between treatments (ALC-CHO vs. ALC-PRO).

~274%) treatments were different to all other time-points within treatments ($P<0.05$). Post-exercise concentrations of EAA and leucine with PRO were elevated above resting values at 1 h (~39%), 2 h (~98%) and 6 h (~61%) time-points, respectively ($P<0.05$). Leucine concentration remained above resting values 2 h (~90%) and 6 h (~102%) post-exercise, and EAA and BCAA were also higher than rest after 6 h recovery (EAA ~77%; BCAA ~38%) in the ALC-PRO treatment ($P<0.05$). Compared to ALC-CHO treatments, AA concentration were higher for ALC-PRO and PRO at 1 h (ALC-PRO: ~115–305%, PRO: ~163–394%), 2 h (~56–168%, ~83–179%) and 6 h (~81–253%, ~75–181%) post-exercise time-points ($P<0.05$). There were no changes in AA concentration in the ALC-CHO treatment.

Intracellular and Plasma Tracer Enrichments

Phenylalanine enrichments showed a stable precursor pool throughout the infusion period in all groups (Figure S1). Linear regression analysis indicated that the intracellular (mean $r^2=0.08$) and plasma (mean $r^2=0.03$) enrichments in ALC-CHO, ALC-PRO and PRO treatments demonstrated isotopic plateau.

Cell Signaling

mTOR-p70S6K. There were main effects for time and treatment for mTOR^{Ser2448} phosphorylation ($P<0.05$, Figure 5A). mTOR phosphorylation increased above rest at 2 h ($P<0.05$) for all treatments (ALC-CHO: ~125%, ALC-PRO: ~157%, PRO: ~297%) and at 8 h ($P<0.05$) for ALC-CHO (~111%) and ALC-PRO (~127%). mTOR phosphorylation with PRO was higher ($P<0.05$) than ALC-CHO (~76%) and ALC-PRO (~54%) at 2 and 8 h post-exercise, and PRO at 8 h post-exercise (~168%).

There were main effects for time and treatment for p70S6K^{Thr389} phosphorylation ($P<0.05$, Figure 5B). p70S6K phosphorylation was greater at 2 h ($P<0.05$) compared to rest and 8 h post–exercise in ALC-PRO (~418–585%) and PRO only (~438–468%). p70S6K phosphorylation was also higher at 2 h

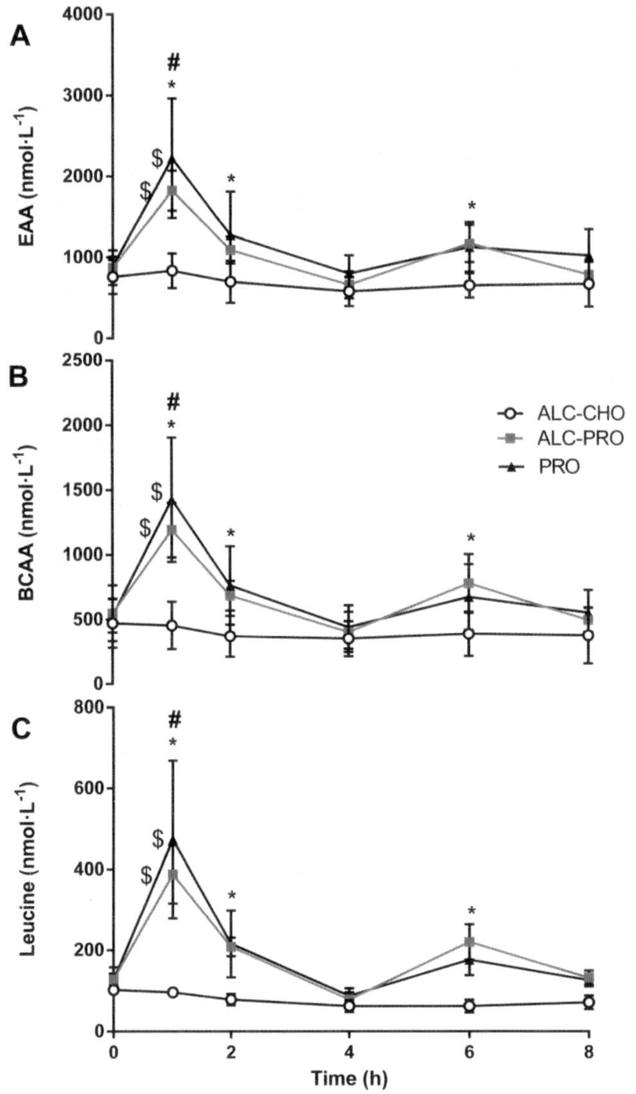

Figure 4. Plasma EAA (A), BCAA (B), leucine (C) concentration following a single bout of concurrent training. EAA – essential amino acids; BCAA – branched-chain amino acids. Data were analysed using a 2-way ANOVA with repeated measures and Student-Newman-Keuls post hoc analysis. Values are mean ± SD. Significant effect of treatment, time and interaction (all P<0.01) for (A), (B), and (C). Significantly different (P<0.05) vs. (#) all timepoints for ALC-CHO and ALC-PRO treatments, (*) vs. rest within treatments, and ($) compared to ALC-CHO.

post-exercise in PRO (~276%) and ALC-PRO (~242%) treatments compared to ALC-CHO treatment (P<0.05).

eEF2-4E-BP1-AMPK. There were decreases in eEF2 phosphorylation (Figure 5C) below rest at 2 h and 8 h post-exercise in ALC-CHO (~66–74%; P<0.05) and ALC-PRO (~61–67%; P< 0.05). No changes in 4E-BP1$^{Thr37/46}$ (Figure 5D) or AMPK^{Thr172} phosphorylation [data not shown] were observed across treatments or times.

Atrogene mRNA expression

There were increases above rest in MuRF-1 mRNA (Figure 6A, P<0.05) at 2 h for all treatments (ALC-CHO: ~404%; ALC-PRO: ~399%; PRO: ~474%). However, there were no differences between treatments, and MuRF1 mRNA returned to resting levels under all conditions after 8 h (P<0.05). There was a main effect for time for atrogin-1 abundance (P<0.05, Figure 6B). Atrogin-1 mRNA expression at 8 h decreased below rest (~37–52%; P<0.05) and 2 h (~46–61%; P<0.05) with all treatments.

Rates of muscle protein synthesis

Rates of myofibrillar FSR were increased above rest (0.025±0.002%·h^{-1}) with ALC-CHO (0.032±0.005%·h^{-1}, ~29%), ALC-PRO (0.039±0.008% h^{-1}, ~57%) and PRO (0.052±0.008%·h^{-1}, ~109%) treatments throughout 2–8 h of recovery (P<0.05; Figure 7). However, compared to PRO alone, there was a hierarchical reduction in myofibrillar FSR with ALC-PRO (24%, P<0.05) and ALC-CHO (37%, P<0.05). ALC-CHO resulted in a lower FSR compared to ALC-PRO (~18%, P<0.05).

Discussion

The first novel finding of this study was that mTOR signaling and rates of myofibrillar protein synthesis (MPS) following concurrent resistance, continuous and intermittent high-intensity exercise, designed to mimic the metabolic profile of many team sports, were impaired during the early (8 h) recovery phase by the ingestion of large amounts (1.5 g•kg^{-1} BM) of alcohol. These outcomes were most evident (37% reduction in rates of MPS) when alcohol was consumed in the absence of post-exercise protein intake, as is likely to occur when intoxication reduces the athlete's compliance to sound recovery practices. However, a second finding was that even when protein was consumed in amounts shown to be optimally effective to stimulate MPS [8] during post-exercise recovery, the intake of alcohol reduced MPS by ~24%, representing only a partial 'rescue' of the anabolic response compared with protein alone.

The alcohol consumption protocol used in the current study, representing the mean intake of alcohol that has been self-reported in several studies of binge drinking practices of team athletes [9,10], elicited blood alcohol concentrations that exceeded the 0.05 g·100 mL^{-1} legal limit for driving in Australia (Figure 1). Although peak post-exercise blood alcohol values were lower than we have previously reported [14], such differences can, in part, be explained by different alcohol ingestion protocols and feeding regimens. The subtle differences in blood alcohol concentration were likely a result of the different macronutrient composition consumed and the aminoacidemia in PRO and ALC-PRO was similar and significantly different to that seen with the carbohydrate treatment (Figure 4).

Despite alcohol having little effect on blood amino acid profiles, myofibrillar FSR was significantly different between treatments (Figure 7). The maximal FSR was measured when protein was the only nutrient ingested, and is similar to other studies incorporating resistance-type exercise with protein feeding [25,27]. However, this study is the first to have measured FSR after consecutive bouts of resistance, continuous and high-intensity exercise when alcohol was consumed during recovery. While several studies examining the effects of alcohol intake have been undertaken in rodents, the relative quantity of alcohol administered in these investigations is several fold higher than in the current human study [18,21,28–30]. Furthermore, there are differences in techniques used to measure rates of protein synthesis in animals versus humans. Notwithstanding these differences, Lang et al. [28] reported a 25% decrease in rates of muscle protein synthesis with alcohol administration in rodents, a value in close agreement with the current study. Our results show alcohol ingestion in humans suppresses the elevated rates of protein synthesis in skeletal muscle induced by exercise and protein ingestion.

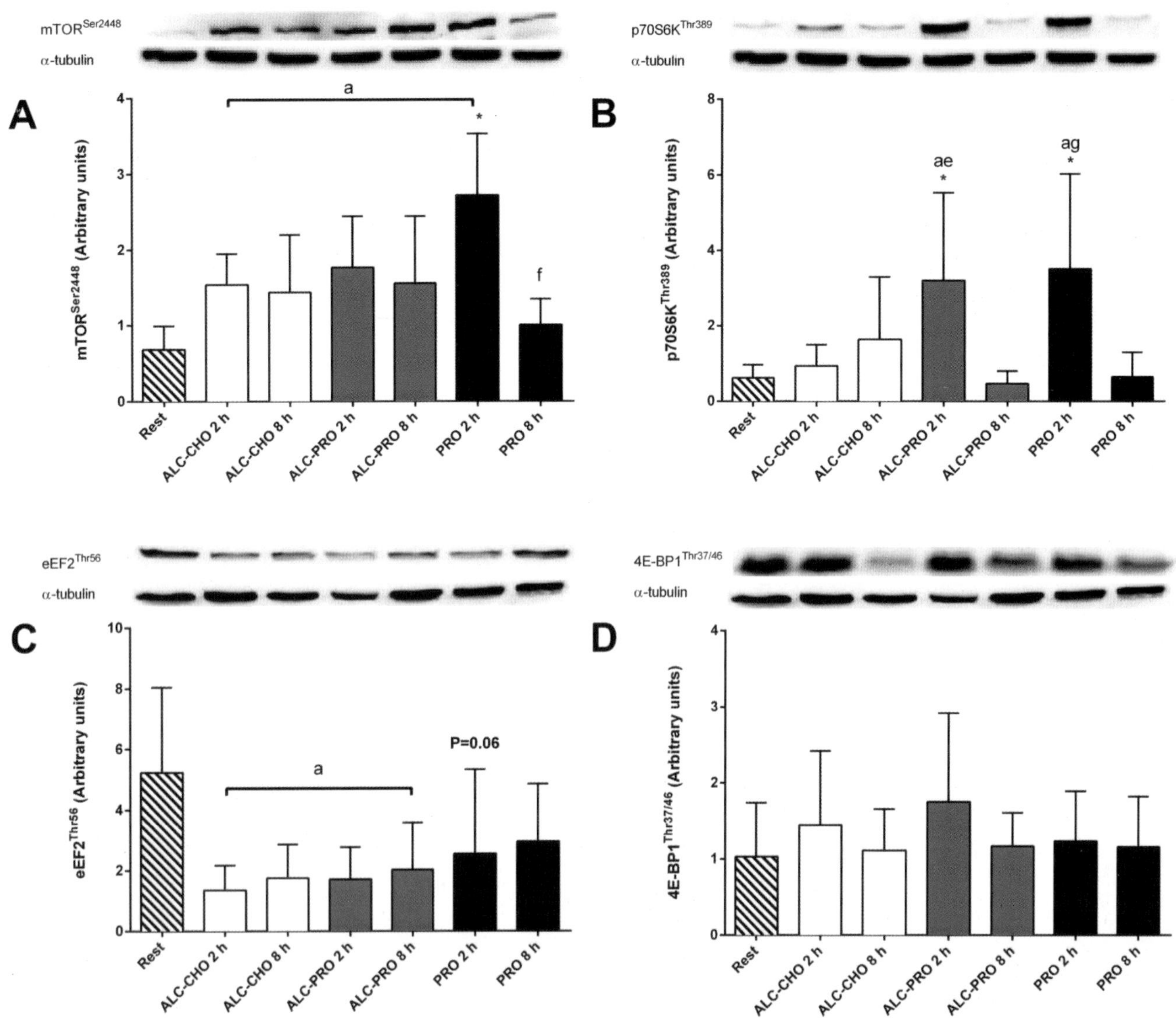

Figure 5. mTOR^{Ser2448} (A), p70S6K^{Thr389} (B), eEF2^{Thr56} (C), 4E-BP1$^{Thr37/46}$ (D) phosphorylation at rest and following a single bout of concurrent training. Images are representative blots for each protein from the same subject and values are expressed relative to α-tubulin and presented in arbitary units. Data were analysed using a 2-way ANOVA with repeated measures with Student-Newman-Keuls post hoc analysis. Values are mean ± SD. Significant effect of time ($P<0.01$) and interaction ($P=0.02$) but not treatment ($P=0.22$) for (A); time ($P<0.01$) and interaction ($P=0.02$) but not treatment ($P=0.46$) for (B); time ($P<0.01$) but not treatment ($P=0.14$) or interaction ($P=0.56$) for (C); no treatment ($P=0.86$), time ($P=0.24$), or interaction ($P=0.77$) effects for (D). Significantly different ($P<0.05$) vs. (a) rest, (e) ACL-PRO 8 h, (f) PRO 2 h, (g) PRO 8 h, and (*) 2 h between treatments.

The mechanistic target of rapamycin complex 1 (mTORC1) is a central node for integrating nutrient (i.e. amino acid) and exercise/contraction signal transduction [31,32]. Post-exercise phosphorylation of mTOR^{Ser2448} was attenuated when alcohol was co-ingested with either carbohydrate or protein compared to protein ingestion alone. Interestingly, there was discordance in phosphorylation responses between mTOR and its downstream signaling targets (p70S6K and 4E-BP1). The mechanism through which alcohol may attenuate mTOR complex 1 activity is still poorly defined. Recent evidence has implicated several upstream regulatory mechanisms of mTOR signaling including the Rag family of GTPases [33,34], phosphatidic acid [35] and the DNA damage response 2 (REDD2) protein [36]. The inhibitory effects of alcohol on mTOR phosphorylation in skeletal muscle have been attributed to increases in the mRNA/protein content of the negative mTOR regulator REDD1 with acute intoxication and that alcohol may also generate greater association of mTOR with raptor to down regulate mRNA translation [20,37]. Thus it is plausible that several mechanisms may act synergistically upstream of mTOR in response to alcohol ingestion to modulate mTOR activity. Nevertheless, our findings indicate that the observed alcohol-induced attenuation of MPS was likely mediated, at least in part, by effects on mTORC1-mediated signaling.

p70S6K enhances translation of mRNAs encoding ribosomal proteins and elongation factors [38] and has been proposed as a 'surrogate' marker associated with rates of muscle protein synthesis [39–42]. Lang and co-workers have previously shown reduced p70S6K signaling following alcohol ingestion in rat skeletal muscle [18,29]. We present new information in human skeletal muscle to demonstrate the exercise and nutrient-induced increase in

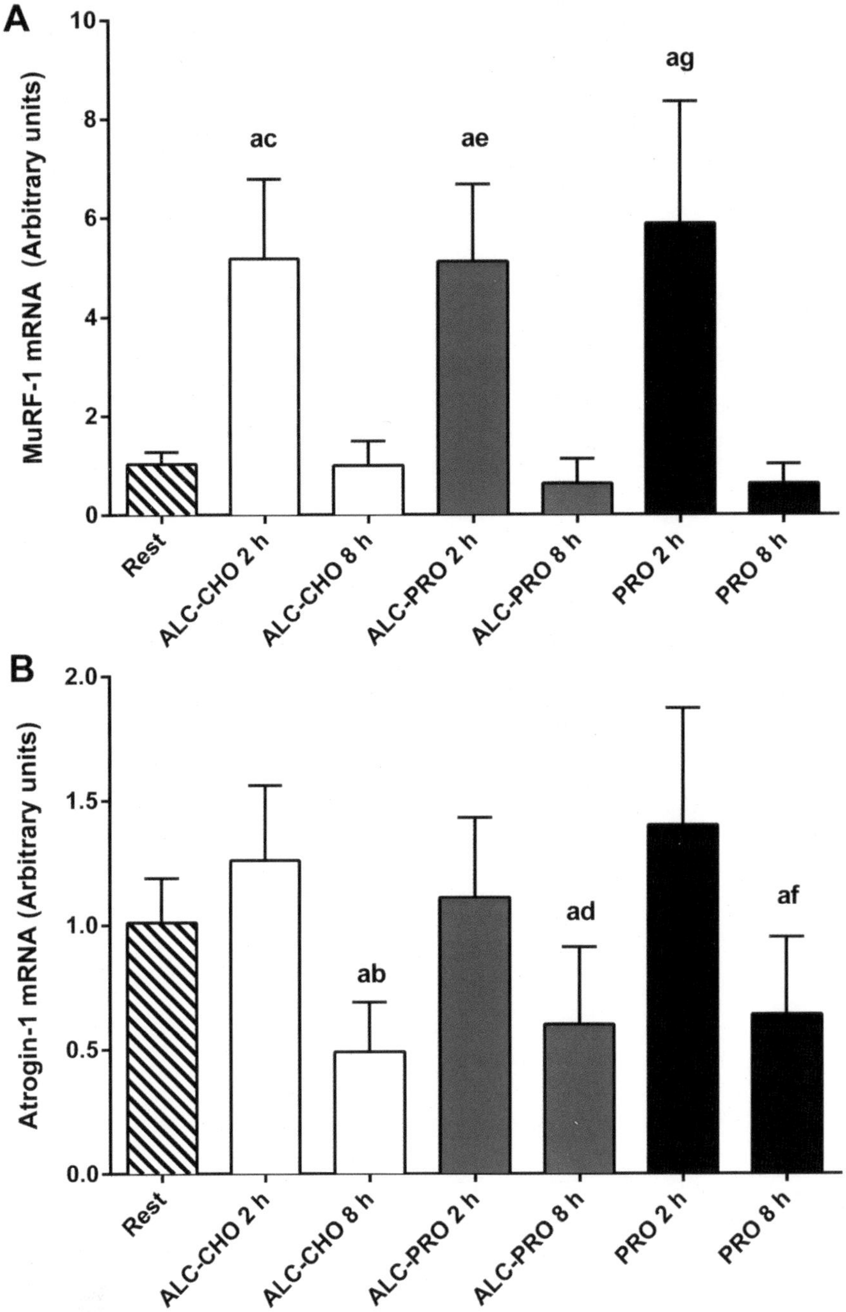

Figure 6. MuRF-1 (A), Atrogin-1 (B) mRNA abundance at rest and following a single bout of concurrent training. Values are expressed relative to GAPDH and presented in arbitrary units (mean ± SD, n = 7). Data were analysed using a 2-way repeated measures ANOVA with Student-Newman-Keuls post hoc analysis. Significantly different ($P<0.05$) vs. (a) rest, (c,e,g) 8 h within treatments, and (b,d,f) 2 h within treatments.

p70S6K phosphorylation is significantly reduced with alcohol ingestion in the absence of the co-ingestion of protein. The discordant mTOR-p70S6K phosphorylation with protein only and protein feedings with alcohol is not unprecedented given we [8] and others [43] have shown that mTOR-S6K phosphorylation often parallels changes in MPS but does not always reflect either the magnitude or duration of the increased MPS signal in humans. An alternate mechanism through which alcohol may limit rates of protein synthesis is endoplasmic reticulum stress and the resultant unfolded protein response. Alcohol consumption generates oxidative stress and inflammation and the potential to disrupt endoplasmic reticulum homeostasis; a consequence of this response is to limit the rate of protein synthesis [44,45]. The lack of change in 4E-BP1$^{Thr37/46}$ phosphorylation following exercise and between treatments contrasts previous findings in rodents [18,20,28]. However, these differences may, in part, be explained by the 2.3 fold greater relative alcohol administration in rodents versus humans. Finally, it must be acknowledged that our data are potentially limited by providing only a single 'snapshot' during recovery and the possibility exists that our muscle biopsy time-points failed to coincide with peak phosphorylation responses of signal transduction. To the best of our knowledge, this is the first

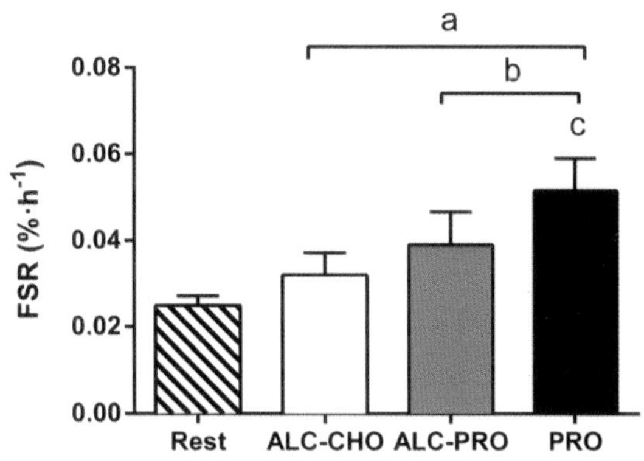

Figure 7. Myofibrillar fractional synthetic rate (FSR) throughout 2–8 h recovery following a single bout of concurrent training. Data were analysed using a 1-way repeated measures ANOVA with Student-Newman-Keuls *post hoc* analysis. Values are mean ± SD expressed as % h^{-1}, n = 8. Significantly different (P<0.05) vs. (a) rest, (b) ALC-CHO, (c) ALC-PRO.

study to investigate the effect of alcohol ingestion following concurrent resistance, continuous and intermittent high-intensity exercise in human skeletal and further studies are needed to better understand the precise mechanisms through which alcohol attenuates human skeletal muscle protein synthesis.

In contrast with the changes in cell signaling, muscle mRNA responses of selected genes associated with muscle proteolysis and catabolism were largely unchanged between treatments. MuRF-1 mRNA expression was elevated 2 h following exercise but had returned to basal levels, by 8 h in all treatments. Whereas, atrogin-1 mRNA expression did not change 2 h following exercise and was significantly lower than rest and 2 h post-exercise at 8 h post-exercise in all treatments. These results contrast findings by Vary and colleagues [30] who found alcohol ingestion to increase MuRF-1 and Atrogin-1 mRNA abundance in rat skeletal muscle. Our data shows protein co-ingested with alcohol following exercise induces comparable increases in atrogene mRNA expression compared to protein ingestion alone in human skeletal muscle. These increases are in agreement with previous findings demonstrating increased atrogene mRNA expression following resistance exercise [46,47]. Although we did not determine rates of muscle protein breakdown, this process is up-regulated in mixed muscle for up to 24 h after resistance exercise in the fasted state [48]. As muscle damaging exercise has previously been reported to decrease GLUT4 translocation and subsequent rates of muscle glycogen resynthesis [49], the possibility that it also may impart a negative effect on protein transporters and rates of protein synthesis cannot be discounted. However, the atrogene results of the current study indicate alcohol ingestion does not exert any additional effects on ubiquitin ligase expression after exercise in human skeletal muscle. Future studies investigating the time course of atrogene expression and direct measures of skeletal muscle proteasome activity and/or protein breakdown following alcohol ingestion in humans are warranted.

In conclusion, the current data provide the novel observation that alcohol impairs the response of MPS in exercise recovery in human skeletal muscle despite optimal nutrient provision. The quantity of alcohol consumed in the current study was based on amounts reported during binge drinking by athletes. However, published reports suggest intakes of some individuals can be significantly greater [9,50], which is of concern for many reasons related to health and safety [13]. Regrettably, there has been difficulty in finding an educational message with alcohol consumption related to sports performance that has resonance with athletes. Given the need to promote protein synthesis that underpins adaptation, repair and regeneration of skeletal muscle the results of the current study provide clear evidence of impaired recovery when alcohol is consumed after concurrent (resistance, continuous and intermittent high-intensity) exercise even in the presence of optimal nutritional conditions. We propose our data is of paramount interest to athletes and coaches. Our findings provide an evidence-base for a message of moderation in alcohol intake to promote recovery after exercise with the potential to alter current sports culture and athlete practices.

Acknowledgments

The authors wish to thank Mr. Stephen Lane, Mr. Joshua Whittaker, Mr. Jong-Sam Lee, Mr. William Manly, and Ms. Eliza Leverett for assistance with experimental trials; Ms. Tracey Rerecich and Mr. Todd Prior for their technical expertise; and the subjects for their time and effort.

Author Contributions

Conceived and designed the experiments: EBP LMB SMP JAH VGC. Performed the experiments: EBP DMC JLA VGC. Analyzed the data: EBP DMC JLA SMP JAH VGC. Contributed reagents/materials/analysis tools: LMB SMP JAH VGC. Wrote the paper: EBP DMC JLA LMB SMP JAH VGC.

References

1. Hawley JA, Burke LM, Phillips SM, Spriet LL (2011) Nutritional modulation of training-induced skeletal muscle adaptations. J Appl Physiol 110: 834–845.
2. Phillips SM (2006) Dietary protein for athletes: from requirements to metabolic advantage. Appl Physiol Nutr Metab 31: 647–654.
3. Stellingwerff T, Maughan RJ, Burke LM (2011) Nutrition for power sports: middle-distance running, track cycling, rowing, canoeing/kayaking, and swimming. J Sports Sci 29: S79–S89.
4. Coffey VG, Jemiolo B, Edge J, Garnham AP, Trappe SW, et al. (2009) Effect of consecutive repeated sprint and resistance exercise bouts on acute adaptive responses in human skeletal muscle. Am J Physiol Regul Integr Comp Physiol 297: R1441–1451.
5. Coffey VG, Moore DR, Burd NA, Rerecich T, Stellingwerff T, et al. (2011) Nutrient provision increases signalling and protein synthesis in human skeletal muscle after repeated sprints. Eur J Appl Physiol 111: 1473–1483.
6. Koopman R, Saris W, Wagenmakers A, van Loon L (2007) Nutritional interventions to promote post-exercise muscle protein synthesis. Sports Med 37: 895–906.
7. Moore DR, Tang JE, Burd NA, Rerecich T, Tarnopolsky MA, et al. (2009) Differential stimulation of myofibrillar and sarcoplasmic protein synthesis with protein ingestion at rest and after resistance exercise. J Physiol 587: 897–904.
8. Areta JL, Burke LM, Ross ML, Camera DM, West DW, et al. (2013) Timing and distribution of protein ingestion during prolonged recovery from resistance exercise alters myofibrillar protein synthesis. J Physiol 591: 2319–2331.
9. Burke L, Read R (1988) A study of dietary patterns of elite Australian football players. Can J Sport Sci 13: 15–19.
10. O'Brien CP (1993) Alcohol and Sport: Impact of social drinking on recreational and competitive sports performance. Sports Med 15: 71–77.
11. Watten R (1995) Sports, physical exercise and use of alcohol. Scand J Med Sci Sports 5: 364–368.
12. Martens MP, Dams-O'Connor K, Beck NC (2006) A systematic review of college student-athlete drinking: Prevalence rates, sport-related factors, and interventions. J Subst Abuse Treat 31: 305–316.

13. O'Brien KS, Ali A, Cotter JD, O'Shea RP, Stannard S (2007) Hazardous drinking in New Zealand sportspeople: level of sporting participation and drinking motives. Alcohol Alcohol 42: 376–382.
14. Burke LM, Collier GR, Broad EM, Davis PG, Martin DT, et al. (2003) Effect of alcohol intake on muscle glycogen storage after prolonged exercise. J Appl Physiol 95: 983–990.
15. Barnes MJ, Mündel T, Stannard SR (2010) Post-exercise alcohol ingestion exacerbates eccentric-exercise induced losses in performance. Eur J Appl Physiol 108: 1009–1014.
16. Barnes MJ, Mündel T, Stannard SR (2011) A low dose of alcohol does not impact skeletal muscle performance after exercise-induced muscle damage. Eur J Appl Physiol 111: 725–729.
17. Kumar V, Frost RA, Lang CH (2002) Alcohol impairs insulin and IGF-I stimulation of S6K1 but not 4E-BP1 in skeletal muscle. Am J Physiol Endocrinol Metab 283: E917–E928.
18. Lang CH, Frost RA, Deshpande N, Kumar V, Vary TC, et al. (2003) Alcohol impairs leucine-mediated phosphorylation of 4E-BP1, S6K1, eIF4G, and mTOR in skeletal muscle. Am J Physiol Endocrinol Metab 285: E1205–E1215.
19. Lang CH, Frost RA, Svanberg E, Vary TC (2004) IGF-I/IGFBP-3 ameliorates alterations in protein synthesis, eIF4E availability, and myostatin in alcohol-fed rats. Am J Physiol Endocrinol Metab 286: E916–E926.
20. Lang CH, Frost RA, Vary TC (2008) Acute alcohol intoxication increases REDD1 in skeletal muscle. Alcohol Clin Exp Res 32: 796–805.
21. Lang CH, Wu D, Frost RA, Jefferson LS, Kimball SR, et al. (1999) Inhibition of muscle protein synthesis by alcohol is associated with modulation of eIF2B and eIF4E. Am J Physiol Endocrinol Metab 277: E268–E276.
22. Hawley JA, Noakes TD (1992) Peak power output predicts maximal oxygen uptake and performance time in trained cyclists. Eur J Appl Physiol Occup Physiol 65: 79–83.
23. Burd NA, Groen BB, Beelen M, Senden JM, Gijsen AP, et al. (2012) The reliability of using the single-biopsy approach to assess basal muscle protein synthesis rates in vivo in humans. Metabolism 61: 931–936.
24. Burke LM, Hawley JA, Wong SH, Jeukendrup AE (2011) Carbohydrates for training and competition. J Sports Sci 29: S17–S27.
25. Camera D, West D, Burd N, Phillips S, Garnham A, et al. (2012) Low muscle glycogen concentration does not suppress the anabolic response to resistance exercise. J Appl Physiol 113: 206–214.
26. Livak KJ, Schmittgen TD (2001) Analysis of relative gene expression data using real-time quantitative PCR and the 2(-Delta Delta C(T)) Method. Methods 25: 402–408.
27. West D, Burd N, Coffey V, Baker S, Burke L, et al. (2011) Rapid aminoacidemia enhances myofibrillar protein synthesis and anabolic intramuscular signaling responses after resistance exercise. Am J Clin Nutr 94: 795–803.
28. Lang CH, Frost RA, Kumar V, Wu D, Vary TC (2000) Impaired protein synthesis induced by acute alcohol intoxication is associated with changes in eIF4E in muscle and eIF2B in liver. Alcohol Clin Exp Res 24: 322–331.
29. Lang CH, Pruznak AM, Deshpande N, Palopoli MM, Frost RA, et al. (2004) Alcohol intoxication impairs phosphorylation of S6K1 and S6 in skeletal muscle independently of ethanol metabolism. Alcohol Clin Exp Res 28: 1758–1767.
30. Vary TC, Frost RA, Lang CH (2008) Acute alcohol intoxication increases atrogin-1 and MuRF1 mRNA without increasing proteolysis in skeletal muscle. Am J Physiol Regul Integr Comp Physiol 294: R1777–R1789.
31. Dreyer HC, Drummond MJ, Pennings B, Fujita S, Glynn EL, et al. (2008) Leucine-enriched essential amino acid and carbohydrate ingestion following resistance exercise enhances mTOR signaling and protein synthesis in human muscle. Am J Physiol Endocrinol Metab 294: E392–E400.
32. Zoncu R, Bar-Peled L, Efeyan A, Wang S, Sancak Y, et al. (2011) mTORC1 senses lysosomal amino acids through an inside-out mechanism that requires the vacuolar H+-ATPase. Science 334: 678–683.
33. Kim E, Goraksha-Hicks P, Li L, Neufeld TP, Guan KL (2008) Regulation of TORC1 by Rag GTPases in nutrient response. Nature cell biology 10: 935–945.
34. Sancak Y, Peterson TR, Shaul YD, Lindquist RA, Thoreen CC, et al. (2008) The Rag GTPases bind raptor and mediate amino acid signaling to mTORC1. Science 320: 1496–1501.
35. O'Neil TK, Duffy LR, Frey JW, Hornberger TA (2009) The role of phosphoinositide 3-kinase and phosphatidic acid in the regulation of mammalian target of rapamycin following eccentric contractions. J Physiol 587: 3691–3701.
36. Miyazaki M, Esser KA (2009) REDD2 is enriched in skeletal muscle and inhibits mTOR signaling in response to leucine and stretch. Am J Physiol Cell Physiol 296: C583–C592.
37. Lang CH, Pruznak AM, Nystrom GJ, Vary TC (2009) Alcohol-induced decrease in muscle protein synthesis associated with increased binding of mTOR and raptor: Comparable effects in young and mature rats. Nutr Metab (Lond) 6: 4.
38. Wang X, Beugnet A, Murakami M, Yamanaka S, Proud CG (2005) Distinct signaling events downstream of mTOR cooperate to mediate the effects of amino acids and insulin on initiation factor 4E-binding proteins. Mol Cell Biol 25: 2558–2572.
39. Baar K, Esser K (1999) Phosphorylation of p70S6k correlates with increased skeletal muscle mass following resistance exercise. Am J Physiol Cell Physiol 276: C120–C127.
40. Burd NA, Holwerda AM, Selby KC, West DW, Staples AW, et al. (2010) Resistance exercise volume affects myofibrillar protein synthesis and anabolic signalling molecule phosphorylation in young men. J Physiol 588: 3119–3130.
41. Fry CS, Drummond MJ, Glynn EL, Dickinson JM, Gundermann DM, et al. (2011) Aging impairs contraction-induced human skeletal muscle mTORC1 signaling and protein synthesis. Skelet Muscle 1: 11–11.
42. Kumar V, Selby A, Rankin D, Patel R, Atherton P, et al. (2009) Age-related differences in the dose–response relationship of muscle protein synthesis to resistance exercise in young and old men. J Physiol 587: 211–217.
43. Atherton PJ, Etheridge T, Watt PW, Wilkinson D, Selby A, et al. (2010) Muscle full effect after oral protein: time-dependent concordance and discordance between human muscle protein synthesis and mTORC1 signaling. Am J Clin Nutr 92: 1080–1088.
44. Deldicque L, Hespel P, Francaux M (2012) Endoplasmic Reticulum Stress in Skeletal Muscle: Origin and Metabolic Consequences. Exercise and Sport Sciences Reviews 40: 43–49.
45. Fernandez-Solà J, Preedy VR, Lang CH, Gonzalez-Reimers E, Arno M, et al. (2007) Molecular and Cellular Events in Alcohol-Induced Muscle Disease. Alcohol Clin Exp Res 31: 1953–1962.
46. Louis E, Raue U, Yang Y, Jemiolo B, Trappe S (2007) Time course of proteolytic, cytokine, and myostatin gene expression after acute exercise in human skeletal muscle. J Appl Physiol 103: 1744–1751.
47. Yang Y, Jemiolo B, Trappe S (2006) Proteolytic mRNA expression in response to acute resistance exercise in human single skeletal muscle fibers. J Appl Physiol 101: 1442–1450.
48. Phillips SM, Tipton KD, Aarsland A, Wolf SE, Wolfe RR (1997) Mixed muscle protein synthesis and breakdown after resistance exercise in humans. Am J Physiol Endocrinol Metab 273: E99–E107.
49. Asp S, Daugaard JR, Richter EA (1995) Eccentric exercise decreases glucose transporter GLUT4 protein in human skeletal muscle. J Physiol 482: 705–712.
50. O'Brien KS, Blackie JM, Hunter JA (2005) Hazardous drinking in elite New Zealand sportspeople. Alcohol Alcohol 40: 239–241.

6

Acute Post-Exercise Myofibrillar Protein Synthesis Is Not Correlated with Resistance Training-Induced Muscle Hypertrophy in Young Men

Cameron J. Mitchell[1], Tyler A. Churchward-Venne[1], Gianni Parise[1], Leeann Bellamy[1], Steven K. Baker[2], Kenneth Smith[3], Philip J. Atherton[3], Stuart M. Phillips[1]*

1 Exercise Metabolism Research Group, Department of Kinesiology, McMaster University, Hamilton, Ontario, Canada, **2** Department of Neurology, School of Medicine, McMaster University, Hamilton, Ontario, Canada, **3** Metabolic and Molecular Physiology Research Group, MRC-ARUK Centre of Excellence for Musculoskeletal Ageing Research, School of Graduate Entry Medicine and Health, Derby, United Kingdom

Abstract

Muscle hypertrophy following resistance training (RT) involves activation of myofibrillar protein synthesis (MPS) to expand the myofibrillar protein pool. The degree of hypertrophy following RT is, however, highly variable and thus we sought to determine the relationship between the acute activation of MPS and RT-induced hypertrophy. We measured MPS and signalling protein activation after the first session of resistance exercise (RE) in untrained men ($n = 23$) and then examined the relation between MPS with magnetic resonance image determined hypertrophy. To measure MPS, young men (24 ± 1 yr; body mass index $= 26.4 \pm 0.9$ kg•m^2) underwent a primed constant infusion of L-[ring-$^{13}C_6$] phenylalanine to measure MPS at rest, and acutely following their first bout of RE prior to 16 wk of RT. Rates of MPS were increased $235 \pm 38\%$ ($P < 0.001$) above rest 60–180 min post-exercise and $184 \pm 28\%$ ($P = 0.037$) 180–360 min post exercise. Quadriceps volume increased $7.9 \pm 1.6\%$ (-1.9–24.7%) ($P < 0.001$) after training. There was no correlation between changes in quadriceps muscle volume and acute rates of MPS measured over 1–3 h ($r = 0.02$), 3–6 h ($r = 0.16$) or the aggregate 1–6 h post-exercise period ($r = 0.10$). Hypertrophy after chronic RT was correlated ($r = 0.42$, $P = 0.05$) with phosphorylation of 4E-BP1$^{Thr37/46}$ at 1 hour post RE. We conclude that acute measures of MPS following an initial exposure to RE in novices are not correlated with muscle hypertrophy following chronic RT.

Editor: Michael Müller, University of East Anglia, United Kingdom

Funding: This work was supported by grants from the National Science and Engineering Research Council (NSERC) of Canada to SMP and GP. CJM and LB were supported by research fellowships from NSERC for this work. The funders had no role in study design, data collection and analysis, decision to publish, or preparation of the manuscript.

* E-mail: phillis@mcmaster.ca

Introduction

Skeletal muscle hypertrophy following resistance training (RT) requires the net addition of new myofibrillar proteins; thus, myofibrillar protein synthesis (MPS) must exceed myofibrillar protein breakdown (MPB). Using contraction-induced phosphorylation as a proxy for activation and activity, signalling pathway proteins in the Akt (PKB)-mTOR pathway have been measured in humans and some [1], but not all [2], have reported correlations between the phosphorylation state of certain proteins and hypertrophy. In larger samples, measures of protein phosphorylation in multiple signaling proteins are not related to the highly variable phenotypic hypertrophic response seen with RT [3]; however, we hypothesized that a stronger relationship would exist between MPS and hypertrophy.

Rates of MPS measured in the fed state have been used to evaluate the effect of exercise and nutritional interventions and their potential to induce muscle hypertrophy following RT [4,5]. Previous work from our lab has shown that responses of MPS measured after resistance exercise with ingestion of milk or soy protein [4] or carbohydrate (Tang et al., 2007) are in alignment with RT-induced muscle hypertrophy during RT program employing similar exercises and post-exercise nutrition in separate groups of subjects [6]. Similarly, we reported that the acute MPS response with: heavy and light-load fatiguing resistance exercise [7], and with differing volumes of resistance exercise [8] were in agreement muscle hypertrophy following 10 wk of RT in a different set of subjects [2]. Taken together, the congruence between acute MPS responses and chronic RT-induced hypertrophy would suggest that measures of acute post-exercise MPS may vary in a similar manner to, and thus be related to, muscle hypertrophy; however, such a possibility has not been tested.

There is a high degree of variability in the hypertrophic response to RT. Typical coefficients of variation of the hypertrophic response measured using muscle fibre size changes in young and old men and women can exceed 100% [2,3,6,9]. There have been attempts to explain this variability in hypertrophy using gene expression [3,10], satellite cell enumeration [9], measures of the hormonal response to exercise [11], and measurement of cell signaling proteins [1,12]. To date, however, there are no published studies addressing the relationship between acute measures of MPS and hypertrophy following RT in the same subjects. Both gene expression [3,10] and satellite cell content [9] have been shown related to hypertrophy in some instances whereas acute post-exercise systemic hormonal responses show no relationship to RT-induced hypertrophy. In humans, protein signaling has only been shown to relate weakly to hypertrophy [13] or in very small sample sizes [1] and is not consistently observed [2,12]. The purpose of this study was to determine if acute myofibrillar protein synthesis measured acutely in training-naïve subjects after their first bout of resistance exercise with protein consumption was related to muscle hypertrophy following 16 weeks of RT.

Methods

Ethics Statement

All participants were informed of the purpose of the study, the experimental procedures involved and all the potential risks involved before obtaining written consent. The protocol and consent form were approved by the Research Ethics Board of Hamilton Health Sciences and McMaster University and complied with all ethical standards for research involving human participants set by the Declaration of Helsinki and by the Canadian Tri-Council statement on ethics in human research (http://www.ethics.gc.ca/eng/policy-politique/initiatives/tcps2-eptc2/Default/).

Subjects

Twenty-three healthy young men (177±2 cm; 84.1±3.5 kg; body mass index =26.4±1.0 kg•m^{-2}; 24±1 yr, means ± SD) participated in the experiment. Subjects were recreationally active but had not engaged in RT within the last year.

Experimental Design

Participants underwent a magnetic resonance imaging (MRI) scan of their right thigh to determine muscle volume and a dual-energy x-ray absorptiometry (DXA) scan to assess whole body fat- and bone-free mass (lean mass). Subjects were then strength tested to determine their maximal isotonic strength, which is traditionally labelled as one repetition maximum (1RM) for all training exercises. At least 5 d following strength testing participants reported to the lab after a 10 h overnight fast for stable isotope infusion. Resting MPS was measured, subjects then completed four sets of 8 repetitions of leg press, leg extension, leg curl and calf press. They then ingested a protein rich beverage containing 30 g of milk protein, 25.9 g of carbohydrates and 3.4 g of fat (Musahi P30, Notting Hill, Australia). Muscle biopsies were then taken at 1, 3 and 6 hours post exercise to measure MPS. Subjects then completed 16 weeks of RT while ingesting the protein rich beverage immediately after their exercise session and with breakfast on non-training days, as previously described in [12] Briefly, participants trained four times weekly with two upper and two lower body workouts. Lower body exercises are described above in the acute exercise session. Upper body exercises consisted of chest press, shoulder press, seated row, lat pulldown, bicep curl and tricep extension. The program was progressive in linear manner moving from 3 sets of 12 repetitions to 4 sets of 6 repetitions. At the end of the training period, MRI, DXA scans, and strength testing were repeated.

Infusion Protocol

On the trial day, participants reported to the lab after an overnight fast having refrained from any strenuous physical activity for at least 3 days. A 20-gauge plastic catheter was inserted into an antecubital vein and a baseline blood sample was obtained. Following the start of a primed constant infusion ofL-[*ring*-$^{13}C_6$] phenylalanine (prime: 2 μmol kg^{-1}; infusion: 0.05 μmol kg^{-1} min^{-1}), participants rested for 3 h before a muscle biopsy was obtained to determine the resting (basal) rate of MPS. Subjects then completed the lower body exercise protocol described above and ingested a protein rich beverage (described above). They then rested in bed for the next 6 h while biopsies (*vastus lateralis*) were taken 1, 3 and 6 h after cessation of the exercise bout.

The drink containing 30 g of milk-based protein was enriched to 6% of the protein phenylalanine content with free [$^{13}C_6$] phenylalanine tracer to minimize disruptions in isotopic steady state, which is an approach we have used numerous times before with good maintenance of isotopic steady-state [14,15]. Biopsies were obtained with a Bergström needle modified for manual suction under local anaesthesia (2% xylocaine). Biopsy samples were blotted and freed of any visible fat and connective tissue, frozen in liquid nitrogen (within ~20 s of being taken from the muscle) and stored at −80°C until further analysis.

Imaging

After arriving at the site of the MRI scanner, subjects rested in the supine position for 1 h prior to scanning to prevent the influence of potential fluid shifts on muscle volume. Subjects were instructed not to engage in any strenuous activity within 24 h of the scanning. MRI scans were performed in a 3-T HD scanner (Signa MRI System; GE Medical, Milwaukee, WI) at the Brain-Body Institute, Imaging Research Centre, St. Joseph's Healthcare (Hamilton, Ontario). Image acquisition was carried out using T1 fluid attenuation inversion recovery in the axial plane with the following parameters: repetition time/echo time =2,100 ms/ 23.8 ms; field of view =25–30 cm; matrix size =512/512 slice thickness =5 mm. Thigh image acquisitions utilized an eight-channel torso coil with two excitations. There was a 10 mm gap between slices. Quadriceps volume was calculated by multiplying the slice area by the distance between slices. Volume was measured from the first slice where the rectus femoris was visible to the first slice where the gluteus maximus was visible. ImageJ software (U. S. National Institutes of Health, Bethesda, MD) was used to determine the area of each slice. Pre- and post-scans were performed at the same time of day and joint angle and leg compression was controlled using a custom built foot frame.

Whole-body DXA scans (QDR-4500A; Hologic, software version 12.31) were carried out pre and post training to determine total body weight, fat mass, and (fat and bone free) lean mass.

Western Blotting

Muscle samples (~40–50 mg) were homogenized on ice in buffer (10 μl mg^{-1} 25 mM Tris 0.5% v/v Triton X-100 and protease/phosphatase inhibitor cocktail tablets (Complete Protease Inhibitor Mini-Tabs, Roche, Indianapolis, IN; PhosSTOP, Roche Applied Science, Mannhein, Germany). Samples were then centrifuged at 15,000 *g* for 10 minutes 4°C. The supernatant was removed and protein concentrations were determined via BCA protein assay (Thermo Scientific, Rockford, IL). Working samples of equal concentration were prepared in Laemmli buffer. Equal amounts (20 μg) of protein were loaded onto 10% or gradient precast gels (BIO-RAD Mini-PROTEAN TGX Gels, Bio-Rad Laboratories, Hercules, CA) for separation by electrophoresis. Proteins were then transferred to a polyvinylidene fluoride membrane, blocked (5% skim milk) and incubated overnight at 4°C in primary antibody: phospho-Akt^{Ser473} (1:1000, Cell Signalling Technology, #4058) phospho-mTOR^{Ser2448} (1:1000, Cell Signalling Technology, #2971), phospho-4E-BP1$^{Thr37/46}$ (1:1000, Cell Signalling Technology, #2855), Phospho-S6$^{Ser240/244}$ Ribosomal protein (1:2000, Cell Signalling Technology, #2215). Membranes were then washed and incubated in secondary antibody (1 h at room temperature) before detection with chemiluminescence (SuperSignalWest Dura Extended Duration Substrate, ThermoScientific, #34075) on a FluorChem SP Imaging system (Alpha Innotech, Santa Clara, CA). Phosphorylation status was expressed relative to α-tubulin (1:2000, Cell Signalling Technology, #2125). Images were quantified by spot densitometry using ImageJ software (US National Institutes of Health).

Isotopic Analyses

As described previously [7] approximately 20 mg (wet weight) of muscle was used to isolate free intracellular amino acids. A separate piece of muscle (~30 mg) was used to isolate, hydrolyse, purify, derivatize and analyse the myofibrillar protein fraction enrichment. The rate of myofibrillar protein synthesis was calculated using the standard precursor–product method as previously described [7]:

$$FSR(\%h^{-1}) = [E_{p2} - E_{P1}/E_{ic} \bullet t^{-1}] \bullet 100$$

Where, FSR is the fractional synthetic rate, E_{p2} and E_{p1} are the protein bound enrichments from muscle biopsies at time 2 (E_{p2}) and plasma proteins or the previous muscle biopsy at time 1 (E_{p1}) and thus their difference is the change in bound protein enrichment between two time points; E_{ic} is the mean intracellular phenylalanine enrichment from biopsies at time 2 and time 1; and t is the tracer incorporation time. The utilization of "tracer naïve" subjects allowed us to use the pre-infusion blood sample (i.e., mixed plasma protein fraction) as the baseline enrichment (E_{p1}) for the calculation of resting MPS. This approach makes the assumption that the baseline ^{13}C enrichment ($\delta^{13}C_{PDB}$) in the blood reflects that of muscle protein; this is an assumption that has been previously [16] and shown to be valid in allowing calculation of a reliable rate of MPS in the fasted state [17,18].

Statistics

Differences in means from pre to post training were compared with parried Student's t-tests. Temporal differences in the phosphorylation of signalling proteins and FSR were compared with one-way repeated measures ANOVA. Relationships between variables were assessed using the Pearson's product moment correlation. All analyses were conducted using SPSS version 20 (IBM Armonk, New York, USA). Alpha was set at $P \leq 0.05$. Means are reported ± SE. A priori sample size calculations revealed that a sample of 23 subjects would be sufficient to detect a relationship accounting 25% of the variance between gains in muscle volume and increases in MPS with 80% power.

Results

Plasma and Muscle Intracellular Free Phenylalanine Enrichment

Intracellular free- phenylalanine precursor enrichments were 0.046±0.003 at rest and 0.066±0.004 throughout the post exercise incorporation period. The slope of a linear regression lines fit through the intracellular enrichments was not significantly different from zero during the post-exercise period ($P>0.05$). Plasma enrichments at 60, 180 and 360 min were 0.070±0.002, 0.075±0.003 and 0.076±0.003, respectively. Linear regression analysis indicated that the slopes of the plasma enrichments were not significantly different from zero ($P>0.05$) and thus an isotopic plateau was achieved and that the use of the steady-state precursor product equation was appropriate.

Muscle Size and Strength

Quadriceps muscle volume increased from 1837±195 to 1970±71 cm^3 (Figure 1A), while whole body fat- and bone-free mass increased from 62.6±2.0 to 64.8±2.1 kg (Figure 1B). Maximal isotonic strength, expressed as 1 RM, increased from 236±15 to 380±15 kg and from 77±4 to 96±4 kg in the leg press (Figure 1C) and chest press (Figure 1D) exercises respectively.

Western Blotting

Phosphorylation of $mTOR^{Ser2448}$ was increased above rest at 1 and 3 h post exercise but had returned to baseline by 6 hours post exercise (Figure 2A). Phosphorylation of Akt^{Ser473} was increased above resting at 1 h post-exercise then returned to baseline by 3 hours post exercise (Figure 2B). Phosphorylation of $4E\text{-}BP1^{Thr37/46}$ was not significantly increased at any time post-exercise ($P = 0.142$; Figure 2C). Phosphorylation of $rpS6^{Ser240/244}$ was elevated above rest at 1,3 and 6 h post-exercise; however, at 6 h post exercise the phosphorylation was reduced compared to 1 and 3 h (Figure 2D). There was a significant correlation between the phosphorylation of 4E-BP1 phosphorylation at 1 h post exercise and the change in muscle volume (r = 0.42, $P = 0.047$, Figure 3B). No correlations were evident between the phosphorylation any of the signalling proteins measured and changes in muscle volume or lean fat-and bone-free mass (data not shown).

Myofibrillar Protein Synthesis

The rate of MPS following resistance exercise was increased compared to rest and was significantly elevated between 1 and 3 h post exercise ($P<0.005$) and from 3 to 6 h post exercise ($P = 0.034$; Figure 4). There was no statistically significant difference between the 1–3 h and the 3–6 h rates ($P = 0.159$). The aggregate response over the entire post-exercise period (1–6 h) was 0.052±0.04%•h^{-1}. There was no correlation between MPS in any of the time periods measured and the change in muscle volume as measured by MRI (data not shown). Figure 3A shows the correlation between MPS measured over the full post exercise infusion period and change in muscle volume (r = 0.01). This comparison is highlighted because it should best reflect the full MPS response after exercise and nutrition. Expressing MPS as a fold change from rest did not results in a correlation with changes in muscle volume over the 1–6 post exercise period (r = −.16, *P> 0.05*). In addition, there was not a significant correlation between the change in fat- and bone-free (lean) mass and the aggregate response of myofibrillar protein synthesis measured over 1–6 h post exercise (r = 0.13).

Discussion

We examined the relationship between the acute fed-state exercise-induced rise in MPS and muscle hypertrophy in the same subject hypothesizing that these variables would be related. Interestingly, we observed no relationship between intra-individual measures of the acute response of MPS following subjects' first exposure to leg resistance exercise and nutrition (which we subsequently had subjects follow throughout their training protocol) and MRI-measured muscle volume or DXA-measured lean body mass. Our finding is actually in agreement with that reported by Mayhew et al. [13] who observed no significant relationship between mixed muscle FSR and hypertrophy in a group of 8 young and 7 older men in which FSR measured 24 h after the first bout of resistance training. It is important for the

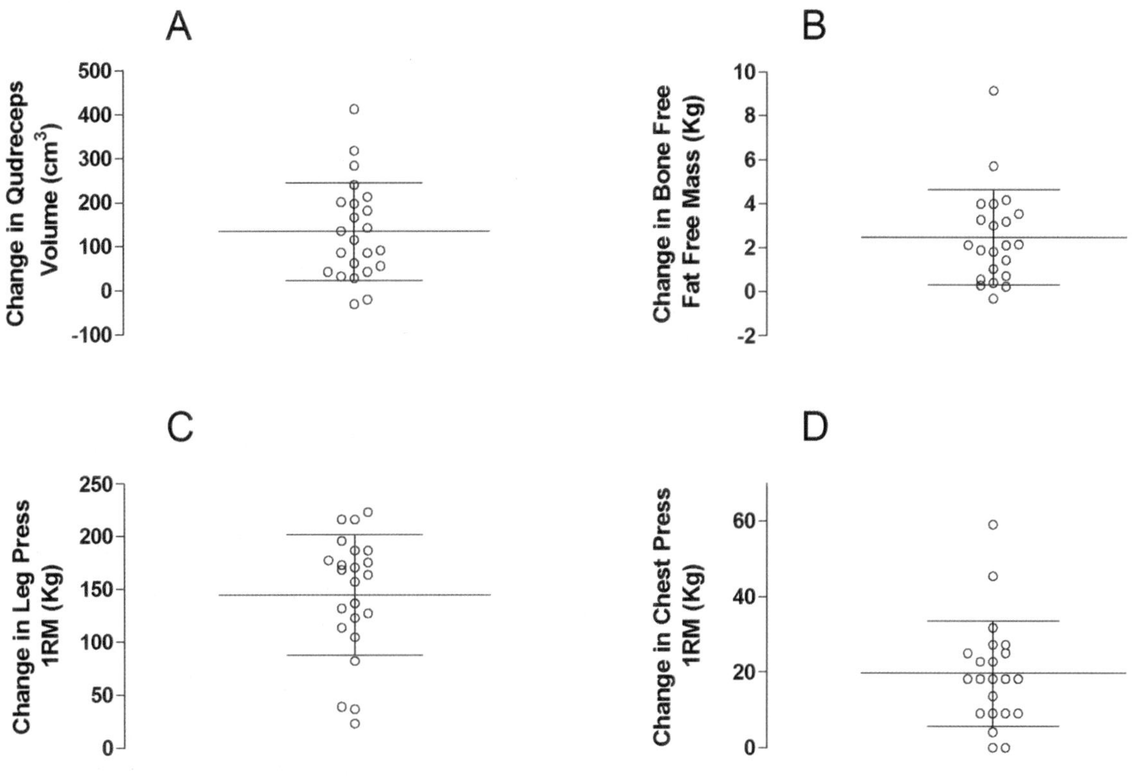

Figure 1. Muscle volume, muscle mass, and strength changes following resistance training. The absolute increase in A) Quadriceps muscle volume determined by MRI, B) Fat free bone free mass determined by DXA, C) Leg press 1RM and D) Chest press 1RM. Each dot represents a single subject, the lines show the group mean change and the standard deviation of the mean. All increases were significantly different from zero (i.e., an increase from pre training $P<0.05$).

reader to note that the present study differed from the Mayhew et al. study in both the timing of the measurement and the feeding state of the subjects. In the present study subjects ingested a protein rich beverage immediately after the first and each subsequent training session whereas in the Mayhew et al study subjects were fasted during the FSR measurement and did not consume supplemental protein during training [13]. The protein rich beverage was ingested during training in order to maximize muscle hypertrophy [19] and reduce heterogeneity in the subjects' diet and was consumed during the measurement of acute FSR so the conditions would be as similar as possible to the training. Although it was not possible to fully control the subjects' diets during the training period previous work has shown that subjects in this type of study consume adequate protein and calories and variation in diet does not explain variation in post training hypertrophy [20]. Diet records collected on a subset of subjects in this study support the previous finding. Similarly differences in habitual activities outside of the study workouts could have impacted hypertrophy however, subjects participated in a maximum of two pre week of sporting activity outside of the study so it is unlikely this had a major impact.

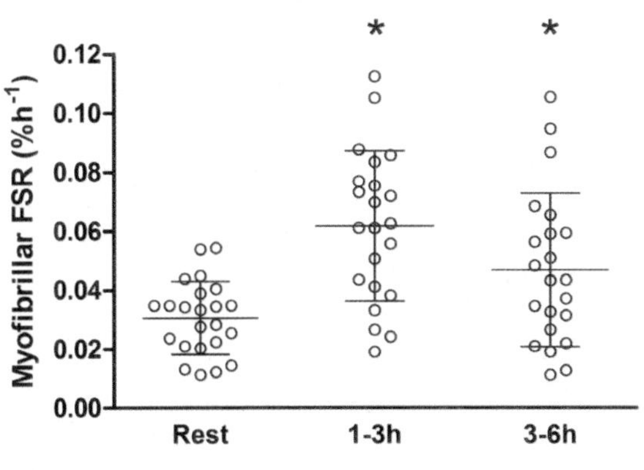

Figure 2. Phosphorylation of anabolic signalizing proteins. The results are expressed as fold changes from rest at 1, 3 and 6 hours after an acute bout of resistance exercise prior to the training period. All changes are normalized to alpha tubulin. A) mTOR phosphorylation at Ser2448, B) Akt phosphorylation at Ser473, C) 4E-BP1 phosphorylation at Thr37/46 and D) rpS6 phosphorylation at Ser240/244. * Significantly different from rest $P<0.05$. † Signficantly different from 1 and 3 hour time points $P<0.05$.

In previous work, acute responses of MPS to differing nutrition [4,6], contraction intensity [2,7], and contraction volume [2,7] were found to align with chronic training-mediated changes in hypertrophy in studies employing roughly equivalent nutritional and/or contractile conditions preformed but in different sets of subjects. The absence of a significant correlation between the acute early measure of MPS in the untrained state and chronic hypertrophy, in the present study, could be explained by a number of subject-specific changes in the MPS response in terms of: magnitude at times later during the training program, specificity of the protein fraction-specific (i.e., myofibrillar vs. non-myofibrillar MPS response), and/or duration of the response of MPS during the course of training, variations in net muscle protein balance due to differential responses in muscle proteolysis. Clearly, however, acute early measures of MPS are not proxy measures for hypertrophy or hypertrophic potential within the same individual.

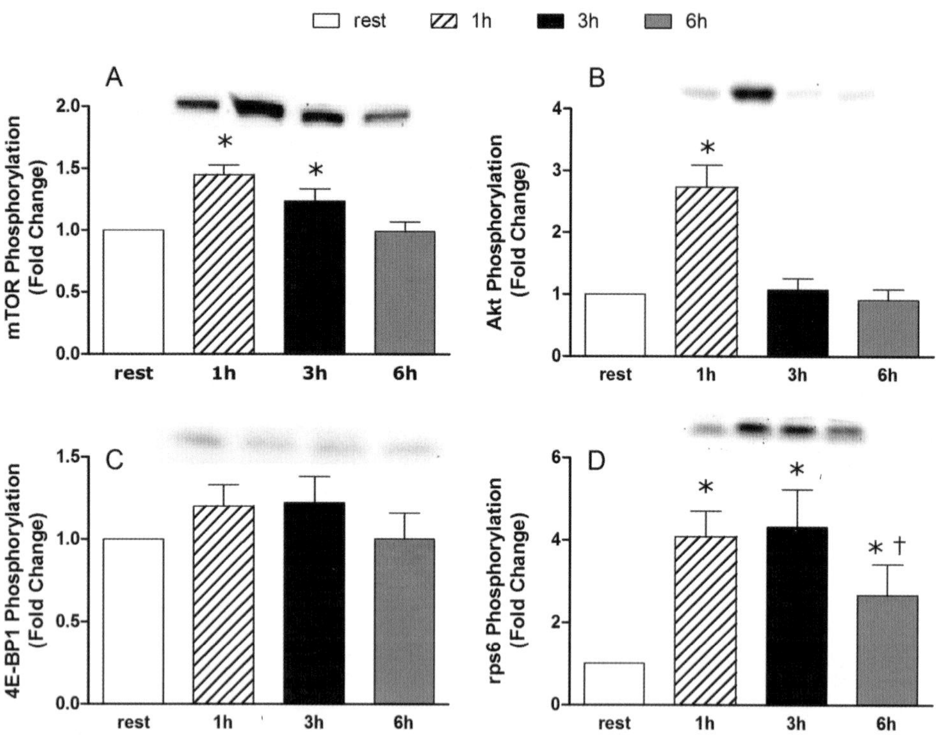

Figure 3. Relationship between muscle hypertrophy and potential correlates. A) The relationship between changes in muscle volume as measured by MRI and the Myofibrillar fractional synthetic rate (FSR) measured from 1 to 6 hours after an acute bout of resistance exercise and nutrition before the start of the resistance training period ($r = 0.10$, $P = 0.67$). B) The relationship between changes in muscle volume as measured by MRI and 4E-BP1 phosphorylation at Thr37/46 measured 1 hour after an acute bout of resistance exercise and nutrition before the start of the resistance training period ($r = 0.42$, $P = 0.05$).

Cross-sectional comparisons of trained with untrained persons show that increases in mixed muscle protein FSR were smaller in magnitude, as were increases in mixed muscle proteolysis, in response to resistance exercise [21]. Tang et al. showed that the mixed muscle protein FSR to a bout of resistance exercise with feeding, performed at the same relative intensity pre- and post-training, produced a slightly higher FSR immediately post exercise (90–270 min post exercise) in the trained state, however, the duration of the response was reduced [22]. In contrast, exercise at the same relative intensity resulted, when combined with feeding, results in a lower mixed muscle protein FSR after training when the same absolute intensity was utilized [23]. When examining myofibrillar as opposed to mixed muscle FSR, there were no differences in acute MPS between the trained and untrained conditions after exercise in the fasted state [24]. Taken together, resistance training appears to reduce the duration, but not the amplitude, of the myofibrillar protein synthetic response. Nonetheless, one conspicuous adaptation with resistance training is a 'refining' of the synthetic response to emphasize synthesis of myofibrillar proteins and reductions in both sarcoplasmic and mitochondrial protein synthesis in response to contraction [24,25]. Further research to delineate if responses of MPS play a role in determining hypertrophy would obviously have to include a more protracted time course of the MPS response and look at whether those gaining more lean mass were able to sustain a greater duration of their MPS response during the RT period. It is possible that high and low responders to RT may have similar acute FSR responses to the first bout of exercise but may significantly diverge in terms of FSR response at a point in the training period. A difference in muscle satellite cell content and the degree of myonuclear addition have been shown to relate to the magnitude of RT-induced hypertrophy [9]. It is conceivable that the individual variation in the change in FSR throughout the training period could be related to the degree of myonuclear addition.

A possibility is that subjects gaining more muscle mass with resistance training had a greater suppression of proteolysis as it is net muscle protein balance (i.e., MPS minus MPB) that would, strictly speaking, determine gains in muscle mass. Work by Glynn and associates shows that there are increases in MPS and reductions MPB in response to a combination of feeding and resistance exercise, however, the magnitude of the changes in MPS is ~4–5 fold greater than the change in MPB [26]. Similar differences in magnitude of the response of MPS relative to MPB have been seen with resistance exercise alone [27]. These data suggest that changes in MPS is the main locus of control and is far more responsive to nutritional and contractile stimuli in regulating, changes in muscle size than MPB. In addition, when measures of mixed muscle protein synthesis and breakdown have been made in the post-exercise period in the same subjects a reasonably good correlation exists between the two variables [21,27] which does not point to a measurable divergence in regulation but rather a link between the two processes. However, we cannot rule out the possibility that changes in protein breakdown could regulate gains in lean mass with resistance training.

The Akt-mTORC-1 pathway is an important regulatory pathway for muscle hypertrophy and is considered necessary for protein synthesis [28]. Phosphorylation of proteins within this pathway such as P70S6K, rpS6 and 4E-BP1 may show stronger relationships with hypertrophy because they are downstream from

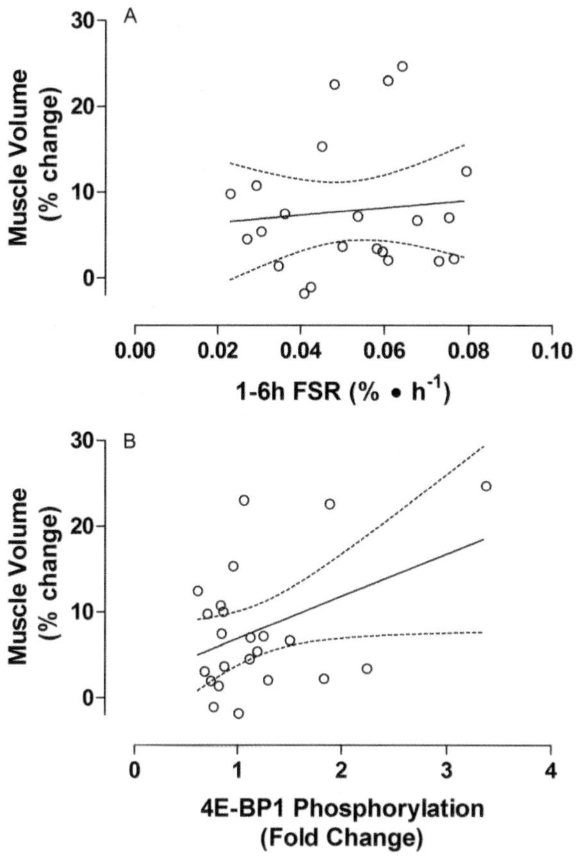

Figure 4. Myofibrillar Protein synthesis. FSR is calculated at rest and after an acute bout of resistance exercise and protein ingestion prior to the start of the resistance training period. The other rates were calculated from 1 to 3 hours and 3–6 hours after the resistance exercises. Each circle, square, and triangle represents a single subject at rest, 1–3 and 3–6 hours post exercises respectively * Significantly different than rest P<0.05.

mTOR in the signalling pathway that culminates in protein translation [13]. There are multiple reports of correlations between P70S6K and hypertrophy in the literature, however, these correlations tend to be weak [12,13] or have a small sample size [1]. Our lab has shown that significant muscle hypertrophy is possible with RT even when there is phosphorylation of P70S6K one hour after the first exercise bout [2], we have also shown that in one study P70S6K phosphorylation six hours after the first exercise bout is weakly related to training mediated hypertrophy [12]. These findings indicate how fickle a single time point measurement can be and provide a justification for our initial hypothesis that dynamic measurement such as MPS would show a greater relationship with hypertrophy.

Previous work from our lab has shown a correlation between acute phosphorylation of 4E-BP1 and myofibrillar FSR after resistance exercise [7]. In the current study we did not, however, see a relationship between FSR and 4E-BP1 phosphorylation but did see a relationship between hypertrophy and 4E-BP1 phosphorylation. Eukaryotic initiation factor 2B epsilon is another member of the Akt-mTOR pathway and has been proposed to be a regulator or variability in human hypertrophy [29]. However, technical limitations did not allow for the measurement of acute phosphorylation status of this target and the small amount of human data available does not suggest a linear relationship between hypertrophy and changes in protein abundance [29]. In a large study with young and old subjects the phosphorylation of multiple proteins in the Akt-mTOR pathway were shown to be unrelated to resistance exercise-induced changes in lean body mass [3]. Because anabolic signaling is transient and measured at discreet time points, and the degree of phosphorylation may not reflect activity it is doubtful that phosphorylation of a single protein could explain a large proportion of the variance in muscle hypertrophy [3].

The results from this study indicate that acute measurements of MPS over 6 hours following exercise and nutrition are not predictive of muscle hypertrophy following 16 weeks of resistance training and supplement ingestion in the same subjects. It is possible that the measures of MPS at later time-points following acute exercise may demonstrate a correlative relationship with muscle hypertrophy. However, the magnitude and duration on the MPS response measured within the same individual appears to change with training [22,24]. It is possible the some subjects may maintain a robust MPS response throughout the training period whereas some subjects may show a diminished MPS response after training. Because data from the present study does not show a relationship between acute measures of MPS and skeletal muscle hypertrophy, it is likely that changes in MPS with training are not uniform between subjects. A systems biology approach incorporating proteomics, genomic, or transcriptomics may be required prospectively to estimate hypertrophy or hypertrophic potential.

Author Contributions

Conceived and designed the experiments: CJM SMP GP. Performed the experiments: CJM SMP LB TAC-V SKB. Analyzed the data: CJM TAC-V KS PJA LB. Contributed reagents/materials/analysis tools: SMP GP KS PJA. Wrote the paper: CJM SMP.

References

1. Terzis G, Georgiadis G, Stratakos G, Vogiatzis I, Kavouras S, et al. (2008) Resistance exercise-induced increase in muscle mass correlates with p70S6 kinase phosphorylation in human subjects. Eur J Appl Physiol 102: 145–152.
2. Mitchell CJ, Churchward-Venne TA, West DW, Burd NA, Breen L, et al. (2012) Resistance exercise load does not determine training-mediated hypertrophic gains in young men. J Appl Physiol 113: 71–77.
3. Phillips BE, Williams JP, Gustafsson T, Bouchard C, Rankinen T, et al. (2013) Molecular Networks of Human Muscle Adaptation to Exercise and Age. PLoS Genet 9: e1003389.
4. Wilkinson SB, Tarnopolsky MA, Macdonald MJ, Macdonald JR, Armstrong D, et al. (2007) Consumption of fluid skim milk promotes greater muscle protein accretion after resistance exercise than does consumption of an isonitrogenous and isoenergetic soy-protein beverage. Am J Clin Nutr 85: 1031–1040.
5. Tang JE, Moore DR, Kujbida GW, Tarnopolsky MA, Phillips SM (2009) Ingestion of whey hydrolysate, casein, or soy protein isolate: effects on mixed muscle protein synthesis at rest and following resistance exercise in young men. J Appl Physiol 107: 987–992.
6. Hartman JW, Tang JE, Wilkinson SB, Tarnopolsky MA, Lawrence RL, et al. (2007) Consumption of fat-free fluid milk after resistance exercise promotes greater lean mass accretion than does consumption of soy or carbohydrate in young, novice, male weightlifters. Am J Clin Nutr 86: 373–381.
7. Burd NA, West DW, Staples AW, Atherton PJ, Baker JM, et al. (2010) Low-load high volume resistance exercise stimulates muscle protein synthesis more than high-load low volume resistance exercise in young men. PLoS One 5: e12033.
8. Burd NA, Holwerda AM, Selby KC, West DW, Staples AW, et al. (2010) Resistance exercise volume affects myofibrillar protein synthesis and anabolic signalling molecule phosphorylation in young men. J Physiol 588: 3119–3130.
9. Petrella JK, Kim JS, Mayhew DL, Cross JM, Bamman MM (2008) Potent myofiber hypertrophy during resistance training in humans is associated with satellite cell-mediated myonuclear addition: a cluster analysis. J Appl Physiol 104: 1736–1742.

10. Davidsen PK, Gallagher IJ, Hartman JW, Tarnopolsky MA, Dela F, et al. (2011) High responders to resistance exercise training demonstrate differential regulation of skeletal muscle microRNA expression. J Appl Physiol 110: 309–317.
11. West DW, Phillips SM (2012) Associations of exercise-induced hormone profiles and gains in strength and hypertrophy in a large cohort after weight training. Eur J Appl Physiol 112: 2693–2702.
12. Mitchell CJ, Churchward-Venne TA, Bellamy L, Parise G, Baker SK, et al. (2013) Muscular and systemic correlates of resistance training-induced muscle hypertrophy. PLoS One 8: e78636.
13. Mayhew DL, Kim JS, Cross JM, Ferrando AA, Bamman MM (2009) Translational signaling responses preceding resistance training-mediated myofiber hypertrophy in young and old humans. J Appl Physiol 107: 1655–1662.
14. Burd NA, Yang Y, Moore DR, Tang JE, Tarnopolsky MA, et al. (2012) Greater stimulation of myofibrillar protein synthesis with ingestion of whey protein isolate v. micellar casein at rest and after resistance exercise in elderly men. Br J Nutr 108: 958–962.
15. Churchward-Venne TA, Burd NA, Mitchell CJ, West DW, Philp A, et al. (2012) Supplementation of a suboptimal protein dose with leucine or essential amino acids: effects on myofibrillar protein synthesis at rest and following resistance exercise in men. J Physiol 590: 2751–2765.
16. West DW, Kujbida GW, Moore DR, Atherton P, Burd NA, et al. (2009) Resistance exercise-induced increases in putative anabolic hormones do not enhance muscle protein synthesis or intracellular signalling in young men. J Physiol 587: 5239–5247.
17. Burd NA, Groen BB, Beelen M, Senden JM, Gijsen AP, et al. (2012) The reliability of using the single-biopsy approach to assess basal muscle protein synthesis rates in vivo in humans. Metabolism 61: 931–936.
18. Burd NA, Pennings B, Groen BB, Gijsen AP, Senden JM, et al. (2012) The single biopsy approach is reliable for the measurement of muscle protein synthesis rates in vivo in older men. J Appl Physiol 113: 896–902.
19. Cermak NM, Res PT, de Groot LC, Saris WH, van Loon LJ (2012) Protein supplementation augments the adaptive response of skeletal muscle to resistance-type exercise training: a meta-analysis. Am J Clin Nutr 96: 1454–1464.
20. Thalacker-Mercer AE, Petrella JK, Bamman MM (2009) Does habitual dietary intake influence myofiber hypertrophy in response to resistance training? A cluster analysis. Appl Physiol Nutr Metab 34: 632–639.
21. Phillips SM, Tipton KD, Ferrando AA, Wolfe RR (1999) Resistance training reduces the acute exercise-induced increase in muscle protein turnover. Am J Physiol 276: E118–124.
22. Tang JE, Perco JG, Moore DR, Wilkinson SB, Phillips SM (2008) Resistance training alters the response of fed state mixed muscle protein synthesis in young men. Am J Physiol Regul Integr Comp Physiol 294: R172–178.
23. Phillips SM, Parise G, Roy BD, Tipton KD, Wolfe RR, et al. (2002) Resistance-training-induced adaptations in skeletal muscle protein turnover in the fed state. Can J Physiol Pharmacol 80: 1045–1053.
24. Kim PL, Staron RS, Phillips SM (2005) Fasted-state skeletal muscle protein synthesis after resistance exercise is altered with training. J Physiol 568: 283–290.
25. Wilkinson SB, Phillips SM, Atherton PJ, Patel R, Yarasheski KE, et al. (2008) Differential effects of resistance and endurance exercise in the fed state on signalling molecule phosphorylation and protein synthesis in human muscle. J Physiol 586: 3701–3717.
26. Glynn EL, Fry CS, Drummond MJ, Dreyer HC, Dhanani S, et al. (2010) Muscle protein breakdown has a minor role in the protein anabolic response to essential amino acid and carbohydrate intake following resistance exercise. Am J Physiol Regul Integr Comp Physiol 299: R533–540.
27. Phillips SM, Tipton KD, Aarsland A, Wolf SE, Wolfe RR (1997) Mixed muscle protein synthesis and breakdown after resistance exercise in humans. Am J Physiol 273: E99–107.
28. Bodine SC, Stitt TN, Gonzalez M, Kline WO, Stover GL, et al. (2001) Akt/mTOR pathway is a crucial regulator of skeletal muscle hypertrophy and can prevent muscle atrophy in vivo. Nat Cell Biol 3: 1014–1019.
29. Mayhew DL, Hornberger TA, Lincoln HC, Bamman MM (2011) Eukaryotic initiation factor 2B epsilon induces cap-dependent translation and skeletal muscle hypertrophy. J Physiol 589: 3023–3037.

7

The Muscle Oxidative Regulatory Response to Acute Exercise Is Not Impaired in Less Advanced COPD Despite a Decreased Oxidative Phenotype

Ilse G. M. Slot[1¶], Bram van den Borst[1¶], Valéry A. C. V. Hellwig[1], Esther Barreiro[2,3], Annemie M. W. J. Schols[1], Harry R. Gosker[1*]

1 Department of Respiratory Medicine, NUTRIM School for Nutrition, Toxicology and Metabolism, Maastricht University Medical Center+, Maastricht, The Netherlands, **2** Pulmonology Department-Muscle and Respiratory System Research Unit (URMAR), Research Institute of Hospital del Mar (IMIM), Department of Experimental and Health Sciences (CEXS), Pompeu Fabra University (UPF), Barcelona Biomedical Research Park (PRBB), Barcelona, Spain, **3** Network of Excellence in Respiratory Research (CIBERES), Institute of Health Carlos III (ISCIII), Bunyola, Majorca, Balearic Islands, Spain

Abstract

Already in an early disease stage, patients with chronic obstructive pulmonary disease (COPD) are confronted with impaired skeletal muscle function and physical performance due to a loss of oxidative type I muscle fibers and oxidative capacity (i.e. oxidative phenotype; Oxphen). Physical activity is a well-known stimulus of muscle Oxphen and crucial for its maintenance. We hypothesized that a blunted response of Oxphen genes to an acute bout of exercise could contribute to decreased Oxphen in COPD. For this, 28 patients with less advanced COPD (age 65±7 yrs, FEV_1 59±16% predicted) and 15 age- and gender-matched healthy controls performed an incremental cycle ergometry test. The Oxphen response to exercise was determined by the measurement of gene expression levels of Oxphen markers in pre and 4h-post exercise quadriceps biopsies. Because exercise-induced hypoxia and oxidative stress may interfere with Oxphen response, oxygen saturation and oxidative stress markers were assessed as well. Regardless of oxygen desaturation and absolute exercise intensities, the Oxphen regulatory response to exercise was comparable between COPD patients and controls with no evidence of increased oxidative stress. In conclusion, the muscle Oxphen regulatory response to acute exercise is not blunted in less advanced COPD, regardless of exercise-induced hypoxia. Hence, this study provides further rationale for incorporation of exercise training as integrated part of disease management to prevent or slow down loss of muscle Oxphen and related functional impairment in COPD.

Editor: Sukesh R. Bhaumik, Southern Illinois University School of Medicine, United States of America

Funding: This study was performed within the framework of the Dutch Top Institute Pharma project T1-201. Partners within this project are Maastricht University Medical Centre+, University Medical Center Utrecht, University Medical Center Groningen, AstraZeneca, Nycomed, GlaxoSmithKline and Danone Research. All the partners approved the manuscript. Dr Gosker was funded by a Netherlands Asthma Foundation grant (NAF 3.2.09.068). The funders had no role in study design, data collection and analysis, decision to publish, or preparation of the manuscript.

* E-mail: h.gosker@maastrichtuniversity.nl

¶ These authors contributed equally to this work.

Introduction

Loss of skeletal muscle oxidative phenotype (Oxphen) is prevalent in chronic obstructive pulmonary disease (COPD) [1-3]. It includes a proportional shift from slow-oxidative type I muscle fibers towards the fast-glycolytic type II fibers, associated with a reduced capacity of oxidative metabolism and in advanced disease also mitochondrial dysfunction [4]. Loss of muscle Oxphen is related to functional impairments, such as a reduction in muscle endurance [4], whole body exercise capacity, and mechanical efficiency [5], and it has been proposed as a driver of cardiovascular and metabolic risk [6] and cachexia [7]. Loss of muscle Oxphen is most prominent in severe COPD, but we recently showed that the process is already ongoing in patients with less advanced COPD [8]. Hence, this earlier stage of the disease is of particular importance to gain mechanistic insight into the onset of Oxphen loss in COPD.

Exercise is an important stimulus for maintenance of muscle Oxphen. Because patients with COPD are physically less active [9], it is tempting to attribute Oxphen loss in these patients to disuse. However, several recent reports could not show such an association between physical activity level and Oxphen [8,10,11]. Physiologically, muscle Oxphen is progressively stimulated and maintained by repeated bouts of exercise through induction of among others peroxisome proliferator-activated receptor (PPAR) coactivator-1α (PGC-1α), PPAR-α and -δ, and mitochondrial transcription factor A (TFAM) [12,13]. We hypothesized that the response of Oxphen regulation to acute bouts of exercise is blunted in COPD, which could contribute to a loss of muscle Oxphen irrespective of physical activity level. To test this hypothesis we compared Oxphen markers and their regulators in muscle biopsies obtained before and after an acute bout of exercise, between less advanced COPD patients and healthy controls who were matched for age and body mass index (BMI).

Hypoxia is known to increase muscle glycolytic capacity relative to oxidative capacity [14,15]. In humans, hypoxic exposure also induces loss of muscle oxidative capacity by reducing mitochondrial volume (reviewed in [16]). Exercise-induced oxygen desaturation even occurs in some patients with less advanced COPD, potentially reflecting or leading to hypoxia in the exercising muscle. Experimental research in mice has shown that exposure to acute hypoxia can also induce oxidative stress in skeletal muscle mitochondria [17]. Indeed, elevated levels of oxidative stress markers have been shown in muscles of COPD patients with chronic hypoxemia [18]. Moreover, enhanced exercise-induced oxidative stress has frequently been observed in muscle of patients with severe COPD [19], particularly in the wasted subgroup [20]. Interestingly, in severe patients, oxidative stress is inversely associated with muscle endurance [21] and *in vitro* permeabilized muscle fibers of patients with severe COPD produce significantly more reactive oxygen species than those of healthy controls [22]. This is possibly related to a fiber-type shift, since studies in rats have shown that mitochondria within type II fibers release significantly more H_2O_2 than those within oxidative fibers [23]. As such, oxygen desaturation and/or muscle oxidative stress could mediate an anticipated blunted Oxphen response in COPD. A secondary objective was therefore to determine the involvement of exercise-induced oxygen desaturation and oxidative stress in the response to an acute exercise bout.

Methods

Ethics statement

Written informed consent was obtained from all subjects and the ethical review board of the Maastricht University Medical Center+ approved the study (08-2-059). The study was registered at www.trialregister.nl as NTR1402.

Patient characteristics

The study population included 28 clinically stable mild to moderate COPD patients (FEV_1 59±16% predicted; P_a,O_2 9.3±1.0 kPa) and 15 healthy controls. Recruitment of patients and controls and exclusion criteria were previously described [8]. Briefly, patients were recruited from the outpatient clinic of Maastricht University Medical Center+ (MUMC+, Maastricht, The Netherlands) and via advertisements in local newspapers. Exclusion criteria were long-term oxygen therapy, oral corticosteroid use, acute exacerbation requiring hospital admission in the past eight weeks, rehabilitation in the past six months and known co-morbidities potentially interfering with study outcome parameters. Healthy controls were recruited via advertising in local newspapers and absence of co-morbidities and airflow limitation was verified through history-taking by a physician, and pulmonary function tests. Healthy controls were matched to COPD patients on age, BMI and sex distribution. Study subjects were carefully characterized regarding body composition, lung function, smoking status and daily physical activity level, as reported previously [8]. The protocol used to determine quadriceps function on a dynamometer was previously described [8]. Briefly, under strong encouragement, subjects performed thirty sequential volitional maximal contractions at an angular velocity of 90°/s. Isokinetic quadriceps endurance was determined as proportional decline in peak torques (relative to the highest peak torque) per repetition (%/rep).

Experimental protocol

To study the response of Oxphen regulators and oxidative stress to acute exercise, subjects performed an incremental load cycle ergometry test. Quadriceps muscle biopsies were obtained directly before and 4 h after the exercise test for Oxphen and oxidative stress analyses to obtain a maximal response of metabolic and oxidative stress-related genes after exercise. During the entire exercise test, oxygen saturation was measured by means of traditional finger pulse oximetry, as well as using a portable continuous-wave near-infrared spectroscopy (NIRS) system to examine oxygen saturation locally at the muscular level. Arterial punctures were performed before exercise and at maximal exertion for gas and lactate analyses.

Acute exercise protocol

All subjects performed an incremental load cycle ergometry test. The rationale for this protocol was to invoke a rapid exercise response in terms of Oxphen regulation particularly in the quadriceps muscle (see below). Peak oxygen uptake ($V'O_{2peak}$) and peak work load were determined as previously described [24]. Anaerobic threshold was determined from ergospirometry data using the v-slope method [25]. Arterial punctures of the radial artery at rest and at $V'O_{2peak}$ were available from $n=19$ COPD patients and $n=11$ healthy subjects. Arterial blood gas and lactate concentrations were analyzed on a Chiron blood gas analyzer 865 (Chiron Diagnostics, Emeryville, CA).

Arterial and peripheral muscle oxygenation

Arterial oxygen saturation was continuously monitored using a finger pulse oximeter. By *post hoc* stratification the patients were divided into those who desaturated during exercise (S_p,O_2 fall ≥ 4%; $COPD_D$, $n=13$) and those who did not (S_p,O_2 fall<4%; $COPD_{ND}$, $n=15$) according to ATS criteria [26]. Quadriceps muscle oxygenation was measured using the PortaMon portable continuous-wave near-infrared spectrophotometer (NIRS, Artinis Medical Systems, Zetten, The Netherlands). The probe was attached with Velcro straps on the *vastus lateralis* of the non-biopsied leg approximately 10 cm proximally from the knee joint, and covered with a black cloth to eliminate environmental light. Measurements started 3 minutes before exercise while the subject was still at rest and continued for 2–5 minutes after the exercise test until the signal had stabilized. Baseline values were established during 3 minutes of unloaded cycling before the incremental exercise test. Tissue oxygenation was measured continuously. Traces were analyzed with OxySoft Software (v2.1.2; Artinis Medical Systems). The tissue saturation index (TSI) was calculated using spatial resolved spectroscopy using the equation below, with $[O_2Hb]$ and $[HHb]$ representing concentrations of oxygenated and deoxygenated hemoglobin/myoglobin.

$$TSI = 100 \times \frac{[O_2Hb]}{[O_2Hb] + [HHb]}$$

Values were reported as change from baseline (Δ). Using mono-exponential curve fitting, the time constant of muscle reoxygenation (tau, τ) was determined from the slope of the TSI curve during the reoxygenation phase. Twelve subjects (4 $COPD_{ND}$, 4 $COPD_D$ patients, and 4 healthy controls) were excluded from further NIRS analyses mainly because their skin fold at the site of the NIRS measurement was greater than 3 cm (which is the operational limit for the NIRS probe), or because the signal was poor or did not show a clear drop in TSI.

Muscle biopsy and analyses

Biopsies were obtained at rest and 4 h after the exercise test from quadriceps muscle (*vastus lateralis*) of the dominant leg from two separate incisions approximately 2 cm apart using the needle biopsy technique [27]. The interval between the exercise test and the second biopsy was chosen after careful study of the literature to obtain a maximal response of metabolic genes after exercise (e.g., [28,29]). Muscle tissue was frozen in melting isopentane precooled in liquid nitrogen and stored in aliquots at −80°C for histology and molecular analyses.

Techniques for sample preparation for analyses of fiber-type composition, gene expression, oxidative stress markers, metabolic enzyme activity as well as the corresponding analyses have been previously described [8]. Briefly, fiber-type composition was determined on 5 μm serial cryosections using antibodies against myosin heavy chain (MyHC) I, MyHC IIa (both from Developmental Studies Hybridoma Bank, University of Iowa, USA), and laminin (Sigma, Zwijndrecht, the Netherlands). Fiber-type classification was aided by myosin ATPase-activity staining with acidic pre-incubation at pH 4.40 [30]. For qRT-PCR, RNA was extracted from 10–30 mg muscle tissue using the ToTALLY RNA^{TM} Kit (Ambion Ltd., Foster City, CA, USA) according to the supplier's protocol, followed by genomic DNA removal with the RNeasy Mini Kit with RNase-free DNase (Qiagen, Venlo, The Netherlands). 400 ng RNA was reverse transcribed to cDNA with anchored oligo(dT) primers according to the supplier's protocol (Transcriptor First Strand cDNA Synthesis kit, Roche Diagnostics, Woerden, The Netherlands). qRT-PCR primers were designed based on Ensembl transcript sequences or selected from literature [31,32] and ordered from Sigma Genosys (Zwijndrecht, the Netherlands), with primer details shown in Table S1 and Table S2 in File S1. Using these analyses, regulators and markers of oxidative and glycolytic metabolism as well as oxidative stress were assessed. Contents of antioxidant enzymes were determined with the western blot protocol using anti-catalase antibody (Calbiochem, San Diego, CA, USA) and anti-manganese superoxide dismutase and anti-Cu/Zn superoxide dismutase antibodies (Santa Cruz Biotechnology, CA, USA). Protein content of oxidative stress markers were identified using antibodies for protein carbonylation (anti-2,4-DNP moiety antibody, Oxyblot kit, Chemicon International Inc., Temecula, CA, USA), total protein nitration (anti-3-nitrotyrosine antibody, Invitrogen, Eugene, OR, USA), and total malondialdehyde (MDA)-protein adducts (anti-MDA antibody, Academy Biomedical Company Inc., Houston, TX, USA). For protein carbonylation, carbonyl groups in the protein side chains were first derivatized to 2,4-dinitrophenylhydrazone (DNP) using the Oxyblot kit (Chemicon International Inc., Temecula, CA, USA) according to the manufacturer's instructions. Exercise responses of gene expression and oxidative stress product variables were summarized with fold inductions, which were calculated by dividing post-exercise values by baseline values. Contents of representative subunits of oxidative phosphorylation (OXPHOS) complexes were determined by western blot using an anti-total OXPHOS antibody cocktail (MS604-300, Abcam, Cambridge, UK) with GAPDH (anti-GAPDH, #2118, Cell Signaling Technology, Leiden, The Netherlands) as a loading control. Metabolic activities for citrate synthase (CS, EC 2.3.3.1) and 3-hydroxyacyl-CoA dehydrogenase (HADH, EC 1.1.1.35) were assayed spectrophotometrically (Multiskan Spectrum; Thermo Labsystems, Breda, The Netherlands) as previously described [33-35]. Absolute CS and HADH activities were normalized to total protein.

Statistics

The assumptions of normality and homogeneity of variances were checked for all experimental groups with the Shapiro-Wilk test and Levene's test. Three different sets of statistical comparisons were made. First, baseline comparisons between the COPD patients and controls were tested using independent Student's *t* test or Mann-Whitney test as appropriate. Comparisons between $COPD_{ND}$, $COPD_D$ and control groups were made using one-way ANOVA (*post hoc* Gabriel), Welch's ANOVA (*post hoc* Games-Howell) or Kruskal-Wallis non-parametric ANOVA (*post hoc* Mann-Whitney U with Bonferroni correction) as appropriate. Discontinuous variables were tested using Fisher's Exact test. These same tests were subsequently employed to analyze differences in exercise-induced response of skeletal muscle metabolic genes and oxidative stress markers *between* the groups (expressed as fold inductions), whereas paired Student's *t* test or Wilcoxon signed-rank test were performed to analyze such changes *within* each study group. Correlations were tested using Pearson's correlation coefficient, or Spearman's ρ in case of non-normally distributed data. Analyses were performed using IBM SPSS Statistics 20.0 (IBM Corp., Armonk, NY). A p-value<0.05 was considered statistically significant.

Results

Pulmonary and anthropometric characteristics

Characteristics of the study subjects are summarized in Table 1. COPD patients had moderate airflow obstruction (FEV_1 59±16). Compared to healthy controls, the COPD patients had a lower resting arterial oxygen saturation (S_p,O_2 96 (95, 97) *vs* 98 (98, 100)%) and daily physical activity level (214 (129, 300) *vs* 328 (276, 489) counts/min). $COPD_D$ patients did not differ from $COPD_{ND}$ patients in terms of pulmonary function indices, but had a lower BMI.

Oxidative phenotype in quadriceps muscle

At baseline, as reported previously [8] and listed in Table 2, Oxphen markers were lower in COPD patients than in controls, which was reflected by lower type I and higher type II fiber proportions, and reduced content of some subunits of the oxidative phosphorylation complexes. Oxphen markers were not different between patients who did or did not desaturate during exercise (Table 2). Moreover, quadriceps endurance was reduced in this COPD cohort (decline in peak torque −1.74 (−2.04, −1.28) in COPD *vs* −1.09 (−1.57, −0.91)%/repetition in healthy controls), but it was not different between $COPD_D$ and $COPD_{ND}$ patients (−1.86 (−2.02, −1.35) in $COPD_D$ *vs* −1.61 (−2.14, −1.25)%/repetition in $COPD_{ND}$).

Cycle ergometry performance

Data from the cycle ergometry test are listed in Table 3. As expected, peak work rate was lower in COPD patients than in controls (72 (56, 96) *vs* 156 (134, 255) Watt). No differences were found between $COPD_D$ and $COPD_{ND}$ patients.

Exercise-induced metabolic gene expression

The acute exercise clearly evoked an upregulation of genes known to be exercise-responsive, including PGC-1α-related co-activator PRC, glycolysis-involved hexokinase II and the master regulator of the hypoxic response, HIF-1α (Figure 1). The COPD patients did not respond differently to exercise than controls regarding expression of genes associated with muscle oxidative metabolism, nor of genes involved in glycolytic metabolism or

Table 1. Main characteristics of subjects.

	Healthy controls	COPD	$COPD_{ND}$	$COPD_D$
N (M/F)	15 (9/6)	28 (16/12)	15 (9/6)	13 (7/6)
Age, y	65±6	65±7	66±7	65±6
Height, cm	170±11	169±9	168±7	169±11
Weight, kg	72±12	71±10	74±10	67±10
BMI, kg/m	24.9±3.3	25.1±2.8	26.4±2.5	23.5±2.3$^{\#}$
FFMI, kg/m	18.0±1.9	17.5±1.8	18.0±2.0	16.9±1.5
Smoking status current/former/never	1/7/7	10/18/0**	7/8/0**	3/10/0*
FEV_1, % predicted	113±15	59±16***	61±13***	56±19***
FVC, % predicted	120±17	104±22*	98±20*	110±24
$D_{L,CO}$, % predicted	95±19	51±16***	55±16***	47±16***
S_{p,O_2} at rest, %	98 (98, 100)	96 (95, 97)***	97 (96, 97)***	95 (94, 98)***
P_{a,O_2} at rest, kPa	12.1±1.1	9.3±1.0***	9.5±0.8***	9.1±1.2***
P_{a,CO_2} at rest, kPa	5.3±0.2	5.2±0.5	5.1±0.5	5.2±0.4
Daily physical activity, counts/min	328 (276, 489)	214 (129, 300)**	208 (140, 278)**	220 (108, 366)

Values are expressed as mean±SD or median (25th percentile, 75th percentile). Abbreviations: BMI, body mass index; FFMI, fat-free mass index; FEV_1, forced expiratory volume in one second; FVC, forced vital capacity; $D_{L,CO}$, diffusion capacity of the lungs for carbon monoxide; Sp,o_2, oxygen saturation measured via pulse oximetry. Significance of difference compared to controls: $^{*}p<0.05$, $^{**}p<0.01$, $^{***}p\leq0.001$. Level of significance $COPD_D$ *vs.* $COPD_{ND}$ patients: $^{\#}p<0.05$.

hypoxia signaling. We also did not observe a different response in $COPD_D$ patients compared to $COPD_{ND}$ patients.

Exercise response of oxidative stress markers

At baseline, oxidative stress-induced protein modification levels such as carbonylation, tyrosine nitration and MDA adducts were not different between COPD patients and controls [8], nor between $COPD_D$ and $COPD_{ND}$ patients (data not shown). After exercise, gene expression levels of heme oxygenase-1 (HO-1) and manganese superoxide dismutase (MnSOD) were increased in both COPD patients and healthy controls (Figure 2A). An exercise response of the antioxidant enzymes was not detected at the protein level as manganese and copper/zinc superoxide dismutase and catalase protein content remained unchanged (Figure 2B). No differential response was shown between $COPD_D$ and $COPD_{ND}$ patients.

Table 2. Main characteristics of *vastus lateralis* muscle fibers.

	Healthy controls	COPD	$COPD_{ND}$	$COPD_D$
Type I proportion, %	62.7 (55.3, 68.3)	39.7 (35.3, 48.6)***	40.3 (35.5, 62.3)*	39.7 (29.8, 47.4)***
Type I/IIa proportion, %	8.1 (4.6, 11.0)	5.6 (2.2, 9.5)	5.3 (3.5, 9.0)	6.4 (1.2, 12.7)
Type IIa proportion, %	25.5 (16.8, 32.4)	40.5 (25.9, 48.9)**	32.0 (24.5, 46.1)*	45.4 (39.7, 55.2)***
Type IIa/IIx proportion, %	1.0 (0.3, 3.4)	3.6 (1.1, 8.1)	4.3 (1.0, 9.4)	3.6 (0.7, 7.4)
Type IIx proportion, %	0.5 (0.0, 2.7)	2.3 (0.5, 9.4)*	2.2 (0.2, 8.8)	3.2 (0.6, 11.0)
Type I fiber CSA, μm^2	8703±1858	8154±2460	8524±2655	7756±2268
Type I/IIa fiber CSA, μm^2	6540±2048	6073±2742	6274±2810	5838±2766
Type IIa fiber CSA, μm^2	7107±2580	7016±2309	7030±2533	7001±2144
Type IIa/IIx fiber CSA, μm^2	7214±3139	5760±2795	6082±3124	5341±2396
Type IIx fiber CSA, μm^2	4694±2613	3792±2032	4375±2192	3257±1799
CS activity, µmol/min/g protein	63±37	54±22	52±24	56±21
HADH activity, µmol/min/g protein	22±9	19±7	19±7	19±6
OXPHOS complex I subunit content, AU	2.0 (1.2, 3.9)	1.5 (0.8, 2.1)	1.6 (1.0, 1.9)	1.2 (0.3, 2.4)
OXPHOS complex II subunit content, AU	2.8 (1.7, 4.3)	2.2 (1.5, 3.6)	2.3 (1.6, 2.5)	2.2 (1.2, 4.2)
OXPHOS complex III subunit content, AU	1.5 (0.7, 2.0)	1.2 (0.8, 1.7)	1.2 (0.9, 1.4)	1.4 (0.7, 1.8)
OXPHOS complex IV subunit content, AU	4.1 (2.8, 8.1)	2.4 (1.1, 3.6)*	2.9 (1.3, 4.1)	1.9 (0.6, 3.3)*
OXPHOS complex V subunit content, AU	0.7 (0.4, 1.1)	0.5 (0.3, 0.7)*	0.5 (0.3, 0.8)	0.6 (0.3, 0.7)

Values are expressed as mean±SD or median (25th percentile, 75th percentile). Abbreviations: CSA, cross-sectional area; CS, citrate synthase; HADH, 3-hydroxyacyl-CoA dehydrogenase; OXPHOS, oxidative phosphorylation; AU, arbitrary units. Significance of difference compared to controls: * $p<0.05$, ** $p<0.01$, *** $p\leq0.001$.

Table 3. Results from the maximal cycle ergometry test.

	Healthy controls	COPD	$COPD_{ND}$	$COPD_D$
Total exercise time, min	10.0 (8.8, 10.6)	7.4 (5.5, 9.4)**	7.5 (5.5, 8.9)*	7.0 (5.7, 9.7)*
Peak work load, Watt	156 (134, 255)	72 (56, 96)***	76 (66, 100)***	66 (53, 96)***
Work load, % predicted	133 (106, 152)	60 (44, 71)***	65 (48, 73)***	57 (37, 69)***
$V'O_{2peak}$, ml/min	1852 (1680, 2785)	1130 (1025, 1406)***	1162 (1075, 1434)***	1084 (901, 1358)***
$V'O_{2peak}$, % predicted	120 (102, 155)	74 (55, 84)***	78 (66, 88)***	64 (51, 74)***
$V'_{E,peak}$, % MVV	66 (61, 80)	85 (81, 94)***	82 (77, 94)**	89 (82, 94)**
HR_{peak}, % HR predicted	100 (97, 106)	78 (68, 89)***	77 (66, 89)**	78 (71, 92)**
$ATV'O_2$, ml/min	1061 (862, 1395)	736 (607, 873)***	776 (601, 875)**	727 (605, 889)**
$S_{p,}O_2$ at $V'O_{2peak}$, %	97 (97, 99)	92 (87, 95)***	94 (93, 96)***	87 (85, 90)$^{***, \#\#\#}$
$\Delta S_{p,}O_2$, %	−1.0 (−2.0, 0.0)	−4.0 (−8.0, −2.3)***	−3.0 (−4.0, 0.0)	−8.0 (−10.0, −6.5)$^{***, \#\#\#}$
$\Delta S_{a,}O_2$, %	0.0 (0.0, 1.0)	−1.0 (−4.0, 0.0)*	−1.0 (−1.8, 1.5)	−4.0 (−10.0, −3.0)$^{**, \#\#}$

Values are expressed as median (25th percentile, 75th percentile). Abbreviations: $V'O_2$, oxygen uptake; V'_E, minute ventilation; MVV, maximal voluntary ventilation, calculated as $FEV_1 \times 37.5$; HR, heart rate; HR predicted calculated as (220 − age); $ATV'O_2$, $V'O_2$ at anaerobic threshold; $S_{p,}O_2$, oxygen saturation measured via pulse oximetry; $S_{a,}O_2$, arterial oxygen saturation. Level of significance of difference *vs.* controls: $^{*}p<0.05$, $^{**}p<0.01$, $^{***}p\leq0.001$. Level of significance of difference $COPD_D$ *vs.* $COPD_{ND}$ patients: $^{\#\#}p<0.01$, $^{\#\#\#}p\leq0.001$.

The increases in HO-1 and MnSOD gene expression did not correlate with exercise-induced oxidative stress-derived products; only MDA-protein adducts were slightly increased (Figure 2C) in $COPD_{ND}$ patients.

Leg muscle desaturation

Although by definition $COPD_D$ patients had significantly reduced end-exercise systemic saturation compared to $COPD_{ND}$ patients and controls, no differences were detected in quadriceps tissue desaturation or time constant of recovery of muscle oxygen saturation among the groups (Table 4). Also, no association was found between systemic and local muscle desaturation (Figure 3). To assess whether the Oxphen response was influenced by muscle oxygen saturation, we tested correlations between Oxphen markers and ΔTSI in the combined group of COPD patients and controls, but did not find significant associations. In addition, we stratified the COPD patients based on the median value of ΔTSI to high (≤−9.1%) and low muscle desaturation (>−9.1%) groups, due to lack of a reference value for muscle desaturation. The response of Oxphen markers was not different between the two groups.

Discussion

The mechanisms leading to loss of muscle Oxphen in COPD thus far remain unclear. We recently showed that the Oxphen loss is not limited to advanced disease but also ongoing in earlier phases of the disease, even in absence of muscle wasting. Potential determinants such as disease-associated persistent systemic inflammation and chronic hypoxia are less likely to be causally involved in this stage. As exercise is a potent Oxphen stimulant we hypothesized that a blunted regulatory Oxphen response to exercise would occur in less advanced COPD, resulting from either exercise-induced hypoxia or oxidative stress, or both. However, we did not demonstrate such a blunted response in quadriceps muscle, regardless of co-occurring oxygen desaturation. Also exercise-induced oxidative stress was not aggravated in these patients with less advanced COPD compared to controls. Moreover, as the COPD patients exercised at an intensity significantly lower than that of healthy controls, it could be argued that, adjusted for absolute intensity, the exercise response was even larger in the patients as compared to the controls. In line, after a constant load test at 80% peak capacity in COPD patients and healthy controls, Steiner *et al.* also did not find significantly different exercise-induced changes in absolute magnitude of the muscle metabolites ATP, inosine monophosphate, phosphocreatine and lactate, despite marked differences in workload between COPD patients and controls [36].

Exercise intensity and response

One explanation for the comparable exercise responses in the COPD patients and healthy controls could be that the induction of Oxphen is not linearly related to exercise intensity but rather determined by a threshold that has to be exceeded to invoke a maximal response. The fact that in our study the anaerobic threshold was reached in all healthy controls and almost all COPD patients would be supportive of this hypothesis. Congruently, in healthy individuals only exercise above the lactate threshold has been shown to significantly induce muscle PGC-1α gene expression [37,38]. In COPD patients, however, exercise both below and above the lactate threshold increased PGC-1α gene expression, although the induction was stronger with the latter [38]. Puente-Maestu *et al.* found increased induction of PGC-1α mRNA in muscle of COPD patients compared to healthy controls after a 45-minutes exercise test at 65% of $V'O_{2peak}$ [38]. Whereas the COPD patients in our study had significantly increased PGC-1α gene expression after exercise compared to baseline, the induction in healthy controls only showed a trend to significance. However, we did not observe a significant difference in the magnitude of the exercise-associated induction between the patients and controls. Puente-Maestu *et al.* found an association of PGC-1α mRNA induction with the amount of ROS that was estimated to be produced during the exercise test [38]. In our study there was no evidence of increased oxidative stress in the quadriceps muscle of COPD patients, which together with the lack of a differential response of PGC-1α mRNA with exercise, is in line with the findings by Puente-Maestu.

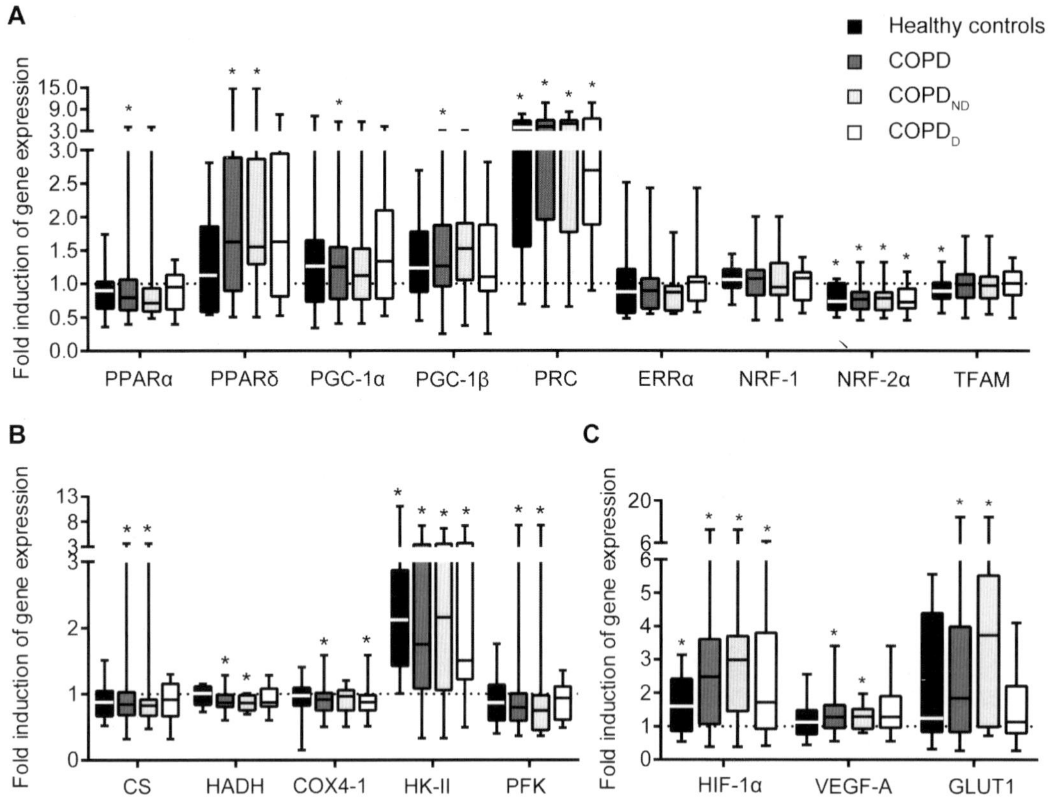

Figure 1. Gene expression responses to exercise are not significantly different between COPD patients and healthy controls, regardless of desaturation status. A Gene expression inductions (post/pre) for regulators of Oxphen. PPAR, peroxisome proliferator-activated receptor; PGC, PPAR gamma co-activator; PRC, PGC-1-related co-activator; ERRα, estrogen-related receptor α; NRF, nuclear respiratory factor; TFAM, mitochondrial transcription factor A. **B** Gene expression inductions for metabolic enzymes involved in citric acid cycle, β-oxidation and glycolysis. CS, citrate synthase; HADH, 3-hydroxyacyl-CoA dehydrogenase; COX4-1, cytochrome *c* oxidase subunit IV isoform 1; HK-II, hexokinase II; PFK, phosphofructokinase muscle isoform. **C** Gene expression inductions of hypoxia-associated targets. HIF-1α, hypoxia-inducible factor 1 alpha; VEGF-A, vascular endothelial growth factor A; GLUT1, glucose transporter 1. Whiskers indicate minimum and maximum values. Level of significance: $^{*}p<0.05$ for post *vs.* pre.

Regulatory gene responses to exercise

Transient induction of PGC-1α gene expression by exercise is well-described (i.e. [13]). Remarkably, in addition to a mild induction of PGC-1α gene expression, we found a strong induction of PRC, a PGC-1-related coactivator involved in mitochondrial respiratory function. Induction of PRC with exercise has been described before in healthy individuals [39], but this is to our knowledge the first time that this marker has been measured in COPD patients in response to acute exercise.

Exercise-induced elevation of HIF-1α gene expression has been proposed to be an important factor in the regulation of adaptive gene responses to exercise [40,41]. In addition to HIF-1α, we found increased expression of some of its target genes, such as VEGF-A, HK-II and GLUT1. The inductions of these genes and PGC-1α and PRC support that there is an ongoing exercise response in the muscle. It is thought that induction of the HIF-1α gene with exercise does not depend on hypoxia *per se*, but may result in increased capillarization and increased glycolytic flux within the mitochondria [40]. Inductions of HIF-1α gene expression have been found to blunt with training [40], and the seemingly stronger inductions of HIF-1α gene expression and its target genes in COPD patients compared to controls could be a reflection of the on average lower physical activity level of the patients.

Exercise-associated hypoxia

In contrast to what we expected, exercise-induced desaturation did not blunt the Oxphen response in COPD patients. This could indicate that acute local hypoxia does not hamper the Oxphen response. Another explanation for the comparable exercise responses between the $COPD_{ND}$ and $COPD_D$ subgroups is that "systemic" oxygen desaturation as measured by finger pulse oximetry does not reflect oxygen desaturation locally in the exercising limb muscle. To define exercise-induced oxygen desaturation, we used the criterion by the American Thoracic Society (ATS), which specifies that the drop in saturation during exercise should be ≥4% [26]. It has also been suggested that desaturation is only clinically relevant when saturation drops below 90% [42], which applied to 12 patients in the current study. However, the outcomes did not change when we used this alternative criterion (results not shown). Indeed, we did not find an association between systemic and skeletal muscle desaturation. The mismatch between systemic and muscle desaturation could be explained by an increased oxygen extraction rate from the systemic circulation to maintain oxygen tension in the muscle but resulting in decreased arterial oxygen saturation in some patients. Nevertheless, we found no significant difference in exercise-induced muscle oxygen desaturation levels among the groups, including the healthy controls, and no associations of muscle desaturation with markers of the Oxphen response.

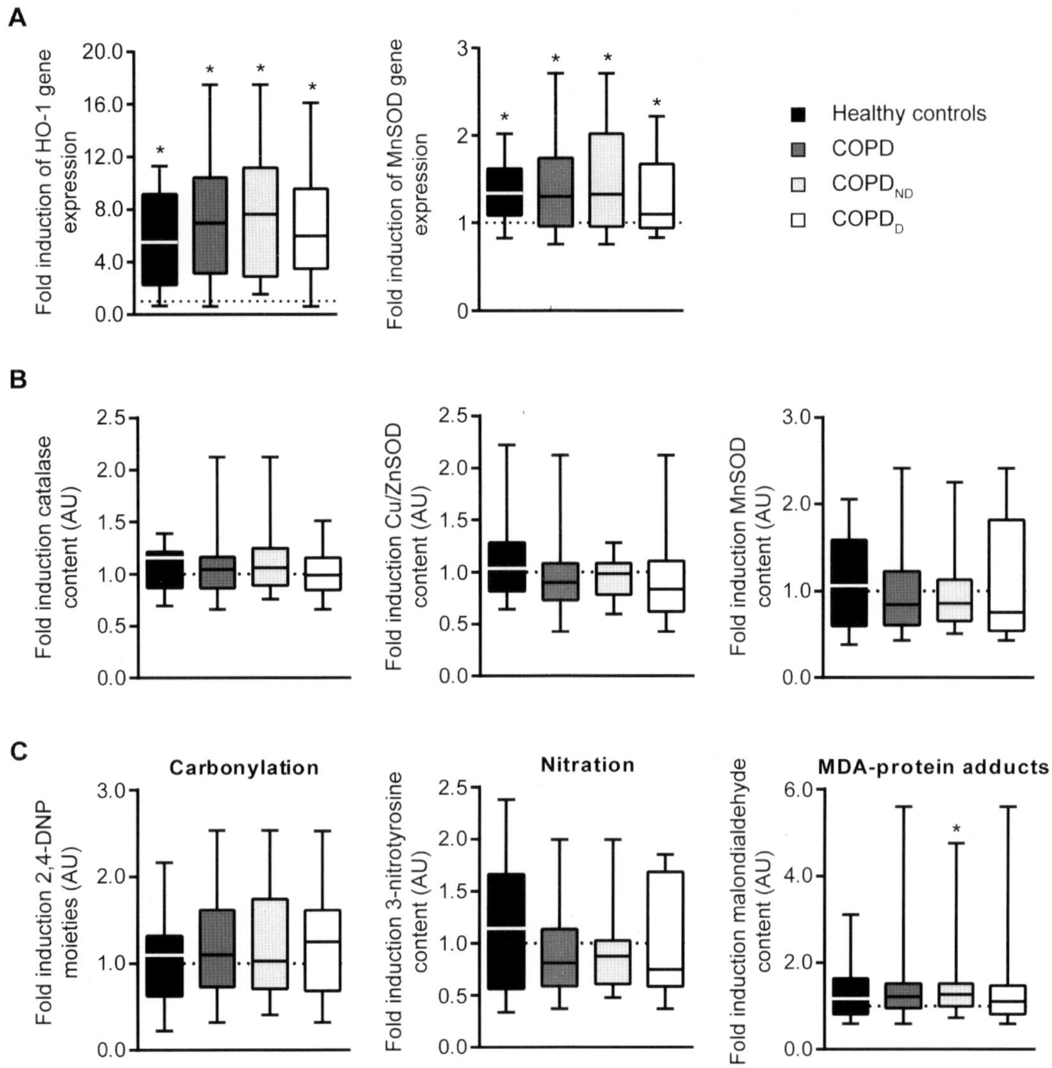

Figure 2. Oxidative stress in quadriceps muscle is only mildly increased in non-desaturating COPD patients; both patients and healthy controls show significant induction of antioxidant genes after exercise. A Box plots of the response of heme oxygenase-1 (HO-1) and manganese superoxide dismutase (MnSOD) genes to exercise presented as fold induction (post/pre). **B** Box plot of the exercise-induced fold inductions of catalase, Cu/ZnSOD and MnSOD content. **C** Box plot of the exercise-induced fold inductions of protein carbonylation, tyrosine nitration and malondialdehyde (MDA)-protein adducts. Whiskers indicate minimum and maximum values. AU, arbitrary units. Level of significance: $^*p<0.05$ for post *vs.* pre.

Exercise-associated oxidative stress response

Previous research in advanced COPD demonstrated an increased resting and exercise-induced oxidative stress response. We also investigated relevant oxidative stress markers in this study

Table 4. Quadriceps desaturation during cycle ergometry.

	Healthy controls	COPD	COPD$_{ND}$	COPD$_D$
ΔTSI, %	−13 (−24, −7)	−9 (−14, −6)	−6 (−14, −5)	−9 (−13, −8)
τ, s	24 (17, 26)	25 (18, 40)	28 (18, 46)	24 (18, 37)

Values are expressed as median (25th percentile, 75th percentile).
Abbreviations: TSI, tissue saturation index; τ, time constant of recovery of muscle oxygen saturation.

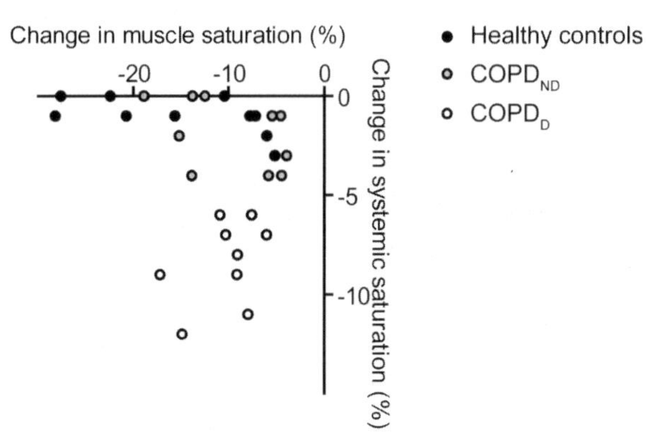

Figure 3. Change in quadriceps muscle saturation during exercise is not associated with systemic desaturation. Reliable muscle saturation data was available for 11 COPD$_{ND}$, 9 COPD$_D$ patients and 11 healthy controls.

to see if a similar enhancement is seen in less advanced COPD, in particular in desaturating patients. No striking differences were observed between COPD patients, subgroups and healthy controls. In contrast Puente-Maestu *et al.* recently described increased exercise-induced oxidative stress in mild to moderate COPD patients, who, similar to those in our study, had a slight loss of muscle Oxphen [43]. However, differences in the intensity of exercise (15 minutes constant work rate at ~65% W_{max} *vs* incremental exercise until exhaustion) and the timing of the muscle biopsy after the exercise test (1 h *vs* 4 h) hamper comparison between our study and theirs.

Although we did not find increased oxidative stress-derived products after exercise, gene expression levels of the antioxidants MnSOD and HO-1 were increased, which is a normal response to exercise [28,44]. The induction of MnSOD and HO-1 gene expression could indicate that the stimulation of the antioxidant system by exercise is not blunted in COPD patients and increased formation of reactive oxygen species by exercise is well-balanced by the antioxidant system [45].

Limitations of the study

A limitation of this study is that only one biopsy was taken after the exercise bout. The timing of the single post biopsy was chosen after careful review of the literature focusing on Oxphen gene expression after exercise, but no inferences can be made regarding differences in the temporal pattern of gene expression changes between COPD patients and controls.

An important constraint of the near-infrared spectroscopy (NIRS) technique is the limited optical penetration depth. As such, subcutaneous fat disturbs or even obstructs the quadriceps NIRS measurement. Therefore, subjects with a large skin fold at the site of the NIRS probe were excluded from the NIRS measurement in our study. We explicitly report this methodological issue as it often seems to be overlooked in the existing literature.

Conclusion

Taken together, the data in this study suggest that patients with less advanced COPD do not have a blunted muscle oxidative regulatory response to acute exercise, regardless of exercise-induced systemic desaturation. This observation, together with a normal oxidative stress response, further supports that incorporation of exercise training as integrated part of COPD management already in early disease could have a pivotal role to prevent or slow down loss of muscle Oxphen and related functional impairment. Further research is needed to investigate if the muscle oxidative regulatory response is blunted in more severe disease stages (i.e. chronic respiratory failure) and disentangle potential contributing factors that may require additional modulation to optimize exercise training in these stages.

Acknowledgments

We thank Kathleen Daenen and Monica Vila-Ubach for their technical support.

Author Contributions

Conceived and designed the experiments: IGMS BvdB VACVH AMWJS HRG. Performed the experiments: IGMS BvdB VACVH EB. Analyzed the data: IGMS BvdB EB AMWJS HRG. Contributed reagents/materials/analysis tools: IGMS BvdB EB AMWJS HRG. Wrote the paper: IGMS BvdB VACVH EB AMWJS HRG.

References

1. Gosker HR, Zeegers MP, Wouters EF, Schols AM (2007) Muscle fibre type shifting in the vastus lateralis of patients with COPD is associated with disease severity: a systematic review and meta-analysis. Thorax 62: 944-949.
2. Maltais F, LeBlanc P, Whittom F, Simard C, Marquis K, et al. (2000) Oxidative enzyme activities of the vastus lateralis muscle and the functional status in patients with COPD. Thorax 55: 848-853.
3. Maltais F, Sullivan MJ, LeBlanc P, Duscha BD, Schachat FH, et al. (1999) Altered expression of myosin heavy chain in the vastus lateralis muscle in patients with COPD. Eur Respir J 13: 850-854.
4. Allaire J, Maltais F, Doyon JF, Noel M, LeBlanc P, et al. (2004) Peripheral muscle endurance and the oxidative profile of the quadriceps in patients with COPD. Thorax 59: 673-678.
5. Layec G, Haseler LJ, Hoff J, Richardson RS (2011) Evidence that a higher ATP cost of muscular contraction contributes to the lower mechanical efficiency associated with COPD: preliminary findings. Am J Physiol Regul Integr Comp Physiol 300: R1142-1147.
6. van den Borst B, Gosker HR, Schols AM (2013) Central fat and peripheral muscle: partners in crime in chronic obstructive pulmonary disease. Am J Respir Crit Care Med 187: 8-13.
7. Remels AH, Gosker HR, Langen RC, Schols AM (2013) The mechanisms of cachexia underlying muscle dysfunction in COPD. J Appl Physiol (1985) 114: 1253-1262.
8. van den Borst B, Slot IG, Hellwig VA, Vosse BA, Kelders MC, et al. (2013) Loss of quadriceps muscle oxidative phenotype and decreased endurance in patients with mild-to-moderate COPD. J Appl Physiol (1985) 114: 1319-1328.
9. Park SK, Richardson CR, Holleman RG, Larson JL (2013) Physical activity in people with COPD, using the National Health and Nutrition Evaluation Survey dataset (2003-2006). Heart Lung 42: 235-240.
10. Gouzi F, Maury J, Molinari N, Pomies P, Mercier J, et al. (2013) Reference values for vastus lateralis fiber size and type in healthy subjects over 40 years old: a systematic review and metaanalysis. J Appl Physiol (1985) 115: 346-354.
11. Natanek SA, Gosker HR, Slot IG, Marsh GS, Hopkinson NS, et al. (2013) Heterogeneity of quadriceps muscle phenotype in chronic obstructive pulmonary disease (Copd); implications for stratified medicine? Muscle Nerve 48: 488-497.
12. Mahoney DJ, Parise G, Melov S, Safdar A, Tarnopolsky MA (2005) Analysis of global mRNA expression in human skeletal muscle during recovery from endurance exercise. FASEB J 19: 1498-1500.
13. Pilegaard H, Saltin B, Neufer PD (2003) Exercise induces transient transcriptional activation of the PGC-1alpha gene in human skeletal muscle. J Physiol 546: 851-858.
14. Itoh K, Itoh M, Ishihara A, Hirofuji C, Hayashi H (1995) Influence of 12 weeks of hypobaric hypoxia on fibre type composition of the rat soleus muscle. Acta Physiol Scand 154: 417-418.
15. Mason SD, Howlett RA, Kim MJ, Olfert IM, Hogan MC, et al. (2004) Loss of skeletal muscle HIF-1alpha results in altered exercise endurance. PLoS Biol 2: e288.
16. Hoppeler H, Vogt M, Weibel ER, Fluck M (2003) Response of skeletal muscle mitochondria to hypoxia. Exp Physiol 88: 109-119.
17. Magalhaes J, Ascensao A, Soares JM, Ferreira R, Neuparth MJ, et al. (2005) Acute and severe hypobaric hypoxia increases oxidative stress and impairs mitochondrial function in mouse skeletal muscle. J Appl Physiol (1985) 99: 1247-1253.
18. Koechlin C, Maltais F, Saey D, Michaud A, LeBlanc P, et al. (2005) Hypoxaemia enhances peripheral muscle oxidative stress in chronic obstructive pulmonary disease. Thorax 60: 834-841.
19. Mercken EM, Gosker HR, Rutten EP, Wouters EF, Bast A, et al. (2009) Systemic and pulmonary oxidative stress after single-leg exercise in COPD. Chest 136: 1291-1300.
20. Barreiro E, Rabinovich R, Marin-Corral J, Barbera JA, Gea J, et al. (2009) Chronic endurance exercise induces quadriceps nitrosative stress in patients with severe COPD. Thorax 64: 13-19.
21. Couillard A, Maltais F, Saey D, Debigare R, Michaud A, et al. (2003) Exercise-induced quadriceps oxidative stress and peripheral muscle dysfunction in patients with chronic obstructive pulmonary disease. Am J Respir Crit Care Med 167: 1664-1669.
22. Picard M, Godin R, Sinnreich M, Baril J, Bourbeau J, et al. (2008) The mitochondrial phenotype of peripheral muscle in chronic obstructive pulmonary disease: disuse or dysfunction? Am J Respir Crit Care Med 178: 1040-1047.

23. Anderson EJ, Neufer PD (2006) Type II skeletal myofibers possess unique properties that potentiate mitochondrial H(2)O(2) generation. Am J Physiol Cell Physiol 290: C844-851.
24. Franssen FM, Broekhuizen R, Janssen PP, Wouters EF, Schols AM (2005) Limb muscle dysfunction in COPD: effects of muscle wasting and exercise training. Med Sci Sports Exerc 37: 2-9.
25. Beaver WL, Wasserman K, Whipp BJ (1986) A new method for detecting anaerobic threshold by gas exchange. J Appl Physiol (1985) 60: 2020-2027.
26. American Thoracic S, American College of Chest P (2003) ATS/ACCP Statement on cardiopulmonary exercise testing. Am J Respir Crit Care Med 167: 211-277.
27. Bergström J (1962) Muscle electrolytes in man. Determination by neutron activation analysis on needle biopsy specimens. A study on normal subjects, kidney patients, and patients with chronic diarrhea. Scand J Clin Lab Invest 14: 1-110.
28. Pilegaard H, Ordway GA, Saltin B, Neufer PD (2000) Transcriptional regulation of gene expression in human skeletal muscle during recovery from exercise. Am J Physiol Endocrinol Metab 279: E806-814.
29. Yang Y, Creer A, Jemiolo B, Trappe S (2005) Time course of myogenic and metabolic gene expression in response to acute exercise in human skeletal muscle. J Appl Physiol (1985) 98: 1745-1752.
30. Ogilvie RW, Feeback DL (1990) A metachromatic dye-ATPase method for the simultaneous identification of skeletal muscle fiber types I, IIA, IIB and IIC. Stain Technol 65: 231-241.
31. Allen D, Winters E, Kenna PF, Humphries P, Farrar GJ (2008) Reference gene selection for real-time rtPCR in human epidermal keratinocytes. J Dermatol Sci 49: 217-225.
32. Vandesompele J, De Preter K, Pattyn F, Poppe B, Van Roy N, et al. (2002) Accurate normalization of real-time quantitative RT-PCR data by geometric averaging of multiple internal control genes. Genome Biol 3: RESEARCH0034.
33. Bergmeyer HU, Gawehn K, Grassl M (1974) 3-Hydroxyacyl-CoA dehydrogenase. In: Bergmeyer HU, editor. Methods of enzymatic analysis. Weinheim; Germany: Verlag Chemie GmbH. pp. 474.
34. Ling KH, Paetkau V, Marcus F, Lardy HA (1966) Phosphofructokinase: I. Skeletal Muscle. Methods Enzymol: Academic Press. pp. 425-429.
35. Shepherd D, Garland PB (1969) Citrate synthase from rat liver. Methods Enzymol: Academic Press. pp. 11-16.
36. Steiner MC, Evans R, Deacon SJ, Singh SJ, Patel P, et al. (2005) Adenine nucleotide loss in the skeletal muscles during exercise in chronic obstructive pulmonary disease. Thorax 60: 932-936.
37. Tobina T, Yoshioka K, Hirata A, Mori S, Kiyonaga A, et al. (2011) Peroxisomal proliferator-activated receptor gamma co-activator-1 alpha gene expression increases above the lactate threshold in human skeletal muscle. J Sports Med Phys Fitness 51: 683-688.
38. Puente-Maestu L, Lazaro A, Tejedor A, Camano S, Fuentes M, et al. (2011) Effects of exercise on mitochondrial DNA content in skeletal muscle of patients with COPD. Thorax 66: 121-127.
39. Russell AP, Hesselink MK, Lo SK, Schrauwen P (2005) Regulation of metabolic transcriptional co-activators and transcription factors with acute exercise. FASEB J 19: 986-988.
40. Lundby C, Gassmann M, Pilegaard H (2006) Regular endurance training reduces the exercise induced HIF-1alpha and HIF-2alpha mRNA expression in human skeletal muscle in normoxic conditions. Eur J Appl Physiol 96: 363-369.
41. Ameln H, Gustafsson T, Sundberg CJ, Okamoto K, Jansson E, et al. (2005) Physiological activation of hypoxia inducible factor-1 in human skeletal muscle. FASEB J 19: 1009-1011.
42. Stoller JK, Panos RJ, Krachman S, Doherty DE, Make B, et al. (2010) Oxygen therapy for patients with COPD: current evidence and the long-term oxygen treatment trial. Chest 138: 179-187.
43. Puente-Maestu L, Tejedor A, Lazaro A, de Miguel J, Alvarez-Sala L, et al. (2012) Site of mitochondrial reactive oxygen species production in skeletal muscle of chronic obstructive pulmonary disease and its relationship with exercise oxidative stress. Am J Respir Cell Mol Biol 47: 358-362.
44. Hollander J, Fiebig R, Gore M, Ookawara T, Ohno H, et al. (2001) Superoxide dismutase gene expression is activated by a single bout of exercise in rat skeletal muscle. Pflugers Arch 442: 426-434.
45. Gosker HR, Bast A, Haenen GR, Fischer MA, van der Vusse GJ, et al. (2005) Altered antioxidant status in peripheral skeletal muscle of patients with COPD. Respir Med 99: 118-125.

8

The Role of Inflammation Resolution Speed in Airway Smooth Muscle Mass Accumulation in Asthma: Insight from a Theoretical Model

Igor L. Chernyavsky[1]*, Huguette Croisier[1], Lloyd A. C. Chapman[2], Laura S. Kimpton[2], Jonathan E. Hiorns[1], Bindi S. Brook[1], Oliver E. Jensen[3], Charlotte K. Billington[4], Ian P. Hall[4], Simon R. Johnson[4]

1 School of Mathematical Sciences, University of Nottingham, Nottingham, United Kingdom, **2** Mathematical Institute, University of Oxford, Oxford, United Kingdom, **3** School of Mathematics, University of Manchester, Manchester, United Kingdom, **4** Department of Therapeutics and Molecular Medicine, University of Nottingham, Nottingham, United Kingdom

Abstract

Despite a large amount of *in vitro* data, the dynamics of airway smooth muscle (ASM) mass increase in the airways of patients with asthma is not well understood. Here, we present a novel mathematical model that describes qualitatively the growth dynamics of ASM cells over short and long terms in the normal and inflammatory environments typically observed in asthma. The degree of ASM accumulation can be explained by an increase in the rate at which ASM cells switch between non-proliferative and proliferative states, driven by episodic inflammatory events. Our model explores the idea that remodelling due to ASM hyperplasia increases with the frequency and magnitude of these inflammatory events, relative to certain sensitivity thresholds. It highlights the importance of inflammation resolution speed by showing that when resolution is slow, even a series of small exacerbation events can result in significant remodelling, which persists after the inflammatory episodes. In addition, we demonstrate how the uncertainty in long-term outcome may be quantified and used to design an optimal low-risk individual anti-proliferative treatment strategy. The model shows that the rate of clearance of ASM proliferation and recruitment factors after an acute inflammatory event is a potentially important, and hitherto unrecognised, target for anti-remodelling therapy in asthma. It also suggests new ways of quantifying inflammation severity that could improve prediction of the extent of ASM accumulation. This ASM growth model should prove useful for designing new experiments or as a building block of more detailed multi-cellular tissue-level models.

Editor: Mohamed Trebak, SUNY College of Nanoscale Science and Engineering, United States of America

Funding: AirPROM 7th European Framework Programme (www.airprom.eu; ILC), Medical Research Council New Investigator Grant G0901174 (www.mrc.ac.uk; BSB & HC), National Centre for the Replacement, Refinement and Reduction of Animals in Research & EPSRC UK Research Council (www.maths-in-medicine.org; all authors). The funders had no role in study design, data collection and analysis, decision to publish or preparation of the manuscript.

* E-mail: Igor.Chernyavsky@nottingham.ac.uk

Introduction

Asthma is a chronic inflammatory disease, characterised by acute inflammatory events during which antigen exposure triggers the production or recruitment of inflammatory cells (mast cells, T-cells, eosinophils, etc.). These cells secrete inflammatory mediators and growth factors which induce acute inflammation and bronchoconstriction of an airway wall over the short term (i.e. minutes to hours) and its remodelling over the long term (i.e. days to months) [1,2].

Airway smooth muscle (ASM) mass increase is an important aspect of both airway remodelling and hyper-responsiveness [3,4]. ASM mass accumulation can be triggered by multiple factors, including inflammation and bronchoconstriction (see Fig. 1). There is ongoing debate regarding the relative contributions of ASM cell proliferation, hypertrophy and recruitment (e.g. via differentiated fibroblasts and myofibroblasts) in asthmatic airways [5–7]. A large number of inflammatory mediators are associated with ASM proliferation *in vitro*, and infiltrating inflammatory cells are a feature of asthma [8]. However, the precise role of these factors in ASM mass accumulation *in vivo* is not well understood [7]. The many factors involved in airway remodelling, combined with the difficulties and risks of invasive airway biopsies in patients with asthma (particularly during exacerbations) and the lack of consensus on animal models and *in vitro* systems, have motivated research on understanding ASM mass increase by non-invasive means, including mathematical modelling [9,10].

Quantitative data on various aspects of lung function and airway inflammation can be used to inform mathematical models. These include [11]: (i) bronchial biopsies, which reveal the amount of airway wall remodelling and allow one to estimate the percentage of proliferating and apoptotic ASM cells; (ii) analyses of inflammatory mediators present in blood and airway sputum differential cell counts; (iii) exhaled nitric oxide concentration measurements, and (iv) lung function tests, in particular forced expiratory volume in one second (FEV_1) recordings. The most direct quantitative information on ASM accumulation, provided by bronchial biopsies, is very limited due to the invasive nature of this procedure. Lung function and inflammatory biomarker measures, however, are more readily performed.

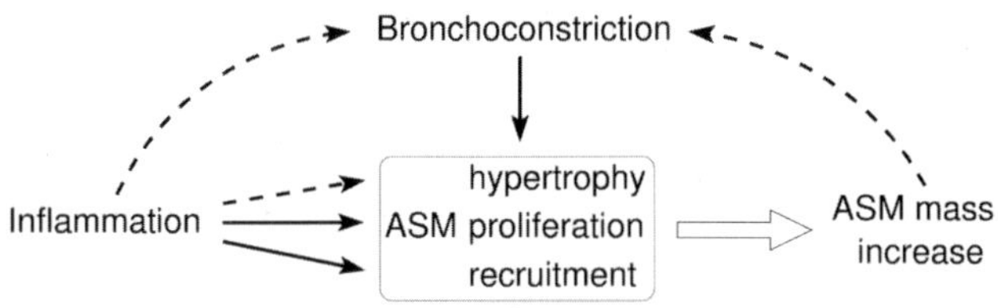

Figure 1. Possible pathways of chronic ASM mass accumulation in asthma (solid lines indicate the mechanisms included in the mathematical model).

In this paper, we focus on developing a simple theoretical model of long-term ASM hyperplasia (proliferation and recruitment) via inflammatory pathways, which has the potential to integrate the information from airway biopsies and inflammatory biomarkers. This model allows possible ASM accumulation scenarios to be explored and suggests possible new targets for diagnosis and prevention of ASM remodelling.

Methods

Model formulation and assumptions

We employ a simple model, schematised in Fig. 2(a), in which we assume ASM cells are either in a proliferative state (which also accounts for recruitment) or a non-proliferative state [12,13]. These are respectively characterized by time-dependent population sizes in an airway wall $p(t)$ and $c(t)$, and the total ASM cell population is denoted $s(t) = p+c$. In the following, "proliferation" refers to both cell replication and recruitment, i.e. it is used as a synonym for hyperplasia.

Switching between the two states is governed by the rates λ_{cp} and λ_{pc}. Proliferation of the p-subpopulation is assumed to follow a logistic law (see S1.1 in Materials S1), with proliferation rate λ_p, and maximal population size ("total capacity") V. The latter implicitly includes the effect of spatial constraints in the airway wall, as well as p-cell apoptosis. For convenience, in the following, all population sizes are normalised by V, so that the maximum total cell population size is $s = 1$. The apoptosis rate of the c-subpopulation, λ_a, is assumed to be much smaller than λ_p ($\lambda_a << \lambda_p$) [14]. We also assume that ASM cells do not remain in the proliferative state for a long time ($\lambda_{pc} >> \lambda_p$).

A third variable, the *inflammatory status* $\mu(t)$, modulates the switching rate λ_{cp} of ASM cells between the non-proliferative and proliferative states (Fig. 2(a,b)). We assume that μ changes in response to environmental stimuli of average magnitude a and average frequency ω and decays with a rate λ_d (the inflammation clearance rate), as illustrated in Fig. 2(c) (see Materials S1 for governing equations). The terminology "inflammatory status" refers in this work to all possible downstream triggers of ASM mass increase, including bronchoconstriction [15,16] (see Fig. 1). Similarly, "exacerbation", or "acute inflammatory event", refers to any substantial rapid increase in the inflammatory status (whether or not this leads to patient hospitalisation).

The way the switching rate λ_{cp} varies as a function of μ, relative to the other rate parameters, is depicted in Fig. 2(b). It is characterised by two thresholds, μ_1 and μ_2, such that:

(1) For $\mu<\mu_1$ (the "healthy" case), λ_{cp} is sufficiently small ($\lambda_a << \lambda_{cp} << \lambda_p << \lambda_{pc}$) for the total ASM cell population to remain approximately stationary (case (1) in Fig. 2(b,d));

(2) For $\mu_1 \leq \mu < \mu_2$ ("mild" inflammation), λ_{cp} is elevated ($\lambda_a << \lambda_{cp} \approx \lambda_p << \lambda_{pc}$) such that the ASM cell population increases on a slow 'remodelling' timescale ($t \approx T >> 1/\lambda_p$, i.e. weeks to months; case (2) in Fig. 2(b,d));

(3) For $\mu \geq \mu_2$ ("severe" inflammation), λ_{cp} is increased further ($\lambda_a << \lambda_p << \lambda_{cp} \approx \lambda_{pc}$), allowing ASM cell population to increase on a fast 'proliferation' timescale ($t \approx 1/\lambda_p$, i.e. days to weeks; case (3) in Fig. 2(b,d)).

Table 1 gives the literature-based values of the model parameters.

We consider both periodic and irregular timing of exacerbation events in the simulations. Given the irregular nature of events that are likely to occur in reality, we seek to explore the impact of this randomness on ASM remodelling. We run a large number of simulations ($N = 1000$), in each of which we allow exacerbation events to occur randomly according to a Poisson process. The resulting fold-increase in ASM mass at 300 days is recorded for each simulation. This may be interpreted as 1000 possible outcomes in an individual subject given the same average characteristics (magnitude and mean frequency) from a given initial state. The outcomes plotted as a histogram then allow quantification of the likelihood of developing severely or moderately remodelled airways. This is analogous to a weather forecast in which a number of different possible outcomes are determined from a given current state.

Solution techniques

We use a combination of analytical techniques (multi-timescale analysis) and computer simulations (with *ode45* MATLAB Runge-Kutta solver) to characterise the dynamics of the ASM cell population growth (see S1.2 in Materials S1 for technical details).

Results

Survey of ASM growth scenarios

The fundamental properties of the model are illustrated in Figure 2(d), where the effect of successive stepwise increases and decreases of the inflammation status μ through the three inflammation regimes (Fig. 2b) is simulated. Over the considered time span (about 1 month in each regime), only severe inflammation (case (3)) leads to substantial growth of the ASM cell population. In the other two cases, the non-proliferative phenotype is predominant and population growth is either negligible (case (1)) or very slow (case (2)). As a consequence, despite μ returning to the initial non-inflammatory value at the end of the considered period (5 months), the ASM cell population size has not decreased to its original value. This feature results from the existence of different timescales in the model and accounts for the persistence of ASM remodelling in asthma beyond acute phases of inflammation (in agreement with a recent chronically-challenged mouse model of asthma [17]). Note that the theoretical model allows for the existence of a very slow decrease in ASM mass in the case of prolonged absence of hyperplastic stimulus (over a timescale of years, thus not apparent in Fig. 2d). Indeed, our model suggests that there is a dynamic balance between state-switching, proliferation and apoptosis in a population of ASM cells: $\lambda_{cp}/\lambda_{pc} \sim \lambda_a/\lambda_p$ (see S1.2 in Materials S1). Such a slow decay in ASM mass has been observed recently in an equine model of asthma (see Discussion and [18]).

Recurrent inflammatory episodes

Figure 3 shows examples of the different proliferation scenarios that can be encountered under a series of regular inflammatory events distributed over about one year, depending on the inflammation magnitude, frequency and resolution rate. When

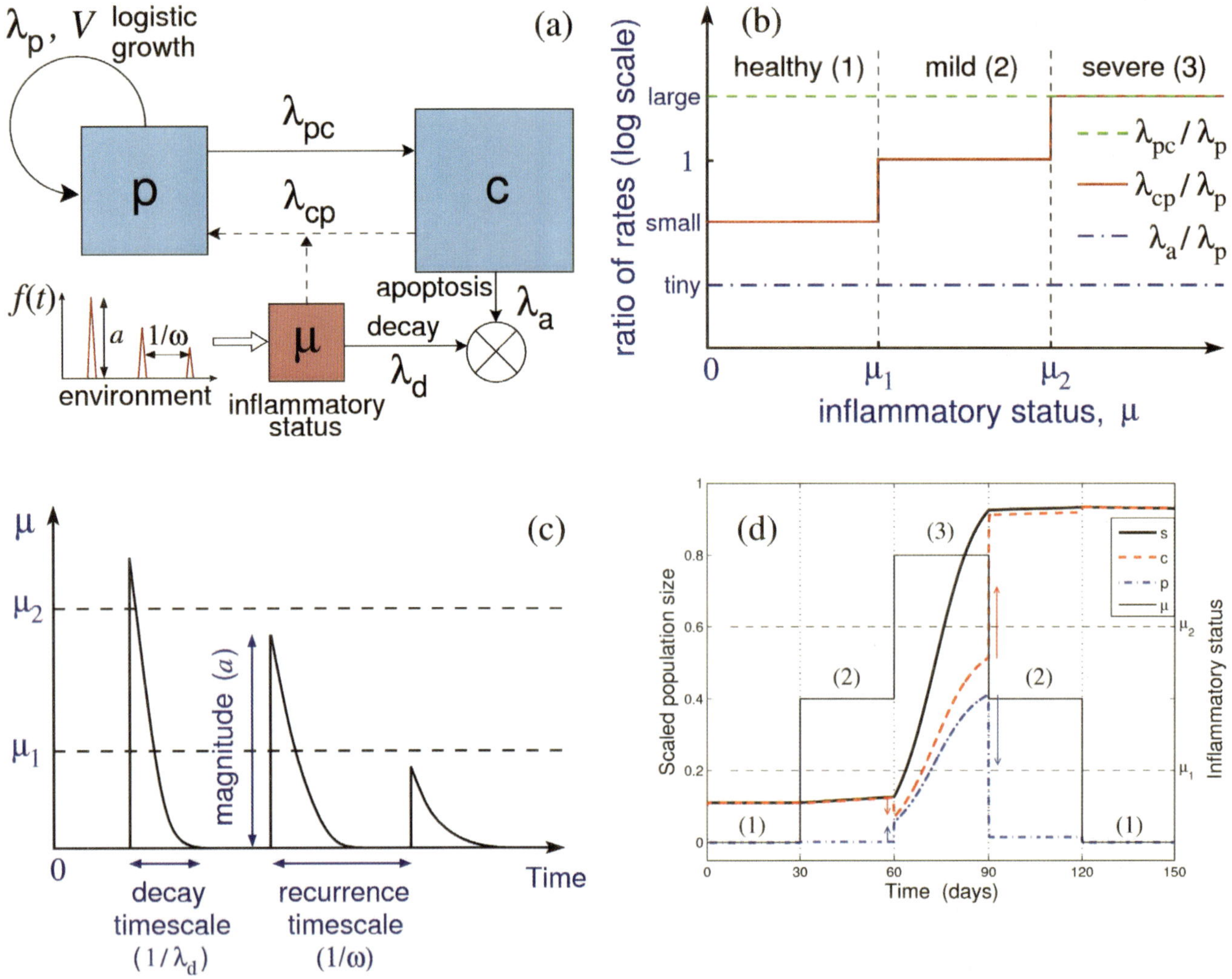

Figure 2. A schematic of the model design. (a) Schematic representation of the model with p being the amount of ASM cells in proliferating state, c the amount of non-proliferative cells and μ the inflammatory status; λ_p is the proliferation rate, λ_a is the apoptosis rate, λ_{cp} and λ_{pc} are the switching rates between non-proliferative and proliferative states, λ_d is the inflammation clearance rate, and $f(t)$ is a time-dependent external inflammatory stimulus. (b) Dependence of the model parameters on the inflammatory status μ (three levels of inflammation are characterised by the thresholds μ_1 and μ_2; see Table 1 for reference values). Rates are plotted on a logarithmic vertical scale. (c) An illustration of the inflammatory status dynamics induced by a series of environmental stimuli such as shown in (a), illustrating graphically the parameters λ_d, a, and ω. (d) A simulation of the ASM cell population response (p, blue dash-dotted; c, red dashed; $s=p+c$, thick black solid) to a stepwise variation in the inflammation status (thin solid); the arrows show the direction of change in the ASM subpopulations. Although the inflammatory status returns to its initial state at the end of the simulation, the total ASM cell population has irreversibly increased, showing thereby "effective" hysteresis. Only the time spent in "severe" regime ($\mu>\mu_2$) contributes to substantial growth (over weeks); however, the "moderate" regime ($\mu_1<\mu<\mu_2$) can also give rise to substantial growth over a longer timescale (months). Note that the proportion of proliferative cells (blue dash-dotted) is significant only during the "severe inflammation" regime (3).

the magnitude of inflammatory events is below the "severe" inflammation threshold μ_2 and the rate of resolution is high, there is no significant ASM mass increase (Fig. 3a); more severe inflammatory events, depending on their magnitude, lead to "moderate" (Fig. 3c) or "severe" (Fig. 3d) long-term ASM mass accumulation. Similarly, changing the frequency of the events from monthly (Fig. 3b) to semi-monthly (Fig. 3c), for the same magnitude and resolution rate, results in about two-fold ASM mass increase.

The outcome of the exacerbation events depends strongly on whether successive inflammatory events accumulate to increase the mean inflammatory status (Fig. 3e) or are independent (Fig. 3(a–d)). In particular, although the frequency and magnitude of inflammatory events are nearly identical in Figs 3(a) and 3(e), the ASM mass remains unchanged in Fig. 3(a) while it increases substantially in Fig. 3(e), due to the slow inflammation resolution.

Figure 4 summarises the possible growth scenarios illustrated in Fig. 3(a–e). The relative fold-increase in ASM population size reached at the end of the observation period (300 days) is plotted as a function of the normalised inflammation resolution rate IR $=\lambda_d/\lambda_p$ (vertical axis), and (on the horizontal axis) the normalised inflammation magnitude a/μ_1 (Fig. 4a) or frequency ω/λ_p (Fig. 4b).

When the inflammation resolution is very slow (small IR $<<1$), the inflammatory status μ accumulates even if individual exacerbations are mild and infrequent, leading to severe increase in ASM mass for a wide range of magnitudes and frequencies (red zones in Fig. 4). Defining the boundaries between "healthy", "moderate" and "severe" outcomes in terms of the isolines for a

Table 1. Literature-based and estimated parameter values used in the ASM growth model.

Parameter	Value	Reference
ASM cell proliferation rate (λ_p) *	$\sim$1/3 days^{-1}	[5,7]
Remodelling time scale (T)	$\sim$100 days	[2]
Time-scale parameter ($\varepsilon = 1/(\lambda_p T)$)	0.02	
Relative $p \to c$ switching rate (λ_{pc}/λ_p)	50 ($\sim\varepsilon^{-1}$)	
Relative $c \to p$ switching rate (λ_{cp}/λ_p)	0.016 ($\sim\varepsilon$) for $\mu<\mu_1$,	
	0.8 ($\sim$1) for $\mu_1<\mu<\mu_2$,	
	40 ($\sim\varepsilon^{-1}$) for $\mu>\mu_2$	
Relative ASM apoptosis rate (λ_a/λ_p)	4×10^{-4} ($\sim\varepsilon^2$)	
Relative severe inflammatory threshold (μ_2/μ_1)	2.5	
Relative inflammatory stimulus magnitude (a/μ_1)	0.1–10	
Relative frequency of inflammatory events (ω/λ_p)	0.1–1 (monthly – weekly)	
Inflammation resolution rate IR = λ_d/λ_p	0.1–10	

(* indicates the values estimated from *in vitro* experiments.)

given long-term fold-increase in ASM mass (the two thick solid lines in Fig. 4(a), corresponding respectively to 2- and 8-fold increase), we see that the chance of an individual being in the "moderate" ASM growth regime, as either the exacerbation magnitude or frequency are increased, drops considerably when the inflammation resolution is slow (IR <1), indicating the possibility of a catastrophic shift straight from the "healthy" to the "severe remodelling" scenario when the inflammation resolution is not fast enough.

For very rapid inflammation resolution (high IR $>>1$), when the individual inflammatory episodes are almost independent of each other, the long-term ASM mass accumulation is determined solely by the total time spent with inflammatory status above the "severe" inflammation threshold ($\mu \geq \mu_2$). Our analysis (see S1.2 in Materials S1) shows that this time is linearly proportional to the exacerbation frequency ω, but the dependence on the relative inflammatory event magnitude a/μ_2 is nonlinear. Hence, the isolines of constant ASM growth are expected to obey IR $\sim (\omega/\lambda_p) \log(a/\mu_2)$ (white dashed lines in Fig. 4; see also S1.2 in Materials S1). This theoretical prediction agrees well with the computed growth isolines (thick black lines in Fig. 4) for IR >1. The model therefore suggests an integral *inflammation severity* (IS) index

$$\frac{(\text{exposure frequency}) \times \log(\text{exposure magnitude})}{(\text{inflammation resolution speed})}$$

(where exposure magnitude is measured relative to the threshold), which has the potential to be used as a predictor of long-term ASM remodelling in the case of moderate-to-fast inflammation resolution. In other words, given the time series of a biomarker of inflammation for a cohort of patients, the model indicates that the IS index computed from these series could correlate with the degree of ASM accumulation in this group.

Individual history effects in ASM growth

For slow recovery from inflammation (IR <1), substantial ASM mass growth can occur even if the inflammatory magnitude lies below the "severe" inflammation threshold ($a<\mu_2$; see e.g. Fig. 3e), in contrast to the fast IR case which requires $a>\mu_2$ for substantial growth. Therefore, the individual history of inflammatory, pro-remodelling events can have a very strong impact on the degree of long-term ASM hyperplasia when successive events can accumulate.

Figure 5 illustrates the importance of history in determining the outcome of a series of inflammatory episodes, when the inflammation resolution is slow. For given inflammation magnitude, frequency and resolution rate, the amount of ASM growth elicited by an inflammatory event depends crucially on the timing of the previous inflammatory events. For example, for regular episodes at a frequency of about once a fortnight (Fig. 5d) and small inflammation magnitude, the inflammatory status lies well within the "moderate inflammation" zone after about 40 days, leading to a "moderate" (less than 3-fold) long-term increase in ASM mass (Fig. 5a). However, when the events occur irregularly (Fig. 5(e,f)) with the same average characteristics as in Fig. 5(d), the individual long-term outcome is much more diverse (Fig. 5(b,c)), due to the possibility of accumulated inflammatory events or prolonged periods of remission.

In order to demonstrate the impact of dangerously frequent exacerbations, Figure 5(g) shows the distribution (histogram) of $N = 1000$ possible outcomes in a given individual at the end of an observation period of 300 days (for a series of random events exemplified in Fig. 5(e,f)). The distribution is bimodal (i.e. has two peaks), with one mode being close to the nearly "healthy" state reached in the absence of randomness (Fig. 5(a,d)), and the other mode corresponding to severe increase in ASM mass (Fig. 5(c,f)). Figure 5(h) shows that an increase of only 25% in the inflammation resolution rate IR can substantially push the mean of the distribution toward the "healthy" mode. This emphasises the importance of individual inflammatory history for prognosis and management of ASM hyperplasia.

We further survey the effect of variability in the timing of acute inflammatory stimuli in Figure 6, which is the analogue of Fig. 4(a) for the case of randomly occurring exacerbation events, and is plotted for a whole range of inflammation resolution rates and magnitudes. Each point in Fig. 6(a) represents the mean long-term fold-increase in ASM mass (at the end of 300 days) for given inflammation characteristics, while each point in Fig. 6(b) represents the variability of the outcome (quantified as the ratio of standard deviation to the mean). Some representative distributions of outcomes are shown in Fig. 6(i–iv).

Figure 6(a) indicates that, at slow resolution rates, the "moderate remodelling" transition zone is larger for random

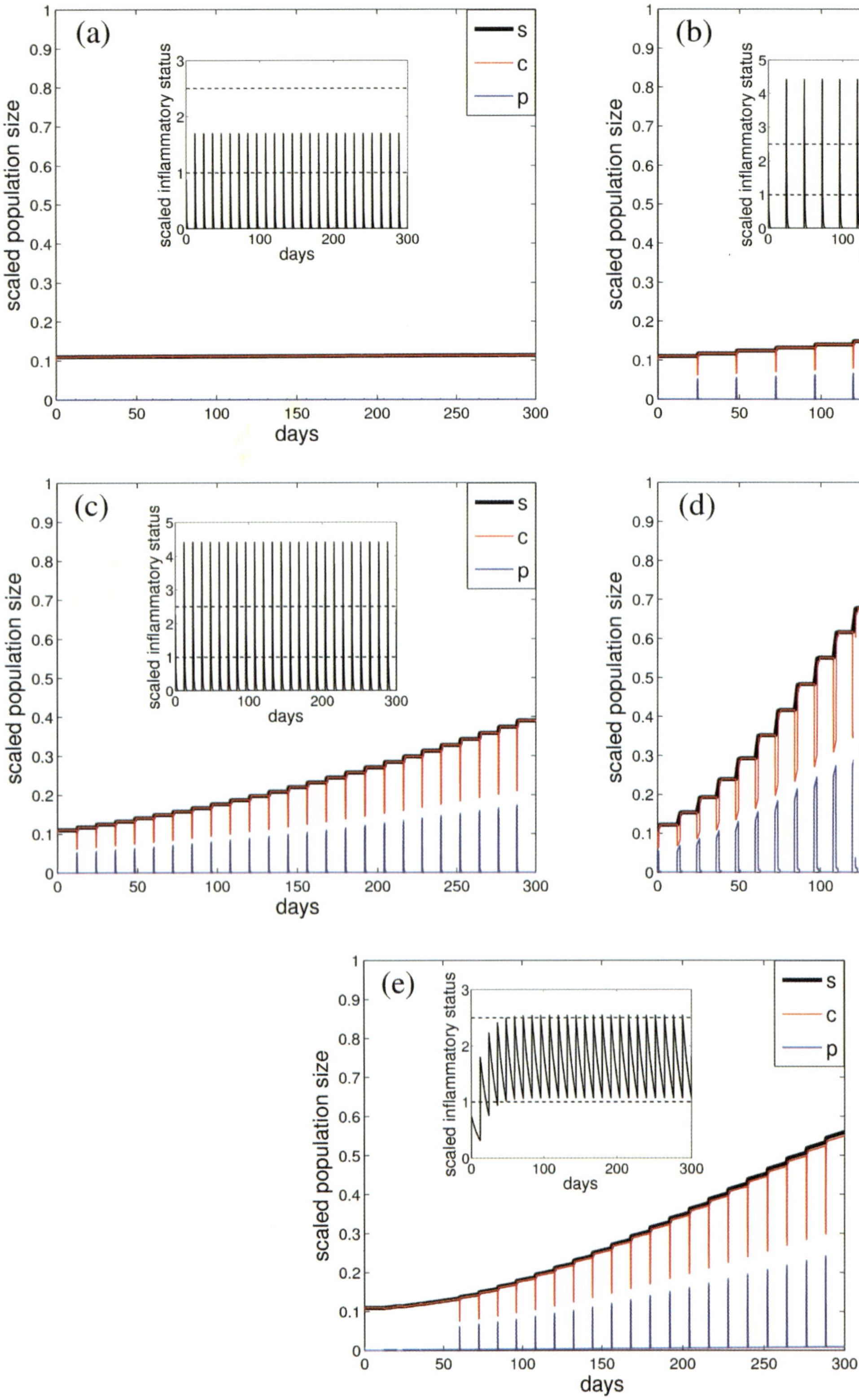

Figure 3. Representative ASM cell population growth dynamics over a period of 300 days, starting from a "healthy" state (c=0.1, p=0.01), for different values of normalised inflammation magnitude a/μ_1, frequency ω/λ_p and inflammation resolution rate λ_d/λ_p: a/μ_1 = {2 (a), 5 (b,c), 8 (d), 1.5 (e)}, ω/λ_p = {0.25 (a,c–e), 0.125 (b)} and λ_d/λ_p = {7 (a), 5 (b,c), 2 (d), 0.22 (e)}. (a,b) show no substantial ASM accumulation, (c,e) show "moderate" and (d) "severe" ASM hyperplasia. The amount of c-cells is depicted by the red line, p-cells (blue) and total population size $s=p+c$ (thick black). Insets plot the corresponding inflammatory status μ (solid black) and the inflammation level thresholds (horizontal dashed lines).

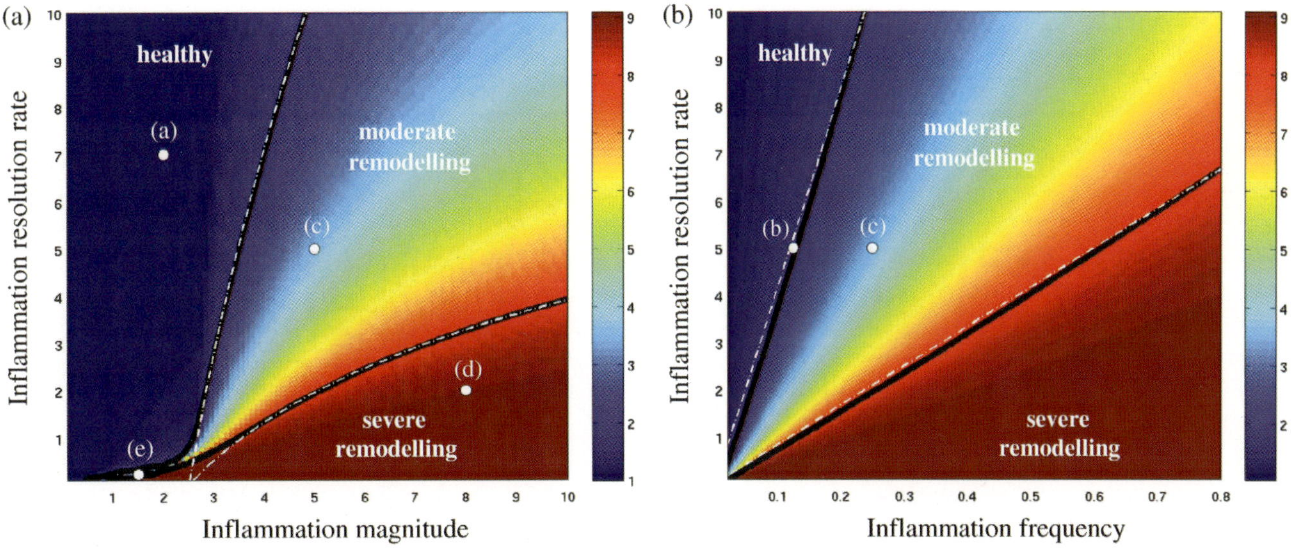

Figure 4. Survey of ASM growth scenarios, showing fold-increase in ASM population size after 300 days (colour scale) as a function of the inflammation resolution rate IR = λ_d/λ_p and (a) inflammation magnitude a/μ_1 (for fixed frequency ω/λ_p = 0.25) or (b) inflammation frequency ω/λ_p (for fixed magnitude a/μ_1 = 5). White dots indicate the growth regimes shown in Fig. 2. Solid black lines are the computed isolines of the 2- and 8-fold ASM growth, which agree with the theoretically predicted dependence $\lambda_d \sim \omega \log a/\mu_2$ (dashed white lines; see Materials S1).

inflammatory episodes (Fig. 6a) than for regular episodes (Fig. 4a). Figure 6(b) shows that the variability of "healthy" and "severe remodelling" outcomes (blue zone in Fig. 6(b)) is very low; uncertainty is mainly concentrated in the "moderate remodelling" zone, and rapidly diminishes as resolution speed increases (Fig. 6b).

The high uncertainty region (yellow-to-red, Fig. 6b) is characterised by a very wide distribution of outcomes, even though some of these distributions (e.g. Fig. 6(iv)) have relatively low mean values of long-term ASM growth. These are therefore as undesirable as high-mean distributions (e.g. Fig. 6(i)) due to a high risk of ending up with "severe" remodelling in the long term.

Discussion

In this work, we have proposed a simple model of inflammation-induced ASM hyperplasia, an important aspect of airway remodelling in asthma. The model assumes that ASM cells can be in one of two states: 'proliferative' (also accounting for the recruitment and differentiation of fibroblasts and myofibroblasts by inflammatory mediators [19]) or 'non-proliferative'. Although the former is usually associated with a synthetic activity, and the latter with a contractile activity, we avoided using this additional terminology here since the synthetic and contractile functions of ASM cells may not be mutually exclusive [20]. Bidirectional switching between the two states is allowed (as observed *in vitro* in both human ASM cells in culture and in human tracheal smooth muscle strips [13,21]), and it is assumed that the level of the inflammatory status μ controls the rate of switching between the two ASM states via the existence of two sensitivity thresholds (Fig. 2b). With the aid of mathematical techniques (see Materials S1), we have shown that this leads to the existence of three corresponding ASM growth regimes (Fig. 2d) and three qualitatively different remodelling outcomes (Figs 4 and 6), matching the classification commonly used in clinical practice [6,22].

The existence of different timescales in the model accounts for several important features of asthma:

i. the persistence of airway remodelling despite the resolution of acute inflammation [1,17], and the correlation of ASM mass with asthma severity rather than with asthma duration [23];
ii. the presence of airway remodelling and abnormal lung function very early in the history of asthma [24];
iii. the very slow decline (of the order of years) in ASM mass in the continued absence of hyperplastic stimuli [18].

Feature (i) can be directly related to Fig. 2(d); feature (ii) can be explained by μ having crossed the severe inflammation threshold, and remained above it a substantial amount of time, early in the disease history; feature (iii) is consistent with the non-negligible role played by apoptosis when the inflammatory status is kept in the healthy range (Fig. 2b) for a sufficiently long time (longer than that considered in Fig. 2(d); see also S1.2 in Materials S1).

Cumulative effects of individual inflammatory history at slow resolution rate

Assuming that inflammatory events are characterised by transient increases in the inflammatory status μ (Fig. 2c), our model predicts that long-term ASM growth is essentially controlled by three parameters: the inflammation resolution speed (IR), the inflammation magnitude (relative to the two sensitivity thresholds μ_1 and μ_2) and the frequency of inflammatory episodes. The severity and frequency of the inflammatory episodes could be targeted to ensure that an asthmatic individual does not fall into the dangerous "severe remodelling" zone (red in Fig. 4). However, our model indicates that faster inflammation resolution could offer a better protection against severe ASM remodelling by increasing the probability of "healthy state" or "moderate" growth (see Figs 4a and 6a).

In addition, irregularity of the occurrence of inflammatory episodes, together with the existence of sensitivity thresholds, lead to a large variability of growth scenarios (see "moderate remodelling" region in Figs 5(b,c) and 6). Thus, one should take into account not only the expected outcome but also the degree of

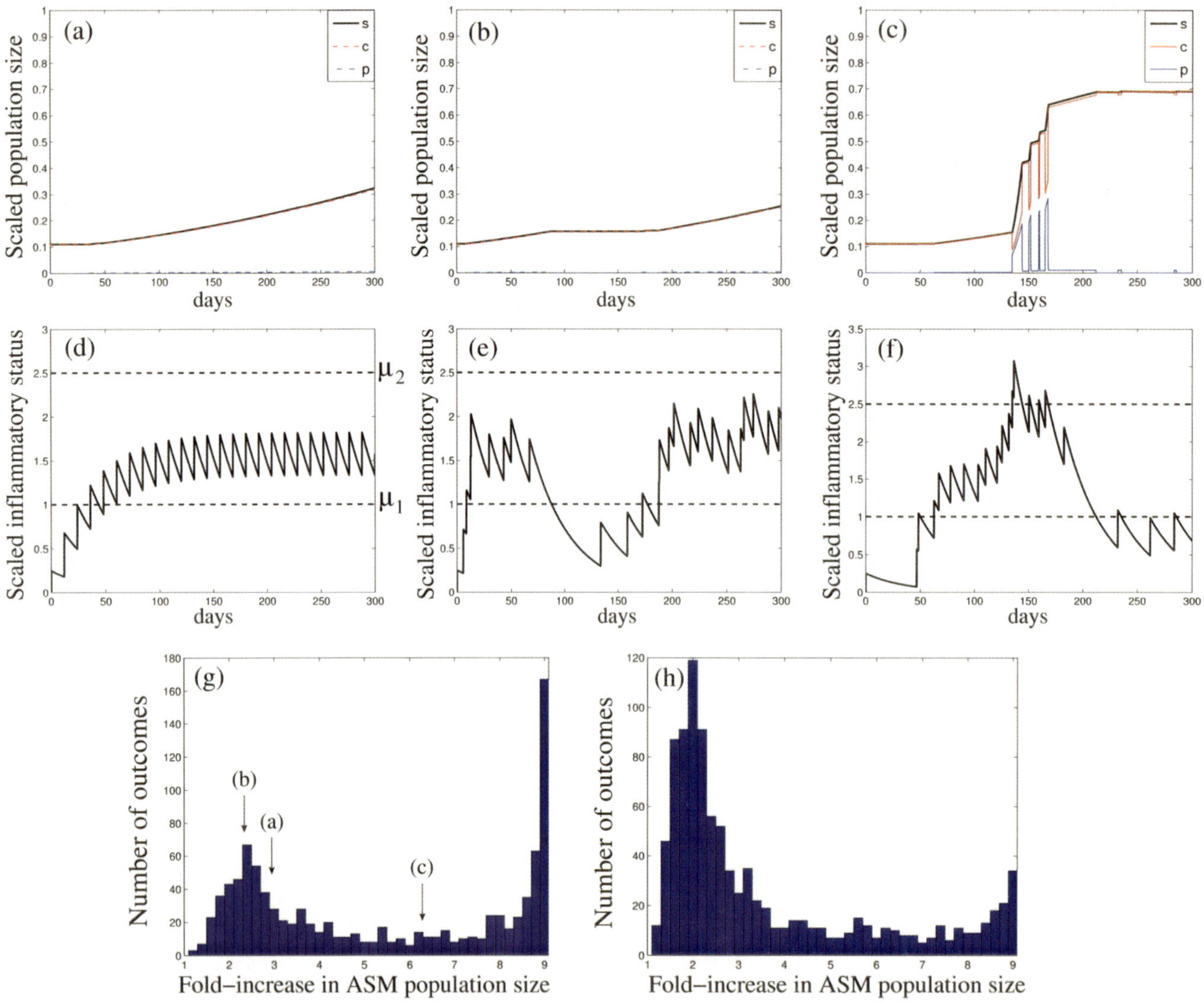

Figure 5. The role of individual inflammation history in the case of slow inflammation resolution (IR <<1). (a–c) ASM population size dynamics (*c*-cells, red; *p*-cells, blue; total population *s*, black) and (d–f) the corresponding inflammatory status evolution (μ, solid black; inflammatory thresholds μ_1 and μ_2, dashed), characterized by the same inflammation resolution rate, magnitude and average stimulus frequency ($\lambda_d/\lambda_p = 0.08$, $a/\mu_1 = 0.5$, $\omega/\lambda_p = 0.25$). (d) Regular series of inflammatory events; (e–f) two realisations of a series of inflammatory events at random times for the same mean frequency (about once a fortnight) as in (d). (g) Distribution of fold-increase in ASM mass after 300 days for a random sequence of inflammatory events with the same characteristics as in panels (b, c); arrows indicate the fold-increase corresponding to (a–c). (h) The distribution of outcomes with an increase of 25% in the inflammation resolution rate ($\lambda_d/\lambda_p = 0.1$). (The outcome histograms (g,h) are computed for $N = 1000$ instances).

uncertainty when deciding on the optimal low-risk treatment strategy (see arrows in Fig. 6a). That means it would be desirable to avoid high outcome variability (Fig. 6b) when navigating towards the "healthy" state by varying the inflammation resolution speed, magnitude or frequency. (Note that another possibility would be to modify the landscape of outcomes itself by elevating the inflammation sensitivity threshold μ_2, thereby "moving the mountain rather than the man"). These results emphasise the importance of individual inflammatory history for prognosis and management of ASM hyperplasia in individuals where slow resolution of inflammation is suspected.

A recent study of a horse model of asthma [18] supports these results by comparing the effect of inflammation resolution speed (modulated by corticosteroids) and the role of frequency and severity of environmental stimuli (by avoidance of antigen exposure). Leclere and colleagues have shown that treatment with corticosteroids gives more rapid (compared to pure antigen avoidance) effects on lung function and ASM remodelling [18], which agrees with our model's prediction of the higher importance of rapid inflammation resolution over stimulus magnitude (see Fig. 6a). This prediction is also supported by the acceleration of ASM mass decline by corticosteroids observed in human peripheral airways after a 6-week treatment [25]. Indeed, the ASM cell population can decrease (very slowly) only when μ is below the mild inflammation threshold (Fig. 2b). The larger the inflammation resolution speed, the sooner this long-term recovery regime can be reached.

Long-term ASM mass accumulation at moderate-to-fast resolution rate

Faster resolution of inflammation decouples individual pro-inflammatory events and thus diminishes the effect of inflamma-

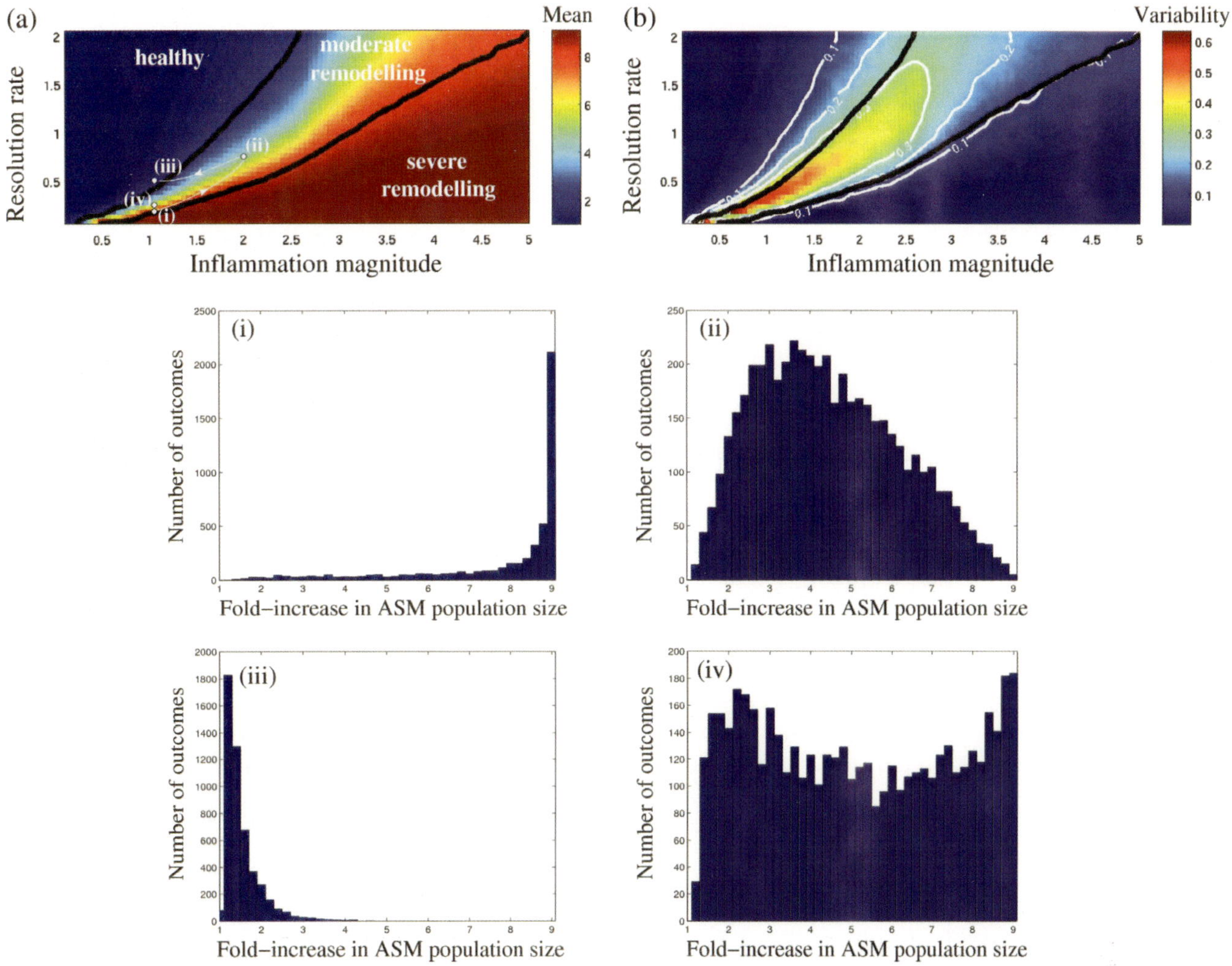

Figure 6. Survey of stochastic ASM growth scenarios in the region of low-to-moderate inflammation resolution rate. (a) Mean fold-increase in the ASM population size at 300 days (colour scale) as a function of inflammation resolution rate IR $=\lambda_d/\lambda_p$ and inflammation magnitude a/μ_1 (*cf.* Fig. 3a). (b) Corresponding uncertainty (colours) quantified as the ratio of SD to the mean; white lines indicate the uncertainty isolines. (Solid black lines in (a,b) show 2- and 8-fold increase in mean; computed for a sample size of $N=500$ random realisations). The parameter dependence of outcome distributions ($N=5000$) are illustrated in (i–iv), indicated by white dots in (a). (Note the variation in vertical scales between panels (i, iii) and (ii, iv)). The quickest transition from (i) to (iii) crosses the high uncertainty region ((iv), red in panel (b)), while a trajectory that bypasses it (white line in (a)) protects against "severe" remodelling outcomes.

tion history in ASM growth. Although this seems to provide greater control over ASM population growth, a mild-to-moderate accumulation of ASM mass over the long term can still occur, provided the magnitude of the exacerbation is above the second threshold μ_2. The model predicts that long-term ASM mass accumulation is proportional to exacerbation frequency but depends less strongly on exacerbation magnitude (see the growth isolines in Fig. 4). The frequency of the pro-inflammatory events could therefore be considered a secondary target, after ensuring rapid resolution of inflammation. The importance of antigen exposure frequency in the degree of airway remodelling has been also confirmed in animal models [26].

Given that resolution of exacerbations can be affected by current therapies [27] and that clinical factors associated with frequent exacerbations are well recognised [28], mechanism-derived links between these factors and exacerbations could be targeted in future studies to prevent airway remodelling.

Model limitations and further development

While accounting for the key features of ASM growth, the proposed model neglects many potentially important factors, such as the detailed pathways governing ASM hyperplasia. However, the kinetic parameters for these pathways remain largely unknown. The generality of our model is also a strength, in that its predictions do not depend on the precise nature of the signalling events (leading to the increase in the "inflammatory status") but only on their dynamical features (magnitude, frequency, resolution speed). In particular, the model is compatible with bronchoconstriction acting as a trigger of airway remodelling [15,16].

We have not included mechanical interaction of the cells between each other and with the extracellular matrix that could affect the growth and apoptosis rates as well as the total capacity V of an airway wall. Our model additionally neglects the spatially heterogeneous and anisotropic growth observed in micrographs and cell hypertrophy. Therefore, the predictions of this ASM growth model are qualitative rather than quantitative.

Extra care should also be taken when interpreting the results of the model in terms of its impact on respiratory lung function. Relative increase in the lumen-narrowing contractile force of an airway wall due to a larger ASM mass could be balanced by a simultaneous increase in the wall stiffness, which may have a constriction-limiting effect [29]. Future models should therefore focus on coupling the mechanics of an airway wall and the ASM population dynamics [29–31].

Further experiments to test the model prediction of the role of inflammation resolution rate in co-cultures of inflammatory and ASM cells or in animal models (such as the studies of Garn and co-workers [17,32]) would be desirable. It would also be of interest to use the model results (in particular, the inflammation severity index) for a detailed statistical analysis of inflammatory status from a time series of inflammatory biomarkers (such as eosinophil counts in sputum or exhaled nitric oxide concentration) and their relation to ASM mass in bronchial biopsies. To our knowledge such longitudinal studies have not yet been performed, due to the difficulties in carrying out repetitive airway biopsies in humans.

Conclusions

We have developed and analysed a theoretical model of ASM mass accumulation driven by a series of exacerbation events. Our model highlights the importance of the resolution speed of inflammation in long-term management of asthma. It exposes the possibility of false security of strict antigen avoidance or reduced sensitivity to inflammatory stimuli. A few accidental exposures or acute exacerbations at impaired resolution can lead to the accumulation of inflammatory status and hence relatively rapid ASM remodelling.

A more robust anti-remodelling strategy could lie in ensuring the rapid clearance of growth or recruitment factors during the post-exacerbation period, thereby protecting against dangerous build-up of these factors, latent ASM mass increase and reducing the risk of severe remodelling.

Acknowledgments

The authors would like to thank all the organisers and participants of the 2011 Mathematics-in-Medicine Study Group (MMSG), in particular, Michelle Baker (University of Nottingham), Dr Anthony M. Holmes (NC3Rs), Dr Joel M. Phillips (University College London) and Thomas J. Snowden (University of Reading) for many discussions that stimulated this study.

Author Contributions

Conceived and designed the experiments: ILC LACC HC BSB OEJ IPH CKB SRJ. Performed the experiments: ILC LACC LSK JEH. Analyzed the data: ILC. Contributed reagents/materials/analysis tools: ILC LACC LSK JEH OEJ. Wrote the paper: ILC HC BSB OEJ CKB SRJ.

References

1. Kariyawasam HH, Aizen M, Barkans J, Robinson DS, Kay AB (2007) Remodeling and airway hyperresponsiveness but not cellular inflammation persist after allergen challenge in asthma. Am J Respir Crit Care Med 175: 896–904.
2. Mauad T, Bel EH, Sterk PJ (2007) Asthma therapy and airway remodeling. J Allergy Clin Immunol 120: 997–1009.
3. Bentley JK, Hershenson MB (2008) Airway smooth muscle growth in asthma: proliferation, hypertrophy, and migration. Proc Am Thorac Soc 5: 89–96.
4. James AL, Elliot JG, Jones RL, Carroll ML, Mauad T, et al. (2012) Airway smooth muscle hypertrophy and hyperplasia in asthma. Am J Respir Crit Care Med 185: 1058–1064.
5. Johnson PRA, Roth M, Tamm M, Hughes M, Ge Q, et al. (2001) Airway smooth muscle cell proliferation is increased in asthma. Am J Respir Crit Care Med 164: 474–477.
6. Hirst SJ, Martin JG, Bonacci JV, Chan V, Fixman ED, et al. (2004) Proliferative aspects of airway smooth muscle. J Allergy Clin Immunol 114: S2–S17.
7. Kaur D, Hollins F, Saunders R, Woodman L, Sutcliffe A, et al. (2010) Airway smooth muscle proliferation and survival is not modulated by mast cells. Clin Exp Allergy 40: 279–288.
8. Brightling CE, Bradding P, Symon FA, Holgate ST, Wardlaw AJ, et al. (2002) Mast-cell infiltration of airway smooth muscle in asthma. N Engl J Med 346: 1699–1705.
9. Baker M, Billington C, Chapman LAC, Chernyavsky IL, Croisier H, et al. (2011) Mathematical modelling of airway smooth muscle cell proliferation and apoptosis in asthma. Reading: Mathematics-in-Medicine Study Group Report. 31 p.
10. Holmes AM, Solari R, Holgate ST (2011) Animal models of asthma: value, limitations and opportunities for alternative approaches. Drug Discov Today 16: 659–670.
11. Contoli M, Bousquet J, Fabbri LM, Magnussen H, Rabe KF, et al. (2010) The small airways and distal lung compartment in asthma and COPD: a time for reappraisal. Allergy 65: 141–151.
12. Halayko AJ, Camoretti-Mercado B, Forsythe SM, Vieira JE, Mitchell RW, et al. (1999) Divergent differentiation paths in airway smooth muscle culture: induction of functionally contractile myocytes. Am J Physiol - Lung Cell Mol Physiol 276: L197–L206.
13. Dekkers BG, Bos IST, Zaagsma J, Meurs H (2012) Functional consequences of human airway smooth muscle phenotype plasticity. Br J Pharmacol 166: 359–367.
14. Markwick LJ, Clements D, Roberts ME, Ceresa CC, Knox AJ, et al. (2012) CCR3 induced-p42/44 MAPK activation protects against staurosporine induced-DNA fragmentation but not apoptosis in airway smooth muscle cells. Clin Exp Allergy 42: 1040–1050.
15. Grainge CL, Lau LCK, Ward JA, Dulay V, Lahiff G, et al. (2011) Effect of bronchoconstriction on airway remodeling in asthma. N Engl J Med 364: 2006–15.
16. Tatler AL, John AE, Jolly L, Habgood A, Porte J, et al. (2011) Integrin αvβ5-mediated TGF-β activation by airway smooth muscle cells in asthma. J Immunol 187: 6094–107.
17. Alrifai M, Marsh LM, Dicke T, Kılıç A, Conrad ML, et al. (2014) Compartmental and temporal dynamics of chronic inflammation and airway remodelling in a chronic asthma mouse model. PLoS ONE 9: e85839.
18. Leclere M, Lavoie-Lamoureux A, Joubert P, Relave F, Setlakwe EL, et al. (2012) Corticosteroids and antigen avoidance decrease airway smooth muscle mass in an equine asthma model. Am J Respir Cell Mol Biol 47: 589–596.
19. Alkhouri H, Hollins F, Moir LM, Brightling CE, Armour CL, et al. (2011) Human lung mast cells modulate the functions of airway smooth muscle cells in asthma. Allergy 66: 1231–1241.
20. Hirota JA, Nguyen TT, Schaafsma D, Sharma P, Tran T (2009) Airway smooth muscle in asthma: Phenotype plasticity and function. Pulm Pharmacol Ther 22: 370–378.
21. Hirst SJ, Twort CHC, Lee TH (2000) Differential effects of extracellular matrix proteins on human airway smooth muscle cell proliferation and phenotype. Am J Respir Cell Mol Biol 23: 335–344.
22. Louis R, Sele J, Henket M, Cataldo D, Bettiol J, et al. (2002) Sputum eosinophil count in a large population of patients with mild to moderate steroid-naive asthma: distribution and relationship with methacholine bronchial hyperresponsiveness. Allergy 57: 907–912.
23. James AL, Bai TR, Mauad T, Abramson MJ, Dolhnikoff M, et al. (2009) Airway smooth muscle thickness in asthma is related to severity but not duration of asthma. Eur Respir J 34: 1040–5.
24. Payne DNR, Rogers AV, Adelroth E, Bandi V, Guntupalli KK, et al. (2003) Early thickening of the reticular basement membrane in children with difficult asthma. Am J Respir Crit Care Med 167: 78–82.
25. Bergeron C, Hauber HP, Gotfried M, Newman K, Dhanda R, et al. (2005) Evidence of remodeling in peripheral airways of patients with mild to moderate asthma: effect of hydrofluoroalkane-flunisolide. J Allergy Clin Immunol 116: 983–9.
26. Allen JE, Bischof RJ, Sucie Chang H-Y, Hirota JA, Hirst SJ, et al. (2009) Animal models of airway inflammation and airway smooth muscle remodelling in asthma. Pulm Pharmacol Ther 22: 455–465.
27. Tattersfield AE, Postma DS, Barnes PJ, Svensson K, Bauer C-A, et al. (1999) Exacerbations of asthma. Am J Respir Crit Care Med 160: 594–599.
28. ten Brinke A, Sterk PJ, Masclee AAM, Spinhoven P, Schmidt JT, et al. (2005) Risk factors of frequent exacerbations in difficult-to-treat asthma. Eur Respir J 26: 812–818.

29. Brook BS, Peel SE, Hall IP, Politi AZ, Sneyd J, et al. (2010) A biomechanical model of agonist-initiated contraction in the asthmatic airway. Respir Physiol Neurobiol 170: 44–58.
30. Byrne H, Preziosi L (2003) Modelling solid tumour growth using the theory of mixtures. Math Med Biol 20: 341–366.
31. Moulton DE, Goriely A (2011) Possible role of differential growth in airway wall remodeling in asthma. J Appl Physiol 110: 1003–1012.
32. Wegmann M, Fehrenbach H, Fehrenbach A, Held T, Schramm C, et al. (2005) Involvement of distal airways in a chronic model of experimental asthma. Clin Exp Allergy 35: 1263–1274.

9

Gene Expression Profiling in Tibial Muscular Dystrophy Reveals Unfolded Protein Response and Altered Autophagy

Mark Screen[1]*, Olayinka Raheem[2], Jeanette Holmlund-Hampf[1], Per Harald Jonson[1], Sanna Huovinen[2,3], Peter Hackman[1], Bjarne Udd[1,2,4]

1 Folkhälsan Institute of Genetics and Department of Medical Genetics, Haartman Institute, University of Helsinki, Helsinki, Finland, **2** Neuromuscular Research Unit, Department of Neurology, University Hospital and University of Tampere, Tampere, Finland, **3** Department of Pathology, Fimlab Laboratories, Tampere University Hospital and University of Tampere, Tampere, Finland, **4** Department of Neurology, Vaasa Central Hospital, Vaasa, Finland

Abstract

Tibial muscular dystrophy (TMD) is a late onset, autosomal dominant distal myopathy that results from mutations in the two last domains of titin. The cascade of molecular events leading from the causative *Titin* mutations to the preterm death of muscle cells in TMD is largely unknown. In this study we examined the mRNA and protein changes associated with the myopathology of TMD. To identify these components we performed gene expression profiling using muscle biopsies from TMD patients and healthy controls. The profiling results were confirmed through quantitative real-time PCR and protein level analysis. One of the pathways identified was activation of endoplasmic reticulum (ER) stress response. ER stress activates the unfolded protein response (UPR) pathway. UPR activation was supported by elevation of the marker genes *HSPA5*, *ERN1* and the UPR specific *XBP1* splice form. However, UPR activation appears to be insufficient to correct the protein abnormalities causing its activation because degenerative TMD muscle fibres show an increase in ubiquitinated protein inclusions. Abnormalities of VCP-associated degradation pathways are also suggested by the presence of proteolytic VCP fragments in western blotting, and VCP's accumulation within rimmed vacuoles in TMD muscle fibres together with p62 and LC3B positive autophagosomes. Thus, pathways controlling turnover and degradation, including autophagy, are distorted and lead to degeneration and loss of muscle fibres.

Editor: Atsushi Asakura, University of Minnesota Medical School, United States of America

Funding: The study received funding from the Folkhälsan Research Foundation, the University of Helsinki, the National Doctoral Program of Musculoskeletal Disorders and Biomaterials. Research grants from the Liv och Hälsa Foundation and Vaasa Central Hospital District Medical Research funds are also acknowledged. The funders had no role in study design, data collection and analysis, decision to publish, or preparation of the manuscript.

* E-mail: mark.screen@helsinki.fi

Introduction

Tibial muscular dystrophy (TMD, OMIM: #600334, Udd myopathy) is an autosomal dominant distal myopathy with a particularly high prevalence in the Finnish population [1–3]. The disease is caused by heterozygous mutations in the last two exons (Mex5-6) of the *Titin (TTN)* gene [4]. Five other phenotypes have been reported to be associated with C-terminal titin mutations: recessive limb-girdle muscular dystrophy type 2J (LGMD2J) [2], dominant hereditary myopathy with early respiratory failure [5,6], recessive early-onset myopathy with fatal cardiomyopathy [7], core myopathy with heart disease [8] and centronuclear myopathy [9]. All Finnish TMD patients reported so far share the 11 bp deletion/insertion FINmaj founder mutation [1,2], which results in C-terminal defects in the M-line region of the sarcomeric titin protein [2]. Several other mutations in the last two exons of *TTN* have been shown to cause TMD in patients of other European populations [4,10,11].

TMD is clinically characterised by atrophy and weakness in the muscles of the anterior compartment of the lower leg (*tibialis anterior*, *extensor hallucis longus* and *extensor digitorum longus*) [3], with typical onset between 35–55 years [12]. Homozygous FINmaj mutations cause the manifestation of the completely different, and much more severe, early onset LGMD2J (OMIM: #608807) [2,3,13]. TMD and LGMD2J patients do not have facial muscle weakness, dysphagia or clinically manifest cardiomyopathy. TMD muscle biopsies show myopathic–dystrophic morphology with rare fibre necrosis and frequent rimmed vacuolated fibres in affected muscles [3,12,14].

Titin molecules are integral to striated muscle structure and function by forming the backbone of the continuous third filament system of the myofibrils. The titin molecule stretches from the Z-disc to the M-line of the sarcomere. One of titin's core functions is to provide muscle elasticity by returning thin and thick filaments to their positions after contractions [15,16]. The last Ig-domain (M10) containing the FINmaj mutation is adjacent to the differentially spliced [17] is7 domain that contains a calpain-3 (CAPN3) binding site [13]. Immunofluorescent (IF) microscopy of homozygous mutant muscles has revealed an absence of C-terminal titin epitopes from at least the three last domains M9, is7 and M10 [2]. Together with the loss of M-line CAPN3 and mislocalization of the C-terminal ligand obscurin, this suggests that the FINmaj mutation leads to a proteolytic cleavage of the titin C-terminus [13,18,19].

As the downstream molecular pathology caused by the FINmaj mutation is still largely unknown, the objective of this study was to identify relevant changes through global expression profiling of affected distal muscles from TMD patients. Significantly changed pathways were identified and confirmed through quantitative real-time PCR and protein level analysis of marker molecules.

Materials and Methods

Ethics statement

All patient biopsies were obtained with written informed consent and according to the Helsinki declaration. The study was approved by the institutional review board of Helsinki University Hospital.

Muscle biopsies

All patients were diagnosed based on DNA mutation testing. Control and patient biopsies were obtained from the distal muscles of male and female patients in a range of ages (37–92; Table 1).

RNA preparation

RNA was extracted from frozen muscles samples using RNAeasy mini kit's (Qiagen, USA) recommended protocol. The RNA quality was assessed using a 2100 Bioanalyzer and the Eukaryote total RNA Nano series II program (Agilent technologies, USA).

Microarray analysis

3 μg of total RNA was used to generate double stranded cDNA. The cRNA was generated using either one- or two-cycle eukaryote target labelling along with controls supplied with the kit (Affymetrix, USA). The samples were biotin labelled and the cRNA randomly fragmented before hybridisation to Affymetrix U133plus2 microarrays following the manufacturer's instructions. The microarray chips were washed and stained using Affymetrix Fluidics Station and scanned using a GeneChip Scanner 3000.

Expression values were determined using Affymetrix Microarray Suite 5.0 and GeneSpring GX version 11.0 (Agilent Technologies, USA) was used for pre-processing the data using the MAS5 algorithm. All probe sets with absent flags were removed from the data. The data was baseline transformed to the median of all samples. Differentially expressed genes were detected using an unpaired *t*-test with unequal variance (Welch correction). *P*-values were corrected using a Benjamini-Hochberg adjustment for multiple testing. Probe sets having a $P<0.05$ and at least a two-fold change were considered to be differentially expressed. The microarray data is available from the GEO website (http://www.ncbi.nlm.nih.gov/geo/) with accession number GSE42806.

Table 1. Summary of patient and control muscle biopsies.

Expression array	qPCR	WB/IF/IHC	Biopsy	Diagnosis	Sex	Age at biopsy	Pathology
T1	rT1		EHL	TMD	M	53	Rimmed vacuoles
T2			GL	TMD	M	62	No rimmed vacuoles
T3			TA	TMD	M	48	Rimmed vacuoles
T4	rT2	TMD 5	EHL	TMD	M	65	Rimmed vacuoles
T5			SOL	TMD	M	52	Rimmed vacuoles
T6			TP	TMD	M	52	No major pathology
T7			TA	TMD	M	52	Rimmed vacuoles
	rT3		EHL	TMD	M	92	Not known
	rT4		TA	TMD	M	73	Rimmed vacuoles
	rT5		TA	TMD	M	78	Rimmed vacuoles
		TMD 1	EHL	TMD	M	62	Rimmed vacuoles
		TMD 2	TA	TMD	M	55	Rimmed vacuoles
		TMD 3	GM	TMD	M	67	Rimmed vacuoles
		TMD 4	EDL	TMD	F	50–55	Rimmed vacuoles
		TMD 6	TA	TMD	M	44	Rimmed vacuoles
C1	rC1		TP	Control	M	76	Normal
C2			EHL	Control	M	76	Normal
C3	rC2		TA	Control	M	80	Normal
C4	rC3		EHL	Control	M	80	Normal
C5			SOL	Control	M	76	Normal
		Ctrl 1	TA	Control	M	37	Normal
		Ctrl 2	TA	Control	F	48	Normal
		Ctrl 3	THP	Control	F	91	Normal

Tibialis anterior (TA), *tibialis posterior* (TP), *gastrocnemius lateralis* (GL), *gastrocnemius medialis* (GM), *soleus* (SOL), *extensor hallucis longus* (EHL), *extensor digitorum longus* (EDL), thigh posterior (THP), immunofluorescence microscopy (IF), western blotting (WB) and immunohistochemistry (IHC). The expression array controls (C1, C2 & C5) and (C3 & C4) were collected from amputation material from the distal lower limb muscles of two individuals.

Pathway Analysis

Pathway analysis was done using Ingenuity Pathway Analysis software (www.ingenuity.com). The significance of each canonical pathway having more affected genes than expected by chance in the data set was determined by the Fisher's exact *t*-test ($P<0.05$).

Quantitative real-time PCR

RNA was extracted from tissue biopsies using a Trizol (Invitrogen, USA) based protocol according to the manufacturer's suggestions. 1 µg of total RNA was reverse-transcribed to cDNA using SuperScript II Reverse Transcriptase (Invitrogen, USA) following the manufacturer's protocol. Quantification of the cDNA was performed using TaqMan based quantitative real-time PCR. The primers and probes used were the spliced form of *XBP1* (Hs00231936_m1), *HSPA5* (Hs00607129_gH), *ERN1* (Hs00980093_m1), *JUN* (Hs99999141_s1), *HSPB1* (Hs03044127_g1) and *GAPDH* (4333764F). 10 µl TaqMan master mix (Applied Biosystems, USA), 0.5 µl 1:10 diluted cDNA and 2 µl of primer and probe set were used in a 20 µl total reaction volume. Amplification and detection were performed using the ABI 7500 system (Applied Biosystems, USA). The PCR thermal conditions were 50°C for 2 min, 95°C for 10 s and 60°C for 1 min. Each sample was performed in triplicate and the expression was normalised to *GAPDH* using standard curves for each gene on the same plate.

Statistical analysis

Statistical significance of the quantitative real-time PCR and western blotting results were calculated using an unpaired *t*-test ($P<0.05$).

Western blotting

Muscle biopsies were homogenized with 19 volumes of sample buffer containing 4 M urea and 4% SDS at 100°C for 5 min. Samples were resolved using 12% SDS-PAGE gels with 4% stacking gels and transferred to PVDF membranes (Bio-Rad Laboratories, USA). Membranes were blocked in TBST 5% milk for 1 h at +4°C. Primary and secondary HPR-conjugated antibodies were incubated at +4°C for 1 h each, followed by 6× TBST (5 min) washes. Antibodies were detected using the SuperSignal West Femto ECL substrate (Pierce, Thermo Scientific, USA) and captured using photographic film. Protein loading was assessed by staining of the post-blotting gel using Bio-Safe Coomassie Stain (Bio-Rad Laboratories, USA). Antibodies used are listed in Table S1. Quantitative analysis of western blotting bands was performed using ImageJ version 1.46f (http://rsb.info.nih.gov/ij/).

Immunohistochemistry and immunofluorescence

Muscle biopsies were snap frozen in liquid nitrogen cooled isopentane to make 6 µm cryosections on SuperFrost (Kindler GmbH, Germany). The sections were fixed in 4% PFA for 10 min, permeabilized in 0.2% Triton X-100 for 10 min, and blocked in 5% BSA for 30 min at room temperature. The DAB immunohistochemistry (IHC) (Universal DAB detection, Ventana, USA) was performed using the BenchMark automated immunostainer following manufacturer's instructions. LAMP2 IHC signal was enhanced using an amplification kit (cat. 760-080, Ventana, USA). Herovici staining (a modified van Gieson stain) on frozen muscle sections was used for identification of the rimmed vacuoles. The immunofluorescence microscopy was performed as described earlier [20]. Antibodies are listed in Table S1.

Results

Expression profiling and pathway analysis

The expression profiles of seven TMD and five control biopsy samples were hierarchically clustered (Fig. 1). Significantly ($P<0.05$) changed probe sets in the TMD samples representing all differentially expressed transcripts are given in Table S2. Ingenuity Pathway Analysis (IPA) showed that endoplasmic reticulum (ER) stress response-, NRF2 mediated oxidative stress-, PTEN-, integrin- and EIF2- signalling pathways were among the most clearly affected pathways in TMD (Fig. 2A, 2B & 2C). There were also a range of pathway changes that have been identified in other myopathies with rimmed vacuoles such as; SAPK/JNK apoptosis- [21], p70S6K- [22,23], protein ubiquitination- [23,24] and mitochondrial dysfunction- [24,25] signalling (Fig. 2B, 2C, & 2D).

Verification of selected expression changes by quantitative real-time PCR

We chose to investigate ER stress response in TMD muscle since this pathway had the highest fraction of genes with significantly changed expression compared to controls. Unfolded protein response (UPR) is the main mechanism used to alleviate the effects of ER stress. HSPB1 proteins are involved in the ER stress response [26], whilst HSPA5 (BIP) [27], ERN1 (IRE1) [28] and the spliced form of XBP1 [29] are involved in the UPR pathway. Significant ($P<0.05$) up-regulation was observed in the expression of *HSPA5* (Fig. 3A), *HSPB1* (Fig. 3B), *ERN1* (Fig. 3C) and the previously described UPR specific *XBP1* splice isoform (Fig. 3D) in TMD samples versus controls.

The SAPK/JNK apoptotic signalling pathway was significantly ($P<0.05$) changed in the TMD samples compared to controls in IPA analysis. We analysed *JUN* (*CJUN*) expression by quantitative real-time PCR, as it is a final stage component of this pathway, and found significantly elevated expression levels of *JUN* in TMD samples (Fig. 3E).

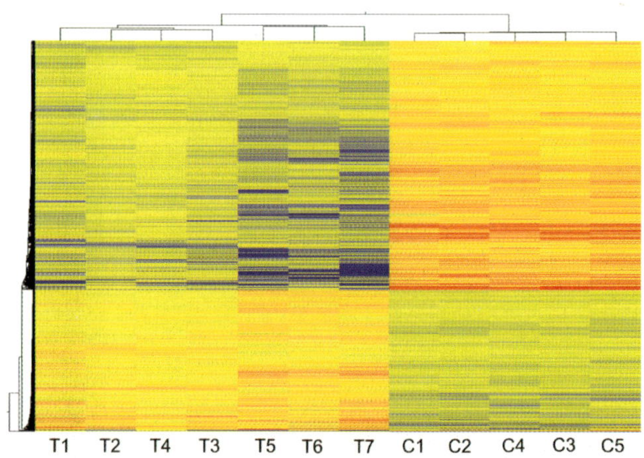

Figure 1. Hierarchal clustering of TMD and control expression profiles. Clustering of differentially expressed probes using centroid linkage and euclidean similarity in GeneSpring GX v11.0. The expression profiles of TMD (T1–T5) and controls (C1–C5) are represented as a heatmap (blue = low expression, red = high expression). A list of significantly changed probes is in Table S2.

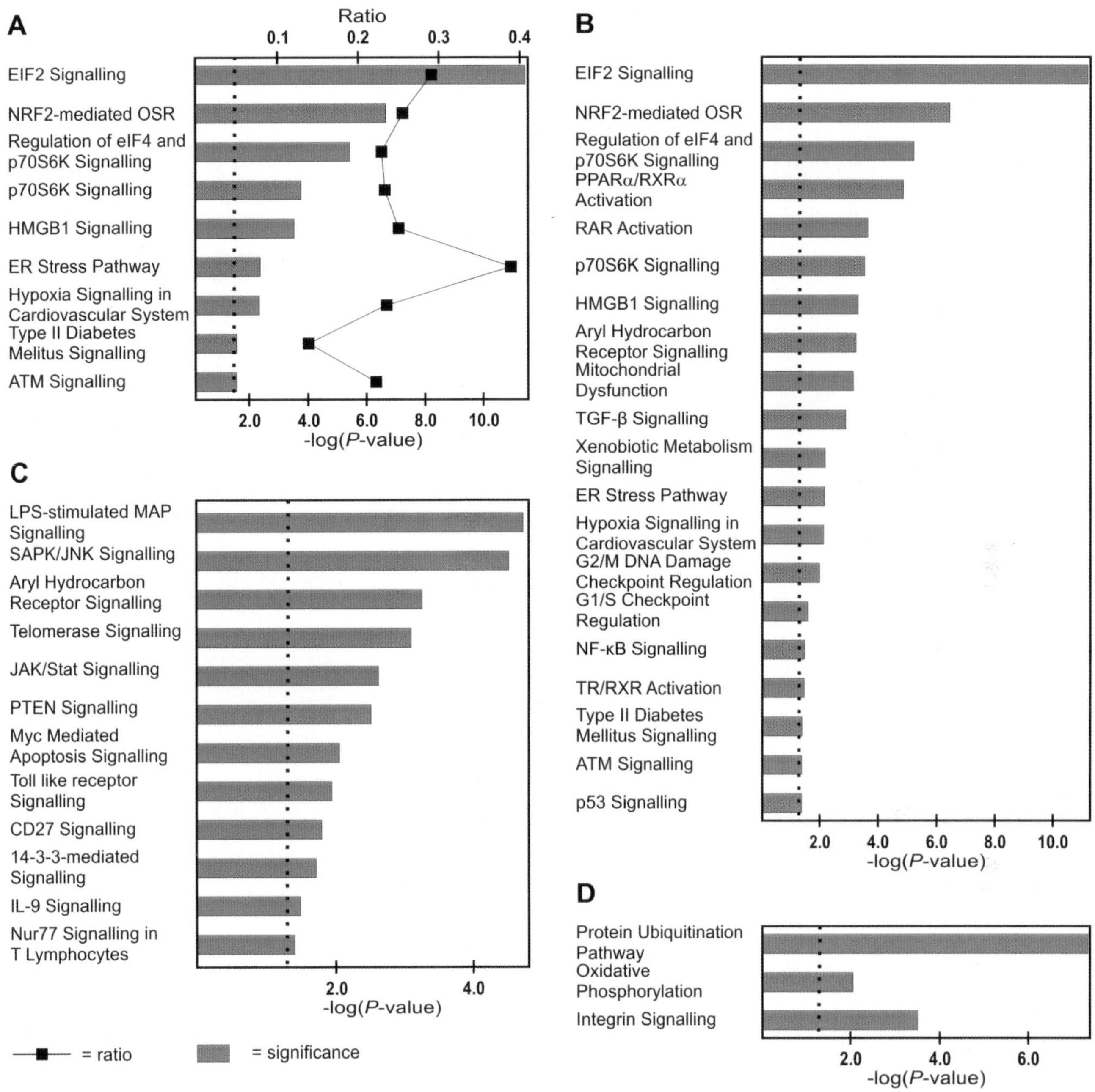

Figure 2. Ingenuity Pathway Analysis of TMD expression profiles. (A) Cell stress pathways affected in TMD also showing the ratio of significantly changed genes versus all genes in the given pathway (oxidative stress response; abbreviated to OSR). (B) Significantly altered cell stress and toxicity pathways, (C) apoptosis pathways, and (D) selected other pathways. The dotted line indicates the statistical significance threshold from a Fisher's exact *t*-test ($P<0.05$).

Analyses of UPR pathway components on the protein level

Numerous rimmed vacuoles were identified in TMD biopsy sections by Herovici staining (Fig. 4A). We observed abnormalities in the ubiquitin-proteasome system (UPS) such as cytoplasmic ubiquitin containing inclusions (Fig. 4B) in the rimmed vacuolated fibres in IHC. We also observed the presence of HSPA5 granular cytoplasmic dots in non-vacuolated fibres by IF microscopy in TMD muscle biopsies (Fig. 5A), which were not observed in controls (Fig. 5B). This was in line with the up-regulation of *HSPA5* we found by quantitative real-time PCR analysis (Fig. 3A). By western blotting HSPA5 levels were increased in two out of five biopsies (Fig. 6A).

Analysis of the ERAD pathway at the protein level

Abnormal or misfolded proteins within the ER are directed into the ER-associated protein degradation (ERAD) pathway. VCP is involved in proteasome-autophagy crosstalk [30,31] and is a core component of the ERAD pathway [32]. In all 5 TMD biopsies tested by IHC, we observed a variable frequency of VCP-positive material connected with rimmed vacuoles (Fig. 4D). Abnormal VCP immunoreactivity was present as bodies in over half of the rimmed vacuoles. VCP labelling was also found in a subset of

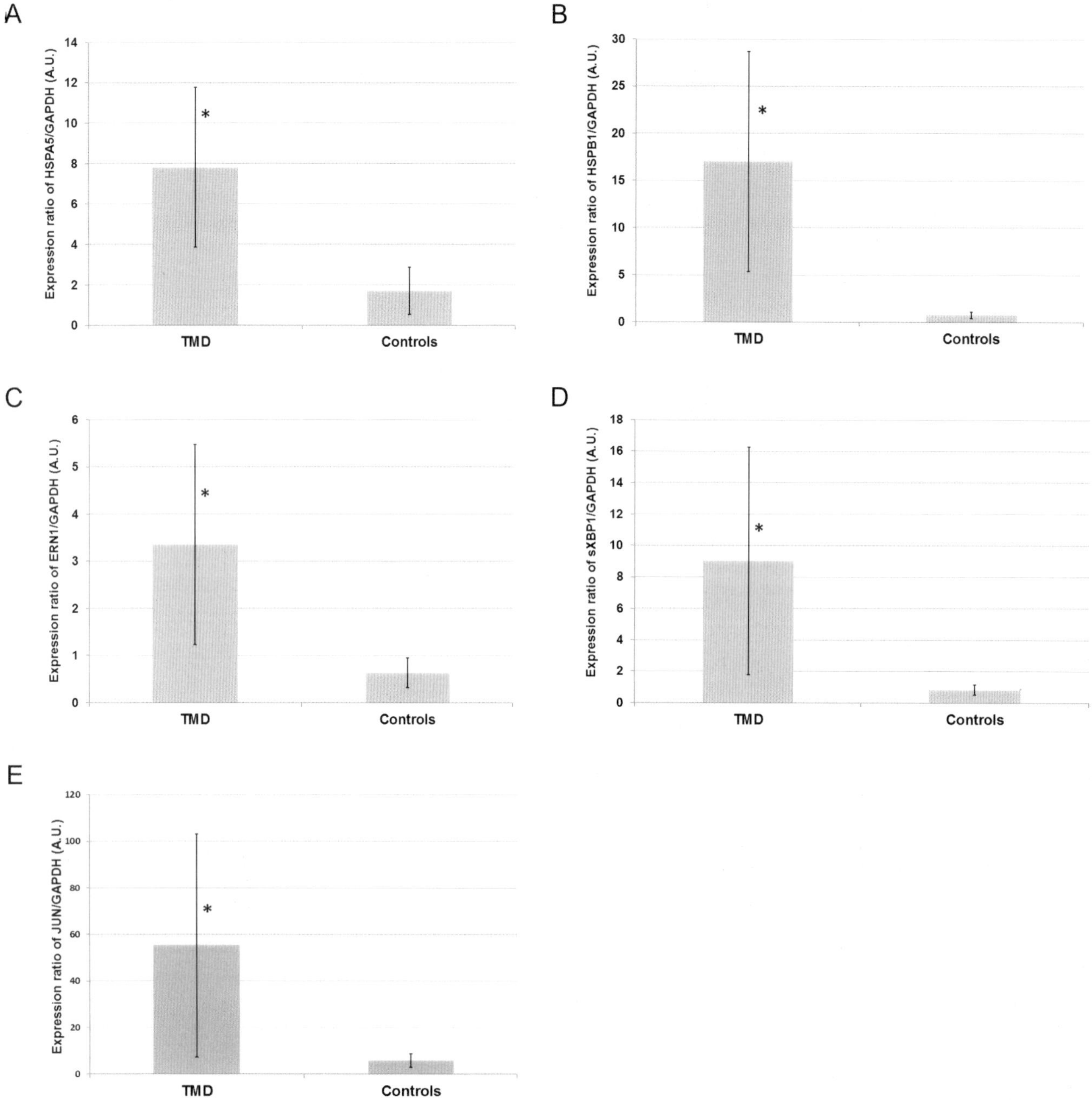

Figure 3. Quantitative real-time PCR analysis of key components of selected pathways. Expression of (A) *HSPA5*, (B) *HSPB1*, (C) *ERN1*, (D) spliced (s) *XBP1*, and (E) *JUN* normalised to *GAPDH* by quantitative real-time PCR from muscle biopsy total RNA (arbitrary units). *Indicates statistical significance in an unpaired *t*-test ($P<0.05$) comparison to the control group. The average and standard deviation of five TMD and three control biopsies each performed in triplicate are shown.

nuclei in control and TMD sections but did not differ between disease and controls samples. Western blotting (Fig. 6B) showed an increase in full length VCP in two TMD samples and an extra band (70 kDa) below the full length VCP in a third sample. Intriguingly, an extra 25-kDa band was observed in three out of five TMD biopsies and not in the controls. These bands were identified as D179-cleaved VCP by staining with a specific antiserum [33] (Fig. 6C). However, by quantification the increased levels of the 25-kDa VCP cleavage product in TMD did not reach statistical significance ($P=0.077$).

Analyses of autophagy pathway components on the protein level

If a protein abnormality cannot be correctly handled and processed through UPR activation using the UPS for degradation, the proteins may be redirected to the autophagic pathway and degraded in the lysosomal system. We observed strong immunoreactivity of the autophagosome marker LC3B in the rimmed vacuoles and in the cytoplasm of very atrophic fibres (Fig. 4C). Accumulation of p62 and the autophagosome marker LC3B have been used to indicate abnormalities in the autophagic degradation pathways [34–36]. We observed p62 immunoreactivity in rimmed

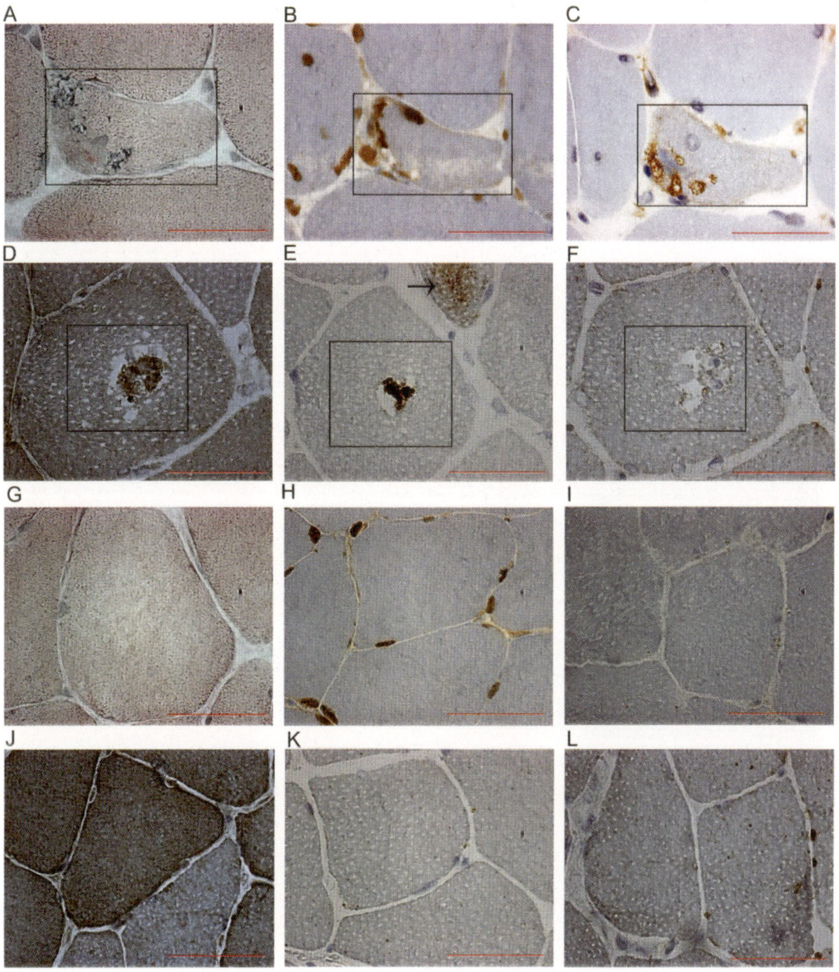

Figure 4. Histology and immunohistochemical analysis of TMD muscle biopsies. (A) Herovici histology staining of TMD muscle sections showing rimmed vacuolar regions within the fibres. (B) Immunohistochemical (IHC) analysis of TMD muscle sections stained for ubiquitin showing localised cytoplasmic ubiquitin containing inclusions in atrophic and rimmed vacuolated fibres and immunoreactivity at the edge of rimmed vacuoles. (C) Autophagosome marker LC3B staining showed strong immunoreactivity within the rimmed vacuolar regions. (D) VCP staining showed immunoreactivity in bodies within a large subset of rimmed vacuoles. (E) p62 staining showed immunoreactivity in rimmed vacuoles and granular immunoreactive dots (shown by an arrow) in an atrophic fibre. (F) Lysosomal protein LAMP2 staining showed no overall increase in rimmed vacuolated fibres. Two separate TMD fibres (A–C and D–F) with rimmed vacuoles in serial sections are shown. Controls of (G) Herovici staining, (H) ubiquitin, (I) LC3B, (J) VCP, (K) p62 and (L) LAMP2 IHC are included for comparison. Sections are from samples TMD 6 and Ctrl 3 in Table 1. Scale bar 50 μm.

vacuoles and granular immunoreactive dots in many atrophic fibres (Fig. 4E). There was no overall increase in immunoreactivity in the lysosomal marker LAMP2 in TMD fibres or within the rimmed vacuoles (Fig. 4F & 5C) when compared to controls (Fig. 4L & 5D).

Discussion

The expression profiling results showed that the samples clustered according to the disease diagnosis as expected. IPA showed that there were differences in distinct molecular pathways between the TMD and the control samples. We were able to confirm selected changes in the studied pathways through quantitative real-time PCR and protein level analysis in the TMD samples.

Pathway analysis indicated a change in the unfolded protein response (UPR) pathway in the TMD samples. This was also suggested by the induction of ER stress response gene *HSPB1* and UPR genes *HSPA5*, *ERN1* and the splice form of *XBP1* in quantitative real-time PCR. The HSPA5 protein also showed restricted areas of increased expression in IF microscopy. Many of the proteins studied showed large variations between samples, and these differences may be due to the patient's biopsy site, disease severity or age at muscle biopsy. UPR activation has been reported in other rimmed vacuolar myopathies with abnormal UPS or lysosomal degradation pathways [37–40], and mildly in a mouse model of desminopathy [41]. This suggests UPR may act as a common protective mechanism during myopathic protein based stress. FINmaj mutated titin appears to cause the activation of UPR and lead to accumulation of ubiquitinated proteins. The increase of ubiquitinated protein components in TMD muscle is unlikely to be related to CAPN3 dysfunction. A secondary CAPN3 defect is present in homozygous LGMD2J, but in heterozygous TMD patients CAPN3 expression, although variable, is typically within the normal range [13].

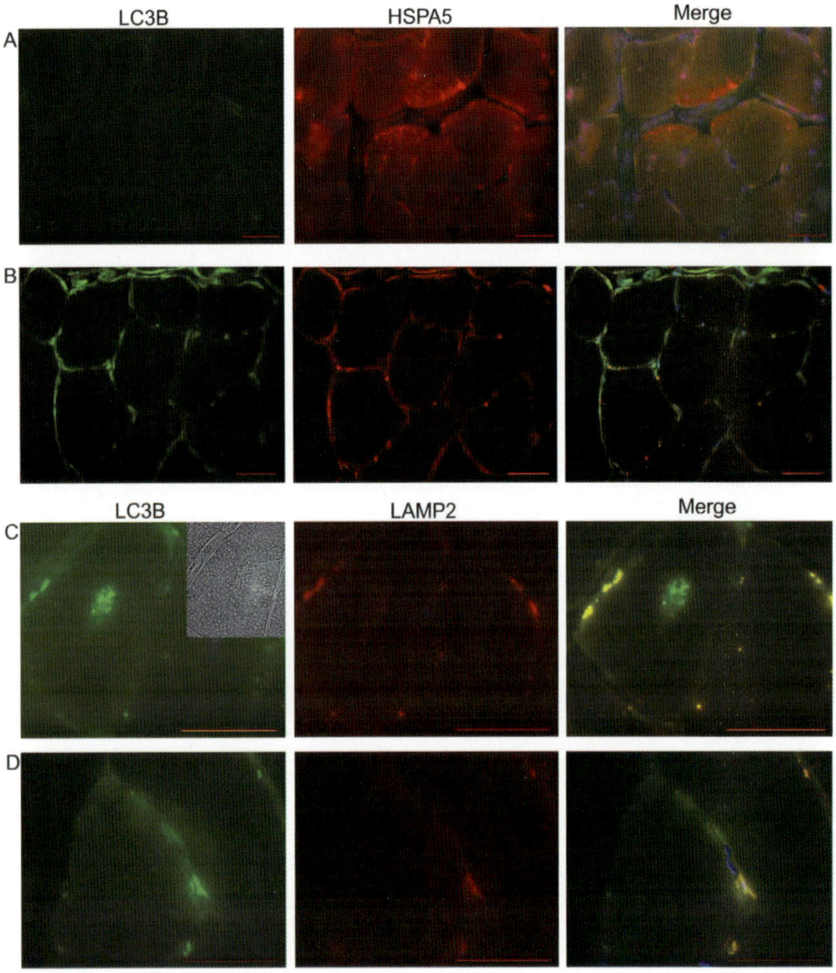

Figure 5. Immunofluorescent microscopy of TMD and control biopsies. (A) HSPA5 staining showed the presence of cytoplasmic granular dots in non-vacuolated TMD muscle fibres. The LC3B channel showed the area has no vacuolated fibres and no autofluorescent material present. (B) A control of HSPA5/LC3B double staining was included for comparison. (C) LAMP2 and LC3B double staining of a TMD muscle fibre showed a representative rimmed vacuole with massive accumulation of LC3B inside and negligible signal from LAMP2 around the edge of the fibre. The top right corner of the LC3B image showed a rimmed vacuole in bright field. (D) A control of LAMP2/LC3B double staining was included for comparison. All images are nuclear counterstained with DAPI (blue signal). Sections are from samples TMD 6 and Ctrl 3 in Table 1. Scale bar 50 μm.

Excess of misfolded proteins in the ER may also activate the ERAD system [42]. A key component of the ERAD pathway is VCP which, among others, retro-translocates unfolded proteins from the ER into the cytosol for degradation by the UPS [43]. Primary mutations in VCP cause a muscle disease with rimmed vacuolar pathology [44,45]. VCP has also been reported to regulate ubiquitin-containing autophagosome maturation during myopathic proteomic stress [30,31], and may therefore be involved in autophagosomal activation in TMD muscle. VCP accumulates inside of rimmed vacuoles suggesting that it may have a role in TMD myopathology with similarities to other neurodegenerative proteinopathies such as VCP-mutated myopathy [44,45]. Western blotting showed an increase in two out of five biopsies and an extra band beneath the full length form in a third biopsy. In addition, we observed unconventional anti-VCP positive bands of approx. 25 kDa in size in 3 of 5 TMD samples. These ~25 kDa bands were subsequently confirmed to be VCP cleavage products by specific antiserum [33]. The expression of these VCP cleavage fragments has been reported to impair degradation by the UPS system in neuroblastoma cells [33], but further studies are required before this pathway can be linked to the pathomechanism of TMD.

The p62 protein acts as an auxiliary autophagy factor by directly binding ubiquitinated proteins and LC3, to facilitate their degradation by autophagy [35]. However, p62 also shuttles ubiquitinated proteins to the proteasome for degradation [46] and has been found in protein aggregates in other neuromuscular and neurodegenerative disorders [47–49]. The accumulation of LC3B positive autophagosome material and p62 within the rimmed vacuolated regions of the degenerative muscle fibres suggests massive activation of compensatory autophagy mechanisms in TMD. Cytoplasmic increase of LAMP2 has been reported in atrophic fibres in other rimmed vacuolar myopathies [50]. However, there was no consistent increase of mature lysosomes based on LAMP2 staining's in atrophic rimmed vacuolated TMD muscle fibres. Apparently the increased induction of autophagy is not paralleled by increased autophagic flux and further processing, which may cause the observed massive increase of LC3B compartments.

JUN, a final stage component of SAPK/JNK apoptosis signalling pathway was significantly increased in quantitative

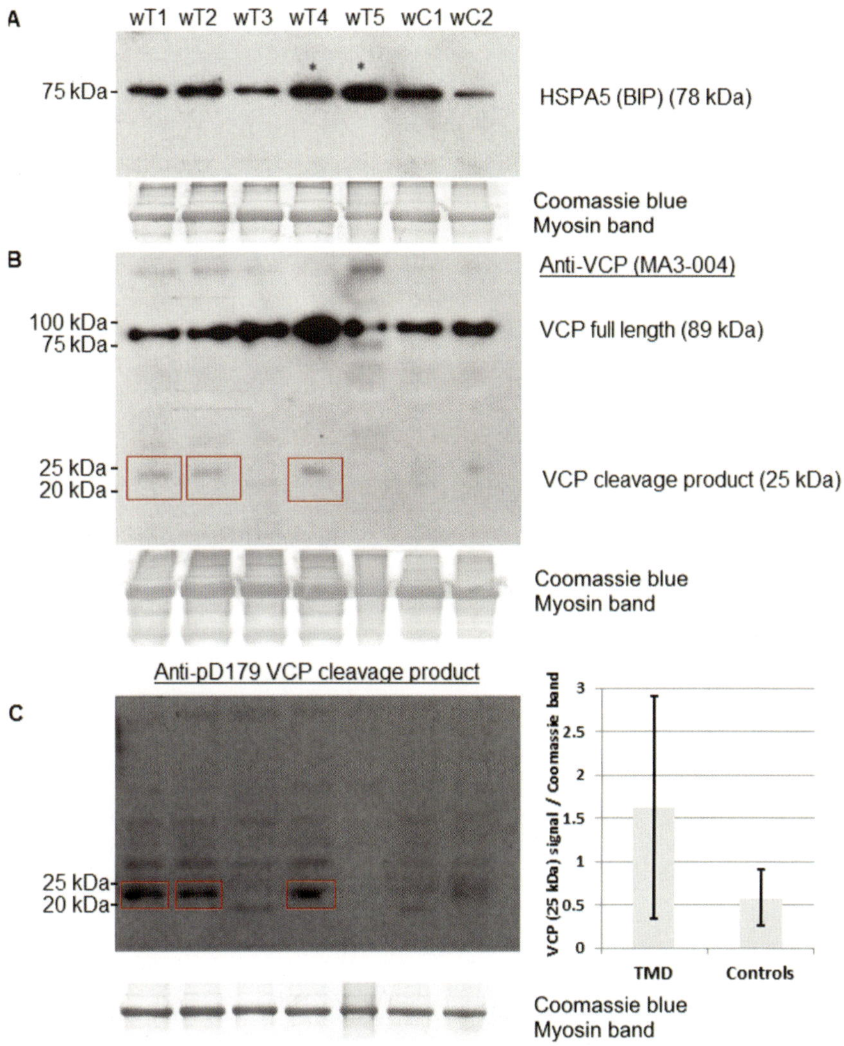

Figure 6. Protein level analysis of UPR and ERAD in TMD biopsies. (A) Western blotting showed HSPA5 increases in two in five samples when compared to controls. (B) Immunoblotting VCP showed an increase in full length VCP in two TMD samples and an extra band (~70 kDa) just below the full length VCP in a third sample. Bands at approx. 25 kDa (red boxes) are observed in three of the TMD samples. (C) Samples were also blotted with p97D179 antiserum specific for VCP cleaved at D179 and show bands at approx. 25 kDa in three of the same samples. Total protein content is shown by the myosin band in Coomassie blue staining and showed equal sample loading. A graph of the quantification of the VCP cleavage product (25 kDa) signals normalised to the Coomassie myosin band showed a trend towards being increased in TMD in a *t*-test ($P = 0.077$).

real-time PCR analysis. In distal myopathy with rimmed vacuoles (DMRV) JUN has been shown to be increased in vacuolated fibres [21]. Nevertheless, whether increased apoptosis leads to a loss of muscle fibres in TMD remains unsettled. A previous study [13] has indicated that apoptosis may not be consistently increased in TMD muscle, although apoptosis is increased in the homozygotic LGMD2J [13] muscle. However, the muscle pathology of LGMD2J is different to TMD and does not show rimmed vacuolar changes.

This study, based on expression profiling and molecular pathology, has identified changes in several subcellular molecular pathways that are apparently involved in the TMD pathomechanism. These include activation of UPR accompanied by increased amounts of ubiquitinated proteins and altered autophagic degradation leading to atrophic and rimmed vacuolated degenerated fibres. Apparently a variety of entries, i.e. different mutant proteins, can result in similar changes in catabolic pathways that control protein turnover. The changes identified in this study are downstream secondary effects of the primary FINmaj mutation in titin. The exact molecular mechanisms that trigger UPR, ERAD and autophagic dysregulation as well as the other abnormally regulated pathways identified in this study need further characterization in order to identify steps that could be therapeutically useful.

Acknowledgments

We are grateful to all the participating patients for their cooperation in this study and to Helena Luque and Hanna-Liisa Kojo for technical assistance and for the gift of p97D179 antiserum from Andréa LeBlanc (McGill University). Matti Kankainen is also acknowledged for his support in bioformatics.

Author Contributions

Conceived and designed the experiments: MS BU. Performed the experiments: MS OR JH. Analyzed the data: MS PHJ PH SH BU. Contributed reagents/materials/analysis tools: SH BU. Wrote the paper: MS PHJ PH BU.

References

1. Udd B, Vihola A, Sarparanta J, Richard I, Hackman P (2005) Titinopathies and extension of the M-line mutation phenotype beyond distal myopathy and LGMD2J. Neurology 64: 636–642.
2. Hackman P, Vihola A, Haravuori H, Marchand S, Sarparanta J, et al. (2002) Tibial muscular dystrophy is a titinopathy caused by mutations in TTN, the gene encoding the giant skeletal-muscle protein titin. Am J Hum Genet 71: 492–500.
3. Udd B (1992) Limb-girdle type muscular dystrophy in a large family with distal myopathy: Homozygous manifestation of a dominant gene? J Med Genet 29: 383–389.
4. Hackman P, Marchand S, Sarparanta J, Vihola A, Pénisson-Besnier I, et al. (2008) Truncating mutations in C-terminal titin may cause more severe tibial muscular dystrophy (TMD). Neuromuscul Disord 18: 922–928.
5. Lange S, Xiang F, Yakovenko A, Vihola A, Hackman P, et al. (2005) The kinase domain of titin controls muscle gene expression and protein turnover. Science 308: 1599–1603.
6. Palmio J, Evila A, Chapon F, Tasca G, Xiang F, et al. (2013) Hereditary myopathy with early respiratory failure: Occurrence in various populations. J Neurol Neurosurg Psychiatry. In press.
7. Carmignac V, Salih MA, Quijano-Roy S, Marchand S, Al Rayess MM, et al. (2007) C-terminal titin deletions cause a novel early-onset myopathy with fatal cardiomyopathy. Ann Neurol 61: 340–351.
8. Chauveau C, Bonnemann CG, Julien C, Kho AL, Marks H, et al. (2013) Recessive TTN truncating mutations define novel forms of core myopathy with heart disease. Hum Mol GenetIn press.
9. Ceyhan-Birsoy O, Agrawal PB, Hidalgo C, Schmitz-Abe K, DeChene ET, et al. (2013) Recessive truncating titin gene, TTN, mutations presenting as centronuclear myopathy. Neurology 81: 1205–1214.
10. Pollazzon M, Suominen T, Penttilä S, Malandrini A, Carluccio MA, et al. (2010) The first italian family with tibial muscular dystrophy caused by a novel titin mutation. J Neurol 257: 575–579.
11. Van den Bergh PY, Bouquiaux O, Verellen C, Marchand S, Richard I, et al. (2003) Tibial muscular dystrophy in a belgian family. Ann Neurol 54: 248–251.
12. Udd B, Partanen J, Halonen P, Falck B, Hakamies L, et al. (1993) Tibial muscular dystrophy. late adult-onset distal myopathy in 66 finnish patients. Arch Neurol 50: 604–608.
13. Haravuori H, Vihola A, Straub V, Auranen M, Richard I, et al. (2001) Secondary calpain3 deficiency in 2q-linked muscular dystrophy: Titin is the candidate gene. Neurology 56: 869–877.
14. Udd B, Haravuori H, Kalimo H, Partanen J, Pulkkinen L, et al. (1998) Tibial muscular dystrophy-from clinical description to linkage on chromosome 2q31. Neuromuscul Disord 8: 327–332.
15. Gautel M, Mues A, Young P (1999) Control of sarcomeric assembly: The flow of information on titin. Ergeb Physiol 138: 97–137.
16. Labeit S, Kolmerer B (1995) Titins: Giant proteins in charge of muscle ultrastructure and elasticity. Science 270: 293–296.
17. Kolmerer B, Olivieri N, Witt CC, Herrmann BG, Labeit S (1996) Genomic organization of M line titin and its tissue-specific expression in two distinct isoforms. J Mol Biol 256: 556–563.
18. Charton K, Danièle N, Vihola A, Roudaut C, Gicquel E, et al. (2010) Removal of the calpain 3 protease reverses the myopathology in a mouse model for titinopathies. Hum Mol Genet 19: 4608–4624.
19. Fukuzawa A, Lange S, Holt M, Vihola A, Carmignac V, et al. (2008) Interactions with titin and myomesin target obscurin and obscurin-like 1 to the M-band: Implications for hereditary myopathies. J Cell Sci 121: 1841–1851.
20. Raheem O, Olufemi S, Bachinski LL, Vihola A, Sirito M, et al. (2010) Mutant (CCTG)n expansion causes abnormal expression of zinc finger protein 9 (ZNF9) in myotonic dystrophy type 2. Am J Pathol 177: 3025–3036.
21. Yan C, Ikezoe K, Nonaka I (2001) Apoptotic muscle fiber degeneration in distal myopathy with rimmed vacuoles. Acta Neuropathol 101: 9–16.
22. Nogalska A, D'Agostino C, Terracciano C, Engel WK, Askanas V (2010) Impaired autophagy in sporadic inclusion-body myositis and in endoplasmic reticulum stress-provoked cultured human muscle fibers. Am J Pathol 177: 1377–1387.
23. Ching JK, Elizabeth SV, Ju J, Lusk C, Pittman SK, et al. (2013) mTOR dysfunction contributes to vacuolar pathology and weakness in valosin-containing protein associated inclusion body myopathy. Hum Mol Genet 22: 1167–1179.
24. Askanas V, Engel WK (2008) Inclusion-body myositis: Muscle-fiber molecular pathology and possible pathogenic significance of its similarity to alzheimer's and parkinson's disease brains. Acta Neuropathol 116: 583–595.
25. Eisenberg I, Novershtern N, Itzhaki Z, Becker-Cohen M, Sadeh M, et al. (2008) Mitochondrial processes are impaired in hereditary inclusion body myopathy. Hum Mol Genet 17: 3663–3674.
26. Ito H, Iwamoto I, Inaguma Y, Takizawa T, Nagata K, et al. (2005) Endoplasmic reticulum stress induces the phosphorylation of small heat shock protein, Hsp27. J Cell Biochem 95: 932–941.
27. Lin H, Masso-Welch P, Di Y, Cai J, Shen J, et al. (1993) The 170-kDa glucose-regulated stress protein is an endoplasmic reticulum protein that binds immunoglobulin. Mol Biol Cell 4: 1109–1119.
28. Chen Y, Brandizzi F (2013) IRE1: ER stress sensor and cell fate executor. Trends Cell Biol 23, 11: 547–555.
29. Yoshida H, Matsui T, Yamamoto A, Okada T, Mori K (2001) XBP1 mRNA is induced by ATF6 and spliced by IRE1 in response to ER stress to produce a highly active transcription factor. Cell 107: 881–891.
30. Ju JS, Fuentealba RA, Miller SE, Jackson E, Piwnica-Worms D, et al. (2009) Valosin-containing protein (VCP) is required for autophagy and is disrupted in VCP disease. J Cell Biol 187: 875–888.
31. Tresse E, Salomons FA, Vesa J, Bott LC, Kimonis V, et al. (2010) VCP/p97 is essential for maturation of ubiquitin-containing autophagosomes and this function is impaired by mutations that cause IBMPFD. Autophagy 6: 217–227.
32. Meyer H, Bug M, Bremer S (2012) Emerging functions of the VCP/p97 AAA-ATPase in the ubiquitin system. Nat Cell Biol 14: 117–123.
33. Halawani D, Tessier S, Anzellotti D, Bennett DA, Latterich M, et al. (2010) Identification of caspase-6-mediated processing of the valosin containing protein (p97) in alzheimer's disease: A novel link to dysfunction in ubiquitin proteasome system-mediated protein degradation. J Neurosci 30: 6132–6142.
34. Weihl CC, Pestronk A (2010) Sporadic inclusion body myositis: Possible pathogenesis inferred from biomarkers. Curr Opin Neurol 23: 482–488.
35. Pankiv S, Clausen TH, Lamark T, Brech A, Bruun JA, et al. (2007) p62/SQSTM1 binds directly to Atg8/LC3 to facilitate degradation of ubiquitinated protein aggregates by autophagy. J Biol Chem 282: 24131–24145.
36. Lee HS, Daniels BH, Salas E, Bollen AW, Debnath J, et al. (2012) Clinical utility of LC3 and p62 immunohistochemistry in diagnosis of drug-induced autophagic vacuolar myopathies: A case-control study. PLoS One 7: e36221.
37. Liewluck T, Hayashi YK, Ohsawa M, Kurokawa R, Fujita M, et al. (2007) Unfolded protein response and aggresome formation in hereditary reducing-body myopathy. Muscle Nerve 35: 322–326.
38. Vattemi G, Engel WK, McFerrin J, Askanas V (2004) Endoplasmic reticulum stress and unfolded protein response in inclusion body myositis muscle. Am J Pathol 164: 1–7.
39. Boito CA, Fanin M, Gavassini BF, Cenacchi G, Angelini C, et al. (2007) Biochemical and ultrastructural evidence of endoplasmic reticulum stress in LGMD2I. Virchows Archiv 451: 1047–1055.
40. Kuga A, Ohsawa Y, Okada T, Kanda F, Kanagawa M, et al. (2011) Endoplasmic reticulum stress response in P104L mutant caveolin-3 transgenic mice. Hum Mol Genet 20: 2975–2983.
41. Lynch JM, Maillet M, Vanhoutte D, Schloemer A, Sargent MA, et al. (2012) A thrombospondin-dependent pathway for a protective ER stress response. Cell 149: 1257–1268.
42. Meusser B, Hirsch C, Jarosch E, Sommer T (2005) ERAD: The long road to destruction. Nat Cell Biol 7: 766–772.
43. Halawani D, Latterich M (2006) p97: The cell's molecular purgatory? Mol Cell 22: 713–717.
44. Watts GDJ, Wymer J, Kovach MJ, Mehta SG, Mumm S, et al. (2004) Inclusion body myopathy associated with paget disease of bone and frontotemporal dementia is caused by mutant valosin-containing protein. Nat Genet 36: 377–381.
45. Palmio J, Sandell S, Suominen T, Penttilä S, Raheem O, et al. (2011) Distinct distal myopathy phenotype caused by VCP gene mutation in a finnish family. Neuromuscul Disord 21: 551–555.
46. Seibenhener ML, Babu JR, Geetha T, Wong HC, Krishna NR, et al. (2004) Sequestosome 1/p62 is a polyubiquitin chain binding protein involved in ubiquitin proteasome degradation. Mol Cell Biol 24: 8055–8068.
47. Olivé M, van Leeuwen FW, Janue A, Moreno D, Torrejon-Escribano B, et al. (2008) Expression of mutant ubiquitin (UBB+1) and p62 in myotilinopathies and desminopathies. Neuropathol Appl Neurobiol 34: 76–87.
48. Nogalska A, Terracciano C, D'Agostino C, King Engel W, Askanas V (2009) p62/SQSTM1 is overexpressed and prominently accumulated in inclusions of sporadic inclusion-body myositis muscle fibers, and can help differentiating it from polymyositis and dermatomyositis. Acta Neuropathol 118: 407–413.
49. Zatloukal K, Stumptner C, Fuchsbichler A, Heid H, Schnoelzer M, et al. (2002) p62 is a common component of cytoplasmic inclusions in protein aggregation diseases. Am J Pathol 160: 255–263.
50. Tsuruta Y, Furuta A, Furuta K, Yamada T, Kira J, et al. (2001) Expression of the lysosome-associated membrane proteins in myopathies with rimmed vacuoles. Acta Neuropathol 101: 579–584.

10

Inflammation-Induced Acute Phase Response in Skeletal Muscle and Critical Illness Myopathy

Claudia Langhans[1,¶], Steffen Weber-Carstens[2,¶], Franziska Schmidt[1], Jida Hamati[1], Melanie Kny[1], Xiaoxi Zhu[1], Tobias Wollersheim[2], Susanne Koch[2], Martin Krebs[2], Herbert Schulz[3], Doerte Lodka[1], Kathrin Saar[3], Siegfried Labeit[4], Claudia Spies[2], Norbert Hubner[3], Joachim Spranger[1,5,6], Simone Spuler[1], Michael Boschmann[1], Gunnar Dittmar[3], Gillian Butler-Browne[7], Vincent Mouly[7], Jens Fielitz[1,8]*

1 Experimental and Clinical Research Center (ECRC), a Cooperation between Max Delbrück Center and Charité Universitätsmedizin Berlin, Campus Buch, Berlin, Germany, **2** Charité Universitätsmedizin Berlin, Campus Virchow and Campus Mitte, Anesthesiology and Operative Intensive Care Medicine, Berlin, Germany, **3** Max Delbrück Center for Molecular Medicine, Berlin, Germany, **4** Universitätsmedizin Mannheim, Mannheim, Germany, **5** Charité Universitätsmedizin Berlin, NeuroCure Clinical Research Center, Berlin, Germany, **6** Charité Universitätsmedizin Berlin, Department of Endocrinology, Diabetes and Nutrition, Berlin, Germany, **7** Institut de Myologie, Institut national de la santé et de la recherche médicale, and L'Université Pierre et Marie Curie Paris, Paris, France, **8** Charité Universitätsmedizin Berlin, Campus Virchow, Cardiology, Berlin, Germany

Abstract

Objectives: Systemic inflammation is a major risk factor for critical-illness myopathy (CIM) but its pathogenic role in muscle is uncertain. We observed that interleukin 6 (*IL-6*) and serum amyloid A1 (*SAA1*) expression was upregulated in muscle of critically ill patients. To test the relevance of these responses we assessed inflammation and acute-phase response at early and late time points in muscle of patients at risk for CIM.

Design: Prospective observational clinical study and prospective animal trial.

Setting: Two intensive care units (ICU) and research laboratory.

Patients/Subjects: 33 patients with Sequential Organ Failure Assessment scores ≥8 on 3 consecutive days within 5 days in ICU were investigated. A subgroup analysis of 12 patients with, and 18 patients without CIM (non-CIM) was performed. Two consecutive biopsies from *vastus lateralis* were obtained at median days 5 and 15, early and late time points. Controls were 5 healthy subjects undergoing elective orthopedic surgery. A septic mouse model and cultured myoblasts were used for mechanistic analyses.

Measurements and Main Results: Early *SAA1* expression was significantly higher in skeletal muscle of CIM compared to non-CIM patients. Immunohistochemistry showed SAA1 accumulations in muscle of CIM patients at the early time point, which resolved later. *SAA1* expression was induced by IL-6 and tumor necrosis factor-alpha in human and mouse myocytes *in vitro*. Inflammation-induced muscular SAA1 accumulation was reproduced in a sepsis mouse model.

Conclusions: Skeletal muscle contributes to general inflammation and acute-phase response in CIM patients. Muscular SAA1 could be important for CIM pathogenesis.

Trial Registration: ISRCTN77569430.

Editor: Jorge I F Salluh, D'or Institute of Research and Education, Brazil

Funding: Funding from the Deutsche forschungsgemeinschaft (FI 965/2-1, FI 965/4-1 and La668/14-1), KFO 192, MyoGrad (Deutsche Forschungsgemeinschaft, GK1631, Université Franco-Allemand [CDFA-06-11] and AFM), Muscular Dystrophy Association, Marie Curie International Reintegration grant, and the Deutsche Gesellschaft für Muskelkranke e. V. all supported this work. The funders had no role in study design, data collection and analysis, decision to publish, or preparation of the manuscript.

* E-mail: jens.fielitz@charite.de

¶ These authors contributed equally to this work.

Introduction

Intensive care unit (ICU)-acquired weakness is a serious complication during critical illness, characterized by loss of muscle mass, preferential atrophy of fast-twitch myofibers and weakness [1–3]. The clinical consequences are prolonged hospital stay and mechanical ventilation, increased hospital mortality, and chronic physical disability [4,5]. Diminished myosin heavy chain (MyHC) content is consistently observed [1,6]. Others and we recently reported that non-excitable muscle membranes indicate patients at risk for critical illness myopathy (CIM) early during the disease process [1,7,8]. CIM deteriorates the disease course and leads to protracted rehabilitation, poor quality-of-life outcomes, and permanent disability [4,5,9]. The suffering and economic impact for the health care system and the society are high [10].

Earlier, we observed disturbed glucose utilization in skeletal muscle from CIM patients caused by insufficient translocation of the glucose transporter GLUT4 to the membrane [11]. Nonetheless, the pathophysiology of CIM is poorly understood [12]. General inflammation with sepsis, immobilization, sedation, hyperglycemia and corticosteroids contribute to CIM [13,14]. Among these the mediators of inflammation interleukin 6 (IL-6) and tumor necrosis factor-alpha (TNF-α) are particularly important [15,16]. Serum levels of IL-6 [14,15] and TNF-α [16] are increased in systemic inflammatory response syndrome and sepsis patients and are associated with increased mortality [14]. Both IL-6 [17,18] and TNF-α [19–21] contribute to muscular atrophy by increasing protein degradation [22,23]. Both cytokines increase the expression of acute phase response proteins, such as serum amyloid A 1 (SAA1) in muscle and other tissues [24]. SAA1 is associated with muscle wasting and atrophy in cachectic mice [25]. In addition, IL-6 and SAA1 cooperate to enhance angiotensin (Ang) II-induced muscle atrophy [26]. However, it is unknown if inflammation induces acute phase response directly in myocytes of critically ill patients which contributes to CIM. We hypothesized that early identification of non-excitable muscle membranes indicative for CIM could be helpful to identify pathways involved in the pathogenesis of CIM. A gene expression array performed on skeletal muscle biopsies from CIM and non-CIM patients drew our attention to increased muscular *SAA1* gene expression indicative for acute phase response in muscle of CIM patients. We investigated factors regulating SAA1 synthesis in skeletal myocytes and tested conservation of this pathway in a sepsis mouse model.

Materials and Methods

Ethics Statement

The institutional review board of the Charité approved the study, and written informed consent was obtained from legal proxy (ICU patients), or the patients themselves (control subjects) (Charité EA2/061/06). The study was registered under http://www.controlled-trials.com, ISRCTN77569430. We specifically included patients at high risk to develop ICU-acquired weakness. Accordingly, critically ill, mechanically ventilated ICU-patients were eligible for inclusion once they showed Sequential Organ Failure Assessment (SOFA) scores ≥8 on three consecutive days within the first five days after ICU admission. In this observational study all patients (n = 33) were treated according to local standard operating procedures [27]. We have reported an analysis on defective glucose utilization in these same patients earlier [11]. All patients received physiotherapy by an experienced physiotherapist starting from day one in ICU. Passive range of motion and active exercise were prescribed daily based on interdisciplinary discussions involving physiotherapists, nurses, ward physicians and consultants, and according to individual patient needs. Study physicians assessed patients' muscle strength according to the Medical Research Council (MRC) score. To be eligible for MRC score evaluation, patients had to be awake (defined as Richmond Agitation Sedation Scale scores of −1, 0, or +1) and to adequately respond to at least three out of five verbal commands as recently reported [8]. Five age- and gender-matched otherwise healthy patients undergoing elective orthopedic surgery permitted muscle biopsies.

Muscle membrane in-excitability after direct muscle stimulation is an accepted marker for early CIM diagnosis and was shown to be associated with later development of ICUAW [1,8,28]. We measured muscle membrane excitability after direct muscle stimulation at day 6 (4–13) in ICU as recently reported [1,8]. Muscle membranes of CIM patients (n = 18) were non-excitable as shown by a reduced compound muscle action potential after direct muscle stimulation (dmCMAP<3 mV), whereas in non-CIM patients (n = 12) muscle membranes (CMAP≥3 mV) were excitable [8,28,29]. For logistical and clinical reasons three patients could not be classified and were consequently not included in comparisons. We took biopsy specimens from *vastus lateralis* muscle in all 33 ICU-patients at median day 5; referred to as early time point. Twenty-two patients were still in the ICU at median day 15, when a second biopsy was performed; referred to as late time point. Serum samples were taken at the second or third day on ICU and stored at −20°C.

Hematoxylin & Eosin and Gomori-trichrome histological staining on cryosections were performed to assess overall muscle pathology as described earlier [30]. Photographs were acquired with a Leica CTR 6500 microscope and a Leica DFC 360 FX digital camera. Further information about animal experiments, Microarray analyses, quantitative real-time RT-PCR (primer sequences are provided in Table S1), immunohistochemistry, ELISA, human and mouse myoblast culture and immunocytochemistry is provided in Methods S1.

Statistical Tests

Non-parametric tests, the Mann-Whitney test to analyze group differences and the Wilcoxon test for dependent samples, were performed. Spearman's rank correlation coefficients were calculated. Data are shown as median with interquartile range (IQR). Student's t-tests and one-way ANOVA analyses were used for PCR data and cell culture experiments. Statistical tests were calculated using SPSS (version 19.0.0.1); box plots were made with the Sigma Plot software (version 12.0). Statistical significance was considered at $P<0.05$.

Results

A Gene Expression Array Analysis Uncovered Increased SAA1 Expression in CIM Muscle

The study design is outlined (Figure 1); data on patient characteristics and further clinical information are presented in Table 1. Patients with non-excitable muscle membrane indicating muscle pathology in CIM developed muscle weakness during ICU treatment, with a median MRC score of 3.0 (interquartile range [IQR], 2.9–3.3), whereas patients with excitable muscle membrane showed a median MRC score of 4.3 (IQR, 3.5–4.8; $P = 0.003$). A non-excitable muscle membrane measured at median day 6 (4/13) was predictive for the development of muscle weakness with a sensitivity and a specificity of 80% each.

To assess very early changes in gene expression, we first performed microarrays. Among 24,133 transcripts, 1,841 genes were differentially expressed in critically ill patients *versus* control patients (5% FDR). The top 30 genes by fold-change increased or decreased in critical illness were revealing (Tables S2 and S3). Additionally, exon expression interaction with the grouping control *versus* CIM patients *versus* non-CIM patients led to a set of 1,948 significant differential expressed transcript clusters (5% FDR). Viewing the top 30 genes by fold change differences between CIM *versus* non-CIM patients implicated several candidates differentially regulated in CIM (Tables S4 and S5). Among these we found serum amyloid A 1 and 4 (*SAA1*, *SAA4*) and therefore reasoned that acute phase response occurred in muscle during critical illness, especially in CIM patients. The data

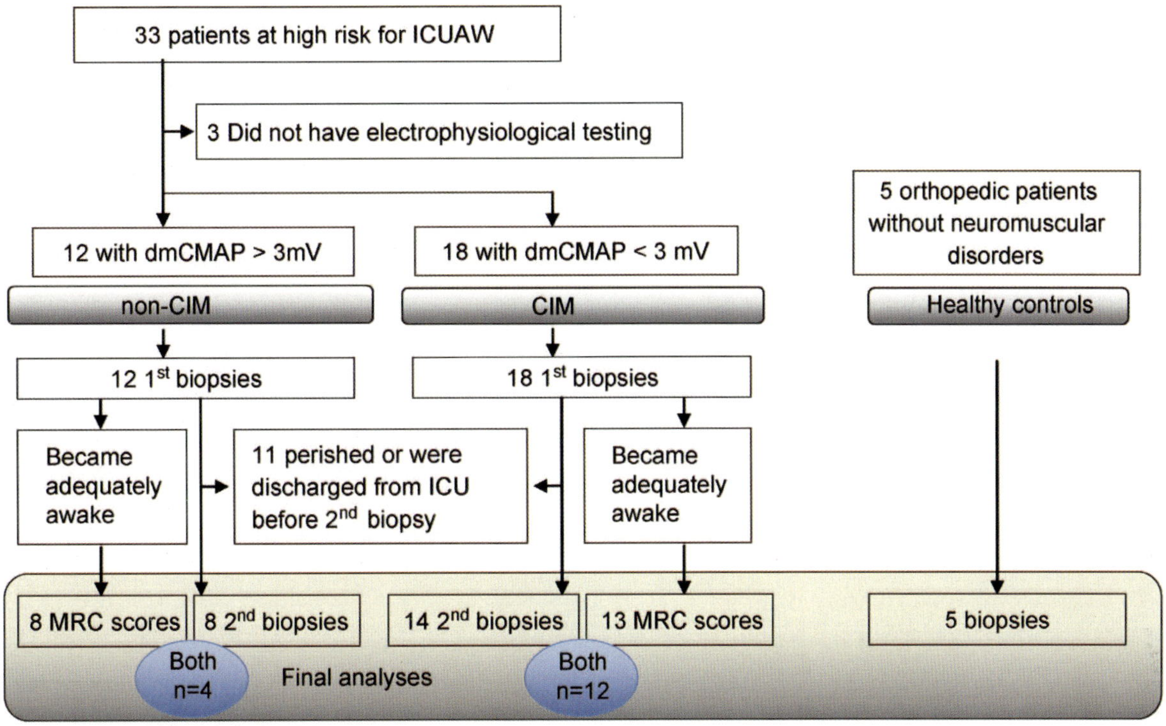

Figure 1. Study protocol.

discussed in this publication have been deposited in NCBI's Gene Expression Omnibus and are accessible through GEO Series accession number GSE53702 (http://www.ncbi.nlm.nih.gov/geo/query/acc.cgi?acc = GSE53702).

RT-PCR analyses on biopsy specimens confirmed the increased *SAA1* (controls: 0.09 (0.09–0.9), ICU-patients early time point: 8.16 (2.42–36.6), $P = 0.005$) and *SAA4* (controls: 0.55 (0.42–1.54), ICU-patients: 8.3 (2.56–29.39), $P = 0.002$) expression levels in critically ill patients. *SAA1* and *SAA4* expression remained unchanged between the early and late biopsy specimen (late time point: *SAA1*:14.77 (4.13–27.2), $P = 0.003$; *SAA4*:16.7 (6.18–40.64), $P = 0.0478$) (Figure 2A). Subgroup analyses showed that *SAA1* and *SAA4* were exclusively increased in CIM patients (*SAA1*:30.6 (7.46–45.8), $P = 0.001$; *SAA4*:22.8 (4.42–51.6), $P = 0.0001$), but remained unchanged in non-CIM (*SAA1*:2.42 (0.53–4.6), $P = 0.15$; *SAA4*:1.64 (1.06–6.64), $P = 0.09$) patients, in the early biopsy specimens (Figure 2B). *SAA1* and *SAA4* expression increased significantly in non-CIM patients (*SAA1*:6.1 (4.99–15.1), $P = 0.012$; *SAA4*:18.4 (8.47–36), $P = 0.018$), and reached the expression level of CIM patients (*SAA1*:19.35 (1.34–67.2), $P = 0.397$ vs. early time point, $P = 0.24$ vs. non-CIM; *SAA4*:16.71 (3.08–70.61), $P = 0.06$ vs. early time point, $P = 0.916$ vs. non-CIM) in the late biopsy specimens. In contrast, no further increase in *SAA1* and *SAA4* expression between the early and late biopsy specimens was observed in CIM patients (Figure 2B).

In addition to electrophysiological testing MRC scoring was possible in 21 out of the 30 ICU patients. In this subgroup, direct muscle stimulation identified weakness with a sensitivity of 80% and a specificity of 83.3%, which is consistent with our recent work [8] (Table S6). Based on MRC scoring (sum score <48 or mean MRC score <4) we performed a subgroup analysis and found an increased *SAA1* expression in patients with (n = 15) compared to patients without clinical evidence of weakness (n = 6) in the early biopsy specimens. *SAA4* expression was not different between both groups. Compared to controls *SAA1* and *SAA4* expression was increased in patients with clinical evidence of weakness at the early time point (Figure S1 and S2). Overall, these findings are consistent with the data shown here for electrophysiological classification of CIM (Figure 2B).

SAA1 Production is Increased Early in Muscle of CIM Patients

We then proceeded to test our hypothesis that SAA1 production is induced in muscle of CIM but not non-CIM patients. Using immunohistochemistry SAA1 protein was found to accumulate in the interstitium, around myofibers, and at the sarcolemma were it co-localized with the membrane-marker laminin (Figure 2C and 2D). CIM patients showed stronger SAA1 accumulation in the early biopsy specimens, compared to non-CIM patients. The same differences, although diminished in SAA1 protein contents, were observed in the late biopsy specimens (Figure S3). These data suggested that high *SAA1* expression translated into a higher SAA1 protein content in skeletal muscle of CIM patients, and that SAA1 was directly synthesized by muscle. Acute phase SAA consist of both SAA1 and SAA2 [24]. Acute phase SAA is associated with generalized inflammation [24]. SAA serum levels were higher in ICU patients than in controls (controls: 333.7 (164.1–433.04), ICU-patients: 606.53 (570.95–631.53), $P < 0.01$). However, SAA serum levels were not increased in CIM compared to non-CIM patients (CIM: 584.9 (560.45–610.34), non-CIM: 631.64 (609.63–650.4), $P < 0.05$) (Figure 3A). These findings suggest that SAA synthesized in the skeletal muscle does not decisively contribute to circulating SAA levels.

Since IL-6 and TNF-α can increase SAA1 [31], we hypothesized that increased muscular IL-6 and/or TNF-α levels could be responsible for higher *SAA1* and *SAA4* expression in CIM patients. We determined *IL-6* and *TNF-α* mRNA expression in biopsy specimens of control and critically ill patients. *IL-6* expression

Table 1. Characterization of critically ill patients.

Parameter	non-CIM-patients dmCMAP≥3mV	CIM-patients dmCMAP<3mV
N	12	18
Age [years]	42.5 (32.5/57.5)	65.5 (41.0/76.0)
Gender [m/f]	7/5 (58.3%/41.7%)	15/3 83.3%/16.7%)
BMI [kg/m^2]	26.0 (23.2/32.5)	27.9 (24.9/31.4)
MRC Score	4.3 (3.5/4.8)	3.0(2.9/3.3)†
Diagnosis [n (%)]		
ARDS	n = 3 (25.0%)	n = 8 (44.4%)
Trauma	n = 4 (33.3%)	n = 2 (11.1%)
Sepsis		n = 7 (38.9%)
CNS	n = 5 (41.7%)	n = 1 (5.6%)
Time point of early biopsy (days after ICU admission)	5.0 (4.0/6.5)	6.0 (4.0/7.0)
Time point of late biopsy (days after ICU admission)	15.0(14.0/16.0)	15.5(14.0/19.0)
Survivors n (%)	12 (100%)	12 (66.7%)
Illness severity at ICU admission		
SOFA	11.0 (9.0/14.0)	11.5 (10.0/14.0)
SAPS-II	53 (42/57)	62 (47/66)
Treatment between ICU-admission and early biopsy		
Norepinephrine [mg/d]	20.0 (8.8/21.7)	12.5 (9.0/24.3)
Patients with median **≥2 organ dysfunctions** until biopsied n (%)	2 (16.7%)	14 (77.8%)†
Patients with **acute renal failure** n (%)	1 (8.3%)	11 (61.1%)*
% of days with **septic shock**	8.3 (0.0/45.0)	45.0 (25.0/71.4)*

ICU indicates intensive care unit; BMI, body mass index; ARDS, acute respiratory distress syndrome; SOFA, Sequential Organ Failure Assessment; SAPS-II, Simplified Acute Physiology Score II; MRC, Medical Research Council; RASS, Richmond Agitation Sedation Scale. Results are expressed as medians with inter-quartile range or as absolute numbers with percentages. Differences are calculated between patients with excitable (non-CIM) and non-excitable (CIM) muscle membrane. Mann-Whitney test.
*$P<0.05$,
$^{\dagger}P<0.01$.

(controls: 1.25 (0.51–1.38), ICU-patients early time point: 5.73 (2.4–9.51), $P<0.0001$), but not that of *TNF-α* (controls: 0.79 (0.34–1.45), ICU-patients early time point: 1.36 (0.96–1.9), $P=0.28$) was elevated in critically ill patients (Figure 3B). Furthermore, no difference in *IL-6* and *TNF-α* expression was found between CIM and non-CIM patients (early time point: *IL-6:* CIM 6.02 (2.74–11.67), non-CIM 5.43 (2.45–7.11), $P=0.175$; *TNF-α:* CIM 1.4 (0.97–1.84), non-CIM 1.31 (1.03–2.08), $P=0.76$) or between the early and late biopsy specimens (late time point: *IL-6:* CIM 8.01 (4.324–10.37), non-CIM 8.92 (3.72–13.46); *TNF-α:* CIM 2.02 (1.15–2.55), non-CIM 1.58 (1.19–2.29), n.s.)(Figure 3B and 3C). These data suggest that inflammation occurred directly in muscle during critical illness.

Muscle biopsies consist of myocyte and non-myocyte cells, such as fibroblasts and endothelial cells. To test if myocytes synthesize SAA1, we performed cell culture experiments using human myocytes which were differentiated into myotubes. Indeed, using real-time RT-PCR we found *SAA1* to be endogenously expressed in myotubes. We treated myotubes with human recombinant IL-6, TNF-α, or both. Both IL-6 and TNF-α increased *SAA1* expression in human myotubes. A combination of IL-6 and TNF-α was more effective than either cytokine alone (Figure 4A). Immunofluorescence staining showed an increase in SAA1 protein (Figure 4B). Lipopolysaccharides (LPS) also mediate muscular atrophy [32]. LPS treatment of human myotubes increased *SAA1* expression (Figure 4C) and protein content (Figure 4D).

To analyze if *SAA1* or *SAA4* expression were directly associated with compound muscle action potential, correlation analyses were performed. We found that *SAA1* and *SAA4* mRNA expression in the early biopsy specimen were inversely correlated with compound muscle action potential after direct muscle stimulation (dmCMAP) (Figure 5). In addition, *SAA1* and *SAA4* expression levels were directly correlated with each other (Figure S4).

Inflammation-induced SAA1 Expression in Muscle is Conserved throughout Species

We next sought to test if inflammation-induced acute phase response in muscle is conserved throughout species. Therefore, we asked if our findings could be reproduced in a mouse model of polymicrobial sepsis. Wild type mice were subjected to the cecal ligation and puncture model (CLP) of sepsis, or a sham procedure, for 24 h [33]. RT-PCR analyses performed on the *gastrocnemius plantaris* and *tibialis anterior* confirmed increased muscular *SAA1* expression during sepsis (Figure 6A). Immunohistochemistry showed that SAA1 protein was increased in myofibers, at the sarcolemma around myofibers and in the interstitium of the *gastrocnemius plantaris* of septic mice (Figure 6B). To investigate if SAA protein was secreted by septic skeletal muscle and was contained in the muscular interstitium, we performed microdialysis in the *vastus medialis* of septic and sham mice 24 h after surgery. Mass-spectrometric analysis of dialysates showed an increase in interstitial SAA1, SAA2 and SAA4 proteins in *vastus*

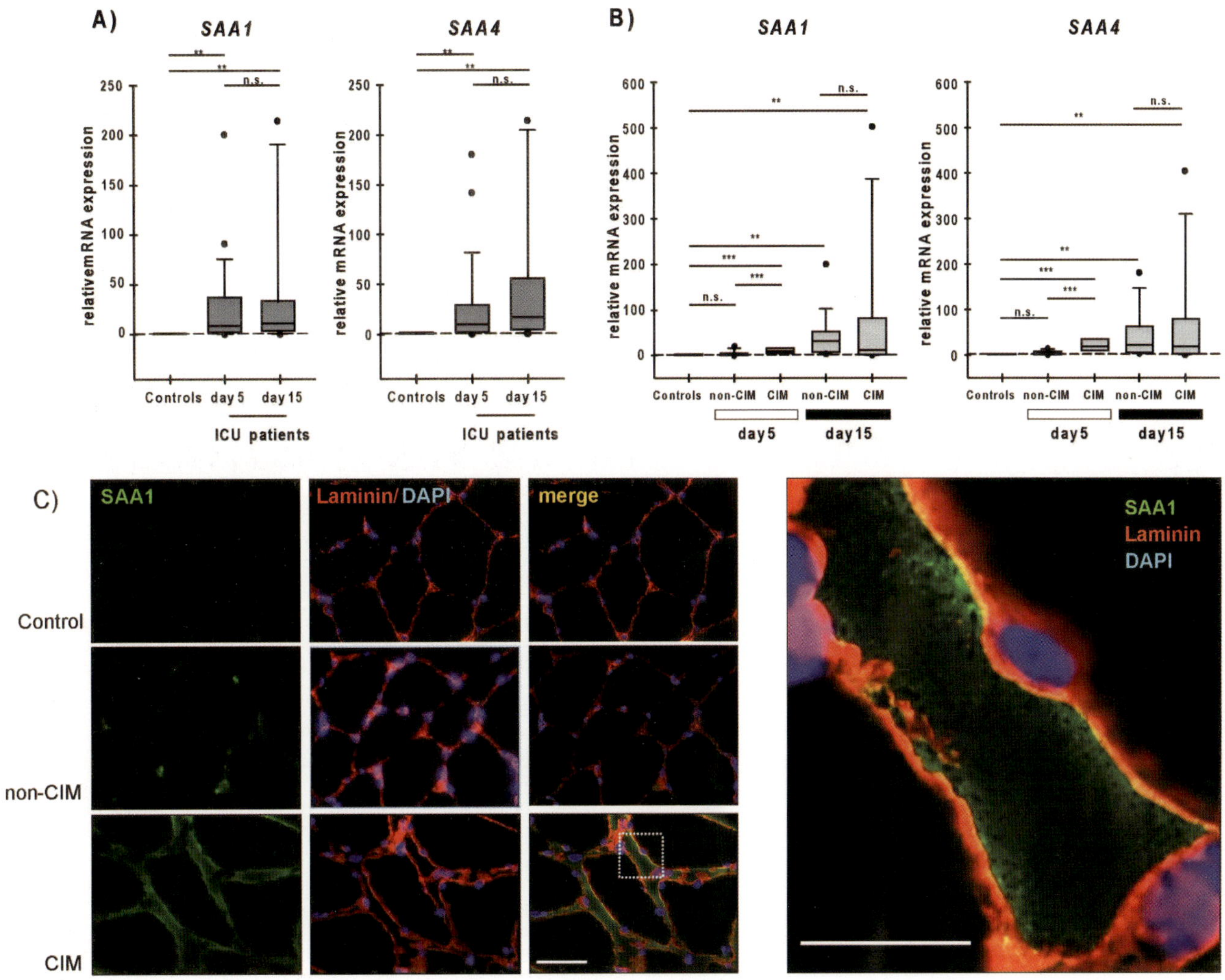

Figure 2. Muscular *SAA1* and *SAA4* expression and accumulation in CIM patients. Control values (no ICU subjects) were set to one and means were indicated as dashed lines. (A) RT-PCR analyses of *SAA1* and *SAA4* expression at early (day 5) and late (day 15) time points in *vastus lateralis* muscle of critically ill patients, and (B) CIM and non-CIM patients. *Glyceraldehyde-3 phosphate dehydrogenase* (*GAPDH*) expression was used as reference. Data are presented as box plots showing median, 25th and 75th percentiles. Wilcoxon tests were performed between early and late biopsy specimens and Mann-Whitney tests for the respective time points and controls. ***$P<0.001$, **$P<0.01$, *$P<0.05$, or n.s. (not statistically significant). (C) Immunohistochemistry of SAA1 (green) and the membrane marker laminin (red) on skeletal muscle biopsy specimens from control subjects, non-CIM and CIM patients. Nuclei were stained with 4′,6-diamidino-2-phenylindole (DAPI; blue); scale bar 50 µm. (D) Higher magnification of the merged picture from CIM patient in (C) to illustrate colocalization of SAA1 (green) and laminin (red) at the cell membrane, accumulation of SAA1 in the interstitium and around myofibers; scale bar 50 µm.

medialis of septic mice (Figure 6C). These data indicate that SAA is not only synthesized, but also secreted by skeletal muscle in response to inflammation. RT-PCR analyses and immunofluorescence stainings revealed that mouse myoblasts differentiated into myotubes also endogenously expressed SAA1. Differentiated myotubes were treated with murine recombinant IL-6 or TNF-α. Both IL-6 and TNF-α increased *SAA1* expression (Figure 6D). Immunofluorescence staining showed an increase in SAA1 protein in those myotubes (Figure 6E). LPS treatment of differentiated mouse myotubes increased *SAA1* expression and protein content (Figure S5A and S5B). These data indicate that inflammation-induced *SAA1* expression in myocytes is conserved throughout species.

Discussion

We found that inflammation caused acute phase response in skeletal muscle of critically ill patients, which was associated with CIM. We demonstrated that early increases in *SAA1* and *SAA4* expression and SAA1 accumulation in muscle are associated with CIM development. *SAA1* was expressed in myocytes *in vitro*. Treatment with IL-6, TNF-α, or LPS increased its expression both in human and mouse skeletal muscle and myocytes. Inverse correlations between early *SAA1* expression and muscle membrane excitability suggest that SAA1 could contribute to the development of CIM.

Few data regarding differences in gene expression between CIM and non-CIM skeletal muscles are available. We relied on an expression array and identified genes that are specifically increased in CIM skeletal muscle at a very early time point after ICU admission. *SAA1* and *SAA4* expression was higher in skeletal

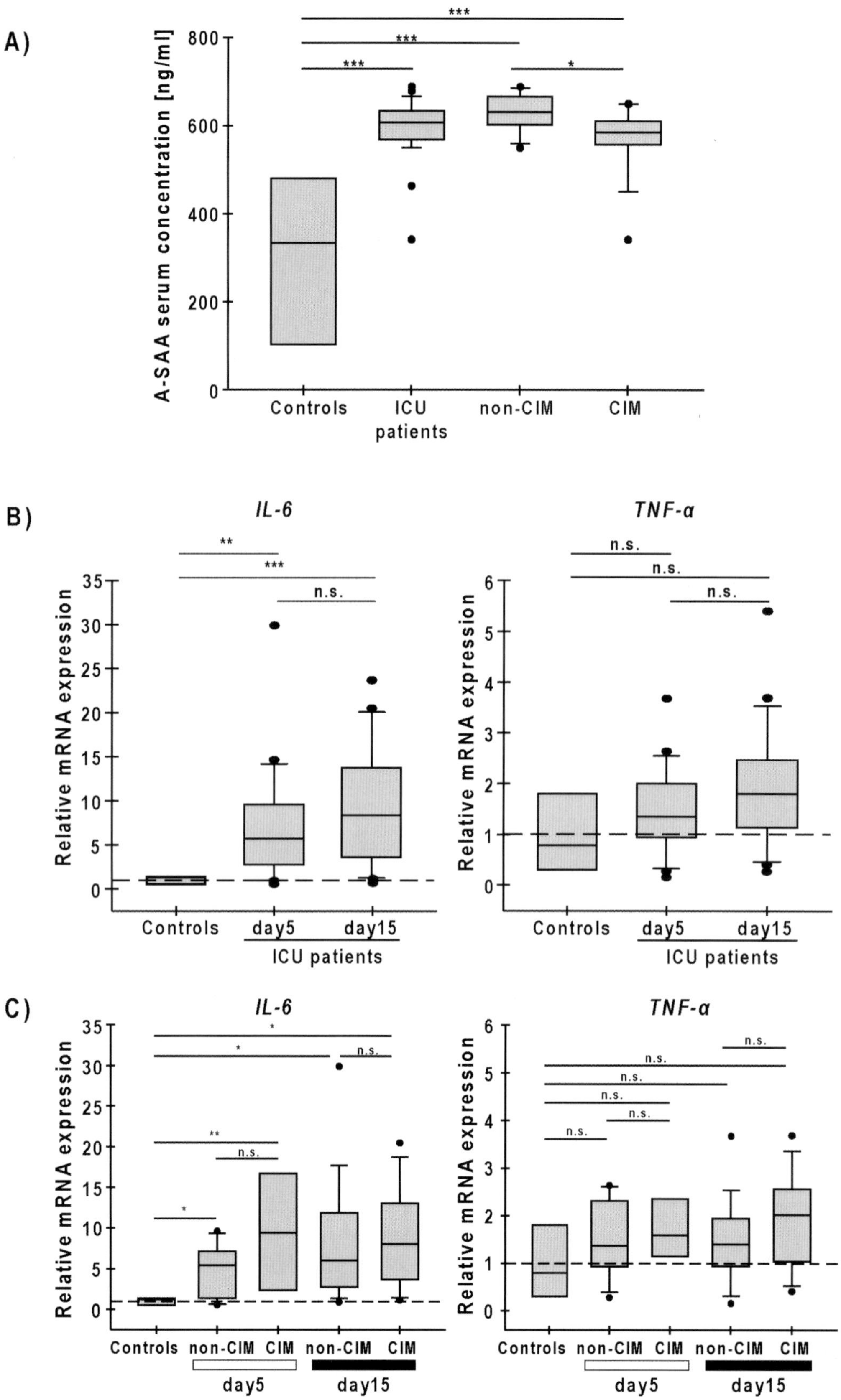

Figure 3. A-SAA serum levels and *IL-6* and *TNF-α* expression in skeletal muscle of critically ill patients. (A) Serum levels of acute phase SAA (A-SAA) measured by ELISA in healthy controls (n=6), critically ill patients (ICUs, n=30), non-CIM (n=19) and CIM (n=11) patients. Serum samples were obtained at days 2 to 3 after ICU admission. **$P<0.01$, *$P<0.05$. (B) RT-PCR analyses of *IL-6* and *TNF-α* expressions in skeletal muscle

from critically ill patients at early (day 5) and late (day 15) time points. *Glyceraldehyde-3 phosphate dehydrogenase* (*GAPDH*) expression was used as reference. (C) RT-PCR analyses of *IL-6* and *TNF-α* expression at early and late time points in CIM and non-CIM patients. Data are presented as box plots showing median, 25th and 75th percentiles. Wilcoxon tests were performed between early and late biopsy specimens and Mann-Whitney tests for the respective time points and controls; $^{***}P<0.001$, $^{**}P<0.01$, $^{*}P<0.05$, or n.s. (not statistically significant).

muscle of CIM patients only in muscle biopsies of the early time point. The rapid and early increase in *SAA1* and *SAA4* expression could be responsible for SAA1 accumulation in the muscle membrane and interstitium of CIM patients, possibly overriding its degradation. SAA1 accumulation coincided with decreased electrical excitability of the muscle membrane measured at median day 6 in CIM patients. At the later time point, *SAA1* and *SAA4* expression were similar in CIM and non-CIM patients and SAA1 accumulation resolved; further supporting the hypothesis that early induction of SAA1 facilitates its accumulation in muscle membrane during inflammation. However, further experiments are needed to elucidate if these aggregates directly affect muscle membrane excitability especially during early critical illness. Our findings also implicate a very early pathomechanism facilitating CIM development right after ICU admission. This hypothesis is strengthened by the rapid increase in SAA1 synthesis and secretion in muscle of septic mice. Based on our findings, we hypothesize that skeletal muscle participates in acute phase responses that self-perpetuate muscle demise during sepsis.

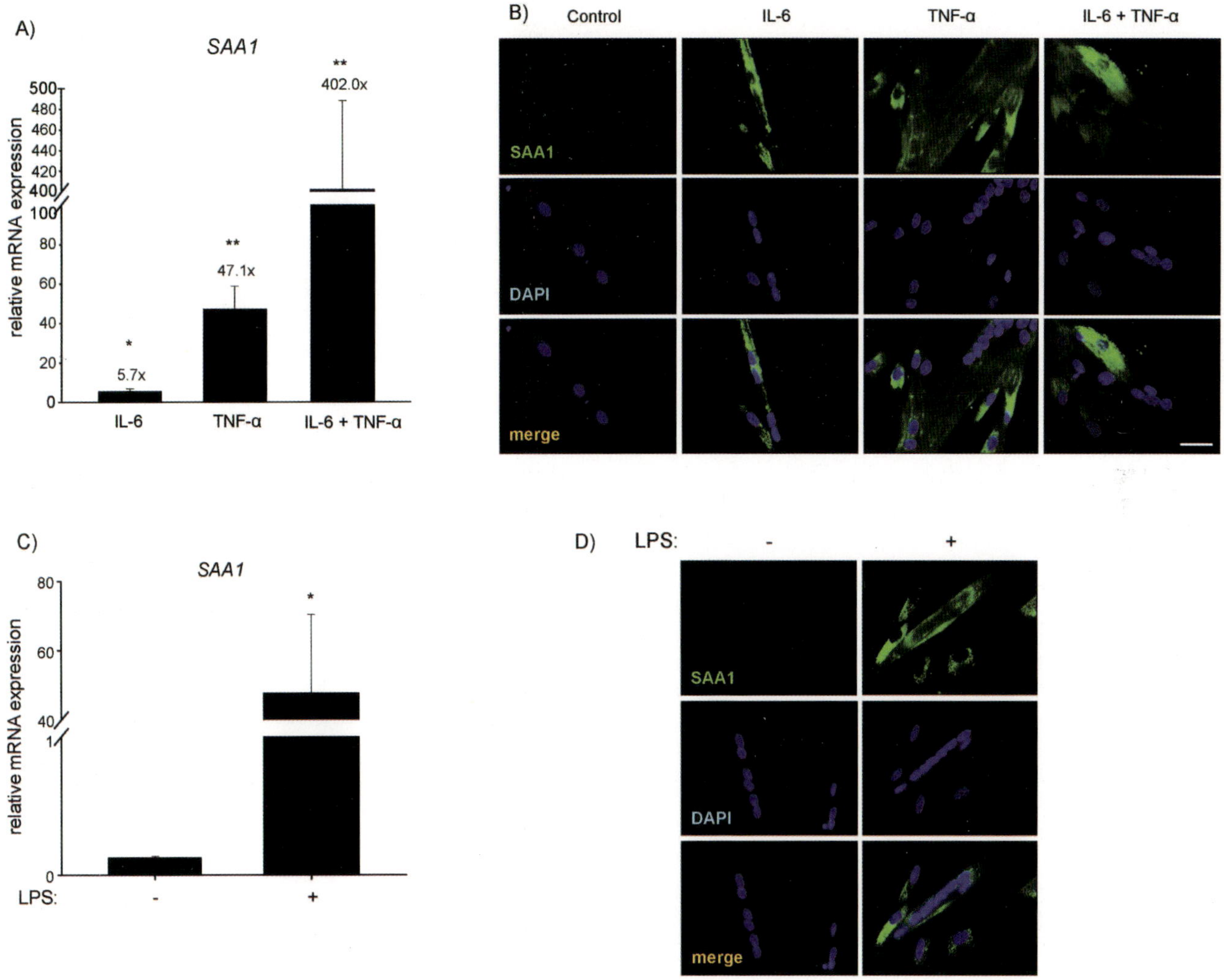

Figure 4. IL-6, TNF-α and LPS increased *SAA1* expression and protein content in human skeletal muscle cells *in vitro*. (A) Differentiated human skeletal myotubes were treated with human recombinant IL-6 (100 ng/ml), TNF-α (10 ng/ml), or a combination of both (IL-6, 100 ng/ml; TNF-α, 10 ng/ml) for 16 h. RT-PCR was used to measure *SAA1* expression, which was normalized to *beta-2-microglobulin* expression. Relative gene expression by fold-induction of *SAA1* expression (above column) is shown. $^{**}P<0.01$, $^{*}P<0.05$. (B) Immunocytochemistry of SAA1 (green) on differentiated human myotubes following treatment with human recombinant IL-6 (100 ng/ml), human recombinant TNF-α (10 ng/ml), and both cytokines (IL-6, 100 ng/ml; TNF-α, 10 ng/ml) together for 16 h is shown. Nuclei were stained with 4′,6-diamidino-2-phenylindole (DAPI; blue); scale bar 50 μm. (C) Human skeletal myotubes were treated with lipopolysaccharide (LPS, 1 μg/ml) for 16 h. RT-PCR was used to measure *SAA1* expression, which was normalized to *Glyceraldehyde-3 phosphate dehydrogenase* (*GAPDH*); $^{*}P<0.05$. (D) Immunocytochemistry of SAA1 (green) on human myotubes following LPS treatment (1 μg/ml) for 16 h. Nuclei were stained with DAPI (blue); scale bar 50 μm.

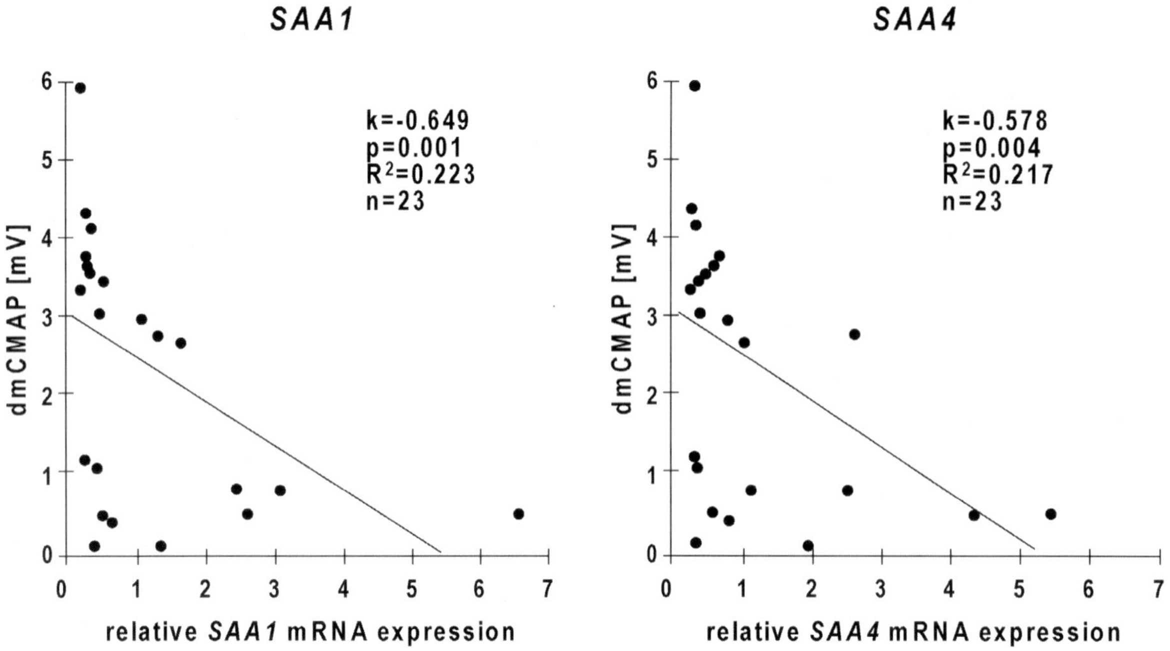

Figure 5. Early *SAA1* expression correlated with muscle membrane excitability of critically ill patients. A multivariate analysis was performed to test, if *SAA1* and *SAA4* expressions were correlated with clinical CIM parameters. *SAA1* (left) and *SAA4* (right) expressions measured in early biopsy specimens were inversely correlated with compound muscle action potential on direct muscle stimulation (dmCMAP).

The SAA family of proteins are sub-classified into acute phase response SAA1 and SAA2 [34], whose expression increases up to 1000-fold during inflammation [26], and SAA4, which is mainly constitutively expressed [35]. However, *SAA4* expression is also increased by inflammatory stimuli in various tissues [36]. Acute phase SAAs are predominantly synthesized and secreted by the liver in response to inflammation [24]. Clinical data suggest markedly increased inflammation in CIM patients [14]. We believe that this increase contributed to the early induction of *SAA1* and *SAA4* expression in muscle. However, for logistical reasons it was impossible to obtain biopsies earlier than five days after ICU admission. Therefore we took advantage of an animal model of polymicrobial sepsis enabling us to investigate much earlier time points of critical illness. With this model we showed that inflammation leads to a rapid increase of SAA1 synthesis in muscle. It also demonstrated that inflammation-induced acute phase response in muscle was conserved throughout species. Conservation of this pathway is also supported by our *in vitro* data showing increased SAA1 synthesis in response to cytokine treatment of murine myocytes. In addition, this mouse model proved to be useful to demonstrate increased SAA1 secretion in the muscular interstitium of septic mice.

The inflammatory cytokines IL-6, TNF-α, and IL-1β all increase hepatic SAA synthesis. However, skeletal muscle apparently also contributes to increased SAA production [26]. Although, *SAA* expression was higher in CIM than in non-CIM patients SAA serum levels were not increased in CIM patients. Possibly, SAA1 accumulations at the sarcolemma and in the interstitium might prevent SAA1's entry into the circulation. Alternatively, SAA1 production in muscle is perhaps only a small fraction of the total SAA produced.

Both TNF-α and LPS increased *SAA1* expression *in vivo* [31,37]. In line with these observations, our data showed that myocytes express *SAA1*, and that IL-6, TNF-α, and LPS all increase its basal expression. Since *IL-6* and *TNF-α* were equally expressed in CIM and non-CIM muscle, muscular IL-6 and TNF-α do not seem to be responsible for increased SAA1 or SAA4 contents in CIM. However, recently we reported that serum IL-6 levels were predictive of CIM [14]. We speculate that increased serum but not muscular IL-6 levels were responsible for increased *SAA1* expression in CIM muscle. A role for both SAA1 and IL-6 in muscular atrophy was recently reported [26]. SAA1 was found to be increased in skeletal muscle of cachectic mice with cancer [25]. In this work, *SAA1* expression correlated with the degree of skeletal muscle wasting and muscular atrophy. IL-6 and SAA1 were also shown to mediate skeletal muscle atrophy induced by AngII [26]. These data, and the findings we report here, implicate that SAA1 contributes to inflammation induced muscular atrophy.

Muscular *TNF-α* expression was unchanged in critically ill patients implicating a minor role of TNF-α in regulation of SAA1 expression. Nevertheless, we investigated the effect of TNF-α on SAA1 expression and protein content in myocytes *in vitro*. First, because *TNF-α* expression follows a time course during inflammation with an early increase and a rapid decrease after the inflammatory stimuli it is possible that the biopsy time point was too late to detect meaningful differences in *TNF-α* expression between CIM and non-CIM patients. Second, TNF-α increases *SAA1* expression in muscle and other tissues [24]. Third, we assumed that TNF-α [19–21] contributes to muscular atrophy in critically ill patients by increasing protein degradation [22,23]. Fourth, it is unknown how much biological active TNF-α is contained in the skeletal muscle of our patients because TNF-α protein levels were not quantitated. Fifth, in general TNF-α serum levels [16] are increased in systemic inflammatory response syndrome and sepsis patients [14]. However, if TNF-α serum levels were elevated in our patients is uncertain.

We also found increased muscular *SAA4* expression in critically ill patients and higher upregulation in CIM muscle at the early time point. Indeed, SAA4 has been described as a minor acute phase reactant [36]. The positive correlation between *SAA1* and

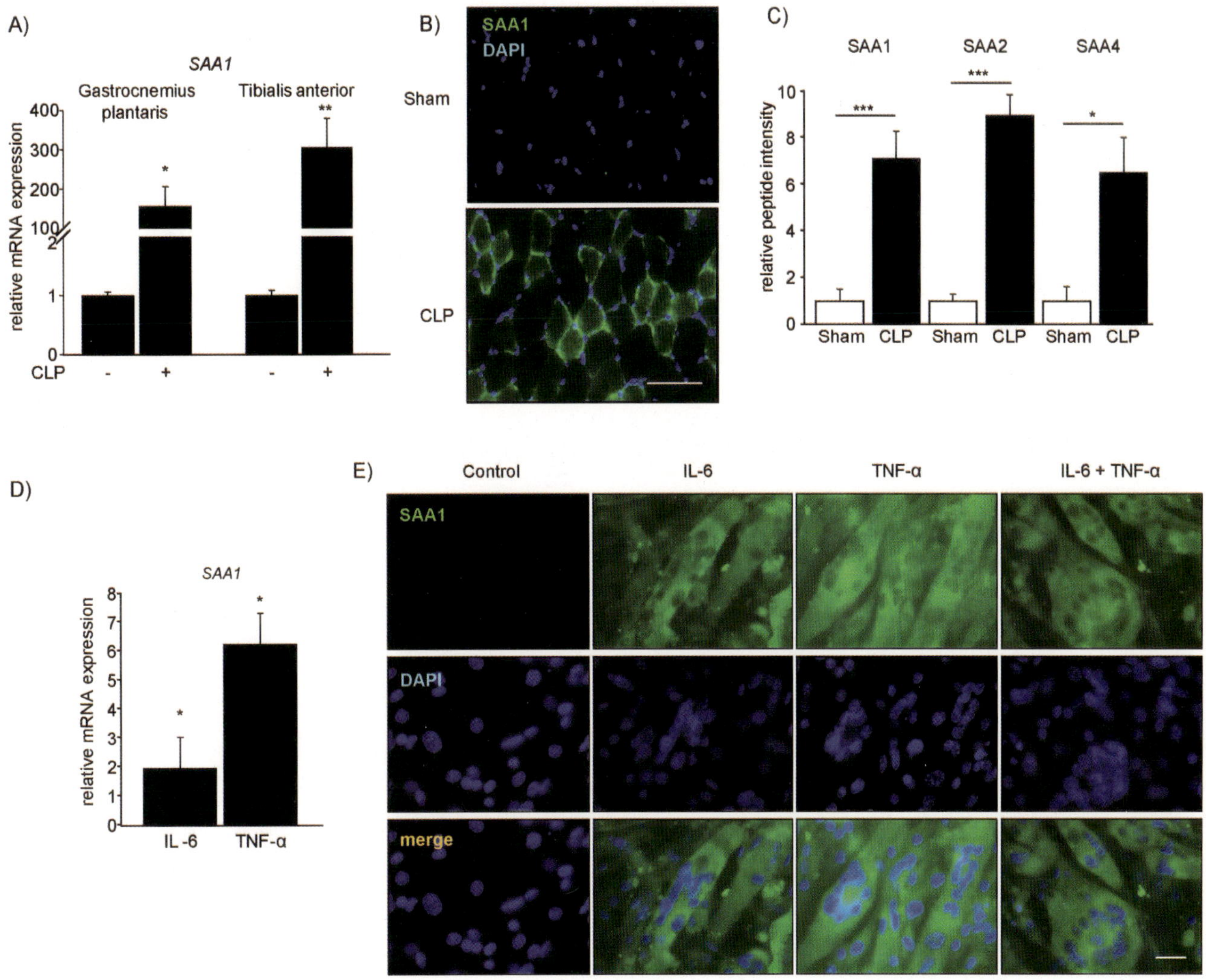

Figure 6. Sepsis and proinflammatory cytokines increase muscular SAA1 expression and protein content *in vivo* and *in vitro*. (A) Polymicrobial sepsis was induced by cecal ligation and puncture (CLP) in mice for 24 h (n = 5). Sham operated mice were used as controls (n = 5). RT-PCR was used to measure *SAA1* expression in *gastrocnemius plantaris* and *tibialis anterior* muscles, which was normalized to *GAPDH* expression. $^{**}P<0.01$, $^{*}P<0.05$. (B) Immunohistochemistry of SAA1 (green) on *gastrocnemius plantaris* muscle of sham and CLP treated mice (24 h treatment). Nuclei were stained with 4′,6-diamidino-2-phenylindole (DAPI; blue); scale bar 50 μm. (C) Mass-spectrometry was used to quantitate SAA1, SAA2 and SAA4 in dialysates of *vastus medialis* of sham (n = 8) and CLP (n = 8) 24 h after surgery. $^{***}P<0.001$, $^{*}P<0.05$. (D) Differentiated mouse skeletal myotubes were treated with murine recombinant IL-6 (100 ng/ml) or murine recombinant TNF-α (10 ng/ml) for 16 h. RT-PCR was used to measure *SAA1* expression, which was normalized to *GAPDH*; $^{*}P<0.05$. (E) Immunocytochemistry of SAA1 (green) on differentiated murine myotubes following treatment with murine recombinant IL-6 (100 ng/ml), murine recombinant TNF-α (10 ng/ml) or a combination of both (IL-6, 100 ng/ml; TNF-α, 10 ng/ml) for 16 h is shown. Nuclei were stained with DAPI (blue); scale bar 50 μm.

SAA4 expression supports a possible common pathway regulating both genes during critical illness.

In these same patients, we recently reported that the glucose transporter GLUT4 a key regulator of glycemic homeostasis in skeletal muscle was trapped at perinuclear spaces of myocytes, most pronounced in patients with CIM, but resided at the sarcolemma in control subjects [11]. Glucose metabolism was not stimulated during euglycemic-hyperinsulinergic clamp. Interestingly, insulin signal transduction was intact and let to activation of Akt. In contrast, p-adenosine monophosphate-activated protein kinase (p-AMPK) was not detectable in CIM muscle. These observations [11] together with the measurement of non-excitable muscle membrane as well as membranous SAA1 accumulation reported here, all occurring early during CIM development, point towards a central role of the myocyte membrane in the pathogenesis of CIM. However, we have not yet identified the pathways that directly interconnect the metabolic disturbances we observed earlier and the inflammatory responses we report here in the same patients. But, avenues to do so certainly exist. For instance, the *SLC2A4* gene encoding GLUT4 is repressed by the inflammatory transcription factor NF-κB [38]. Thus, increased inflammation in CIM skeletal muscle could have let to an activation of the inflammation mediator NF-κB mediating downregulation of GLUT4. Finally, SAA is a known marker for insulin resistance [39].

We conclude that skeletal muscle contributes to general inflammation and acute-phase response in CIM patients. Differences in muscular SAA1 expression and content could be important for CIM pathogenesis.

Limitations

We used muscle membrane excitability to differentiate between CIM and non-CIM patients. MRC scores could not be assessed for all patients mainly due to the fact that not all patients became awake during the study period. Therefore, the number of patients diagnosed with weakness based on MRC scoring is smaller compared to electrophysiological testing. Although, muscle membrane in-excitability after direct muscle stimulation is an accepted marker for early CIM diagnosis and correlates with ICUAW, membrane in-excitability and weakness are not synonymous [1,8,28]. However, direct muscle stimulation identified weakness with a sensitivity and specificity of 80% each, which is consistent with our recent work [8]. We conclude that electrophysiological testing is useful to predict weakness in patients who are not assessable by clinical measurements of muscle strength.

To get insights into early molecular changes in skeletal muscle caused by critical illness biopsies from the very beginning of the disease, preferably from day 1 if not hours after the onset of critical illness, are needed. However, according to German law and the ethic committee a legal proxy must give his or her informed consent before a muscle biopsy can be performed. Usually this process takes 3 to 5 days. At this time point molecular pathways leading to myopathy are already activated. Nevertheless, we identified early and specific changes in gene expression in the skeletal muscle of patients developing CIM. For the same reason, quantitation of *IL-6* and *TNF-α* expression might not be representative for the initial disease phase. Our findings that IL-6 and TNF-α increased SAA1 gene expression and protein content in human and mouse myotubes do not mean that they account for the observed changes in SAA1 expression and content between CIM and non-CIM patients; but we can also not exclude their involvement. The discrepancy between *IL-6* and *TNF-α* expression in human skeletal muscle, and the results of our cell culture and animal work in terms of SAA1 expression might be explained by differences in timing; early biopsies were performed at median day 5, animal experiments were performed after 24 hours of sepsis and cytokine treatment was performed for 16 hours *in vitro*. In addition, despite its association with CIM we did not prove that SAA1 is causatively linked to CIM development. Because we hypothesize that molecular changes in muscle of critically ill patients occur early during the disease process and based on the fact that it is difficult to obtain biopsy specimens much earlier than 3 days after onset of critical illness we think that cell culture and animal experiments are required to investigate mechanisms of inflammation induced muscle atrophy. Extrapolation of *in vivo* and *in vitro* data to the human situation needs to be done with caution.

Supporting Information

Figure S1 Muscular *SAA1* expression in patients with ICU-acquired weakness (ICUAW) according to dmCMAP or MRC scoring. RT-PCR analyses of *SAA1* expression at the early time point in *vastus lateralis* muscle of critically ill patients with (A) excitable (n = 12) and non-excitable (n = 18) muscle membrane and (B) MRC score ≥ (n = 6) or <4 (n = 15) are shown. Control values (no ICU subjects) were set to one. *Glyceraldehyde-3 phosphate dehydrogenase* (*GAPDH*) expression was used as reference. Data are presented as box plots showing median, 25th and 75th percentiles.

Figure S2 Muscular *SAA4* expression in patients with ICU-acquired weakness (ICUAW) according to dmCMAP or MRC scoring. RT-PCR analyses of *SAA4* expression at the early time point in *vastus lateralis* muscle of critically ill patients with (A) excitable (n = 12) and non-excitable (n = 18) muscle membrane and (B) MRC score ≥ (n = 6) or <4 (n = 15) are shown. Control values (no ICU subjects) were set to one. *Glyceraldehyde-3 phosphate dehydrogenase* (*GAPDH*) expression was used as reference. Data are presented as box plots showing median, 25th and 75th percentiles.

Figure S3 SAA1 accumulations were found in the skeletal muscle of CIM patients at the late time point. Representative immunohistochemistry for SAA1 (green) and laminin (red) for the late time point of control subjects, CIM and non-CIM patients. Nuclei were stained with 4′,6-diamidino-2-phenylindole (DAPI; blue); scale bar 50 μm.

Figure S4 *SAA1* and *SAA4* expression were positively correlated with each other.

Figure S5 (A) Mouse skeletal myotubes were treated with lipopolysaccharide (LPS, 1 μg/ml) for 16 h. RT-PCR was used to measure *SAA1* expression, which was normalized to *Glyceraldehyde-3 phosphate dehydrogenase* (*Gapdh*); **P*<0.05. (B) Immunocytochemistry of SAA1 (green) on murine myotubes following LPS treatment (1 μg/ml) for 16 h. Nuclei were stained with 4′,6-diamidino-2-phenylindole (DAPI; blue); scale bar 50 μm.

Table S1 Primer pairs for RT-PCR are shown. SAA indicates serum amyloid A; GAPDH, glyceraldehyde-3-phosphate dehydrogenase; Hs, Homo sapiens; Mm, Mouse musculus.

Table S2 Top 30 genes increased in vastus lateralis of ICU patients.

Table S3 Top 30 genes decreased in vastus lateralis of ICU patients.

Table S4 Top 30 genes increased in vastus lateralis of CIM compared to non-CIM patients.

Table S5 Top 30 genes decreased in vastus lateralis of CIM compared to non-CIM patients.

Table S6 Direct muscle stimulation identified weakness with a sensitivity of 80% and a specificity of 83.3%.

Methods S1 Details about electrophysiological measurements, muscle biopsies, microarray analyzes and quantitative real-time PCR, the animal model of polymicrobial sepsis by cecal ligation and puncture surgery, mass spectrometry, immunohistochemistry and ELISA, and human and murine myoblast culture, RT-PCR, and immunofluorescence are provided.

Acknowledgments

We thank Friedrich C. Luft for helpful advice on the manuscript. We thank Janine Woehlecke, Sibylle Schmidt, Josefine Ruβ and Anika Lindner for excellent technical assistance. We are grateful for the patience and courage of our patients and their consenting relatives.

Author Contributions

Conceived and designed the experiments: CL, SWC, FS, JH, M. Kny, XZ, DL, SS, JS, MB, GD, JF. Performed the experiments: CL, SWC, FS, JH, M. Kny, XZ, DL, SS, JS, MB, GD, JF, HS, KS, NH, SL, TW, SK, M. Krebs CS. Analyzed the data: CL, SWC, FS, JH, M. Kny, XZ, DL, SS, JS, MB, GD, JF, HS, KS, NH, GD, SL, GBB, VM, TW, SK, M. Krebs, CS. Contributed reagents/materials/analysis tools: SL. Wrote the paper: CL, SWC, FS, JH, M. Kny, DL, JF.

References

1. Bierbrauer J, Koch S, Olbricht C, Hamati J, Lodka D, et al. (2012) Early type II fiber atrophy in intensive care unit patients with nonexcitable muscle membrane. Crit Care Med 40: 647–650.
2. Lefaucheur JP, Nordine T, Rodriguez P, Brochard L (2006) Origin of ICU acquired paresis determined by direct muscle stimulation. J Neurol Neurosurg Psychiatry 77: 500–506.
3. Bolton CF, Young GB, Zochodne DW (1993) The neurological complications of sepsis. Ann Neurol 33: 94–100.
4. De Jonghe B, Sharshar T, Lefaucheur JP, Authier FJ, Durand-Zaleski I, et al. (2002) Paresis acquired in the intensive care unit: a prospective multicenter study. Jama 288: 2859–2867.
5. Herridge MS, Tansey CM, Matte A, Tomlinson G, Diaz-Granados N, et al. (2011) Functional disability 5 years after acute respiratory distress syndrome. N Engl J Med 364: 1293–1304.
6. Helliwell TR, Wilkinson A, Griffiths RD, McClelland P, Palmer TE, et al. (1998) Muscle fibre atrophy in critically ill patients is associated with the loss of myosin filaments and the presence of lysosomal enzymes and ubiquitin. Neuropathol Appl Neurobiol 24: 507–517.
7. Callahan LA, Supinski GS (2009) Sepsis-induced myopathy. Crit Care Med 37: S354–367.
8. Weber-Carstens S, Koch S, Spuler S, Spies CD, Bubser F, et al. (2009) Nonexcitable muscle membrane predicts intensive care unit-acquired paresis in mechanically ventilated, sedated patients. Crit Care Med 37: 2632–2637.
9. Ali NA, O'Brien JM Jr, Hoffmann SP, Phillips G, Garland A, et al. (2008) Acquired weakness, handgrip strength, and mortality in critically ill patients. Am J Respir Crit Care Med 178: 261–268.
10. Kress JP, Herridge MS (2012) Medical and economic implications of physical disability of survivorship. Semin Respir Crit Care Med 33: 339–347.
11. Weber-Carstens S, Schneider J, Wollersheim T, Assmann A, Bierbrauer J, et al. (2012) Critical Illness Myopathy and GLUT4 - Significance of Insulin and Muscle Contraction. Am J Respir Crit Care Med.
12. Friedrich O (2006) Critical illness myopathy: what is happening? Curr Opin Clin Nutr Metab Care 9: 403–409.
13. Winkelman C (2010) The role of inflammation in ICU-acquired weakness. Crit Care 14: 186.
14. Weber-Carstens S, Deja M, Koch S, Spranger J, Bubser F, et al. (2010) Risk factors in critical illness myopathy during the early course of critical illness: a prospective observational study. Crit Care 14: R119.
15. Damas P, Ledoux D, Nys M, Vrindts Y, De Groote D, et al. (1992) Cytokine serum level during severe sepsis in human IL-6 as a marker of severity. Ann Surg 215: 356–362.
16. Waage A, Halstensen A, Espevik T (1987) Association between tumour necrosis factor in serum and fatal outcome in patients with meningococcal disease. Lancet 1: 355–357.
17. Tsujinaka T, Fujita J, Ebisui C, Yano M, Kominami E, et al. (1996) Interleukin 6 receptor antibody inhibits muscle atrophy and modulates proteolytic systems in interleukin 6 transgenic mice. J Clin Invest 97: 244–249.
18. Zimmers TA, McKillop IH, Pierce RH, Yoo JY, Koniaris LG (2003) Massive liver growth in mice induced by systemic interleukin 6 administration. Hepatology 38: 326–334.
19. Adams V, Mangner N, Gasch A, Krohne C, Gielen S, et al. (2008) Induction of MuRF1 is essential for TNF-alpha-induced loss of muscle function in mice. J Mol Biol 384: 48–59.
20. Anker SD, Clark AL, Kemp M, Salsbury C, Teixeira MM, et al. (1997) Tumor necrosis factor and steroid metabolism in chronic heart failure: possible relation to muscle wasting. J Am Coll Cardiol 30: 997–1001.
21. Phillips T, Leeuwenburgh C (2005) Muscle fiber specific apoptosis and TNF-alpha signaling in sarcopenia are attenuated by life-long calorie restriction. Faseb J 19: 668–670.
22. Zamir O, Hasselgren PO, Kunkel SL, Frederick J, Higashiguchi T, et al. (1992) Evidence that tumor necrosis factor participates in the regulation of muscle proteolysis during sepsis. Arch Surg 127: 170–174.
23. Goodman MN (1991) Tumor necrosis factor induces skeletal muscle protein breakdown in rats. Am J Physiol 260: E727–730.
24. Uhlar CM, Whitehead AS (1999) Serum amyloid A, the major vertebrate acute-phase reactant. Eur J Biochem 265: 501–523.
25. Bonetto A, Aydogdu T, Kunzevitzky N, Guttridge DC, Khuri S, et al. (2011) STAT3 activation in skeletal muscle links muscle wasting and the acute phase response in cancer cachexia. PLoS One 6: e22538.
26. Zhang L, Du J, Hu Z, Han G, Delafontaine P, et al. (2009) IL-6 and serum amyloid A synergy mediates angiotensin II-induced muscle wasting. J Am Soc Nephrol 20: 604–612.
27. Dellinger RP, Levy MM, Rhodes A, Annane D, Gerlach H, et al. Surviving Sepsis Campaign: International Guidelines for Management of Severe Sepsis and Septic Shock: 2012. Crit Care Med 41: 580–637.
28. Rich MM, Teener JW, Raps EC, Schotland DL, Bird SJ (1996) Muscle is electrically inexcitable in acute quadriplegic myopathy. Neurology 46: 731–736.
29. Koch S, Spuler S, Deja M, Bierbrauer J, Dimroth A, et al. (2011) Critical illness myopathy is frequent: accompanying neuropathy protracts ICU discharge. J Neurol Neurosurg Psychiatry 82: 287–293.
30. Fielitz J, Kim MS, Shelton JM, Latif S, Spencer JA, et al. (2007) Myosin accumulation and striated muscle myopathy result from the loss of muscle RING finger 1 and 3. J Clin Invest 117: 2486–2495.
31. Zhang N, Ahsan MH, Purchio AF, West DB (2005) Serum amyloid A-luciferase transgenic mice: response to sepsis, acute arthritis, and contact hypersensitivity and the effects of proteasome inhibition. J Immunol 174: 8125–8134.
32. Doyle A, Zhang G, Abdel Fattah EA, Eissa NT, Li YP (2011) Toll-like receptor 4 mediates lipopolysaccharide-induced muscle catabolism via coordinate activation of ubiquitin-proteasome and autophagy-lysosome pathways. Faseb J 25: 99–110.
33. Rittirsch D, Huber-Lang MS, Flierl MA, Ward PA (2009) Immunodesign of experimental sepsis by cecal ligation and puncture. Nat Protoc 4: 31–36.
34. Lowell CA, Potter DA, Stearman RS, Morrow JF (1986) Structure of the murine serum amyloid A gene family. Gene conversion. J Biol Chem 261: 8442–8452.
35. de Beer MC, de Beer FC, Gerardot CJ, Cecil DR, Webb NR, et al. (1996) Structure of the mouse Saa4 gene and its linkage to the serum amyloid A gene family. Genomics 34: 139–142.
36. Steel DM, Sellar GC, Uhlar CM, Simon S, DeBeer FC, et al. (1993) A constitutively expressed serum amyloid A protein gene (SAA4) is closely linked to, and shares structural similarities with, an acute-phase serum amyloid A protein gene (SAA2). Genomics 16: 447–454.
37. Foyn Bruun C, Sletten K, Marhaug G (1998) Mouse serum amyloid A (SAA) proteins isolated by two-dimensional electrophoresis: characterization of isotypes and the effect of separate and combined administrations of cytokines, dexamethasone and lipopolysaccharide (LPS) on serum levels and isotype distribution. Clin Exp Immunol 111: 231–236.
38. Furuya DT, Neri EA, Poletto AC, Anhe GF, Freitas HS, et al. (2013) Identification of nuclear factor-kappaB sites in the Slc2a4 gene promoter. Mol Cell Endocrinol 370: 87–95.
39. Filippin-Monteiro FB, de Oliveira EM, Sandri S, Knebel FH, Albuquerque RC, et al. (2012) Serum amyloid A is a growth factor for 3T3-L1 adipocytes, inhibits differentiation and promotes insulin resistance. Int J Obes (Lond) 36: 1032–1039.

11

Novel *TCAP* Mutation c.32C>A Causing Limb Girdle Muscular Dystrophy 2G

Amirtharaj Francis[1], Balaraju Sunitha[2], Kandavalli Vinodh[1], Kiran Polavarapu[3], Shiva Krishna Katkam[1], Sailesh Modi[3], M. M. Srinivas Bharath[4], Narayanappa Gayathri[2], Atchayaram Nalini[3]*, Kumarasamy Thangaraj[1]*

1 CSIR-Centre for Cellular and Molecular Biology, Hyderabad, India, **2** Department of Neuropathology, National Institute of Mental Health and Neurosciences, Bengaluru, India, **3** Department of Neurology, National Institute of Mental Health and Neurosciences, Bengaluru, India, **4** Department of Neurochemistry, National Institute of Mental Health and Neurosciences, Bengaluru, India

Abstract

TCAP encoded telethonin is a 19 kDa protein, which plays an important role in anchoring titin in Z disc of the sarcomere, and is known to cause LGMD2G, a rare muscle disorder characterised by proximal and distal lower limb weakness, calf hypertrophy and loss of ambulation. A total of 300 individuals with ARLGMD were recruited for this study. Among these we identified 8 clinically well characterised LGMD2G cases from 7 unrelated Dravidian families. Clinical examination revealed predominantly proximo - distal form of weakness, scapular winging, muscle atrophy, calf hypertrophy and foot drop, immunoblot showed either complete absence or severe reduction of telethonin. Genetic analysis revealed a novel nonsense homozygous mutation c.32C>A, p.(Ser11*) in three patients of a consanguineous family and an 8 bp homozygous duplication c.26_33dupAGGTGTCG, p.(Arg12fs31*) in another patient. Both mutations possibly lead to truncated protein or nonsense mediated decay. We could not find any functionally significant *TCAP* mutation in the remaining 6 samples, except for two other polymorphisms, c.453A>C, *p.(=)* and c.-178G>T, which were found in cases and controls. This is the first report from India to demonstrate *TCAP* association with LGMD2G.

Editor: Maurilio Sampaolesi, Stem Cell Research Institute, Belgium

Funding: This study was funded by Department of Science and Technology (DST) Government of India (F.No. SR/SO/HS-16/2009) and KT was supported by CSIR Network project - GENESIS (BSC0121), Government of India. The funders had no role in study design, data collection and analysis, decision to publish, or preparation of the manuscript.

* Email: thangs@ccmb.res.in (KT); atchayaramnalini@yahoo.co.in (AN)

Introduction

The seventh form of Autosomal Recessive Limb-Girdle Muscular Dystrophy (LGMD2G; OMIM 601954) is caused by genetic variations in the telethonin gene (also named as *TCAP* or titin-cap gene) (NM_003673.3). LGMD2G has been mapped to chromosome 17q12 [1]. LGMD2G was first described from Brazil [2]; subsequently it was reported from China [3], Moldavia [4], and Portugal [5]. Onset of this disease is usually in the second decade, with predominant pelvic girdle weakness and associated distal weakness with foot drop [2]. About50% of the cases are known to have calf hypertrophy and 40% are known to lose independent ambulation during the third or fourth decade [1].

Telethonin is amongst the most abundant nuclear mRNA transcribed in skeletal muscle and encodes for a 19 kDa protein consisting of 167 amino acids [6]. The protein is located in the Z-disc of sacromere, the basic functional contractile unit in the skeletal and cardiac muscles [6,7,8]. Telethonin plays an important role in the sarcomeric assembly as it joins the two antiparallel titin (Z1-Z2) domains together through beta strand crossing and represents the strongest protein–protein interaction observed so far [9,10,11,12]. Telethonin is also known for its interaction with other Z-disc proteins of sarcomeric assembly such as LIM protein (MLP) [13], Ankrd2 [14], myostatin [15], potassium channel B-subunit minK [16], protein kinase D [17], murine double minute2 (MDM2) [18],and calsarcin [19]. Thus, *TCAP* is expected to play a very important role in the sarcomeric assembly.

It has been demonstrated that the *TCAP* knockout mouse resulted in a modest increase in passive muscle stiffness and shared many of the features of LGMD 2G phenotype [20]. Looking at the functional importance of telethonin in muscles, we have analysed *TCAP* in eight patients of Dravidian origin (south-India) in order to identify *TCAP* mutations in LGMD2G.

Materials and Methods

Subjects

This study was approved by the Institutional Ethical Committee (IEC) of Centre for Cellular and Molecular Biology, Hyderabad, India and National Institute of Mental Health and Neurosciences, Bangalore, India. The subject recruitment and sample collection were done after obtaining written informed consent/assent forms

Table 1. Primer sequence used for the TCAP amplification.

Name	Forward	Reverse	Annealing temp
TCAP 1F	TTCTGCTTCCCACTTTATGAAAA	AGAAGGGAGAGTGCAACCAC	55
TCAP 2F	GTGAGGGTGACTGGGGACTA	GAAATTTCTCCAGGGCTTCA	54
TCAP 3F	GAGAGCAAAGGGGAACCAC	ACCCTCCCTTTGGGAACTC	55
TCAP 4F	GCCATGGCTGCTTTGTAGT	TGGGGTGTACCCATTAGCTC	54

from all participants. In this prospective study (February 2010 to September 2012) a total of 300 patients with features of ARLGMD were prospectively evaluated by the principal investigator (AN) at the National Institute of Mental Health and Neurosciences. Of these 300 cases, 246 patients were confirmed to have various forms of ARLGMD based on characteristic clinical phenotype, biochemical and histopathological analysis. IB was performed sequentially based on the IHC results to confirm the type of ARLGMD.

Sequence analysis of TCAP gene was undertaken in the eight cases which were found to be LGMD2G based on immunoblotting. All patients hailed from South India and shared the ethnic origin (Dravidian linguistic group). Family members, wherever available, were included in the analysis. Among these 7 families, one (F50) had two more affected siblings. Family (F111) also had one affected sibling (F111-2), who was available for clinical examination and genetic analysis, but muscle biopsy was not done. In total, we have studied 8 patients and 49 related family members. The inclusion criteria for the index cases were: clinical phenotype consistent with LGMD2G, elevated creatine kinase (CK) level, and loss or severe reduction of telethonin expression in IB studies. One hundred and sixty seven control samples, after ruling out muscular dystrophy or family history of muscular dystrophy, were recruited for comparison purpose.

Histopathology and Immunohistochemistry (IHC)

Muscle biopsy. Open biopsy from the quadriceps femoris or biceps brachii muscle was performed in 280 patients. Samples were flash frozen in isopentane chilled in liquid nitrogen. Serial

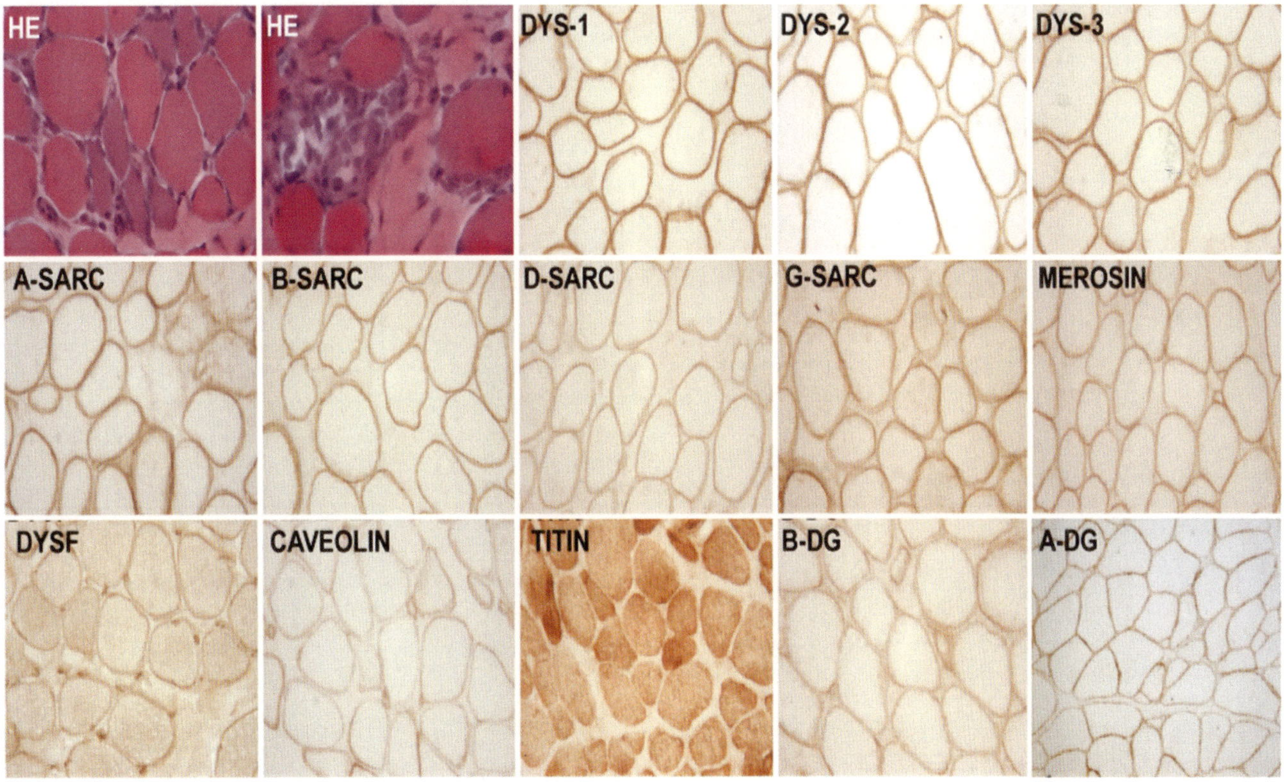

Figure 1. Transversely cut skeletal muscle tissue stained for Haematoxylin and eosin (HE) shows variation in fiber diameter clusters of basophilic regenerating fibers and myophagocytosis. Immunolabeling to antibodies against dystrophin (dys1,dys2,dys3) sarcoglycans (alpha-A, beta-B, delta-D, gamma-G, merosin, dysferlin (DYSF), caveolin, beta dystroglycan (B-DG), alpha dystroglycan (A-DG) shows uniform labeling along the sarcolemma and positive sarcoplasmic labeling to titin. X400

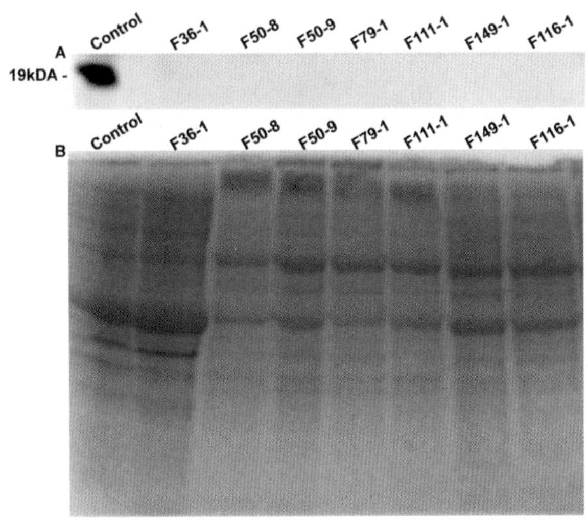

Figure 2. Western blot analysis of telethonin protein in muscle biopsies of control and telethoninopathy patients. A. Telethonin western Blot: Lane C corresponds to non-dystrophic positive control which shows telethonin band at 19 kDa. Lanes 1–7 corresponding to the Telethoninopathy patient samples, shows complete absence of the telethonin band. **B.** Coomassie stained SDS PAGE (15%) profile of total muscle extract from the samples.

frozen sections were stained with hematoxylin and eosin (HE), modified gomoritrichome (MGT), succinic dehydrogenase (SDH), nicotinamide adenine dinucleotide (NADH-TR), succinic dehydrogenase–cytochrome C oxidase (SDH-COX), and adenosine triphosphatase (ATPase pH 9.4,4.6).

Antibodies. IHC staining was carried out on fresh frozen sections using monoclonal antibodies against dystrophin (1,2,3), sarcoglycans (α,β,δ,γ), dysferlin, caveolin-3, titin, merosin (α2 laminin) (Novocastra Laboratories, Newcastle, UK) and α-dystroglycan (Santacruz Biotechnology, Santacruz, CA, USA) as primary and HRP tagged NOVO linked as secondary antibody (Novocastra Laboratories, Newcastle, UK).

Preparation of protein extracts, SDS-PAGE and immunoblot

Frozen muscle tissue (20 mg) was minced in 20 volumes of extraction buffer (75 mM Tris-HCl, pH 6.8, 15% SDS, 20% glycerol, 5% dithiothreitol and 0.001% bromophenol blue), homogenized and sonicated for 30 seconds (6 x 5s).The extract was boiled at 95°C for 5 minutesfollowed by centrifugation at 12000 rpm for 10 minutes. 10 µl of the supernatant was subjected to size fractionation using 15% SDS-PAGE followed by western blot using anti-Telethonin antibody (monoclonal antibody G-11, Santacruz Biotech) [21]. For myosin profile (loading control), protein extracts were run on 6% SDS-PAGE and stained with coomassie brilliant blue. To avoid artifactual protein degradation, which might reduce telethonin signal, precaution was taken to preserve the integrity of the biopsies and to maintain optimal protein loading and gel transfer conditions.

Muscle MR Imaging

Muscle MRI was performed as a multi-sequence imaging protocol using a 1.5-T scanner (Magnetom, AERA, Siemens). Sections were obtained from axial planes including a T1-weighted spin-echo sequence (repetition time –918 msec, echo time 9.7 msec) and a short-time inversion recovery (STIR) sequence (repetition time 4020 msec, echo time 99 msec, inversion time 150 msec), in 10-mm slices. Involvement of all thigh and lower leg muscles was staged according to the intensity of the increased signals depicting fatty infiltration and STIR sequences for myoedema. Images were analyzed for signs of muscle degeneration, edema and normal/abnormal muscle bulk (hypertrophy, atrophy). Muscles evaluated on MRI: At *pelvis*: gluteus maximus, medius, minimus, piriformis, iliopsoas; *Thighs*: vastusmedialis, intermedius and lateralis, gracilis, sartorius, adductor muscles, tensor fasciae latae, rectus femoris, semimembranosus, semitendinosus, biceps femoris; *Lower legs*: tibialis anterior, extensor hallucis longus, peroneii, soleus, popliteus, extensor digitorum longus, medial and lateral head of gastrocnemius, tibialis posterior. The fibro-fatty replacement was evaluated on T1sequences by applying Mercuri score [22]; and myoedema was evaluated on STIR sequences by using a specific new oedema score [23].

Genetic analysis of *TCAP*

About 5.0 ml of peripheral blood sample from each participant was collected in EDTA vacutainers. DNA was isolated according to the protocol described in our earlier study [24]. The coding region, including exon-intron boundaries and the UTR regions of Telethonin gene were amplified using 4 sets of primers. The sequence of primers and the conditions used for amplification are given in Table 1. PCR was performed in 0.2 ml thin-walled tubes using 50.0 ng of genomic DNA, 10 pmol of each primer, 200 µM of dNTPs, PCR buffer containing 1.5 mM $MgCl_2$, and 2 units of AmpliTaqGold (Perkin Elmer). Amplified products were evaluated using 2% agarose gel electrophoresis. PCR products were purified by treating with exonuclease I and Shrimp alkaline phosphatase (Amersham, Piscataway, NJ) at 37°C and 80°C for 15 minutes each. Sequencing of PCR products was carried out using 100.0 ng (2.0 µl) of PCR product and 4 pmol (1.0 µl) of primer (forward and reverse in separate reactions), and 4.0 µl of BigDye Terminator ready mixture (Applied Biosystem, Foster city, USA). Cycle sequencing was carried out in a GeneAmp 9600 thermal cycler (Applied Biosystem, Foster city, USA) employing the following conditions: 30 cycles at 96°C for 10 seconds, 50°C for 5 seconds, and 60°C for 4 minutes. PCR amplicons were purified using the protocol described in our earlier study [25], dissolved in 10 µl of 50% Hi-Di formamide and analyzed using ABI 3700 automated DNA analyzer (Perkin Elmer). The sequences obtained were aligned with NCBI Reference Sequence: NG_008892.1 (gene)/NM_003673.3 (mRNA) using the Auto-Assembler software to identify the sequence variations.

Results

Clinical features

Based on the combined IHC and IB results, the commonest form of ARLGMD was LGMD 2B (Dysferlin) in 82/246 (33.33%); followed by 2I (FKRP) in 51/246 (20.73%), 2C-F (gamma, alpha, beta and delta sarcoglycan) in 35/246 (14.23%), 2A (calpain-3) in 25/246 (10.16%), and 2G (Telethonin) in 8/246 (3.25%). The remaining cases (45/246-18.30%) remained unclassified.

The age of onset of LGMD2G cases ranged from 5 to 40 years (mean ±SD, 12.38±11.35) and the mean age at evaluation and mean duration of illness were 22.8±14.2, (9–52 years) and

Table 2. Clinical features and Muscle Histopathology findings of patients with LGMD-2G.

Clinical features								
Parameter/Patient ID	F36-1	F50-1	F79-1	F97-1	F111-1	F111-2	F149-1	F116-1
Age at presentation (Yrs)	52	10	9	21	17	14	30	15
Gender	F	M	F	M	F	F	M	M
Place of origin	AP	KA	KA	TN	KE	KE	TN	KA
Onset (Yrs)	12	2	4	9	10	5	23	3
Presenting symptom	Difficulty in running fast; waddling	Difficulty in running fast	Slow in walking	Difficulty in running fast	Toe walking	Exertion induced muscle pain	Toe walking	Toe walking
Hypertrophy	absent	Calves	Triceps, calves	absent	Calves	Calves	absent	Absent
Scapular winging	Moderate	Moderate	Mild	Absent	Severe	Moderate	Mild	Severe
Facial weakness	absent	present	absent	absent	absent	absent	absent	Absent
Contractures	Ankle	Ankle	Ankle	Ankle, Hips	Ankle	Ankle	Ankle	Ankle
Deltoids	3-	5	4	4	4	4	4	4-
Pectorals	4	3-	4	4+	4	4	4	4+
Biceps brachii	4	4+	4	4	4	4	4	4-
Triceps	4	4-	3+	4	4	4	4	3+
Distal UL	5	5	5	5	5	5	5	5
Glut. Medius	3	3	2	3	2	3	1	5
Hip adductors	1	2	2	3+	1	1	1	2
Iliopsoas	3-	3	2	3+	1	3	1	3-
Glut maximus	1	2	2	3+	1	3	1	2
Quadriceps	3-	4	4+	3+	1	3	1	3-
Hamstrings	1	3+	3	5	1	3	3	3+
Tibialis Anterior	5	3+	4+	5	1	3	4+	4
Gastrocnemius	4	5	5	5	2	3+	4+	5
CK (IU/L)	1057	3729	1325	1583	719	9283	1281	1649
MDFRS Scoring	90	101	93	116	67	80	72	99
Disability	Dependent	Independent	Independent	Independent	Dependent	Independent	Dependent	Dependent
Muscle Histopathology findings								
Fascicular architecture	Severely effaced	Normal	Mild to moderately effaced	normal	Mild/moderate	-	Mild to moderate	Mild to moderate
Myofibril shape and size	Round fibers with marked variation	Round to Polygonal,/ mild variation in size	Round/mild	polygonal	Round/mild variation	-	Round to polygonal/ Mild variation	Round/marked variation
Myophagocytosis/ Necrotic fibers	absent	absent	present/present	absent/absent	present/absent	-	absent/absent	Present

Table 2. Cont.

Muscle Histopathology findings								
Endomysial fibrosis/Adipose tissue infiltration	Marked/marked	Mild to moderate/absent	Mild to moderate/absent	Absent/absent	Marked/marked	-	absent/mild to moderate	absent/mild to mod
Regenerating fibers	absent	absent	absent	absent	absent	-	present	Absent
Hypertrophy	absent	absent	present	absent	present	-	absent	Present
Atrophy	yes present	absent	present/present	present	present	-	absent	Present
Splitting/internal nuclei	present/occasional	present/occasional	present/occasional	absent/absent	present/ occasional	-	present/ occasional	present/present
Inflammation	absent	absent	absent	absent	absent	-	mild	Absent
Lobulated fibers	occasional	occasional	absent	occasional	absent	-	absent	Moth eaten fibers and lobulated fibers
Ragged red and blue fibers	present/absent	absent	absent	absent	absent	-	absent	Absent
Rimmed vacuoles	absent	absent	absent	absent	absent	-	absent	Absent

Yrs-Years; F-Female; M-Male; KA-Karnataka; TN-Tamilnadu; AP-Andhra Pradesh; EDB-Extensor digitorumbrevis; TA-Tibialis anterior; CK-Creatine kinase; MDFRS-Muscular dystrophy functional rating scale; Note: Biopsy was not done for patient F111-2 (sibling of patient F111-1).

8.50±6.87 (2–23 years), respectively. Gender distribution was equal. CK value ranged from 718 to 9253 IU/L (mean ± SD, 2574.4±2847.52). The clinical features and histopathological findings of the patients are presented in Table 2. IB studies in 7 patients (Biopsy not done for F111-2) showed normal expression of dystrophin, dysferlin, calpain-3 and all four sarcoglycans with complete or partial absence of telethonin on IB (Fig 1-2). A majority of patients had the typical phenotype with predominantly a proximo - distal form of involvement, scapular winging, muscle atrophy, presence of calf hypertrophy and foot drop and slowly progressive in most cases.

Muscle MRI findings

MRI findings of the patient, 97-1 (Fig 3), revealed: At Pelvis: gluteus maximus showed stage 2b fatty infiltration and iliopsoas showed stage 2a involvement. Rectus femorus was atrophied; At thighs: global atrophy of muscles of all three compartments. Sartorius, gracilis, semitendinosus and short head of biceps were spared and also hypertrophied. In the anterior compartment vastus, intermedius showed severe atrophy. Myoedema was mainly seen in the anterior compartment and more on the left side. In the posterior compartment, stage 2b myoedema was seen only on the left side; At legs: Atrophy of tibialis anterior, extensor digitorum longus, extensor hallucis longus, flexor hallucis longus, flexor digitorum longus was noted. Medial head of gastrocnemius was hypertrophied. Soleus appeared to be atrophied on left side and preserved on right side. Myoedema was noted only in gastrocnemius and soleus muscles. MRI staging of the affected individual muscles are listed in table 3.

Sequence analysis

The *TCAP* gene was analysed in ten patients (including two affected siblings from family F50), belonging to seven unrelated families. We have identified four different mutations that included; one novel and three reported variations (www.dmd.nl). Mutation numbering was based on *TCAP* cDNA with sequence position 1 being the A in the first ATG codon. The novel mutation (c.32C> A) (Fig 4C) is a nonsense substitution in the first exon, which introduces a stop codon (TCG to TAG) in three patients (homozygous mutant) of a consanguineous family (F50) (Table 4). All the unaffected family members were either heterozygous or homozygous for the alternate allele (Fig 4A). None of the control samples had this mutation.

The second variation is an eight base pair duplication in the first exon (c.26_33dupAGGTGTCG), (Fig 4F) which leads to an amino acid change from 12th codon and terminates at 31stcodon, resulting in the formation of a truncated protein in one of the patients (F97-1) (Table 4). Both the parents, two brothers, and the grandfather were found to be heterozygous for this duplication and were unaffected (Fig 4B). This mutation was not found in the control samples. Two other mutations; c.453A> C; *p.(=)* in exon2and c.-178G>T of the 5′ UTR region; were polymorphic and found in all the patients, their relatives, and control samples.

Discussion

For the first time in India, we have performed a comprehensive analysis of LGMD2G, a rare muscle disease caused by telethonin protein deficiency encoded by the *TCAP* gene. The clinical manifestations in all our patients was classical, with a phenotype consisting of mild to moderate limb girdle muscle weakness, significant thigh and anterior leg atrophy with weakness, mild

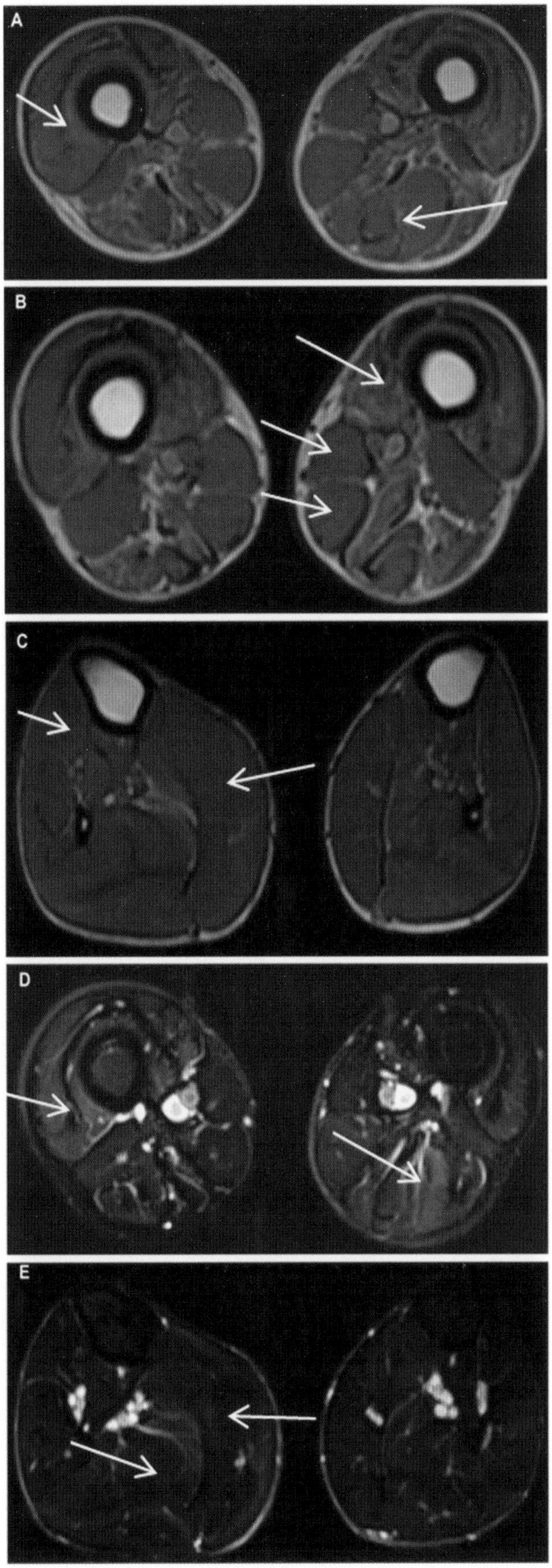

Figure 3. Muscle MRI of patient F97-1. A. T1W image showing global atrophy of muscles of anterior compartment, medial compartment and posterior compartment of thigh. Biceps femoris long head shows stage 3 fatty infiltration. Short head of biceps femoris, sartorius and gracilis are hypertrophied; **B**. shows severely atrophied vastus intermedius muscle, Mercurie stage 2b infiltration of vastus medialis muscle. Short head of biceps femoris, sartorius and gracilis are hypertrophied; **C**. Tibilialis anterior, extensor hallucis longus and extensor digitorum longus are atrophied (right more than left). On right side the medial head of gastrocnemius is hypertrophied and lateral head is atrophied. Left soleus is atrophied. Mild fatty infiltration of soleus muscle is noted in left side. Striking asymmetry is present; **D**. STIR image of thigh shows asymmetrical myoedema pattern. On the right side there is stage 3a myoedema and on the left side it is stage 2a. There is stage 2b myodema noted in the posterior compartment on left side; **E**. Myoedema mainly seen in gastrocnemius and soleus muscle. Stage 2b on right side and stage 2a on left side.

scapular winging and calf hypertrophy. The mutational analysis revealed one novel and three reported substitutions.

The c.32C>A, p.(Ser11*) mutation is a novel, nonsense change and exists in the N-terminal region of the gene. Serine in the codon 11 was replaced by premature translational termination codon and it may lead to nonsense mediated decay or truncated protein. This mutation was found in a patient born to consanguineous parents (F50-1). The proband was a 10 year old boy and was the ninth child born to a first cousins marriage. He presented with exertion induced calf muscle pains and progressive toe walking from eight years of age, progressive pectoral girdle, arm and lower limb proximal muscle wasting with weakness, scapular winging and mild foot drop. There was significant global wasting of the thigh and anterior leg muscles with hypertrophied calves and tip toe walking. Biceps muscle biopsy revealed a dystrophic changes. He had two sisters (F50-8 and F50-9) with similar phenotype, both of who had this mutation in the homozygous condition (Fig 4A). The case F50-8, aged 25 years, attained wheelchair bound state at 21 years of age and the case F50-9 is ambulant at 17 years of age. All three affected individuals of a family had the same mutation, were affected by eight years of age and showed similar phenotype. The father, one sister, one brother, one paternal uncle, and a maternal aunt were heterozygous for this mutation and were unaffected. The other unaffected brother, sister, and maternal uncle did not have the mutation (Fig 4A). This clearly shows the recessive pattern of the disease and pathogenicity associated with the mutation c.32C>A.

Frame shift variation c.26_33dupAGGTGTCG, (eight base pair duplication) in the first exon observed in a 21 year old proband (Fig 5) leads to an amino acid change from 12th codon and terminates the reaction at 31st codon, p.(Arg12fs31*). This may result in a truncated protein or nonsense mediated decay. The c.26_33dupAGGTGTCG has been reported in three unrelated Chinese families [26] and ours is the fourth family from Asia, but the first from India. This mutation is consistent with previous reports [3,26] confirming that homozygous individuals have the typical LGMD2G phenotype. This patient (F97-1) presented with motor disabilities since early childhood with inability to run fast. By the age of 10 he had progressive generalized wasting and lower limb proximal muscle weakness. He was slender built, had moderate scapular winging, mild calf hypertrophy and contractures at the hips and ankles (Fig 5). There

Table 3. MRI staging of the individual muscles of lower limb for presence of fatty infiltration and myoedema.

Muscle	Mercurie staging		Myoedema staging		Atrophy		Hypertrophy	
	Right	Left	Right	Left	Right	Left	Right	Left
Gluteus maximus	2b	2b	0	0	Yes	Yes		
Iliopsoas	2a	2a	0	0	Yes	Yes		
Tensor facia lata	0	0	0	0	No	No		
Vastuslateralis	0	0	3a	0	Yes	Yes		
Vastusintermedius	1	1	3a	0	Yes	Yes		
Vastusmedialis	2b	2b	2a	0	Yes	Yes		
Rectus femoris	0	0	0	0	Yes	Yes		
Sartorius	0	0	0	0	No	No	Yes	Yes
Gracilis	0	0	0	0	No	No	Yes	Yes
Semimembranous	2b	2b	0	2b	Yes	Yes		
Semitendinosus	0	0	0	2b	No	No	Yes	Yes
Biceps long head	3	3	0	1	Yes	Yes		
Biceps short head	0	0	0	2b	No	No	Yes	Yes
Adductor brevis	1	1	0	0	Yes	Yes		
Adductor longus	1	1	0	0	Yes	Yes		
Adductor magnus	3	3	0	0	Yes	Yes		
Tibialis anterior	0	1	0	0	Yes	Yes		
Tibialis posterior	0	0	0	0	Yes	Yes		
Peroneus longus	0	0	0	1	No	No		
Soleus	0	1	2b	2a	Yes	Yes		
Gastrocnemius medialis	0	0	2b	2a	No	No	Yes	No
Gastrocnemius lateralis	0	0	2b	2a	Yes	Yes		
Extensor digitorumlongus	0	1	1	0	Yes	Yes		
Extensor hallucislongus	0	1	1	0	Yes	Yes		
Flexor digitorumlongus	0	1	1	1	yes	yes		
Flexor hallucislongus	0	1	1	1	yes			

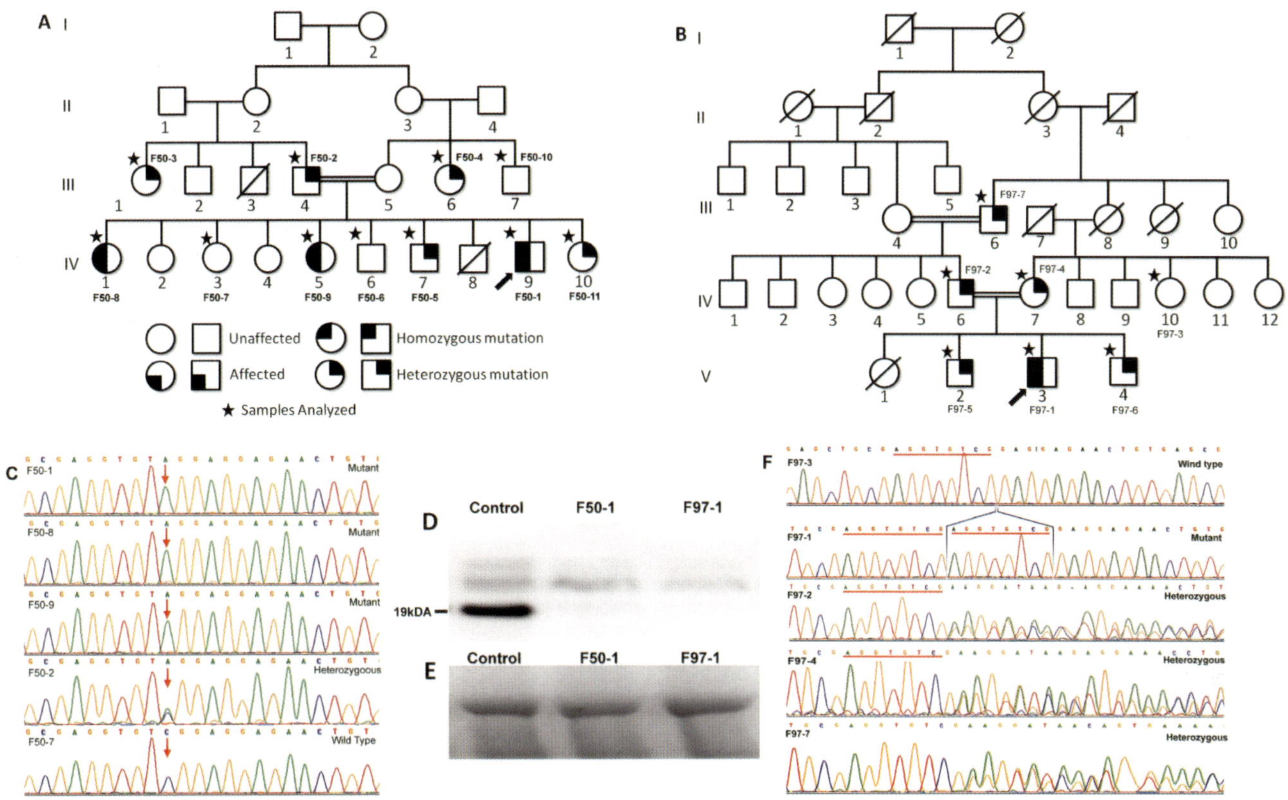

Figure 4. Mutational analysis of TCAP gene. A&B. Pedigree of F50 & F97 families respectively and the arrow indicates the proband; C. Electrophorogram representing heterozygous, homozygous and wild type c.32C>A mutation from family F50; Arrow indicates the polymorphic site; D. IB representing absence of telethonin band in F50-1 and F97-1; (E). Represents myosin bands of F50-1 and F97-1; (F). Electrophorogram representing homozygous, heterozygous and wild type c.26_33dupAGGTGTCG mutation in family F97.

was MRC grade 4- weakness of the gluteus maximus, iliopsoas, quadriceps and hamstrings with mild asymmetry. Foot dorsiflexors were grade 3+ and other groups had normal power with elevated CK level and normal ECG and 2D ECHO. EMG was myopathic, nerve conductions were normal, pulmonary function tests showed moderate restrictive abnormality, and biceps muscle biopsy revealed dystrophic features. Parents, two brothers, and the grandfather were found to be heterozygous and unaffected.

Both, c.32C>A and c.26_33dupAGGTGTCG, mutations lead to truncation of the telethonin protein. Interestingly, all of the mutations reported (p.Gln35*, g.637–640del2, p.Trp25*, c.26_33dupAGGTGTCG), so far, in the *TCAP* gene in LGMD2G have been either nonsense or frame shift variation, which either gives rise to a truncated protein or terminates protein synthesis [2,4,27,28]. To this list, we are adding a novel nonsense mutation.

Out of the eight patients studied, few had significant degree of toe walking from the onset of illness and this feature has been described earlier. [4]. In the previous reports, the onset of illness ranged between 2–15 years of age, with muscle weakness in all limbs, calf hypertrophy, and marked weakness of distal anterior leg muscles [29,30]. Our patients also had similar age of onset and a comparable pattern of muscle involvement. Even though it is reported that *TCAP* is necessary for the cardiomyocyte's stretch sensor and the structural organization of the cardiac sarcomere [31,32,33], none of our cases had evidence of clinical or echocardiographic evidence of cardiac dysfunction at the time of clinical evaluation. Muscle biopsy has been reported to show dystrophic features with or without rimmed vacuoles [4,27]. In our study, rimmed vacuoles were not noted in any case.

Certain muscle MRI findings observed in one of our proband's (case- 97-1) were comparable to those reported in a previous report [5]. Clinical examination revealed marked global atrophy of thigh muscles and atrophy of muscles in the anterior compartment of the leg. MRI showed a comparable pattern with atrophy of muscles in all three compartments of the thigh and anterior leg muscles. Sartorius, gracilis, semitendinosus, short head of biceps and medial head of gastrocnemius were spared and also hypertrophied. Anterior tibialis, extensor hallucis longus and extensor digitorum longus muscles showed prominent atrophy. The gastrocnemius muscles were slightly atrophic. Symmetry was noted in all the features. Only one previous report on a 50 year old Portuguese patient, describes the MRI findings of the muscles of the thighs and legs [5]. Myoedema was observed in anterior thigh and posterior leg muscles, which were relatively less affected. These features are unique and have not been reported so far. The Portuguese patient had demonstrated a homozygous nonsense c.157C>T (p.Gln53*) mutation in exon 2 of the TCAP gene, as

Table 4. Description of genetic analysis of *TCAP* gene.

Patient ID	Nucleotide change	Protein change	State
F36-1	c.-178G>T	NA	Homozygous
	c.453A>C	p.(=)	Homozygous
F50-1	***c.32C>A**	**p.(Ser11*)**	Homozygous
	c.-178G>T	**NA**	Heterozygous
	c.453A>C	p.(=)	Heterozygous
F50-8	***c.32C>A**	**p.(Ser 11*)**	Homozygous
	c.-178G>T	**NA**	Homozygous
	c.453A>C	p.(=)	Homozygous
F50-9	***c.32C>A**	**p.(Ser 11*)**	Homozygous
	c.-178G>T	NA	Homozygous
	c.453A>C	p.(=)	Homozygous
F79-1	c.-178G>T	NA	Homozygous
	c.453A>C	p.(=)	Homozygous
F97-1	**c.26 -33 Dup**	p. (Arg12fs31*)	Homozygous
	c.-178G>T	NA	Homozygous
	c.453A>C	p.(=)	Homozygous
F111-1	c.-178G>T	NA	Heterozygous
	c.453A>C	p.(=)	Heterozygous
F111-2	c.-178G>T	NA	Heterozygous
	c.453A>C	p.(=)	Heterozygous
F149-1	c.-178G>T	NA	Homozygous
	c.453A>C	p.(=)	Homozygous
F116-1	c.-178G>T	NA	Homozygous
	c.453A>C	p.(=)	Homozygous

*Novel mutation.

described among Brazilian patients [1]. We have identified a 8 bp duplication c.26_33dupAGGTGTCG, which is reported among Chinese patients [26].Although LGMD2G may have phenotypic characteristics ofLGMD-2A, 2B, the sarcoglycanopathies and distal myopathies with rimmed vacuoles (DMRV), it could be well differentiated from these disorders noting that LGMD-2A usually does not have thigh atrophy or rimmed vacuoles. LGMD-2B has predominantly posterior leg muscle weakness with calf muscle wasting, sarcoglycanopathies do not have foot drop or rimmed vacuoles, DMRV have progressive anterior leg muscle wasting and weakness with sparing of quadriceps. In comparison, in LGMD2G there is presence of significant atrophy of the thigh muscles including quadriceps and significant involvement of anterior tibialis. The predominant involvement of pelvic girdle muscles with calf hypertrophy observed in LGMD2G resembles the phenotype of some LGMD-2I. However, in 2G patients the thigh muscles are severely affected along with tibialis anterior weakness and wasting [29,30]. Thus, patients in the present series had the typical phenotypes described in LGMD2G and the genetic analysis confirms the same in two cases.

It has been reported that at least 25% of families and 40% of the isolated cases have no detectable mutation in any of the reported LGMD genes [34]. In agreement to this, we did not find any genetic variation in the telethonin gene in the remaining six IB confirmed cases. However, all of them showed partial or complete absence of telethonin on IB. This may be due to the secondary reduction of *TCAP* protein by some other Z-disk gene and probably involves a combination of genetic factors, since no protein in the Z-disc can be considered as an island separated from the others [35]. Many human diseases however, can be expected to be genetically heterogeneous caused by any one of several genes. The autosomal recessive limb-girdle muscular dystrophies represent a heterogeneous group of diseases which may be characterised by one or more autosomal loci. Further investigations may help in identification of additional genes responsible for LGMD2G.

In conclusion, we report LGMD2G cases for the first time from India. In this study, among the eight Indian LGMD2G patients, we found two telethonin mutations which include a novel c.32C>A mutation and a reported c.26_33dupAGGTGTCG duplication; both may be responsible for the formation of a truncated protein or nonsense mediated decay. Further investigation is needed to find the unknown factor for the telethonin deficiency in the remaining six cases.

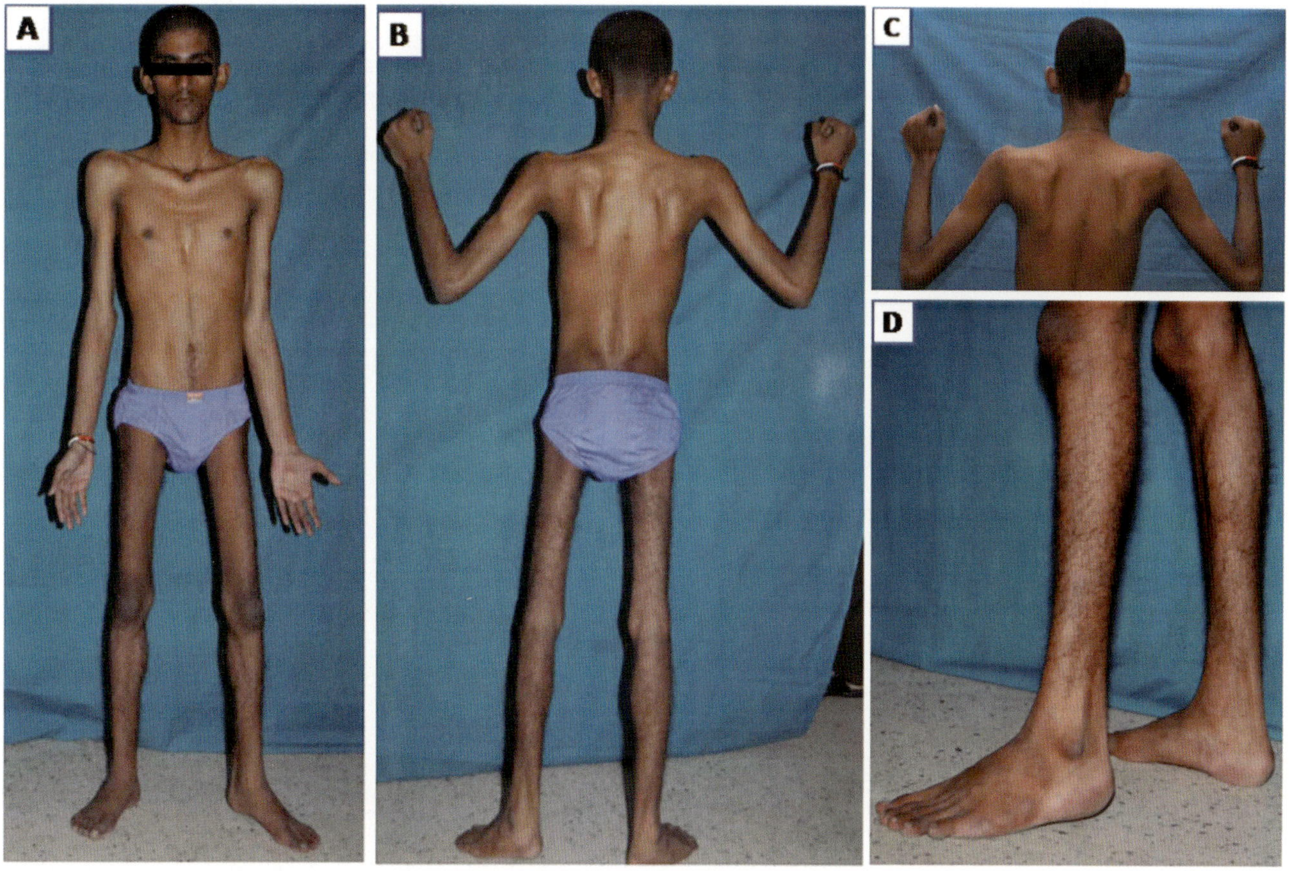

Figure 5. Clinical phenotype of patient F97-1. A. Slender habitus, B. Generalised poor muscle mass, global wasting of thigh muscles, C. moderate scapular winging, D. mild clf hypertrophy with minimal ankle contracture.

Acknowledgments

Authors are thankful to the patients for their participation in the study.

Author Contributions

Conceived and designed the experiments: AF AN KT. Performed the experiments: AF KV BS SKK. Analyzed the data: AF KV BS KP SKK MMSB SM NG AN KT. Contributed reagents/materials/analysis tools: AF AN KT. Wrote the paper: AF AN KT. Clinical Investigaion: SM KP AN.

References

1. Moreira ES, Wiltshire TJ, Faulkner G, Nilforoushan A, Vainzof M, et al. (2000) Limb-girdle muscular dystrophy type 2G is caused by mutations in the gene encoding the sarcomeric protein telethonin. Nat Genet 24: 163–166.
2. Moreira ES, Vainzof M, Marie SK, Sertie AL, Zatz M, et al. (1997) The seventh form of autosomal recessive limb-girdle muscular dystrophy is mapped to 17q11-12. Am J Hum Genet 61: 151–159.
3. Yee W, Pramono Z, Tan C, Kathiravelu P, Lai P (2007) G.P.8.15 Limb girdle muscular dystrophy 2G and novel TCAP mutations in ethnic Chinese. Neuromuscular disorders: NMD 17: 814.
4. Olive M, Shatunov A, Gonzalez L, Carmona O, Moreno D, et al. (2008) Transcription-terminating mutation in telethonin causing autosomal recessive muscular dystrophy type 2G in a European patient. Neuromuscul Disord 18: 929–933.
5. Negrao L, Matos A, Geraldo A, Rebelo O (2010) Limb-girdle muscular dystrophy in a Portuguese patient caused by a mutation in the telethonin gene. Acta Myol 29: 21–24.
6. Valle G, Faulkner G, De Antoni A, Pacchioni B, Pallavicini A, et al. (1997) Telethonin, a novel sarcomeric protein of heart and skeletal muscle. FEBS Lett 415: 163–168.
7. Mason P, Bayol S, Loughna PT (1999) The novel sarcomeric protein telethonin exhibits developmental and functional regulation. Biochem Biophys Res Commun 257: 699–703.
8. McNally EM, Pytel P (2007) Muscle diseases: the muscular dystrophies. Annu Rev Pathol 2: 87–109.
9. Bertz M, Wilmanns M, Rief M (2009) The titin-telethonin complex is a directed, superstable molecular bond in the muscle Z-disk. Proc Natl Acad Sci U S A 106: 13307–133310.
10. Gao M, Lee E, Band AMR Case Study: Titin Ig domains.
11. Knoll R, Buyandelger B (2013) Z-disc transcriptional coupling, sarcomeroptosis and mechanopoptosis. Cell Biochem Biophys 66: 65–71.
12. Lee EH, Gao M, Pinotsis N, Wilmanns M, Schulten K (2006) Mechanical strength of the titin Z1Z2-telethonin complex. Structure 14: 497–509.
13. Knoll R, Hoshijima M, Hoffman HM, Person V, Lorenzen-Schmidt I, et al. (2002) The cardiac mechanical stretch sensor machinery involves a Z disc complex that is defective in a subset of human dilated cardiomyopathy. Cell 111: 943–955.
14. Kojic S, Medeot E, Guccione E, Krmac H, Zara I, et al. (2004) The Ankrd2 protein, a link between the sarcomere and the nucleus in skeletal muscle. J Mol Biol 339: 313–325.
15. Nicholas G, Thomas M, Langley B, Somers W, Patel K, et al. (2002) Titin-cap associates with, and regulates secretion of, Myostatin. J Cell Physiol 193: 120–131.
16. Furukawa T, Ono Y, Tsuchiya H, Katayama Y, Bang ML, et al. (2001) Specific interaction of the potassium channel beta-subunit minK with the sarcomeric protein T-cap suggests a T-tubule-myofibril linking system. J Mol Biol 313: 775–784.
17. Haworth RS, Cuello F, Herron TJ, Franzen G, Kentish JC, et al. (2004) Protein kinase D is a novel mediator of cardiac troponin I phosphorylation and regulates myofilament function. Circ Res 95: 1091–1099.

18. Tian LF, Li HY, Jin BF, Pan X, Man JH, et al. (2006) MDM2 interacts with and downregulates a sarcomeric protein, TCAP. Biochem Biophys Res Commun 345: 355–361.
19. Frey N, Olson EN (2002) Calsarcin-3, a novel skeletal muscle-specific member of the calsarcin family, interacts with multiple Z-disc proteins. Journal of Biological Chemistry 277: 13998–14004.
20. Markert CD, Meaney MP, Voelker KA, Grange RW, Dalley HW, et al. (2010) Functional muscle analysis of the Tcap knockout mouse. Hum Mol Genet 19: 2268–2283.
21. Zardini E, Franciotta D, Melzi d'Eril GV (1993) Detection of dystrophin with a modified western blot technique in muscle tissue extracts. Clin Chem 39: 915.
22. Mercuri E, Pichiecchio A, Allsop J, Messina S, Pane M, et al. (2007) Muscle MRI in inherited neuromuscular disorders: past, present, and future. J Magn Reson Imaging 25: 433–440.
23. Carlo B, Roberta P, Roberto S, Marina F, Corrado A (2006) Limb-girdle muscular dystrophies type 2A and 2B: clinical and radiological aspects. Basic Appl Myol 16: 17–25.
24. Thangaraj K, Joshi MB, Reddy AG, Gupta NJ, Chakravarty B, et al. (2002) CAG repeat expansion in the androgen receptor gene is not associated with male infertility in Indian populations. J Androl 23: 815–818.
25. Thangaraj K, Ramana GV, Singh L (1999) Y-chromosome and mitochondrial DNA polymorphisms in Indian populations. Electrophoresis 20: 1743–1747.
26. Waddell L, Lek M, Bahlo M, Bromhead C, Jones K, et al. (2012) GP 41 The identification of LGMD2G (TCAP) in Australia. Neuromuscular Disorders 22: 831–832.
27. Vainzof M, Moreira ES, Suzuki OT, Faulkner G, Valle G, et al. (2002) Telethonin protein expression in neuromuscular disorders. Biochim Biophys Acta 1588: 33–40.
28. Waddell LB, Tran J, Zheng XF, Bonnemann CG, Hu Y, et al. (2011) A study of FHL1, BAG3, MATR3, PTRF and TCAP in Australian muscular dystrophy patients. Neuromuscul Disord 21: 776–781.
29. Bonnemann C, Bushby K (2004) The limb-girdle muscular dystrophies. In: Engel AG; Franzini Armstrong A, editors Myology 3rd McGraw-Hill: p. 1077–1121.
30. Fischer D, Walter MC, Kesper K, Petersen JA, Aurino S, et al. (2005) Diagnostic value of muscle MRI in differentiating LGMD2I from other LGMDs. J Neurol 252: 538–547.
31. Bos JM, Poley RN, Ny M, Tester DJ, Xu X, et al. (2006) Genotype-phenotype relationships involving hypertrophic cardiomyopathy-associated mutations in titin, muscle LIM protein, and telethonin. Mol Genet Metab 88: 78–85.
32. Hayashi T, Arimura T, Itoh-Satoh M, Ueda K, Hohda S, et al. (2004) Tcap gene mutations in hypertrophic cardiomyopathy and dilated cardiomyopathy. J Am Coll Cardiol 44: 2192–2201.
33. Zhang R, Yang J, Zhu J, Xu X (2009) Depletion of zebrafish Tcap leads to muscular dystrophy via disrupting sarcomere-membrane interaction, not sarcomere assembly. Hum Mol Genet 18: 4130–4140.
34. Blandin G, Marchand S, Charton K, Daniele N, Gicquel E, et al. (2013) A human skeletal muscle interactome centered on proteins involved in muscular dystrophies: LGMD interactome. Skelet Muscle 3: 3.
35. Faulkner G, Lanfranchi G, Valle G (2001) Telethonin and other new proteins of the Z-disc of skeletal muscle. IUBMB Life 51: 275–282.

12

Conditioning Increases the Gain of Contraction-Induced Sarcolemmal Substrate Transport in Ultra-Endurance Racing Sled Dogs

Michael S. Davis[1]*, Arend Bonen[2], Laelie A. Snook[2], Swati S. Jain[2], Kenneth Bartels[3], Raymond Geor[4], Karsten Hueffer[5]

1 Department of Physiological Sciences, Oklahoma State University, Stillwater, Oklahoma, United States of America, **2** Department of Human Health and Nutritional Sciences, University of Guelph, Guelph, Ontario, Canada, **3** Department of Veterinary Clinical Sciences, Oklahoma State University, Stillwater, Oklahoma, United States of America, **4** Department of Large Animal Clinical Science, Michigan State University, East Lansing, Michigan, United States of America, **5** Department of Veterinary Medicine, University of Alaska-Fairbanks, Fairbanks, Alaska, United States of America

Abstract

Endurance exercise relies on transsarcolemmal flux of substrates in order to avoid depletion of intramuscular reserves. Previous studies of endurance trained sled dogs have shown a remarkable capacity of these dogs to adapt rapidly to endurance exercise by decreasing the utilization of intramuscular reserves. The current study tested the hypothesis that the dogs' glycogen-sparing phenotype is due to increased sarcolemmal transport of glucose and fatty acids. Basal and exercise-induced transport of glucose and fatty acids into sarcolemmal vesicles was evaluated in racing sled dogs prior to and after 7 months of exercise conditioning. Sarcolemmal substrate transport capacity was measured using sarcolemmal vesicles and radiolabelled substrates, and transporter abundance was measured using Western blot quantification in whole muscle homogenates and the sarcolemmal vesicle preparations. Conditioning resulted in increased basal and exercise-induced transport of both glucose and palmitate. Neither acute exercise nor conditioning resulted in changes in muscle content of GLUT4 or FAT/CD36, but conditioning did result in decreased abundance of both transporters in the sarcolemmal vesicles used for the basal transport assays, and this decrease was further amplified in the vesicles used for the exercise-induced transport assays. These results demonstrate conditioning-induced increases in sarcolemmal transport of oxidizable substrates, as well as increased gain of exercise-induced sarcolemmal transport of these substrates. These results further indicate that increased sarcolemmal transport of oxidizable substrates may be due to either an increased intrinsic capacity of the existing transporters or to a different population of transporters from those investigated.

Editor: Dmitri Boudko, Rosalind Franklin University, United States of America

Funding: These studies were supported by grants from United States Department of Defense Army Research Office Division of Life Sciences (W911NF-09-1-0549) and by the Natural Sciences and Engineering Research Council of Canada (AB), The Heart and Stroke Foundation of Ontario (AB), the Canadian Institutes of Health Research (AB), and the Canada Research Chair program. A. Bonen, PhD, FRSC, was the Canada Research Chair in Metabolism and Health. Swati S. Jain was the recipient of an NSERC Canadian Graduate Scholarship. The funders had no role in study design, data collection and analysis, decision to publish, or preparation of the manuscript.

* Email: michael.davis@okstate.edu

Introduction

Metabolizable substrate uptake in skeletal muscle is regulated in order to meet the dual roles of the tissue of energy storage during periods of overall positive energy balance and energy expenditure during muscular work. Diffusion of the key metabolizable substrates across the sarcolemma is either limited (fatty acids) or virtually non-existent (glucose), and therefore sarcolemmal expression of substrate-specific transporters provides a key point of regulation [1,2]. Dynamic expression of transporters such as GLUT4 and fatty acid translocase (FAT)/CD36, controlled by the appropriate intracellular and extracellular signals, provides a mechanism for a large range of transsarcolemmal flux that is responsive to acute changes in the need for metabolizable substrate uptake. Both GLUT4 and FAT/CD36 are stored intracellularly, but will translocate to the sarcolemma during periods of contraction or insulin stimulation. In both cases, increased transsarcolemmal flux of their respective substrates occurs with increased sarcolemmal localization of these transporters.

Endurance-trained racing sled dogs have been shown to sustain large caloric expenditures during competition (nearly 12,000 kcal/day or over 4000 kJ/kg$^{0.75}$/day) [3], indicating a tremendous capacity to transport oxidizable substrates into working muscle cells. However, this capacity appears to be highly dynamic and capable of rapid increases within the context of a single multiday exercise challenge. In previous studies in which trained racing sled dogs performed daily controlled exercise sessions, the dogs initially depleted intramuscular glycogen and triglyceride, but transitioned from glycogen-depleting to glycogen-sparing over 96 hrs of continued intermittent exercise [4,5]. With the overall workload (speed, distance, duration, load) held constant, we hypothesized that the overall energetic requirements of the exercise were similarly constant and that the sparing of intramuscular glycogen was made possible by increased availability of blood-borne oxidative substrates. Therefore, we conducted a set of experiments to test the hypothesis that the development of a glycogen-sparing, fatigue-resistant phenotype is the result of increased sensitivity of exercise-induced translocation of substrate transporters to the sarcolemma.

Materials and Methods

This study was carried out in strict accordance with the recommendations in the Guide for the Care and Use of Laboratory Animals of the National Institutes of Health. The protocol was approved by the Institutional Animal Care and Use Committee of Oklahoma State University (Permit Number: 27-2956). All surgery was performed as described under general anesthesia, post-operative pain management was provided to all subjects, and all efforts were made to minimize suffering.

Thirty-seven mature sled dogs were used in the study, and assigned randomly into one of 5 groups. Six dogs were examined as unconditioned sedentary controls, and had not had any compulsory exercise for at least 4 months. Eight additional unconditioned dogs were examined immediately following a treadmill standardized exercise test (25 min at 6.5 mph and 4.5% incline). Eight dogs were examined as conditioned sedentary controls and had completed a full season (7 months) of endurance conditioning and racing, including a single 1000 mile race completed approximately 2 weeks prior to the examination, but had not undergone any compulsory exercise for at least 96 h prior to examination. Eight dogs with the same conditioning, racing, and recent exercise history were examined immediately following the same treadmill standardized exercise test as used for the unconditioned dogs. Seven dogs with the same conditioning and racing history were also examined after completing a multiple-day exercise session of 400 miles in 4 days, followed 6 hr later by a treadmill standardized exercise test.

Muscle biopsies were obtained from all dogs and prepared for the isolation of sarcolemmal vesicles. General anesthesia was induced and maintained using intravenous propofol; dogs completing a treadmill standardized exercise test were anesthetized within 2 min of completion of the exercise. Approximately 1 g of muscle was obtained through aseptic excisional biopsy from the gracilis muscle. Giant sarcolemmal vesicles were prepared as described by Luiken *et al.* [6]. Muscle was cut into thin strips and incubated for 1 hr at 34°C with shaking (100 rpm) in a solution of 140 mM KCl/10 mM MOPS (pH 7.4) with collagenase VII (150 units/ml) and aprotinin (10 mg/ml). The muscle was washed with additional volumes of KCl/MOPS containing 10 mM EDTA and the supernatants collected. Percoll, KCl and aprotinin were added to the supernatants to a final concentration of 3.5%, 28 mM and 10 μg/ml, respectively. The supernatant was placed as the bottom layer of a density gradient under 3 mL of 4% Nycodenz (middle layer) and 1 mL KCl/MOPS (upper layer), and centrifuged at 60 xg for 45 min at 25°C. The vesicles were harvested from the interface of Nycodenz and KCl/MOPS, washed with KCl/MOPS, and pelleted by centrifugation at 9000 xg for 10 min. The resulting pellet was resuspended in KCl/MOPS to a final protein concentration of 1.25 μg/ml.

Palmitate and glucose uptake were measured simultaneously according to previously-published techniques [6] by adding 40 μl of a reaction solution containing 14 μM palmitate (including 0.3 μCi of ^{14}C-palmitate, Sigma Aldrich NEC534050UC, specific activity 850 mCi/mmol) and 5 mM glucose (including 0.3 μCi of ^{3}H-3-O-methylglucose, Sigma Aldrich NET379001MC, specific activity: 80.2 Ci/mmol), and 0.1% bovine serum albumin in KCl/MOPS to 40 μL of vesicle solution containing 50 μg of protein (final transport volume 80 μL). Substrate uptake was terminated after 15 s by adding 1.4 ml of ice-cold KCl/MOPS containing 2.5 mM HgCl and 0.1% bovine serum albumin. The reaction tubes were centrifuged in a microfuge at maximum speed for 1 min, and the supernatant removed. The radioactivity in the tip of the tube was measured to determine vesicle uptake. A subset of vesicles that were mixed with the radio-substrate solution were disrupted using 3X freeze/thaw cycles prior to centrifugation to quantify the amount of non-specific substrate binding (i.e., binding to the vesicles without transport).

Whole muscle (50–60 mg) was homogenized using a Polytron in ice cold buffer (1 mL) containing Tris (50 mM), Triton X-100 (1% v/v), EGTA (1 mM), EDTA (1 mM), NaF (50 mM), sodium β-glycerol phosphate (10 mM), sodium pyrophosphate (5 mM), DTT (2 mM), sodium orthovanadate (1 mM), phenylmethylsulfonyl fluoride (1 mM), and aprotinin, leupeptin, and pepstatin A (10 μg/mL each). After homogenization, the solution was sonicated (15 s) and rocked for 30 min at 4°C. The solution was centrifuged at 1,500 xg for 15 min at 4°C and the supernatant collected. Protein concentration was determined by the Bradford method, the sample was combined with Lamelli buffer and 20 μg of protein was loaded for SDS-PAGE.

The protein concentration of the giant sarcolemmal vesicle samples was determined by the BCA method, the sample combined with Lamelli buffer and 10 μg of protein was loaded for SDS-PAGE. Proteins were separated by electrophoresis on a 7.5% SDS-polyacrylamide gel and transferred to a polyvinylidene difluoride membrane. Membranes were blocked for 1 h at room temperature (RT) in TBS-T containing 7.5% bovine serum albumin (BSA). Membranes were incubated overnight at 4°C in the appropriate primary antibody in TBS-T containing 7.5% BSA. Antibodies for GLUT4 was from Chemicon (Temecula, CA). Antibodies for FAT/CD36 (MO25) were gifts from N.N. Tandon. Membranes were incubated for 1 h (RT) with the corresponding secondary antibody, and the immune complex detected with enhanced chemiluminescence (PerkinElmer Life Science, Boston, MA) and quantified by densitometry (Chemi-Genius2 Bioimaging, SynGene, Cambridge, UK). An internal standard was included on all blots and the relative densitometry values for the samples were expressed as a percentage of the standards on the corresponding gels. All blots were stained with Ponceau S (Sigma, Missiauga, ON) to ensure equal loading of protein.

The effect of conditioning on basal (unstimulated) transport or transporter expression was evaluated by comparing biopsy data obtained from rested unconditioned and rested conditioned dogs. The effect of conditioning on exercise-stimulated transport or transporter expression was determined by comparing data from post-exercise biopsies from unconditioned and conditioned dogs. The effect of treadmill exercise was determined by comparing basal and post-exercise biopsies in dogs with similar conditioning states. Finally, the effect of sustained multiday exercise on exercise-stimulated transport or transporter expression was evaluated by comparing biopsies from post-exercise conditioned dogs and post-exercise multiday exercise dogs. All comparisons were performed using a Student's t-test and $p<0.05$ was considered significant.

Results

Western blot assays for abundance of sarcolemmal transporters in whole muscle were performed on tissues from 5 rested unconditioned dogs, 8 post-exercise unconditioned dogs, 8 rested conditioned dogs, 8 post-exercise conditioned dogs, and 7 post-exercise conditioned dogs following the 4 day exercise session. Insufficient tissue was obtained to prepare sarcolemmal vesicles in some instances, and therefore transport data were only obtained in some of the subjects. Sarcolemmal transport assays were performed on 4 rested unconditioned dogs, 3 post-exercise unconditioned dogs, 3 rested conditioned dogs, 4 post-exercise conditioned dogs, and 6 post-exercise conditioned dogs following the 4 day exercise session. Western blot assays for abundance of sarcolemmal transporters on the sarcolemma (using the sarcolemmal vesicles) were performed on samples from 6 rested unconditioned dogs, 8 post-exercise unconditioned dogs, 7 rested conditioned dogs, 8 post-exercise conditioned dogs, and 7 post-exercise conditioned dogs following the 4 day exercise session.

Multiday exercise did not result in a change in contraction-induced sarcolemmal transport of either glucose or palmitate when compared to similarly-conditioned dogs that were rested prior to treadmill exercise (Glucose: 7.35 (SD 5.26) vs 5.41 (SD 4.05) μmol/mg protein/15 sec, $p=0.28$; Palmitate: 32.91 (SD 5.31) vs 27.27 (SD 7.20) pmol/mg prot/15 sec, $p=0.10$) (Figures 1-2); therefore the data from these groups were combined for further evaluation of the effects of conditioning on sarcolemmal substrate transport.

Conditioning resulted in increased basal and contraction-stimulated glucose and palmitate transport. Basal transport of glucose increased 270% (0.84 (SD 0.25) vs 3.15 (SD 0.48) nmol/mg protein/15 sec, $p<0.01$) (Figure 1) and basal transport of palmitate increased by 60% (14.42 (SD 4.07) vs 22.48 (SD 1.59) pmol/mg prot/15 sec, $p=0.03$) (Figure 2). Contraction stimulated transport of glucose increased 550% (0.95 (SD 0.43) vs 6.19 (SD 4.40) nmol/mg protein/15 sec, $p=0.04$) (Figure 1) and contraction-stimulated transport of palmitate increased almost 100% (14.90 (SD 3.01) vs 29.52 (SD 6.83) pmol/mg prot/15 sec, $p<0.01$) (Figure 2). The standardized exercise test resulted in signficant increases in glucose and palmitate uptake in the conditioned dogs ($p=0.03$ and <0.01, respectively), but not in the unconditioned dogs ($p=0.36$ and 0.42, respectively).

There were no significant changes in transporter abundance in the whole muscle homogenates from any of the groups (Figures 3-4). In the sarcolemmal vesicles, conditioning resulted in decreased presence of GLUT4 and FAT/CD36 at the plasma membrane in rested dogs ($p=0.02$ and 0.03, respectively) and in post-exercise dogs ($p<0.01$ in both) (Figures 5-6). There was no effect of multiday exercise on contraction-mediated sarcolemmal levels of either transporter ($p=0.26$ for both), and there was no significant effect of contraction on sarcolemmal levels of either transporter within a conditioning state (GLUT4 unconditioned $p=0.15$, conditioned $p=0.33$; FAT/CD36 unconditioned $p=0.26$, conditioned $p=0.36$) (Figures 5-6).

Discussion

The physiological limitations to exercise performance can be different for different types of exercise. In the case of prolonged submaximal exercise, the availability of macromolecular oxidizable substrates such as glucose and fatty acid can be limiting. Intramuscular stores of these substrates are finite, and if a given exercise intensity results in the reliance on these stores, then that exercise intensity can not be performed for prolonged periods. Conversely, in order to perform such exercise for prolonged periods, an alternate strategy for the provision of oxidizable substrates is necessary. Our previous studies of racing Alaskan sled dogs have suggested that dogs conditioned for ultra-endurance competition – races that span multiple days – develop just such an alternative strategy when performing exercise that would otherwise rely on finite stores of intramuscular substrate. Our primary hypothesis was simple – that the dogs rapidly increase their capacity for sarcolemmal transport of blood-borne substrates. The results of our studies partially support our original hypothesis, but also provide some unusual findings that raise questions regarding the metabolic strategy of a racing sled dog to meet its energetic demands.

The specific phenomenon that we sought to explain with this series of experiments was the rapid conversion from a glycogen-depleting to a glycogen-sparing phenotype described in our previous studies [4,5]. In our previous studies, the exercise challenges were conducted after approximately 4 months of conditioning but no multiday race, compared to the current study in which the dogs had completed 7 months of conditioning and multiple races, ranging from 300 miles to 1000 miles. It is possible, perhaps even likely, that the metabolic strategy present in the conditioned dogs of the current study was similar to the exercise-induced glycogen-sparing phenotype present at the end of the previous studies and as a result, the additional 400-mile exercise challenge imposed in this study was not sufficiently stressful, from a metabolic perspective, to induce any further adaptation. This aspect of the experimental design was unavoidable due to the greater invasiveness of the biopsy technique required for sarcolemmal vesicle preparation, but serves as a caution that the magnitude of conditioning may not be comparable between the current study and previous studies of endurance sled dogs.

A season of aerobic conditioning resulted in a significant increase in the resting (basal) sarcolemmal transport of both glucose and palmitate. The increased basal transport of glucose and palmitate are unlikely to be due to the effects of post-prandial insulin since at the time of examination, the dogs had not been fed for at least 12 h. It is also unlikely to be due to residual effects of acute exercise as the dogs had been rested for at least 96 h and previous studies have shown that 96 h following a prolonged, glycogen depleting exercise bout, muscle glycogen concentrations have returned to baseline values [5]. It is possible that the increase in basal transport measured in this study is not present *in vivo*. Although expression of sarcolemmal GLUT4 is considered the rate-limiting step for muscle glucose uptake at rest, phosphorylation of intracellular glucose by hexokinase II is believed to be the rate-limiting step during exercise [1]. It is possible that in highly-conditioned dogs, the latter regulatory approach predominates even at rest. In this scenario, sarcolemmal transport of glucose is limited by down-regulation or inhibition of hexokinase II, resulting in increased intracellular concentrations of glucose and loss of the trans-sarcolemmal concentration gradient. Sarcolemmal flux of glucose would thus be reduced despite increased expression of transporters on the sarcolemma. Alternatively, the measured increase in basal substrate uptake suggests an increased metabolic activity of the muscle. The nature of this increased activity, if it exists, is unknown. Lacking a recent history of strenuous exercise that might induce a conditioning response, we would not expect increased metabolic activity secondary to *de novo* protein synthesis. Rather, the most likely explanation would be increased energetic costs of maintenance of the conditioned phenotype, which also could also help explain why such a phenotype is not maintained when it is not needed during deconditioning. However, the magnitude of the substrate transport increases are substantial (3-fold increase in glucose transport and ~50% increase in fatty acid transport), making it unlikely to be explained entirely by increased metabolic requirements of the conditioned muscle.

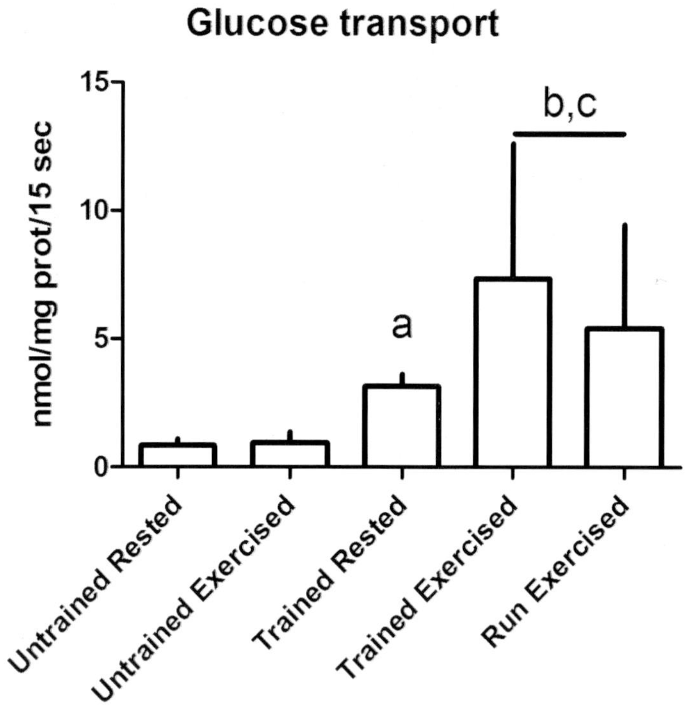

Figure 1. Transport rate of glucose across sarcolemmal vesicles. Data displayed as mean and standard deviation. Untrained Rested n = 4, Untrained Exercised n = 3, Trained Rested n = 3, Trained Exercised n = 4, Run Exercised n = 6. a: significantly different from Untrained Rested, p = 0.0029; b: significantly different from Untrained Exercised, p = 0.035; c: significantly different from Trained Rested, p = 0.029.

The effect of exercise on substrate transport was profoundly affected by conditioning. With the translocation of both GLUT4 and FAT/CD36 being contraction-mediated [7,8], resulting in increased substrate transport [9], the lack of an exercise effect on substrate transport in unconditioned dogs was somewhat surprising. However, the intensity of our exercise test was relatively modest by the standards of even unconditioned sled dogs, whose initial conditioning activities may last 2-3 h at speeds 50% greater than our exercise test and while pulling a load. Exercise-induced translocation of GLUT4 increases as the duration of the exercise challenge increases [9], so the 20 min of exercise used in this study may not have been sufficiently strenuous to stimulate increased transarcolemmal movement of substrate. That the same modest intensity exercise resulted in large increases in substrate transport in conditioned dogs suggests that an increase in the gain of contraction-mediated substrate uptake is a major feature of endurance conditioning in dogs. Our finding of increased sarcolemmal transport of glucose during submaximal exercise in response to endurance conditioning is in contrast to a similar study in humans which found decreased sarcolemmal glucose transport [10]. Fatty acid transport was not measured in that study, but presumably the sarcolemmal transport of fatty acids increased to fuel the exercise challenge. It is possible that the increase in sarcolemmal transport capacity of glucose is misleading as the increased permeability of the sarcolemma to glucose may be offset by insufficient hexokinase II activity to maintain a large diffusion gradient for glucose [11]. However, a similar regulatory point for fatty acids has not been described and the increase in the gain of contraction-mediated fatty acid transport reported here is consistent with the general conclusion that endurance training increases fatty acid utilization at moderate workloads.

Endurance conditioning did not increase the abudance of either GLUT4 or FAT/CD36 in skeletal muscle. Previous studies in humans [12,13], rats [14], and horses [15] have documented increased skeletal muscle content of GLUT4 following exercise conditioning, as well as increased FAT/CD36 in humans [16] and horses [17]. While surprising, these results are in agreement with our unpublished data showing a lack of upregulation of the corresponding genes during endurance conditioning in sled dogs. These data suggest that regulation of sarcolemmal substrate transport in dogs is accomplished more through alterations in the intrinsic activity of the components of substrate transport pathways, rather than synthesis and turnover of the components themselves.

Perhaps the most intriguing result from this study is the apparent lack of concordance between the substrate sarcolemmal transport data and the data relating to the sarcolemmal abundance of the putative transporters of these substrates. Numerous studies have reported concurrent increases in sarcolemmal expression of substrate-specific transporters and increased sarcolemmal transport of those substrates [1,18], and this body of work is sufficiently robust to support the general conclusion that increases in sarcolemmal transport of specific substrates is the result of increased numbers of transporters expressed on the sarcolemma. The results presented herestand in stark contrast to this conclusion. In fact, to a large degree the changes transport data and transporter abudance data are opposite; the detected abundance of the transporters goes down as transport increases. Two possible explanations exist. First, that the transporters we selected to represent glucose and fatty acid transport (GLUT4 and FAT/CD36, respectively) are not the prevailing transporters for these substrates in these dogs and instead other, unmeasured transporters are responsible for the changes in substrate flux

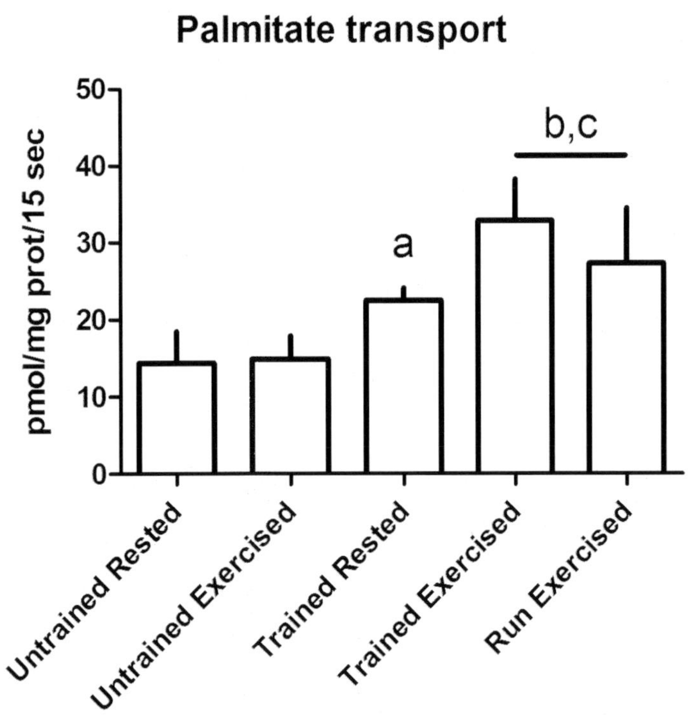

Figure 2. Transport rate of palmitate across sarcolemmal vesicles. Data displayed as mean and standard deviation. Untrained Rested n = 3, Untrained Exercised n = 4, Trained Rested n = 2, Trained Exercised n = 4, Run Exercised n = 6. a: significantly different from Untrained Rested, p = 0.031; b: significantly different from Untrained Exercised, p = 0.0015; c: significantly different from Trained Rested, p = 0.0091.

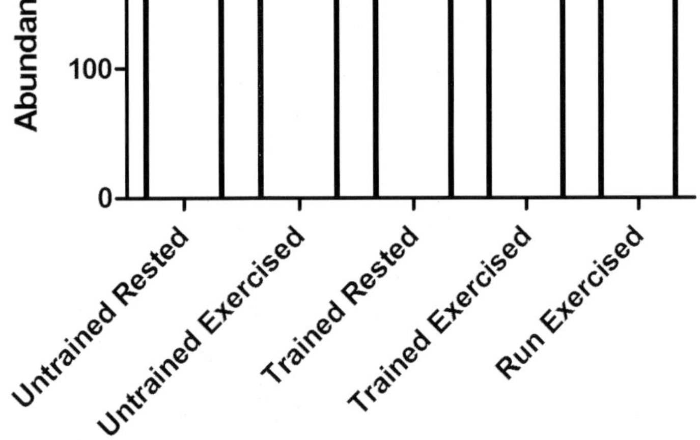

Figure 3. GLUT4 abundance in whole muscle homogenates. Transporter was quantified using Western blot, and abundance is expressed as arbitrary optical density units. Data displayed as mean and standard deviation. Untrained Rested n = 5, Untrained Exercised n = 8, Trained Rested n = 8, Trained Exercised n = 8, Run Exercised n = 7.

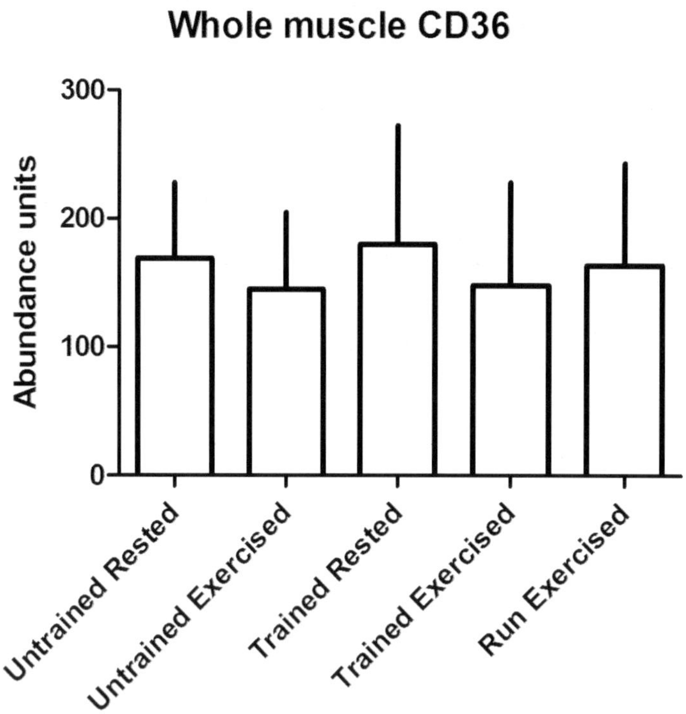

Figure 4. FAT/CD36 abundance in whole muscle homogenates. Transporter was quantified using Western blot, and abundance is expressed as arbitrary optical density units. Data displayed as mean and standard deviation. Untrained Rested n = 5, Untrained Exercised n = 8, Trained Rested n = 8, Trained Exercised n = 8, Run Exercised n = 7.

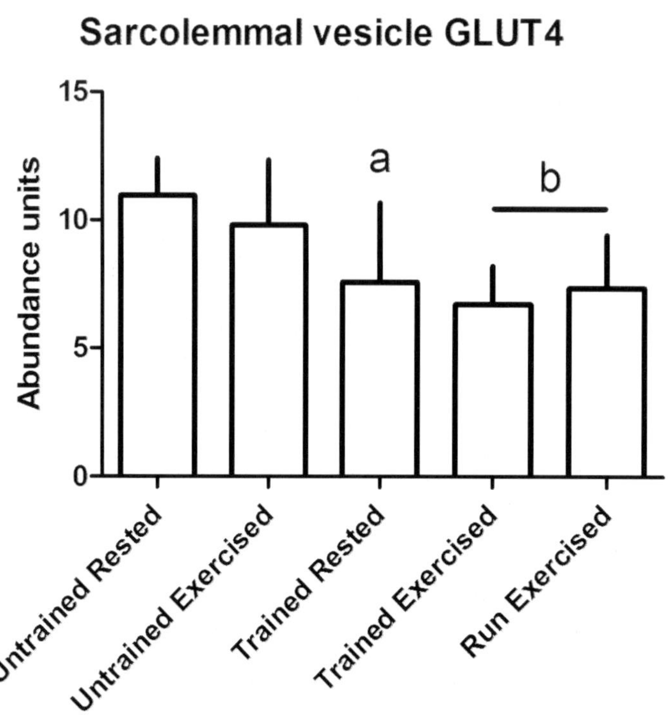

Figure 5. Plasma membraneGLUT4 abundance. Transporter was quantified using Western blot, and abundance is expressed as arbitrary optical density units. Data displayed as mean and standard deviation. Untrained Rested n = 6, Untrained Exercised n = 8, Trained Rested n = 7, Trained Exercised n = 8, Run Exercised n = 7. a: significantly different from Untrained Rested, p = 0.015; b: significantly different from Untrained Exercised, p = 0.0025.

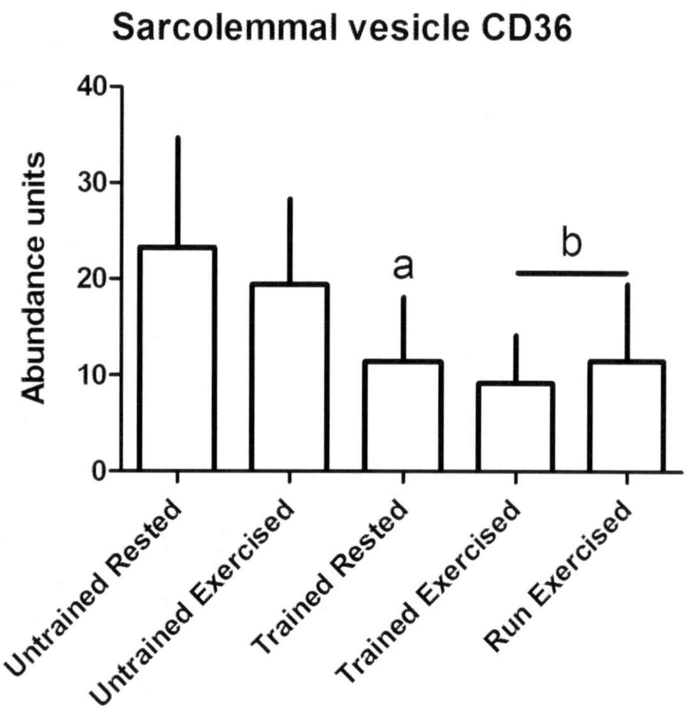

Figure 6. Plasma membraneFAT/CD36 abundance. Transporter was quantified using Western blot, and abundance is expressed as arbitrary optical density units. Data displayed as mean and standard deviation. Untrained Rested n = 6, Untrained Exercised n = 8, Trained Rested n = 6, Trained Exercised n = 8, Run Exercised n = 7. a: significantly different from Untrained Rested, p = 0.030; b: significantly different from Untrained Exercised, p = 0.0048.

resulting from conditioning and exercise. Of all the identified fatty acid transport proteins, FAT/CD36 is the logical vehicle for dynamically-regulated fatty acid transport across the sarcolemma given its high capacity relative to the other fatty acid transport proteins [19] and the fact that its expression on the sarcolemma is upregulated by muscle contraction [7]. Similarly, GLUT4 is the most abundant glucose transporter identified in skeletal muscle and, like FAT/CD36, demonstrates increased sarcolemmal expression in response to muscle contraction [8]. Certainly, there are other possible transporters for both glucose and fatty acids, but unfortunately we lacked the sample volume to perform an exhaustive characterization of all possible transporters.

A second possibility is that the selected transporters undergo post-translational modification that increases the intrinsic activity of the transporters, thus requiring fewer transporters on the sarcolemmal to meet the metabolic demands of the contracting muscle. Phosphorylation of GLUT4 reduces the intrinsic activity of the transporter and one of the effects of insulin (in addition to stimulating transporter translocation to the cell membrane) is to dephosphorylate GLUT4 to increase intrinsic activity [20]. This effect can be inhibited by high intracellular calcium and by palmitate [21]. Reduced intrinsic activity of GLUT4 by high cytoplasmic ATP also has been suggested by molecular modelling [22]. There is also evidence to suggest that association of glyceraldehyde-3-phosphate dehydrogenase with the GLUT4 transporter increases the intrinsic activity of the latter [23,24]. Less is known regarding the intrinsic activity of FAT/CD36, but there is some evidence that increased fatty acid transport activity of this transporter is related to its association with calveolae and lipids rafts [25]. Lack of concordance between substrate transport and transporter abundance in contracting muscle has been previously reported for lactate flux and monocarboxylate transporters [26], presumably due to a change in the intrinsic activity of these transporters, establishing at least the fact that such a change in the intrinsic activity of other transporters is a tenable possibility.

Our study demonstrates that endurance conditioning in racing sled dogs results in increased capacity for sarcolemmal transport of oxidizable substrates, but raises the possibility that in vivo, this transport capacity may be in excess of demand and actual transsarcolemmal flux of these substrates are regulated elsewhere in the transport pathway. Furthermore, our data suggests, albeit indirectly, that the increased transport capacity is due to modification of existing transporters instead of de novo synthesis of new transporters. Direct demonstration of this feature of exercise conditioning on substrate metabolism will be the focus of additional studies.

Acknowledgments

The authors gratefully acknowledge the participation of Aliy Zirkle and Allen Moore of SP Kennels and Jake Berkowitz of Apex Kennels in the performance of this research.

Author Contributions

Conceived and designed the experiments: MSD AB LAS SSJ KB. Performed the experiments: MSD AB LAS SSJ KB RG KH. Analyzed the data: MSD AB LAS SSJ. Contributed reagents/materials/analysis tools: MSD AB KH. Contributed to the writing of the manuscript: MSD AB LAS SSJ KB RG KH.

References

1. Richter EA, Hargreaves M (2013) Exercise, GLUT4, and skeletal muscle glucose uptake. Physiol Rev 93: 993–1017. 93/3/993 [pii]; doi:10.1152/physrev.00038.2012
2. Bonen A, Campbell SE, Benton CR, Chabowski A, Coort SL, et al. (2004) Regulation of fatty acid transport by fatty acid translocase/CD36. Proc Nutr Soc 63: 245–249.
3. Hinchcliff KW, Reinhart GA, Burr JR, Schreier CJ, Swenson RA (1997) Metabolizable energy intake and sustained energy expenditure of Alaskan sled dogs during heavy exertion in the cold. Am J Vet Res 58: 1457–1462.
4. McKenzie E, Holbrook T, Williamson K, Royer C, Valberg S, et al. (2005) Recovery of muscle glycogen concentrations in sled dogs during prolonged exercise. Med Sci Sports Exerc 37: 1307–1312.
5. McKenzie EC, Hinchcliff KW, Valberg SJ, Williamson KK, Payton ME, et al. (2008) Intramuscular triglyceride and glycogen utilization during prolonged repetitive exercise by Alaskan sled dogs. Am J Vet Res In press.
6. Luiken JJ, Turcotte LP, Bonen A (1999) Protein-mediated palmitate uptake and expression of fatty acid transport proteins in heart giant vesicles. J Lipid Res 40: 1007–1016.
7. Bonen A, Luiken JJ, Arumugam Y, Glatz JF, Tandon NN (2000) Acute regulation of fatty acid uptake involves the cellular redistribution of fatty acid translocase. J Biol Chem 275: 14501–14508. 275/19/14501 [pii].
8. Ren JM, Semenkovich CF, Gulve EA, Gao J, Holloszy JO (1994) Exercise induces rapid increases in GLUT4 expression, glucose transport capacity, and insulin-stimulated glycogen storage in muscle. J Biol Chem 269: 14396–14401.
9. Kristiansen S, Hargreaves M, Richter EA (1997) Progressive increase in glucose transport and GLUT-4 in human sarcolemmal vesicles during moderate exercise. Am J Physiol 272: E385–E389.
10. Richter EA, Jensen P, Kiens B, Kristiansen S (1998) Sarcolemmal glucose transport and GLUT-4 translocation during exercise are diminished by endurance training. Am J Physiol 274: E89–E95.
11. Halseth AE, Bracy DP, Wasserman DH (1998) Limitations to exercise- and maximal insulin-stimulated muscle glucose uptake. J Appl Physiol (1985) 85: 2305–2313.
12. Phillips SM, Han XX, Green HJ, Bonen A (1996) Increments in skeletal muscle GLUT-1 and GLUT-4 after endurance training in humans. Am J Physiol 270: E456–E462.
13. Hardin DS, Azzarelli B, Edwards J, Wigglesworth J, Maianu L, et al. (1995) Mechanisms of enhanced insulin sensitivity in endurance-trained athletes: effects on blood flow and differential expression of GLUT 4 in skeletal muscles. J Clin Endocrinol Metab 80: 2437–2446. doi:10.1210/jcem.80.8.7629239
14. Ploug T, Stallknecht BM, Pedersen O, Kahn BB, Ohkuwa T et al. (1990) Effect of endurance training on glucose transport capacity and glucose transporter expression in rat skeletal muscle. Am J Physiol 259: E778–E786.
15. McCutcheon LJ, Geor RJ, Hinchcliff KW (2002) Changes in skeletal muscle GLUT4 content and muscle membrane glucose transport following 6 weeks of exercise training. Equine Vet J Suppl 199–204.
16. Talanian JL, Holloway GP, Snook LA, Heigenhauser GJ, Bonen A, et al. (2010) Exercise training increases sarcolemmal and mitochondrial fatty acid transport proteins in human skeletal muscle. Am J Physiol Endocrinol Metab 299: E180–E188. ajpendo.00073.2010 [pii]; doi:10.1152/ajpendo.00073.2010
17. Kitaoka Y, Mukai K, Aida H, Hiraga A, Masuda H, et al. (2012) Effects of high-intensity training on lipid metabolism in Thoroughbreds. Am J Vet Res 73: 1813–1818. doi:10.2460/ajvr.73.11.1813
18. Koonen DP, Glatz JF, Bonen A, Luiken JJ (2005) Long-chain fatty acid uptake and FAT/CD36 translocation in heart and skeletal muscle. Biochim Biophys Acta 1736: 163–180. S1388-1981(05)00216-7 [pii]; doi:10.1016/j.bbalip.2005.08.018
19. Nickerson JG, Alkhateeb H, Benton CR, Lally J, Nickerson J, et al. (2009) Greater transport efficiencies of the membrane fatty acid transporters FAT/CD36 and FATP4 compared with FABPpm and FATP1 and differential effects on fatty acid esterification and oxidation in rat skeletal muscle. J Biol Chem 284: 16522–16530. M109.004788 [pii]; doi:10.1074/jbc.M109.004788
20. Begum N, Leitner W, Reusch JE, Sussman KE, Draznin B (1993) GLUT-4 phosphorylation and its intrinsic activity. Mechanism of Ca(2+)-induced inhibition of insulin-stimulated glucose transport. J Biol Chem 268: 3352–3356.
21. Alkhateeb H, Chabowski A, Glatz JF, Luiken JF, Bonen A (2007) Two phases of palmitate-induced insulin resistance in skeletal muscle: impaired GLUT4 translocation is followed by a reduced GLUT4 intrinsic activity. Am J Physiol Endocrinol Metab 293: E783–E793. 00685.2006 [pii]; doi:10.1152/ajpendo.00685.2006
22. Mohan S, Sheena A, Poulose N, Anilkumar G (2010) Molecular dynamics simulation studies of GLUT4: substrate-free and substrate-induced dynamics and ATP-mediated glucose transport inhibition. PLoS One 5: e14217. doi:10.1371/journal.pone.0014217
23. Klip A (2009) The many ways to regulate glucose transporter 4. Appl Physiol Nutr Metab 34: 481–487. h09-047 [pii]; doi:10.1139/H09-047
24. Zaid H, Talior-Volodarsky I, Antonescu C, Liu Z, Klip A (2009) GAPDH binds GLUT4 reciprocally to hexokinase-II and regulates glucose transport activity. Biochem J 419: 475–484. BJ20081319 [pii]; doi:10.1042/BJ20081319
25. Su X, Abumrad NA (2009) Cellular fatty acid uptake: a pathway under construction. Trends Endocrinol Metab 20: 72–77. S1043-2760(09)00003-4 [pii]; doi:10.1016/j.tem.2008.11.001
26. Tonouchi M, Hatta H, Bonen A (2002) Muscle contraction increases lactate transport while reducing sarcolemmal MCT4, but not MCT1. Am J Physiol Endocrinol Metab 282: E1062–E1069.

13

Upregulation of Immunoproteasome Subunits in Myositis Indicates Active Inflammation with Involvement of Antigen Presenting Cells, CD8 T-Cells and IFNγ

Khetam Ghannam[1], Lorena Martinez-Gamboa[1], Lydia Spengler[1], Sabine Krause[2], Biljana Smiljanovic[1], Marc Bonin[1], Salyan Bhattarai[1], Andreas Grützkau[3], Gerd-R. Burmester[1], Thomas Häupl[1*❡], Eugen Feist[1❡]

1 Department of Rheumatology and Clinical Immunology, Charité University Hospital, Berlin, Germany, **2** Friedrich Baur Institute, Ludwig Maximilians University, Munich, Germany, **3** German Arthritis Research Center, Berlin, Germany

Abstract

Objective: In idiopathic inflammatory myopathies (IIM) infiltration of immune cells into muscle and upregulation of MHC-I expression implies increased antigen presentation and involvement of the proteasome system. To decipher the role of immunoproteasomes in myositis, we investigated individual cell types and muscle tissues and focused on possible immune triggers.

Methods: Expression of constitutive (PSMB5, -6, -7) and corresponding immunoproteasomal subunits (PSMB8, -9, -10) was analyzed by real-time RT-PCR in muscle biopsies and sorted peripheral blood cells of patients with IIM, non-inflammatory myopathies (NIM) and healthy donors (HD). Protein analysis in muscle biopsies was performed by western blot. Affymetrix HG-U133 platform derived transcriptome data from biopsies of different muscle diseases and from immune cell types as well as monocyte stimulation experiments were used for validation, coregulation and coexpression analyses.

Results: Real-time RT-PCR revealed significantly increased expression of immunoproteasomal subunits (PSMB8/-9/-10) in DC, monocytes and CD8+ T-cells in IIM. In muscle biopsies, the immunosubunits were elevated in IIM compared to NIM and exceeded levels of matched blood samples. Proteins of PSMB8 and -9 were found only in IIM but not NIM muscle biopsies. Reanalysis of 78 myositis and 20 healthy muscle transcriptomes confirmed these results and revealed involvement of the antigen processing and presentation pathway. Comparison with reference profiles of sorted immune cells and healthy muscle confirmed upregulation of PSMB8 and -9 in myositis biopsies beyond infiltration related changes. This upregulation correlated highest with STAT1, IRF1 and IFNγ expression. Elevation of T-cell specific transcripts in active IIM muscles was accompanied by increased expression of DC and monocyte marker genes and thus reflects the cell type specific involvement observed in peripheral blood.

Conclusions: Immunoproteasomes seem to indicate IIM activity and suggest that dominant involvement of antigen processing and presentation may qualify these diseases exemplarily for the evolving therapeutic concepts of immunoproteasome specific inhibition.

Editor: Frederick Miller, National Institutes of Health, United States of America

Funding: German Research Foundation grant DFG FE470/3-1; German Research Foundation grant DFG GRK1631 (MyoGrad); EU IMI grant BeTheCure, contract no 115142-2; European Science Foundation, grant EUMYONET. The funders had no role in study design, data collection and analysis, decision to publish, or preparation of the manuscript.

* Email: thomas.haeupl@charite.de

❡ These authors contributed equally to this work.

Introduction

Idiopathic inflammatory myopathies (IIM) are a heterogenous group of muscle diseases characterized by inflammatory infiltrates in the skeletal muscle. Three major diseases are defined: dermatomyositis (DM), polymyositis (PM), and inclusion body myositis (IBM). The main autoimmune response in DM resembles a microangiopathy affecting skin and muscle tissue. In polymyositis and inclusion body myositis, cytotoxic CD8+ T cells invade muscle fibers. All of the invaded fibers and numerous non-invaded fibers express increased amounts of major histocompatibility complex class I (MHC-I) molecules [1]. In fact, the presence of MHC-I/CD8+ complex is considered as a characteristic immunopathological marker of PM and IBM [2]. Continuous upregulation of expression of MHC class I molecules in muscle fibers is thought to induce an endoplasmic reticulum stress response with accumulation of misfolded glycoproteins and activation of nuclear factor kappa B (NF-κB). As a consequence, MHC-I/CD8+ complexes may form and perpetuate an autoinflammatory response [3].

The ubiquitin-proteasome system (UPS) is a 26S, non-lysosomal, multicatalytic, and multisubunit complex involved in the ubiquitin-dependent, selective intracellular degradation of proteins [4]. In this way, the proteasome plays a central role in the activation of transcription factors such as NF-κB [5]. Furthermore, it is involved in the generation of peptides presented by the MHC-I to the antigen receptors of cytotoxic T cells [6,7], and thus, is involved in the regulation of the inflammatory response. Many studies suggest that the proteasome participates in muscle fiber degradation in various physiological and pathological conditions and may therefore also play an important role in myositis [8,9].

The 26S proteasome is composed of a proteolytically active core, namely the 20S proteasome, and one or two 19S regulator complexes. The 20S or constitutive proteasome is a cylindrical particle that consists of four rings, each composed of seven different subunits. The outer two rings are formed by seven alpha-type subunits (PSMA1–PSMA7), while the inner two rings contain seven beta-type subunits (PSMB1–PSMB7) [6]. The proteolytically active sites are limited to three constitutive beta subunits, proteasome subunit beta type 5-PSMB5, proteasome subunit beta type 6-PSMB6 and proteasome subunit beta type 7-PSMB7.[10]. Importantly, under the influence of the pro-inflammatory cytokine IFNγ, the structure and the catalytic properties of the constitutive proteasome are modified by substitution of the catalytic subunits PSMB5, PSMB6 and PSMB7 with three catalytic immunosubunits proteasome subunit beta type 8-PSMB8, proteasome subunit beta type 9-PSMB9 and proteasome subunit beta type 10-PSMB10 respectively, leading to the formation of the so-called immunoproteasome. This process is considered to strongly influence the production of peptides for antigen presentation by MHC class I as well as the immune response [11–13]. As IFNγ is also secreted in IIM [14], the immunoproteasomal system may also contribute to pathomechanisms in myositis. Recently, mutations in human were detected in proteasome subunit PSMB8, which cause joint contractures, muscle atrophy, microcytic anemia, and panniculitis-induced lipodystrophy syndrome in addition to other autoinflammatory syndromes [15–18]. Impaired immunoproteasome assembly and decreased proteolytic activity have been confirmed in some of these diseases. On the other hand, elevated levels of circulating proteasomes as well as autoantibodies against several proteasomal subunits have been detected in patients with autoimmune myositis and other autoimmune disorders [19,20]. Moreover, it has also been shown that anti-proteasome autoantibodies derived from patients with connective tissue diseases, including a patient with polymyositis, were capable of blocking the stimulation of the catalytic proteasome core complex by the proteasome activator PA28, consisting of the subunits alpha (PSME1) and beta (PSME2) [21]. Additionally, an upregulation of some proteasomal genes has been shown in PBMCs of patients with systemic autoimmune disorders including patients with PM [22].

Based on the existing but so far indirect assumption of an involvement of the proteasome system in the pathogenesis of IIM, we investigated the expression of all catalytic proteasome subunits in inflammatory and non-inflammatory myopathies in order to search for an activation of the 20S core complex in patients with autoimmune myositis. Results were validated and comprehensively screened in a large panel of disease related as well as cell type and stimulation specific transcriptome data sets in order to confirm our results and to identify induction mechanisms and the regulatory network for the immune proteasome subunits.

Materials and Methods

Ethics Statement

The study was performed in accordance with the 1964 Declaration of Helsinki and approved by the "Charité University Medicine ethics committee I of Charité Campus Mitte" and patients provided written consent to participate in the study.

Patients and healthy donors

Expression of proteasome subunits was investigated in 17 patients with idiopathic inflammatory myopathies (IIM), including polymyositis (PM, n = 5), dermatomyositis (DM, n = 5), and overlap-syndromes with myositis (OM, n = 7) (8 male, 9 female, mean age 54.3 years, age range 22–72 years). Patients were selected based on typical clinical symptoms, laboratory and/or muscle biopsy findings, which were indicative for the different groups of myopathies. Patients with PM and DM fulfilled the classification criteria according to Bohan and Peter [23,24]. For details of diagnosis and clinical parameters see supplementary table S1. Autoantibody screening was performed according to diagnostic standards including ANA in indirect immunofluorescence on HEp2 cells. Depending on the result of the ANA pattern, further differentiation of the antibody reactivity was performed for detection of ENA using ELISA. Furthermore, a profile of myositis specific autoantibodies including anti-Jo1-, anti-SRP-, anti-Mi2, anti-PM/Scl and anti-U1RNPantibodies as well as anti-proteasomal antibodies was analyzed in each suspected case of myositis. Controls included 7 patients with different non-inflammatory myopathies (NIM, 4 male, 3 female, mean age 48.7 years, age range 35–59 years). Time and patient matched samples of muscle biopsies and blood were taken from 14 patients. Control samples from 15 healthy donors (HD, 2 male, 13 female, mean age 45 years, age range 27–56 years without clinical signs of disease, no clinical signs of muscular weakness, no medication) included only blood and no muscle biopsies. All patients were diagnosed at the Department of Rheumatology and Clinical Immunology, Charité – University Medicine Berlin and informed consent was obtained from all subjects.

Isolation of peripheral blood mononuclear cells (PBMCs) and cellular subsets

PBMCs were collected by Ficoll density gradient centrifugation (Biochrom, Germany) and divided into two fractions. One was used for separation of dendritic cells (DCs) by Magnetic Cell Separation (MACS) using the Blood Dendritic Cell Isolation Kit-II (Miltenyi Biotec, Germany), the other for isolation of T lymphocytes (CD4+, CD8+), B lymphocytes (CD19+), and monocytes (CD14+) by fluorescence activated cell sorting (FACS) with a FACS DiVa Flow Cytometer (BD, Germany).

Collection of muscle biopsies

Muscle tissues were stabilized in RNA later (Qiagen, Germany) to avoid RNA degradation and were stored at −70°C. For RNA isolation, biopsies were ground with a pestle and mortar in the presence of liquid N_2 to protect RNA against degradation. Disrupted samples were then added to lysis buffer containing β-mercaptoethanol.

RNA isolation, reverse transcription into cDNA and real-time reverse transcriptase-polymerase chain reaction (real time RT-PCR)

RNA was isolated from muscle tissues and blood cells using the NucleoSpin RNA/Protein kit (Macherey-Nagel, Germany). First-

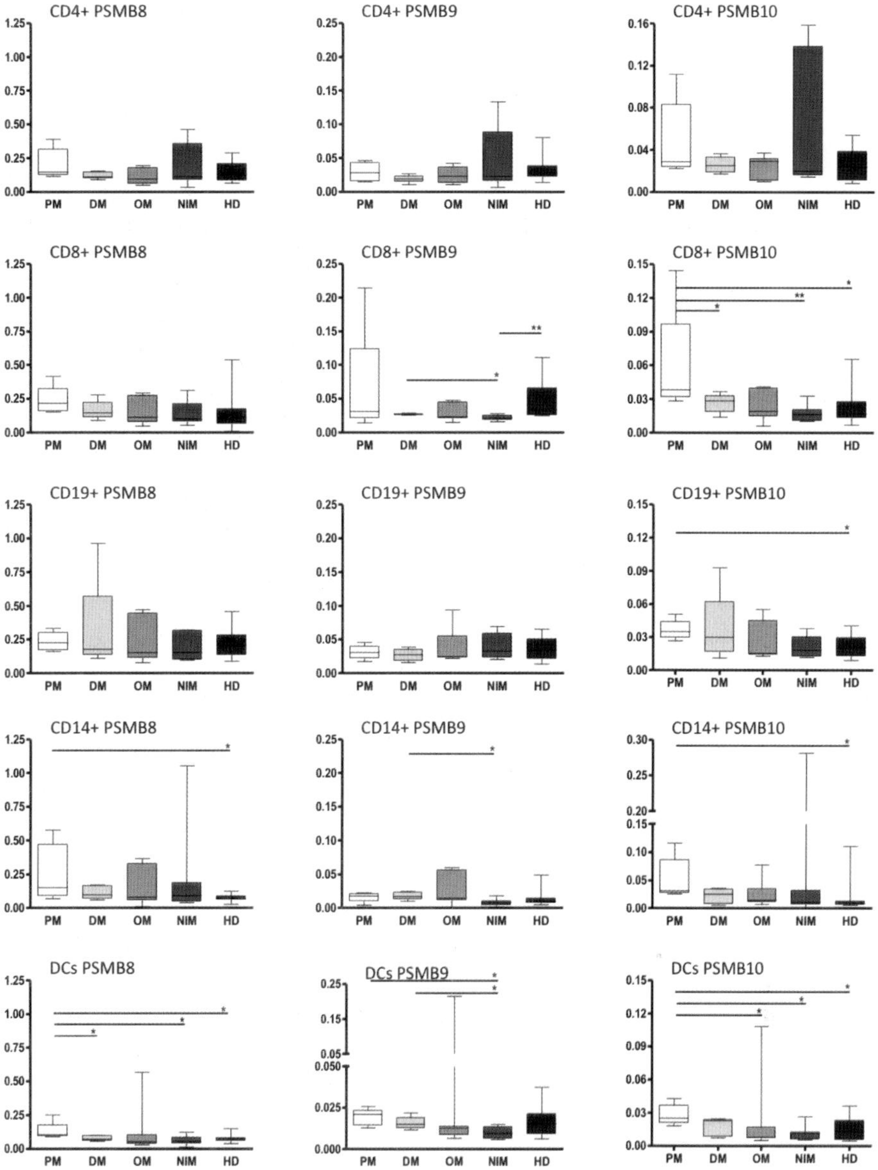

Figure 1. Expression of immunoproteasomal subunits in immune cells: Gene expression of immunoproteasomal subunits (PSMB8–10) in CD4+, CD8+, CD19+, CD14+ and DCs of patients with myopathies (PM, DM, OM, NIM) and controls (HD). Data are shown as relative expression normalized to beta actin. Box plots indicate percentiles 0, 25, 50, 75 and 100. Groups were compared by Mann-Whitney U test and statistical significance is indicated for $p<0.05$ (*) and $p<0.01$ (**). Significantly higher expression of PSMB8 was observed in CD14+ cells and DC of PM patients compared to HD or DM, NIM and HDs, respectively. PSMB9 was increased in CD8+ and CD14+ of DM and in DCs of PM and DM patients compared to NIM. PSMB10 was found increased in PM patients compared to DM, NIM and HD in CD8+, compared to HD in CD19+ and CD14+ cells and compared to OM, NIM, and HD in DCs.

strand cDNA was synthesized using the SuperScript III First-Strand Synthesis System for RT-PCR (Invitrogen, Germany) according to the instructions of the manufacturer.

Forward and reverse primers of proteasome subunits PSMB5, PSMB6, PSMB7, PSMB8, PSMB9 and PSMB10 for real time RT-PCR were designed as described elsewhere [25].

Amplification reactions contained SYBR Green PCR Master Mix (Applied Biosystems), 200 nM forward and reverse primers for each gene and cDNA. Real-time PCR was performed in triplicates using the ABI prism 5700 Sequence Detection System (Applied Biosystems).

Relative expression of the target compared to the house keeping gene beta-actin was determined as $R = \frac{E^{CT_{house-keeping-gene}}}{E^{CT_{target-gene}}}$ [26], with E representing the amplification efficiency of the respective primer system. Mann-Whitney U-test was applied for group comparisons (figures 1, 2, 3).

Western blot analysis

Muscle biopsies were minced in the presence of radioimmuno-precipitation assay (RIPA) lysis buffer. PBMCs were used as positive control and treated with the same lysis buffer. 30 µg of total protein from tissue homogenate or cell lysate were loaded and fractionated by 15% sodium dodecyl sulfate polyacrylamide gel

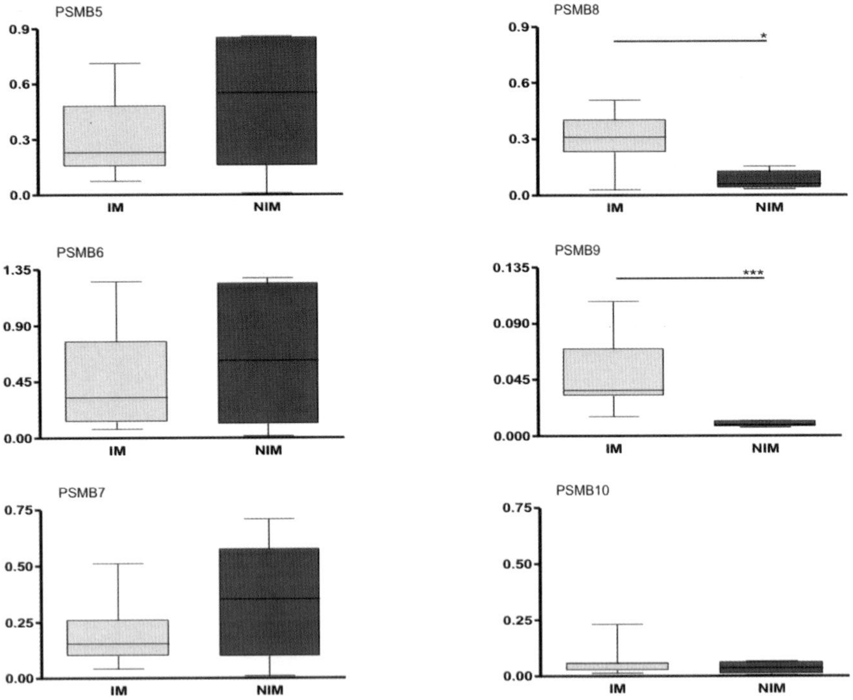

Figure 2. Expression of catalytic proteasomal subunits in muscle: Gene expression analysis of constitutive and immunoproteasomal subunits (PSMB5–10) in muscle biopsies of patients with inflammatory myopathies (IM) and patients with non inflammatory myopathies (NIM). Data are shown as relative expression normalized to beta actin. Box plots indicate percentiles 0, 25, 50, 75 and 100. Groups were compared by Mann-Whitney U test and statistical significance is indicated for $p<0.05$ (*), $p<0.01$ (**) and $p<0.001$ (***). Comparing to NIM, mean relative expression levels in IM revealed 4-fold for PSMB8 [0.302 ± 0.139 and 0.075 ± 0.041] and about 5-fold increase for PSMB9 [0.049 ± 0.029 and 0.009 ± 0.002] but less than 2-fold for PSMB10 [0.065 ± 0.064 and 0.036 ± 0.022].

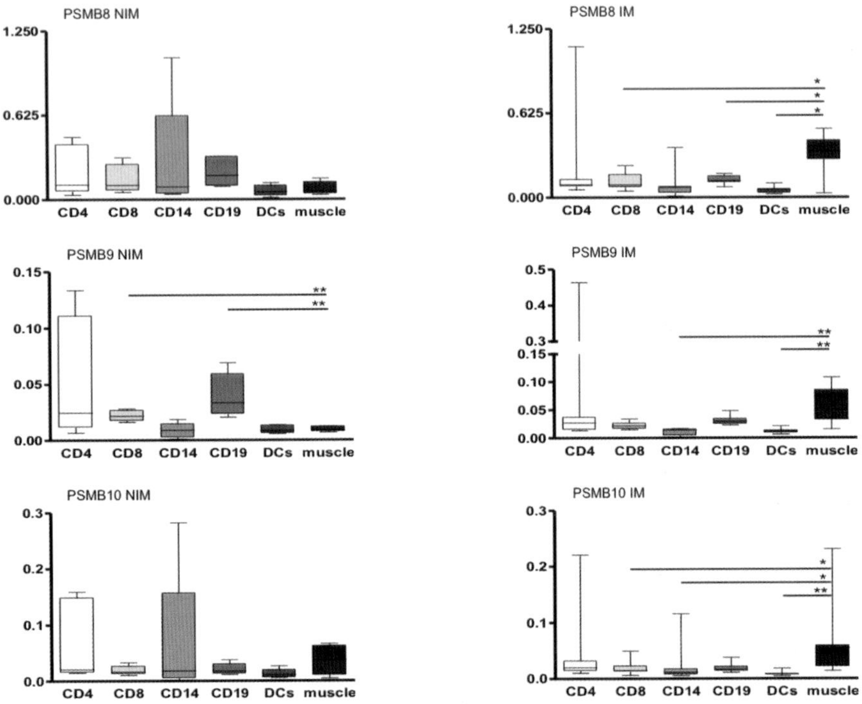

Figure 3. Comparison of immunoproteosomal subunit expression between paired samples from isolated cells and muscle tissue: Gene expression analysis of immunoproteasomal subunits (PSMB8–10) in muscle biopsies vs. CD4+, CD8+, CD14+, CD19+, and DCs from patients with inflammatory myopathies (IM) and patients with non-inflammatory myopathies (NIM). Data are shown as relative expression normalized to beta actin. Box plots indicate percentiles 0, 25, 50, 75 and 100. Groups were compared by Mann-Whitney U test and statistical significance is indicated for $p< 0.05$ (*) and $p<0.01$ (**).

electrophoresis. After transfer to a polyvinylidene fluoride (PVDF) membrane, the blots were incubated overnight at 4°C with monoclonal antibodies against proteasome PSMB8 or proteasome PSMB9, both diluted 1:1000 (Enzo Life Sciences, USA). Staining was performed with polyclonal rabbit anti mouse immunoglobulins conjugated with horseradish peroxidase (1:1000; Dako, Denmark) and visualised by enhanced electrochemiluminescence Pierce ECL Western Blotting Substrate (Thermo Scientific, USA) (figure 4). For quantification relative to a housekeeping gene, beta actin was detected using the same procedure and mouse anti-beta actin diluted 1:10,000 as primary antibody (Sigma, USA). Quantification on western blot images was performed with the intensity histogram function of Adobe Photoshop (Munich, Germany).

Microarray data and statistical analysis

For validation, transcriptome data of muscle biopsies were collected from the open access database Gene Expression Omnibus (GEO, http://www.ncbi.nlm.nih.gov/geo/). The selection included muscle tissue biopsies from different types of IIM, non-inflammatory myopathies, septic patients, volunteers after IL-6 infusion and healthy controls as well as purified dendritic cells from peripheral blood (GSE2044, GSE3112, GSE5370, GSE39454, GSE3307, GSE13205, GSE10685 and GSE23618; table S2). Own data included transcriptomes of stimulated monocytes (GSE38351) [27] and sorted immune cell populations (CD14+ monocytes, CD15+ granulocytes, CD4+ T-cells, CD8+ T-cells, CD19+ B-cells and CD56+ NK-cells, each n = 3; GSE58173) from peripheral blood of healthy donors, generated after RNA extraction, amplification and hybridization to Affymetrix GeneChip HG-U133 Plus 2.0 arrays according to standard protocols to minimize influence on gene expression by sorting [28]. All data were analysed in the BioRetis database (www.bioretis.de) using standard algorithms [29]. Selection of differentially expressed genes was performed by "default increased" filtering in BioRetis [29]. Probesets were ranked by an equally weighted sum-score for "SLR" and "frequency of increase" in disease compared to control (table S3).

Signals were quantile normalized for evaluation of cell infiltration and correlation analysis (figure 5). Percentage of immune cell infiltration was estimated using tissue and cell type specific marker probesets by comparing the reference transcriptomes of each individual cell type and healthy muscle tissue with each other (figure 6). To assess the maximum of infiltration related signal intensity for the immunoproteasome transcripts in each myositis biopsy a linear model of relationship between signal intensity and percentage of infiltration was applied. The highest expected signal (S_{exp}) related to infiltration was calculated as $S_{exp} = S_{max} \cdot P_{inf}$ with P_{inf} as the percentage of all non-muscle cell types (infiltrated cells) and S_{max} as the maximum signal observed in the reference transcriptomes of any of the purified immune cells from healthy donor. The median of log-transformed and z-normalized signals of all 1209 myositis related probesets was used for scoring and sorting of the samples (myositis score).

Results

Dendritic and monocytic cells of the peripheral blood are the leading cell type for immunoproteasome upregulation in myositis

Relative quantification of proteasomal subunit expression by real time RT-PCR revealed a myositis related significant increase of at least one of the immunoproteasomal subunits PSMB8, PSMB9 and/or PSMB10 in all investigated cellular subsets except CD4+ (figure 1). DCs were the leading subset with differences in all immunoproteasomal subunits followed by monocytes, CD8+

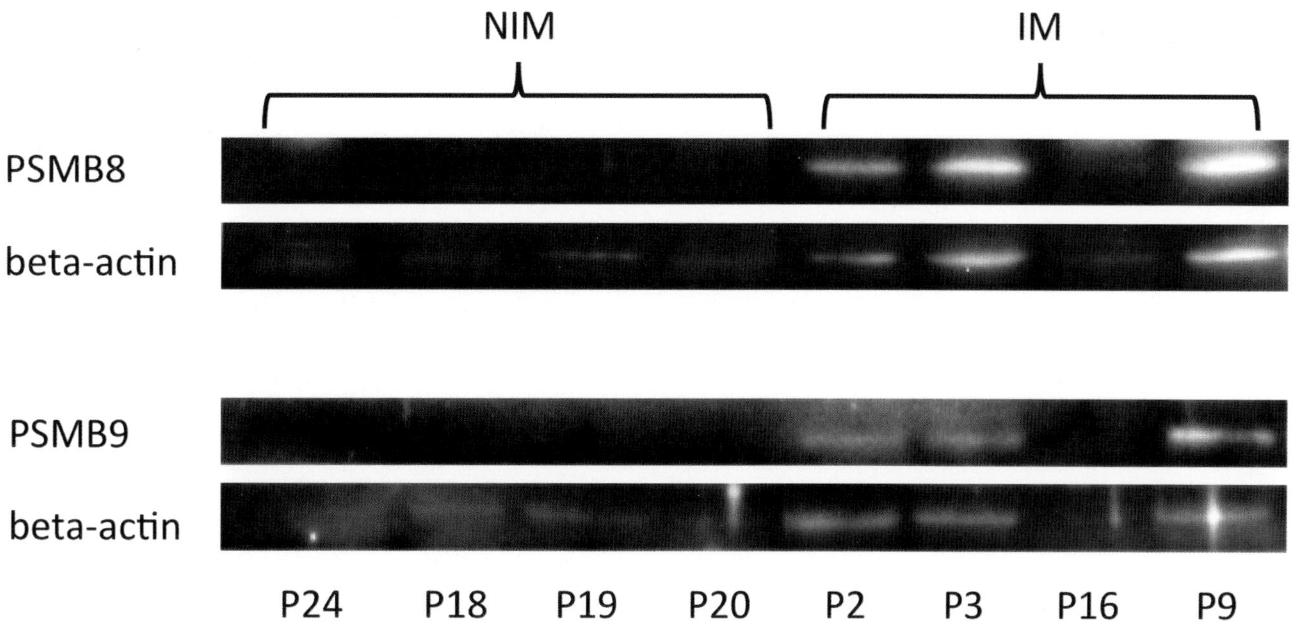

Figure 4. Protein expression of the immunoproteasome subunits PSMB8 and PSMB9 relative to beta actin in IM and NIM. The protein expression of the two subunits was analyzed by western blot in muscle biopsies from four non-inflammatory myopathies (NIM) and four inflammatory myopathies (IM). Intensity of chemiluminescent signals for PSMB8 and PSMB9 was normalized to corresponding signals of the housekeeping protein beta actin, which was detected in a second staining procedure on the same membrane. Only IM samples revealed PSMB8 and -9 protein expression.

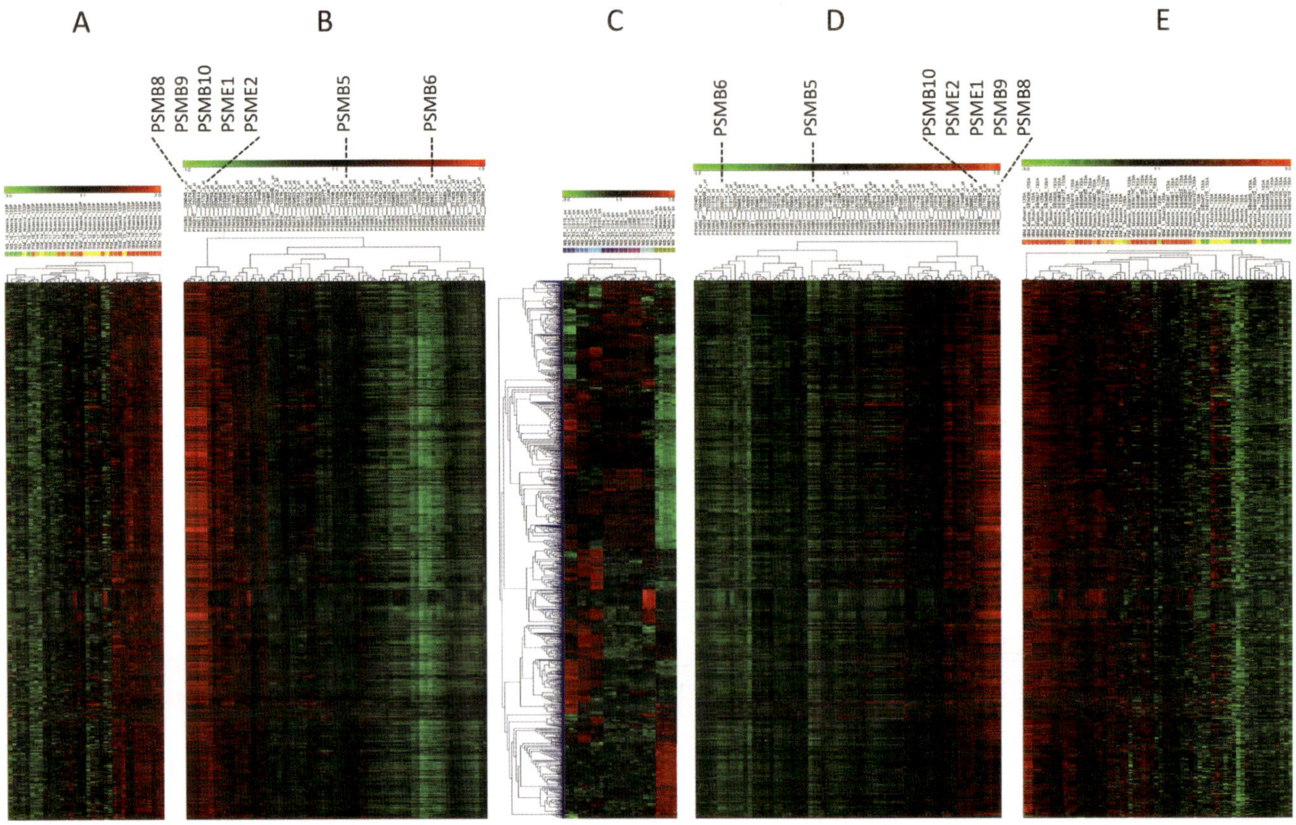

Figure 5. Correlation of proteasome subunit expression with myositis signatures and overlap with immune cell infiltration: Expression of all proteasome units were investigated in transcriptome data of muscle biopsies referenced in table S2 and were correlated with genes increased in myositis muscle tissue. The heatmap of the probeset signal intensities (A) is opposed to the heatmap of the gene by gene correlation matrix (B) in 133P array experiments. Identical analysis in 133A arrays are shown in D and E. Expression of the 1209 probesets in reference transcriptomes of purified immune cells from the blood of healthy donors served as basis for clustering by probesets and cell types (C). Identification of cell type specific transcriptional patterns in the 1209 probesets demonstrates the extent of overlap of these probesets with immune cell related transcripts. Myositis samples include IBM (red), PM (orange), DM (yellow), NM (necrotizing myopathy)/IM (inflammatory myopathy) (light green) and HD (green). Immune cell types include neutrophils (dark blue), monocytes (blue), dendritic cells (light blue), CD4+ T-cells (dark violet), CD8+ T-cells (violet), NK-cells (light violet), B-cells (cyan), and healthy muscle (moss-green). A detailed graph with all probesets labelled is presented in supplemental material (figure S4).

and finally CD19+ lymphocytes. Differences were most prominent in PM and to a lower extent in DM patients when compared to non-inflammatory myopathies (NIM) and healthy donors (HD). Differences between immunoproteasomal and corresponding constitutive subunits were especially found between PSMB8 and PSMB5 in all investigated peripheral blood cell types of all patients (figure S1) and HD (data not shown).

Immunoproteasomal subunit expression is higher in IIM than NIM muscle biopsies and indicates a substitution of constitutive subunits

In all patients with inflammatory myopathies (IM) including PM, DM and OM, immunoproteasomal subunits PSMB8 and PSMB9 were significantly increased when compared to NIM patients (figure 2). In contrast, PSMB10 was less increased in IM patients compared to NIM and not statistically significant. The ratios between immunoproteasomal and corresponding constitutive subunits (PSMB8/PSMB5, PSMB9/PSMB6 and PSMB10/PSMB7) in IM [1.79, 0.35 and 0.42, respectively] compared to non-inflammatory biopsies [0.94, 0.1 and 0.18, respectively] indicate an imbalance and suggest substitution of constitutive by immunoproteasomal subunits in patients with IIM.

Immunoproteasomal subunit expression in IIM is higher in muscle compared to donor matched immune cells of peripheral blood

In paired samples of blood and tissue from 7 IM and 6 NIM patients collected at the same time, real time RT-PCR revealed significant increase of immunoproteasomal subunits in muscle compared to blood cells only in IM. In contrast, in NIM, expression of immunoproteasomal subunits was higher in most blood cell types compared to muscle tissue (figure 3). Constitutive subunits were higher expressed in all muscle biopsies from IM and NIM when compared to any cell type of the blood (data not shown).

Regulation of PSMB8 and PSMB9 protein in myopathy patients

To confirm that the elevated transcriptional activity is also translated into protein, PSMB8 and PSMB9 proteins were investigated in muscle tissue of representative patients with

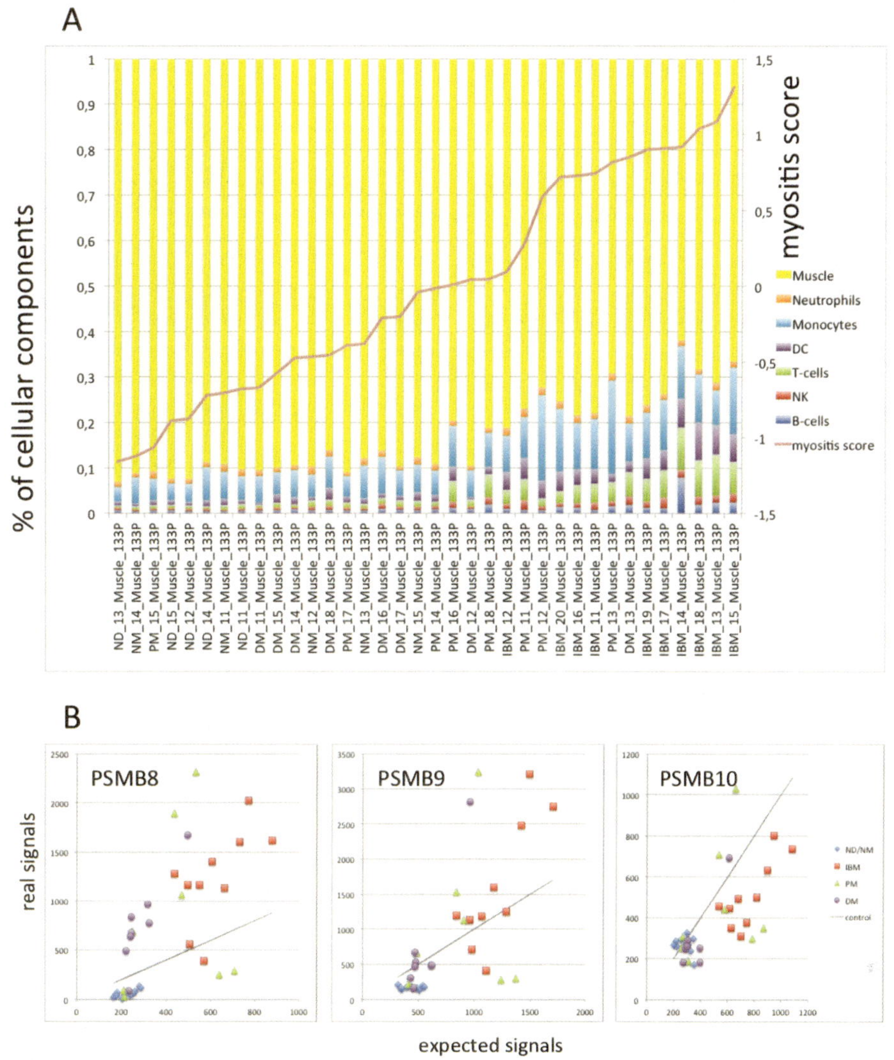

Figure 6. Quantification of cellular infiltration and confirmation of PSMB8/-9 gene activation in myositis muscle samples: Transcriptome data referenced in table S2 were re-investigated. A) Cell type infiltration was quantified based on the expression of cell specific marker transcripts (figure S5). Signal ratios between muscle biopsy and purified cell type were calculated for each cell type specific transcriptional markers. Taking the median of the ratios in each cell specific marker set and scaling their sum to 100% revealed an estimate of the cellular composition. Increase of monocyte, dendritic cell and T-cell transcription patterns corresponds to the molecular myositis score. (ND = normal donor; NM = necrotizing myopathy). B) The maximum of infiltration related signal intensity was calculated as described in materials and methods. Comparing these expected intensities (x-axis) with real intensities (y-axis) in each sample, PSMB8 and PSMB9 are higher expressed than expected in the majority of IBM and several of the PM muscle. In DM, PSMB8 expression also exceeds the expected signal intensity, although on a lower level. One out of the 8 DM samples (DM_13) showed consistently a pattern similar to the highly inflamed IBM samples. All other conditions including controls remained below the expected intensity. For PSMB10, the increased signal intensity in several samples of IBM seems to correspond to the level of infiltration.

dermatomyositis (P2 and P3), polymyositis (P9), overlap syndrom (P16) and non-inflammatory muscle diseases (P18, P19, P20, P24). Western blot analysis revealed equal or higher protein detection intensities of PSMB8 compared to actin in the patients with inflammatory muscle diseases and slightly weaker intensities for PSMB9. In all samples investigated from non-inflammatory diseases both immunoproteasomal subunits were not visible as a distinct band (figure 4). Intensities determined for PSMB8/-9 relative to actin were also significantly lower in NIM than in IIM. Correlation between immunoproteasomal protein and RNA transcript expression, both as relative quantities compared to actin protein or transcript, revealed high correlation coefficients of R = 0.90 for PSMB8 and R = 0.80 for PSMB9.

Transcriptome data for validation and pathophysiologic classification of defined transcripts

To validate these results and to characterize the importance of immunoproteasomes in myositis compared to other molecular mechanisms, we investigated open access transcriptome data of muscle biopsies from patients with IIM and NIM as well as from healthy donors. Transcriptomes from different types of immune cells and stimulation experiments with IFN, TNF and LPS were selected to address functional interpretation (table S2).

Immunoproteasomal subunits PSMB8/-9 are leading candidates in the pathophysiology of IIM muscle inflammation. Muscle transcriptomes from patients with IBM, PM and DM were compared to healthy controls and revealed 1209 probesets equal to 927 genes, which were upregulated in at least one of the myositis diseases (table S3) as a molecular correlate of disease activity. PSMB8 ranked at position 9 and PSMB9 at position 58 out of the 927 genes when scored for magnitude and consistency of increase. Based on these 1209 probesets, IIM samples did not cluster by disease specific patterns but overall intensity of molecular changes. High molecular activity was most frequent in IBM followed by PM and DM muscle biopsies. This was observed independently for both 133A and 133P data sets (figure 5A, 5E, S2). Of all known proteasomal subunits, PSMB8/-9 as well as their activator subunits PSME1 and -2 [30] correlated best with the 1209 probesets while most of the constitutively expressed subunits including PSMB5 and -6 were inversely correlated. This was again independently observed in 133A and 133P datasets (figure 5B and 5D). Characterizing the panel of 1209 probesets with DAVID (http://david.abcc.ncifcrf.gov/) revealed that almost each gene annotated to the antigen processing and presentation pathways of MHC-I and II was included (figure S3).

Transcription of PSMB8/-9 is actively up-regulated in IIM muscle tissue. Investigating gene expression for the 1209 probesets in reference signatures of healthy muscle and immune cell populations uncovers that the majority is also part of the physiologic expression in immune cells and is sufficiently specific to correctly cluster the immune cell profiles (figure 5 C tree of clustered samples). Thus, these transcripts could be unregulated but passively transported by cell infiltration into muscle or also upregulated by additional gene activation (figure 5). Such active upregulation seems to occur for transcripts specific for healthy muscle (bottom of figure 5 C), which were increased in myositis. A magnification of figure 5 with detailed description of genes is provided in figure S4.

Compared to immune cells, there is no relevant expression of immunoproteasomes in healthy muscle. Selection of optimized cell type specific marker transcripts (figure S5) disclosed quantitatively the cell type specific transcriptional activities in the muscle biopsies, which were besides muscle especially related to T-cells, monocytes and dendritic cells and corresponded to the overall molecular change in myositis muscle transcriptomes (myositis score; figure 6 A). Comparing real expression levels of immunoproteasome subunits in myositis with intensities expected from immune cell infiltration demonstrated that PSMB8/-9 were actively upregulated in patients with IBM, PM and DM, especially when high expression levels not only of the immunoproteasomal subunits but also of genes differentially expressed in inflammatory myopathies compared to healthy muscle were observed and thus were indicative for high molecular disease activity (figure 6 B). PSMB10 expression, however, matched with expected intensities, which indicated no additional upregulation.

Transcription factors STAT1 and IRF1 correlate with upregulation of PSMB-8 and -9 expression in IIM and in IFN stimulated monocytes. Regulatory mechanisms for immunoproteasomes in myositis were searched by correlation of transcription factors defined by GO:0003700 with PSMB8/-9 in all muscle biopsy samples. This revealed STAT1, IRF1, TRIM22 and IRF9 as potential regulators, which were predominantly increased in IBM, but also present in many PM and several DM samples. PSMB5/-6 were not or inversely correlated. In different healthy donor immune cell types and healthy muscle, correlation between PSMB8/-9 and these transcription factors was much weaker. However, monocytes stimulated with TNF, LPS, IFNα2 or IFNγ revealed highest correlation between PSMB8/-9 and STAT1 followed by IRF1 (table S4). This was related to IFNα2 and IFNγ. In contrast, TNF suppressed both transcription factors and PSMB8/-9, while LPS induced both transcription factors but suppressed PSMB8/-9 expression (table S4).

In IIM, IFNγ but not type-1 IFN correlate with PSMB8/-9 expression and T-cell markers including CD8. Although both types of interferons may induce PSMB8/-9 [27], in myositis muscle transcriptomes only IFNγ was significantly increased with dominance in IBM (74% increased change call, 4.9-fold increased) and correlated with PSMB8/-9. These analyses were separately performed with 133P and 133A data sets and independently confirmed each other (figure 7). To trace the cellular origin, signals of IFNγ in myositis were correlated with all cell type specific marker transcripts and the median of all correlation coefficients per cell type was calculated. IFNγ expression correlated best with T-cells (133P: $R = 0.78$; 133A: $R = 0.62$) and CD8 (133P: $R = 0.80$; 133A: $R = 0.69$) followed by dendritic cells (133P: $R = 0.66$; 133P: $R = 0.57$) in both, 133A and 133P datasets. NK-cell association was also high in 133P ($R = 0.54$) but much lower in 133A datasets ($R = 0.17$).

Immunoproteasome activation is specific for IIM but not non-inflammatory myopathies. Reanalysis of muscle transcriptomes from 12 different muscle diseases (GSE3307) with non-inflammatory myopathies except from juvenile dermatomyositis (JDM) revealed upregulation of PSMB8/-9 only in samples from JDM and in one out of four samples from limb girdle muscular dystrophy 2I (LGMD2I). Furthermore, muscle biopsies from healthy donors after IL-6 infusion (GSE10685) or patients with sepsis induced multiple organ failure (GSE13205) did not reveal any increase of the immunoproteasome expression, indicating that expression of PSMB8/-9 in muscle is specific for IIM.

Discussion

With this first comprehensive analysis of muscle biopsies and blood derived immune cells in myositis on the catalytic subunits of the proteasome, we could demonstrate a central role of immunoproteasomes in the inflammatory process of IIM including IBM, PM and DM on transcriptional as well as protein expression level. We identified PSMB8/-9 upregulation only in combination with infiltration of antigen presenting cells and associated with the expression of IFNγ and CD8 accompanied by T-cell infiltration in biopsies of inflamed muscle. This perfectly integrates into current concepts of IIM pathophysiology and extends these towards a strong involvement of mechanisms and modulations of antigen processing.

IIM are of unknown aetiology and present with characteristic upregulation of MHC-class I and II molecules [1,31], which was also detectable in the myositis transcriptome data. Antigen presentation is affected by replacement of constitutive with immunoproteasomal subunits [13]. In this study, we observed that physiologic expression of the immunoproteasome subunits in healthy controls was not only restricted to professional antigen presenting cells but found in all subtypes of peripheral blood immune cells. Healthy muscle tissue in contrast expressed only constitutive subunits while immunoproteasome expression was negligible. Immunoproteasomal processing is especially linked to the MHC-I pathway [13]. Thus, it is important that in our investigation transcription was highly correlated with protein production of immunopreteasomes and also associated with the histological finding of MHC-I protein upregulation in muscle tissue of the analyzed IIM samples.

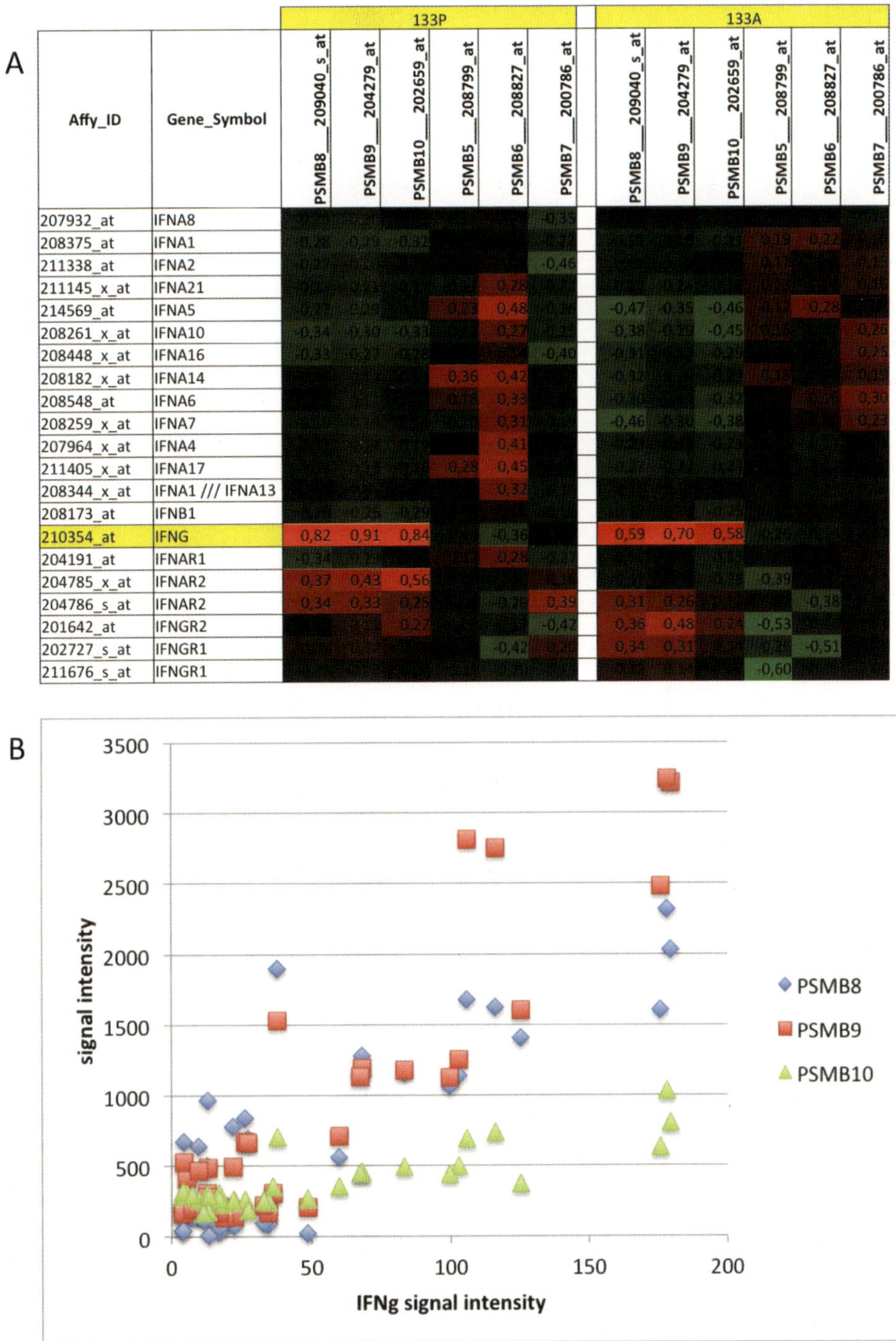

Figure 7. Correlation of immunoproteasome with IFN and IFNR expression in myositis muscle tissue: Transcriptome data referenced in table S2 were re-investigated. A) Correlation analysis was performed for 133P and 133A datasets independently. Only IFNγ revealed high correlation coefficients with PSMB8, PSMB9 and PSMB10. The corresponding constitutively expressed subunits PSMB5-7 were not or even negatively correlated. B) Comparing the association of IFNγ with PSMB8, -9 and -10 for each sample individually, the increase was much higher for PSMB8/-9 compared to PSMB10 as described before (figure 6).

Our reanalysis of the myositis transcriptomes revealed that molecular changes of active inflammation were mainly associated with an increase of immune cell transcriptome signatures and interestingly independent from clinical diagnosis. Immunoproteasome subunit expression in IIM was upregulated especially in DC and monocytes of the peripheral blood but also in muscle, where PSMB8/-9 correlated with the molecular changes of inflammation and thus infiltration of immune cells. The increase of PSMB8/-9 expression in IIM was higher than the level expected by infiltration of immune cells and was also higher in total biopsy material with an immune cells fraction below 40% compared to any of the purified (100%) donor matched immune cells from peripheral blood. This clearly indicates that these immunoproteasomal transcripts must be upregulated in one or more of the cell types of inflamed muscle.

Recently, transcriptomes obtained from type I and II IFN stimulated monocytes [27] revealed similar expression patterns of immunoproteasomal subunits with upregulation of PSMB8/-9 but not -10, suggesting the involvement of type I and/or type II IFN triggers on PSMB8/-9 regulation in inflamed muscle tissues. IFNγ was reported to induce MHC-II and enhance MHC-I expression in affected muscles of PM and DM patients [32]. Recently, an IFNα signature and influence is discussed especially in DM but also in PM [33]. In contrast, a role of IFNγ triggering is assumed especially in IBM [34]. In this study, we could identify in the myositis transcriptomes only IFNγ but not IFNα as a predominant trigger for PSMB8/-9, which also correlated with the expression of STAT1 and IRF-1. Both transcription factors were also reported to mediate IFNγ induced PSMB9 expression in murine macrophages [35]. Interestingly, IFNγ production by T-cells was reported to depend on immunoproteasomes [36]. Especially in IBM the link of MHC-I with immunoproteasomal units suggests an important role for antigen processing via PSMB8 and -9 dependent mechanisms. This may be induced by misfolded protein from fiber degradation or suspected retroviral or viral triggers in this type of myositis [37] and thereby contribute to CD8+ T-cell triggering, expansion and IFNγ production.

Thus, immunoproteasomes and antigen processing seem to be pivotal in molecular pathomechanisms of myositis and may serve particularly as biomarker of myositis activity. This is further supported by the lack of immunoproteasome activation in our reanalysis of muscle transcriptomes from non-inflammatory myopathies [38], patients with severe inflammatory syndroms like sepsis [39] or conditions related to high IL-6 levels in the circulation [40].

This important association of immunoproteasome upregulation with myositis activity raises the discussion, whether these diseases qualify as a model for therapeutic targeting of immunoproteasomes. Inhibitors are currently developed and tested with controversial effects [41,42]. Application of the PSMB8 selective inhibitor PR-957 in experimental arthritis or colitis could reduce cytokine production and attenuate disease activity [43,44]. On the other hand, the recently described mutations c.224C>T (p.Thr75Met) [15], G201V [16], G197V [17] and c.405C>A [18] in PSMB8 were all associated with decreased subunit activity and different inflammatory syndroms, suggesting that immunoproteasome suppression may cause additional effects depending on dosage and cell type involvement. Studies in PSMB8/-9 deficienct mice suggested that inflammation induced immunoproteasome expression in tissue may also prevent CD8+ T-cell mediated autoimmunity [45].

Knowing that immunoproteasomes modulate antigen processing with effects on MHC-I peptide presentation [46], intracellular protein homeostasis [47] and CD8 T-cell responses [48] especially in mixed proteasomes [49], immunoproteasome inhibition may be a double-edged sword. Influencing antigen processing and presentation may reduce CD8+ T-cell triggering through MHC-I but may also increase toxicity by accumulating misfolded proteins.

In summary, our results support the hypothesis that the proteasome system is activated and contributes to a perpetuating crosstalk between antigen-presenting cells and T-cells via immunoproteasome generated peptides and IFNγ. Assuming altered autoantigen processing as driving mechanism, suppression of the immunoproteasome could be a promising therapeutic concept. Therefore, further studies are needed that focus on antigens and peptides, which are specifically processed by immunoproteasomes in IIM as well as on mechanisms of suppressing or modulating antigen processing and presentation.

Supporting Information

Figure S1 High expression levels of PSMB8 compared to PSMB5 in all isolated cells: Gene expression of constitutive (PSMB5-7) and immunoproteasomal subunits (PSMB8-10) in CD4+, CD8+, CD19+, CD14+, DCs and muscles of all patients. Data are shown as relative expression normalized to beta actin. Box plots indicate percentiles 0, 25, 50, 75 and 100.

Figure S2 Differences in upregulation of myositis related genes between IBM, PM, DM, NM and IM: All 1209 probesets were sorted by a sum-score for magnitude and frequency of increase in myositis. The heat map presents each disease group by the mean values of the signal intensity in all samples of the group. Combined scoring according to analysis on the 133A and 133P platform demonstrates that the strongest increase is observed in IBM followed by PM and DM, while IM and NM were closest to healthy control. This pattern was observed in 133A samples as well as in 133P samples independently of combined scoring (A and B) or scoring based on each individual platform (C and D).

Figure S3 Identification of genes involved in MHC-I and MHC-II antigen processing and presentation pathways: The 1209 probesets upregulated in myositis were uploaded into the DAVID database (http://david.abcc.ncifcrf.gov/) for functional annotation. All genes highlighted with a red star are included in the 1209 probesets.

Figure S4 This is the corresponding image to figure 5 in the manuscript. It lists all gene names and is provided as an additional jpg-file "Figure_S4" for further magnification (http://www.charite-bioinformatik.de/supplementary_data/immunoproteasomes/04_Sj9CPykssy0xPLMnMz0vMAfGjzOLNLU_Figure_S4.jpg).

Figure S5 Cell type specific transcripts and corresponding changes of gene expression in myositis: Cell type specific transcripts were determined from transcriptomes of monocytes, neutrophils, CD1+ dendritic cells, T-cells, B-cells, NK-cells and muscle tissue by filtering for cell type specific transcripts with signal level >2000 in the population of interest, < 200 in all other populations and a fold change of >20 if possible. In the heatmap on the right side, there is some overlapping expression in the different types of phagocytic cells and in the different lymphocyte populations. CD4+ and CD8+ T-cells do not allow the establishment of a transcript pattern that will distinguish them from other cell types and at the same time will differentiate between these two T-cell subpopulations. In the heatmap on the left side, all myositis transcriptomes were mapped to these marker panels and samples were sorted by intensity of change in the 1209 "myositis genes". This was performed using the median of log-transformed and z-normalized signals of all 1209 probesets for each sample as a score (myositis score). Sorting myositis samples from the lowest score on the left side (predominantly normal donor samples) to the highest score on the right side (predominantly IBM samples), there is an increase especially of transcripts related to monocytes, dendritic cells and T-cells corresponding to the severity of myositis with a corresponding decrease of muscle specific transcripts. (Figure S5 is also provided as an additional separate jpg-file for further magnification: http://www.charite-bioinformatik.de/supplementary_data/immunoproteasomes/yMDI2dDbwsPIJdDBwNDNwCjLzDgowsDIEK_Figure_S5.jpg).

Table S1 Clinical data of patients with DM, PM, OM and NIM.

Table S2 Collection of transcriptome data from the Gene Expression Omnibus repository: These transcriptome data were used for analysis of the role of immunoproteasomes in inflammatory and non-inflammatory muscle diseases compared to other genes differentially expressed in myositis.

Table S3 Probesets and genes identified as upregulated in IBM, PM and/or DM with signal intensities and molecular scores: Datasets of GSE2044, GSE3112, and GSE39454 were used to identify molecular changes in IBM, PM and DM compared to healthy muscle biopsies. Data generated with the different platforms HG-U133A (133A) and HG-U133Plus 2.0 (133P) were analysed separately to avoid technical bias. Each disease entity was compared to healthy controls. Selection of differentially expressed probesets was based on the frequency of change in pairwise comparisons between arrays from two different groups, on signal log ratio (SLR), on t-test statistics and on cut-off for absolute signal intensities combined to a default filtering as provided in BioRetis. Probesets, which were upregulated in the same disease in both platforms, were selected and combined from all diseases to a total of 1209 probesets/927 genes. To score these probesets by dominance of increase, the frequency of change call for all pairwise comparisons and the SLR were z-normalized across all selected probesets and then scaled to the maximum of "1". The sum of both normalized values was used for ranking, thus identifying genes with the best sum-score for "highly increased" and "most frequently increased" in disease compared to control in the top ranks. These probesets were sorted by a sum-score for magnitude and frequency of increase. See file "Table_S3.xls" accessible via: http://www.charite-bioinformatik.de/supplementary_data/immunoproteasomes/Tcx8DAP8zJzMDIKSjY3M_R2cDA3YCQ_nD9_Table_S3.xls. 1. sheet "probesets" with the list of the 1209 probesets sorted by the composed score of SLR and change call. 2. sheet "genes" with the list of the 927 genes sorted by the composed score of SLR and change call. 3. sheet "PSM 133P" with signals for all proteasomal units of the 133P arrays. 4. sheet "PSM 133A" with signals for all proteasomal units of the 133A arrays. Data of all microarrys and group comparisons are available in BioRetis (www.bioretis.com).

Table S4 Correlation of PSMB8 and PSMB9 expression in myositis with transcriptions factors: Correlation coefficients on the basis of signal values from myositis muscle biopsies (columns A1–A4), immune cells (B1–B2) and cytokine stimulated monocytes (C1–C2) are presented in combination with the z-normalized signal values of purified immune cells (columns D1–D21), healthy muscle profiles (E1–E5), cytokine stimulated monocytes (F1–F22), muscle biopsies based on 133P arrays (G1–G36) and 133A arrays (H1–H62); (see file Table_S4.xls download link: http://www.charite-bioinformatik.de/supplementary_data/immunoproteasomes/KFQlWFwAVoDPCrACAxzA0UDfzyM_N1W_ID_Table_S4.xls).

Acknowledgments

We thank Toralf Kaiser and Jenny Kirsch from the Deutsches Rheuma-Forschungszentrum, Flow cytometry Core Facility in Berlin for technical assistance in cell sorting. The authors have no commercial or other associations to disclose.

Author Contributions

Conceived and designed the experiments: EF KG TH G-RB SK. Performed the experiments: KG LM-G BS MB SB LS AG. Analyzed the data: TH KG MB SB BS EF LM-G. Contributed reagents/materials/analysis tools: EF TH AG BS MB SB LS SK. Wrote the paper: KG TH EF G-RB LM-G SK BS AG SB MB LS.

References

1. Dalakas MC, Hohlfeld R (2003) Polymyositis and dermatomyositis. Lancet 362: 971–982.
2. Dalakas MC (2004) Inflammatory disorders of muscle: progress in polymyositis, dermatomyositis and inclusion body myositis. Curr Opin Neurol 17: 561–567.
3. Dalakas MC (2006) Mechanisms of disease: signaling pathways and immunobiology of inflammatory myopathies. Nat Clin Pract Rheumatol 2: 219–227.
4. Rechsteiner M, Hoffman L, Dubiel W (1993) The multicatalytic and 26S proteases. J Biol Chem 268: 6065–6068.
5. Muratani M, Tansey WP (2003) How the ubiquitin-proteasome system controls transcription. Nat Rev Mol Cell Biol 4: 192–201.
6. Coux O, Tanaka K, Goldberg AL (1996) Structure and functions of the 20S and 26S proteasomes. Annu Rev Biochem 65: 801–847.
7. Groettrup M, Soza A, Kuckelkorn U, Kloetzel PM (1996) Peptide antigen production by the proteasome: complexity provides efficiency. Immunol Today 17: 429–435.
8. Kumamoto T, Fujimoto S, Ito T, Horinouchi H, Ueyama H, et al. (2000) Proteasome expression in the skeletal muscles of patients with muscular dystrophy. Acta Neuropathol 100: 595–602.
9. Mitch WE, Goldberg AL (1996) Mechanisms of muscle wasting. The role of the ubiquitin-proteasome pathway. N Engl J Med 335: 1897–1905.
10. Groll M, Ditzel L, Lowe J, Stock D, Bochtler M, et al. (1997) Structure of 20S proteasome from yeast at 2.4 angstrom resolution. Nature 386: 463–471.
11. Aki M, Shimbara N, Takashina M, Akiyama K, Kagawa S, et al. (1994) Interferon-gamma induces different subunit organizations and functional diversity of proteasomes. J Biochem 115: 257–269.
12. Boes B, Hengel H, Ruppert T, Multhaup G, Koszinowski UH, et al. (1994) Interferon gamma stimulation modulates the proteolytic activity and cleavage site preference of 20S mouse proteasomes. J Exp Med 179: 901–909.
13. Kuckelkorn U, Frentzel S, Kraft R, Kostka S, Groettrup M, et al. (1995) Incorporation of major histocompatibility complex–encoded subunits LMP2 and LMP7 changes the quality of the 20S proteasome polypeptide processing products independent of interferon-gamma. Eur J Immunol 25: 2605–2611.
14. Lundberg IE, Nyberg P (1998) New developments in the role of cytokines and chemokines in inflammatory myopathies. Curr Opin Rheumatol 10: 521–529.
15. Agarwal AK, Xing C, DeMartino GN, Mizrachi D, Hernandez MD, et al. (2010) PSMB8 encoding the beta5i proteasome subunit is mutated in joint contractures, muscle atrophy, microcytic anemia, and panniculitis-induced lipodystrophy syndrome. Am J Hum Genet 87: 866–872.
16. Arima K, Kinoshita A, Mishima H, Kanazawa N, Kaneko T, et al. (2011) Proteasome assembly defect due to a proteasome subunit beta type 8 (PSMB8) mutation causes the autoinflammatory disorder, Nakajo-Nishimura syndrome. Proc Natl Acad Sci U S A 108: 14914–14919.
17. Kitamura A, Maekawa Y, Uehara H, Izumi K, Kawachi I, et al. (2011) A mutation in the immunoproteasome subunit PSMB8 causes autoinflammation and lipodystrophy in humans. J Clin Invest 121: 4150–4160.
18. Liu Y, Ramot Y, Torrelo A, Paller AS, Si N, et al. (2012) Mutations in proteasome subunit beta type 8 cause chronic atypical neutrophilic dermatosis with lipodystrophy and elevated temperature with evidence of genetic and phenotypic heterogeneity. Arthritis Rheum 64: 895–907.
19. Egerer K, Kuckelkorn U, Rudolph PE, Ruckert JC, Dörner T, et al. (2002) Circulating proteasomes are markers of cell damage and immunologic activity in autoimmune diseases. J Rheumatol 29: 2045–2052.
20. Feist E, Dörner T, Kuckelkorn U, Schmidtke G, Micheel B, et al. (1996) Proteasome alpha-type subunit C9 is a primary target of autoantibodies in sera of patients with myositis and systemic lupus erythematosus. J Exp Med 184: 1313–1318.
21. Brychcy M, Kuckelkorn U, Hausdorf G, Egerer K, Kloetzel PM, et al. (2006) Anti-20S proteasome autoantibodies inhibit proteasome stimulation by proteasome activator PA28. Arthritis Rheum 54: 2175–2183.
22. Krause S, Kuckelkorn U, Dörner T, Burmester GR, Feist E, et al. (2006) Immunoproteasome subunit LMP2 expression is deregulated in Sjogren's syndrome but not in other autoimmune disorders. Ann Rheum Dis 65: 1021–1027.

23. Bohan A, Peter JB (1975) Polymyositis and dermatomyositis (second of two parts). N Engl J Med 292: 403–407.
24. Bohan A, Peter JB (1975) Polymyositis and dermatomyositis (first of two parts). N Engl J Med 292: 344–347.
25. Morawietz L, Martinez-Gamboa L, Scheffler S, Hausdorf G, Dankof A, et al. (2009) Expression of proteasomal immunosubunit beta1i is dysregulated in inflammatory infiltrates of minor salivary glands in Sjogren's syndrome. J Rheumatol 36: 2694–2703.
26. Pfaffi MW (2001) A new mathematical model for relative quantification in real-time RT–PCR. Nucleic Acids Res v.29(9): e45.
27. Smiljanovic B, Grün JR, Biesen R, Schulte-Wrede U, Baumgrass R, et al. (2012) The multifaceted balance of TNF-alpha and type I/II interferon responses in SLE and RA: how monocytes manage the impact of cytokines. J Mol Med (Berl) 90: 1295–1309.
28. Smiljanovic B, Grün JR, Steinbrich-Zollner M, Stuhlmüller B, Häupl T, et al. (2010) Defining TNF-alpha- and LPS-induced gene signatures in monocytes to unravel the complexity of peripheral blood transcriptomes in health and disease. J Mol Med (Berl) 88: 1065–1079.
29. Menssen A, Edinger G, Grün JR, Haase U, Baumgrass R, et al. (2009) SiPaGene: A new repository for instant online retrieval, sharing and meta-analyses of GeneChip expression data. BMC Genomics 10: 98.
30. Ahn JY, Tanahashi N, Akiyama K, Hisamatsu H, Noda C, et al. (1995) Primary structures of two homologous subunits of PA28, a gamma-interferon-inducible protein activator of the 20S proteasome. FEBS Lett 366: 37–42.
31. Jain A, Sharma MC, Sarkar C, Bhatia R, Singh S, et al. (2007) Major histocompatibility complex class I and II detection as a diagnostic tool in idiopathic inflammatory myopathies. Arch Pathol Lab Med 131: 1070–1076.
32. Kalovidouris AE (1992) The role of cytokines in polymyositis: interferon-gamma induces class II and enhances class I major histocompatibility complex antigen expression on cultured human muscle cells. J Lab Clin Med 120: 244–251.
33. Greenberg SA, Higgs BW, Morehouse C, Walsh RJ, Kong SW, et al. (2012) Relationship between disease activity and type 1 interferon- and other cytokine-inducible gene expression in blood in dermatomyositis and polymyositis. Genes Immun 13: 207–213.
34. Ivanidze J, Hoffmann R, Lochmuller H, Engel AG, Hohlfeld R, et al. (2011) Inclusion body myositis: laser microdissection reveals differential up-regulation of IFN-gamma signaling cascade in attacked versus nonattacked myofibers. Am J Pathol 179: 1347–1359.
35. Brucet M, Marques L, Sebastian C, Lloberas J, Celada A (2004) Regulation of murine Tap1 and Lmp2 genes in macrophages by interferon gamma is mediated by STAT1 and IRF-1. Genes Immun 5: 26–35.
36. Rockwell CE, Monaco JJ, Qureshi N (2012) A critical role for the inducible proteasomal subunits LMP7 and MECL1 in cytokine production by activated murine splenocytes. Pharmacology 89: 117–126.
37. Ferrer I, Martin B, Castano JG, Lucas JJ, Moreno D, et al. (2004) Proteasomal expression, induction of immunoproteasome subunits, and local MHC class I presentation in myofibrillar myopathy and inclusion body myositis. J Neuropathol Exp Neurol 63: 484–498.
38. Bakay M, Wang Z, Melcon G, Schiltz L, Xuan J, et al. (2006) Nuclear envelope dystrophies show a transcriptional fingerprint suggesting disruption of Rb-MyoD pathways in muscle regeneration. Brain 129: 996–1013.
39. Fredriksson K, Tjader I, Keller P, Petrovic N, Ahlman B, et al. (2008) Dysregulation of mitochondrial dynamics and the muscle transcriptome in ICU patients suffering from sepsis induced multiple organ failure. PLoS One 3: e3686.
40. Mortensen OH, Andersen K, Fischer C, Nielsen AR, Nielsen S, et al. (2008) Calprotectin is released from human skeletal muscle tissue during exercise. J Physiol 586: 3551–3562.
41. Huber EM, Basler M, Schwab R, Heinemeyer W, Kirk CJ, et al. (2012) Immuno- and constitutive proteasome crystal structures reveal differences in substrate and inhibitor specificity. Cell 148: 727–738.
42. Verbrugge SE, Assaraf YG, Dijkmans BA, Scheffer GL, Al M, et al. (2012) Inactivating PSMB5 mutations and P-glycoprotein (multidrug resistance-associated protein/ATP-binding cassette B1) mediate resistance to proteasome inhibitors: ex vivo efficacy of (immuno)proteasome inhibitors in mononuclear blood cells from patients with rheumatoid arthritis. J Pharmacol Exp Ther 341: 174–182.
43. Muchamuel T, Basler M, Aujay MA, Suzuki E, Kalim KW, et al. (2009) A selective inhibitor of the immunoproteasome subunit LMP7 blocks cytokine production and attenuates progression of experimental arthritis. Nat Med 15: 781–787.
44. Basler M, Dajee M, Moll C, Groettrup M, Kirk CJ (2010) Prevention of experimental colitis by a selective inhibitor of the immunoproteasome. J Immunol 185: 634–641.
45. Zaiss DM, Bekker CP, Grone A, Lie BA, Sijts AJ (2011) Proteasome immunosubunits protect against the development of CD8 T cell-mediated autoimmune diseases. J Immunol 187: 2302–2309.
46. Kloetzel PM, Ossendorp F (2004) Proteasome and peptidase function in MHC-class-I-mediated antigen presentation. Curr Opin Immunol 16: 76–81.
47. Seifert U, Bialy LP, Ebstein F, Bech-Otschir D, Voigt A, et al. (2010) Immunoproteasomes preserve protein homeostasis upon interferon-induced oxidative stress. Cell 142: 613–624.
48. Chen W, Norbury CC, Cho Y, Yewdell JW, Bennink JR (2001) Immunoproteasomes shape immunodominance hierarchies of antiviral CD8(+) T cells at the levels of T cell repertoire and presentation of viral antigens. J Exp Med 193: 1319–1326.
49. Zanker D, Waithman J, Yewdell JW, Chen W (2013) Mixed Proteasomes Function To Increase Viral Peptide Diversity and Broaden Antiviral CD8+ T Cell Responses. J Immunol 191: 52–59.

14

Calcium Homeostasis in Myogenic Differentiation Factor 1 (MyoD)-Transformed, Virally-Transduced, Skin-Derived Equine Myotubes

Marta Fernandez-Fuente[1], Cesare M. Terracciano[2], Pilar Martin-Duque[3], Susan C. Brown[4], Georges Vassaux[5], Richard J. Piercy[1]*

1 Comparative Neuromuscular Diseases Laboratory, Department of Clinical Sciences and Services, Royal Veterinary College, London, United Kingdom, **2** Laboratory of Cell Electrophysiology, Imperial College London, Myocardial Function, National Heart and Lung Institute, Hammersmith Hospital, London, United Kingdom, **3** Universidad Francisco de Vitoria, Facultad de Ciencias Biosanitarias: Pozuelo de Alarcón (Madrid), Madrid, Spain, **4** Comparative Biomedical Sciences, Royal Veterinary College, London, United Kingdom, **5** Laboratoire TIRO, UMRE 4320, iBEB, DSV, Commissariat a' l'Energie Atomique, Nice, France

Abstract

Dysfunctional skeletal muscle calcium homeostasis plays a central role in the pathophysiology of several human and animal skeletal muscle disorders, in particular, genetic disorders associated with ryanodine receptor 1 (RYR1) mutations, such as malignant hyperthermia, central core disease, multiminicore disease and certain centronuclear myopathies. In addition, aberrant skeletal muscle calcium handling is believed to play a pivotal role in the highly prevalent disorder of Thoroughbred racehorses, known as Recurrent Exertional Rhabdomyolysis. Traditionally, such defects were studied in human and equine subjects by examining the contractile responses of biopsied muscle strips exposed to caffeine, a potent RYR1 agonist. However, this test is not widely available and, due to its invasive nature, is potentially less suitable for valuable animals in training or in the human paediatric setting. Furthermore, increasingly, RYR1 gene polymorphisms (of unknown pathogenicity and significance) are being identified through next generation sequencing projects. Consequently, we have investigated a less invasive test that can be used to study calcium homeostasis in cultured, skin-derived fibroblasts that are converted to the muscle lineage by viral transduction with a MyoD (myogenic differentiation 1) transgene. Similar models have been utilised to examine calcium homeostasis in human patient cells, however, to date, there has been no detailed assessment of the cells' calcium homeostasis, and in particular, the responses to agonists and antagonists of RYR1. Here we describe experiments conducted to assess calcium handling of the cells and examine responses to treatment with dantrolene, a drug commonly used for prophylaxis of recurrent exertional rhabdomyolysis in horses and malignant hyperthermia in humans.

Editor: Atsushi Asakura, University of Minnesota Medical School, United States of America

Funding: This work has been funded by Horserace Betting Levy Board. The funders had no role in study design, data collection and analysis, decision to publish, or preparation of the manuscript.

* Email: rpiercy@rvc.ac.uk

Introduction

Skeletal muscle contraction involves highly specialised and tightly regulated mechanisms that convert electrochemical signals to mechanotransduction. A crucial element within this machinery is the interaction between sarcolemmal voltage-gated L-type Ca^{2+} channels (dihydropyridine receptors - DHPR) and sarcoplasmic Ca^{2+} channels - mainly ryanodine receptors (RYR1). Upon depolarization of the skeletal muscle transverse tubule (T-tubule) membrane, DHPRs interact with RYR1, activating a massive release of calcium from the sarcoplasmic reticulum (SR) into the cytoplasm. This conversion of an electrical to a chemical signal (a Ca^{2+} transient) is essential for excitation–contraction coupling (ECC): calcium released into the cytoplasm during ECC-initiation enables contraction of myofibrils via ATP hydrolysis from myosin ATPases following a calcium-dependent conformational change in the troponin-tropomyosin complex [1–3]. Relaxation, following myofibre contraction, occurs with calcium re-uptake by the SR via Ca^{2+} ATPase (SERCA1) pumps. Gradual depletion of SR calcium storage activates a calcium entry pathway through the plasma membrane known as store-operated calcium entry (SOCE) that can be activated during intensive exercise [4–6]. In addition, relatively small amounts of calcium can enter muscle cells through a prolonged voltage-dependent (excitation) -coupled calcium entry mechanism (ECCE) [7].

Several human and animal myopathies are associated with dysfunction of skeletal muscle calcium regulation. These include malignant hyperthermia (MH), a life-threatening form of rhabdomyolysis associated with use of volatile anaesthetic and certain neuromuscular blocking agents that occurs in humans [8,9], dogs [10,11] and horses [12,13], and in porcine stress syndrome, a disorder that leads to major losses to the pork industry due to its association with poor quality (pale, soft, exudative) meat [14,15].

Both MH and porcine stress syndrome are associated with RYR1 mutations, as are the human muscle disorders, central core disease (CCD), multiminicore disease (MmD), certain nemaline rod-associated myopathies and some centronuclear myopathies [16–24]. In CCD, evidence suggests 2 possible pathophysiological mechanisms: RYR1-associated calcium leakage [25] and uncoupling of DHPR-RYR1 [23,26,27]. Brody disease (a myopathy associated with recessive mutations in SERCA1 and delayed muscle relaxation) is reported in humans and cattle [28–30]. In addition, some human patients are reported with phenotypes suggestive of calcium handling defects, including MH, but without detectable mutations in RYR1 or other related genes [31]. Similarly, an inherited and apparent calcium handling defect that affects 5–7% of Thoroughbred racehorses worldwide, known as recurrent exertional rhabdomyolysis (RER) [32–34], shares pathophysiological features with MH, but mutations in RYR1, SERCA1 and DHPR have been excluded [35]. A likely-identical disorder also occurs in Standardbred racehorses with a similar prevalence [36]. RER in horses is widely treated prophylactically with orally-administered dantrolene, an RYR1-antagonist that at high doses can induce transient paresis [37] but that reduces severity of exercise-induced muscle damage in some affected horses [38]. Dantrolene is also used to treat episodes of MH in humans, conceivably by reducing voltage dependent (excitation) coupled calcium entry [7,39] but the mechanism of action in each species is poorly understood.

The RYR1 cDNA's large size (~15 kb) traditionally made mutational analysis (and consequent study of the downstream effect of defects in the gene), extremely labour intensive. With the advent of next generation sequencing technologies it is feasible rapidly to sequence the entire gene; however, and consequently, many single nucleotide polymorphisms (SNPs) have been found in RYR1 and without some functional assessment, it is sometimes difficult to determine their pathogenicity, if any [40,41].

Functional assessment of MH in humans and RER in horses traditionally relied on *in vitro* contraction testing (IVCT) of isolated strips of skeletal muscle when exposed to caffeine and other agents [42]. Furthermore, diagnosis in other calcium-related human disorders, such as CCD and MmD still relies heavily on muscle biopsy [43]. However, muscle biopsy in general, and the IVCT (which requires an open biopsy) in particular, are relatively invasive. Consequently, clinicians and researchers have looked for alternative cell culture systems that can model calcium handling *in vitro*, with a view to gaining insight into disease pathophysiology, accurate diagnosis and for investigation of novel treatments. This has been achieved in cultured myoblasts (derived from muscle biopsy specimens) [44,45], but a system that instead utilises fibroblasts derived from small skin biopsy samples [46,47], is attractive, because the sampling method is less invasive, and the primary cells are more robust in culture than myoblasts. Several groups, including our own have converted skin derived fibroblast-like cells to muscle cells (myotubes) in culture, utilising viral transduction with muscle-specific transcription factors [48,49]. For example, calcium handling - specifically caffeine and chloro-m-cresol responses - has been studied in human skin-derived fibroblasts-converted to myotubes through forced (adenovirally-mediated) expression of MyoD [46,50–53]. The method is especially attractive in the paediatric setting and in animals where the more invasive muscle biopsy, might affect value or influence athletic training.

Despite previously published work, there has been very little functional analysis of skin-derived myotubes in relation to RYR1-associated physiology; therefore, an in-depth analysis of their excitation-calcium release dynamics seems essential if they are to be used in confirming or characterising the phenotype of patients in whom RYR1 mutations or a defect in calcium handling is suspected. Validation of the use of virally-transduced, skin-derived fibroblasts in assessment of human and animal myopathies is extremely important, since this *in vitro* approach has great potential in both clinical diagnostic and research settings. In our earlier work, we reported a lentivirus-based system that converted cultured equine skin-derived fibroblasts to myotubes through expression of equine MyoD [48]. More recently, we reported the generation of an adenoviral vector expressing (equine) MyoD that also transforms both equine and human skin-derived fibroblasts to myotubes [49]. Here we describe a comprehensive characterisation of this system, in the context of the modelling of skeletal muscle calcium homeostasis in horses.

Materials and Methods

Animals and cell culture

Primary equine fibroblast-like cells were derived from skin biopsy samples collected under local anaesthesia with sterile 4 mm disposable punch instruments, from the left side of the mid neck crest in 2, two-year-old, Thoroughbred racehorse geldings. Muscle biopsy samples were obtained from 2 three-year-old Thoroughbred geldings, euthanased for reasons unrelated to this study. The procedure was approved by the Royal Veterinary College local Ethics' committee and was performed with adherence to a Home Office Project license (PPL 70/6523) according to the Animal (Scientific Procedures) Act 1986 of the United Kingdom. Horses were selected on the basis of their being normal on physical examination and through their never having been observed to have a clinically-detectable episode of RER during their racing career; subclinical RER was considered highly unlikely on the basis of plasma creatine kinase and aspartate amino transferase activities remaining within normal laboratory limits when tested approximately fortnightly throughout an entire racing season (data not shown).

Skin samples were collected into sterile tissue culture growth medium (see below) and transported to the laboratory and maintained at 4°C. Within 24 hours, biopsy specimens were cut into 1-mm cubes with a sterile scalpel blade and placed into the centre of 3.5 cm tissue culture dishes containing culture medium and incubated at 37°C in an incubator containing 5% CO_2. Skin and muscle samples were routinely cultured in normal growth medium consisting of Dulbecco modified Eagle medium, 10% foetal bovine serum (FBS; PAA), penicillin-streptomycin (1 U/mL and 1 μg/mL, respectively; Life Technologies) and 2 mM L-glutamine (Life Technologies). Within 5–7 days, spindle-shaped cells were readily visible migrating outward from the minced tissue. Cells were passaged routinely (fewer than 10 times) until cell numbers were high enough for subsequent experiments.

Equine cells (passage<5) and human embryonic kidney cell line (293T) cells were routinely cultured in normal growth medium (as above). 20% FBS-containing media was used for primary myoblast culture (as derived and described previously [49]) prior to their differentiation.

Virus production and myogenic conversion

Adenovirus particles expressing bicistronic eqMyoD cDNA and eGFP from the same CMV promoter, were produced using the system developed by the Vogelstein lab [54] as we previously described [49]. Viral titre was determined (through infection of 293T cells) to be 2.4×10^9 infectious units/ml; particles were stored in aliquots at −80°C until use.

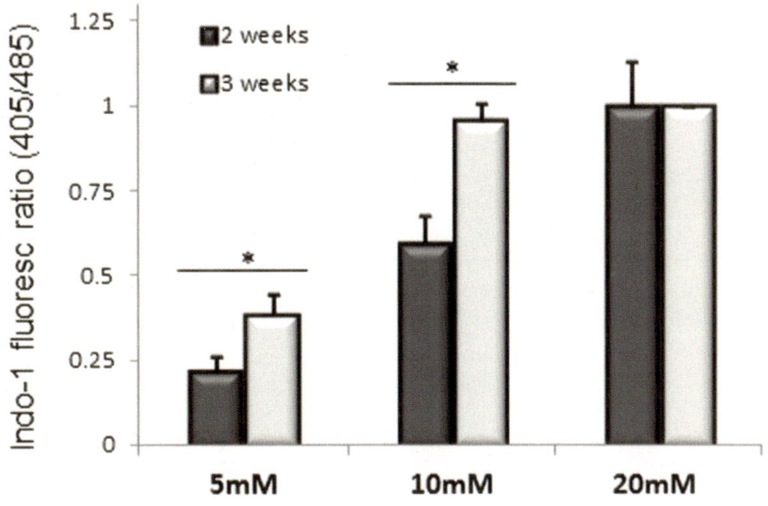

Figure 1. Caffeine dose response. Histogram of Indo-1 response to increasing concentrations of caffeine in adenovirally-transduced equine myotubes. Results show mean (+/−1 SEM) derived from 40 myotubes from 2 control horses sequentially exposed to 5, 10 and 20 mM caffeine at 2 and 3 weeks' differentiation.

Matrigel (1:1000, Becton-Dickinson)–coated, glass-bottomed 3.5 cm diameter dishes (MatTek Corporation) were seeded with 5×10^4 equine skin fibroblast–like cells/well and transduced with the adenovirus (multiplicity of infection (MOI) of 5) [49] in a final volume (50 μL drop) on the central glass coverslip for 4 hours after which virus-containing medium was replaced by 2 ml fresh growth medium. 48 hours after infection, medium was replaced with differentiation medium (MegaCell; Sigma), 2% FBS, penicillin-streptomycin (1 U/ml and 1 μg/ml, respectively), L-glutamine (2 mM; Sigma), 1x Non-essential Amino acids (Sigma) and beta mercaptoethanol (0.7 μl/100 ml, Sigma). Approximately 1 week after infection, the cells' morphological characteristics had changed, becoming more elongated with the formation of myotubes. 14–21 days later, cells were used for assessment of calcium homeostasis by fluorescence.

Calcium measurements

Myotubes (either 14 or 21 days following transduction), were loaded with Indo-1 AM (Molecular Probes) at a concentration of 10 μM for 20 min at 37°C and then incubated for at least 1 h in normal growth medium in order to ensure complete intracellular de-esterification of Indo1-AM. Cells were subsequently analyzed while being superfused with normal Tyrode solution (140 nM NaCl, 6 mM KCl, 10 mM glucose, 10 mM HEPES, 1 mM Mg_2Cl and 2 mM $CaCl_2$; pH 7.4) and at a constant temperature of 37°C. After 5 min accommodation, cells were excited at 360 nm using a 100 W xenon lamp (Nikon); cellular fluorescence signals were recorded simultaneously at 405 nm (F405) and 485 nm (F485) using photomultiplier tubes (PMT, PTI814 Thorn EMI). Background fluorescence subtraction was routinely performed using a cell-free region as zero fluorescence. Changes in cytoplasmic calcium concentration were expressed as changes in

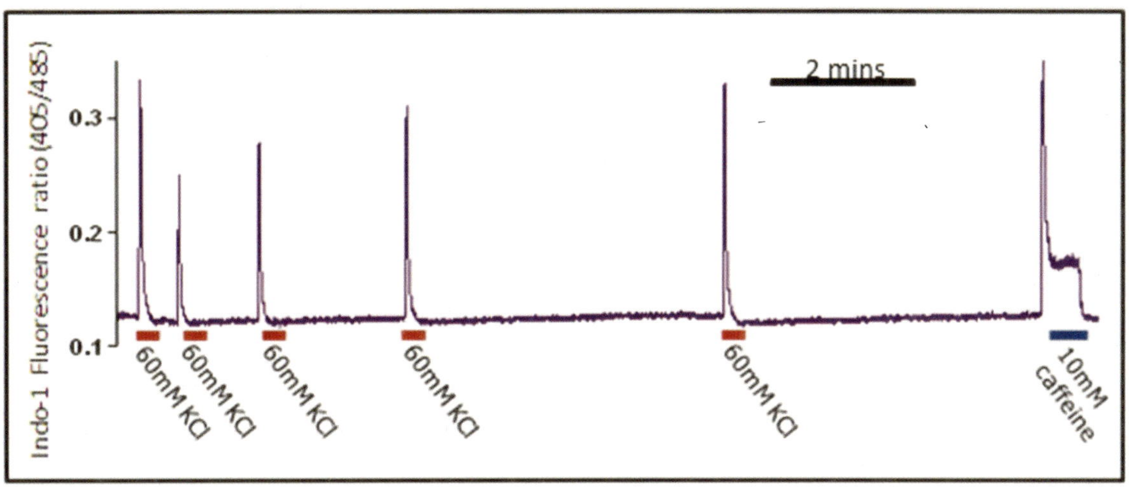

Figure 2. Depolarisation with KCl. Representative experiment where skin-derived equine myotubes were subjected repeatedly to depolarization with 60 mM KCl (red line). 10 mM caffeine responses (blue line) are shown for comparison. Note that responses are reproducible and near maximal within approximately 4 minutes.

the ratio (R = F405/F485) thereby avoiding the influence of photobleaching.

Cells were exposed to calcium-modifying agents through use of a solenoid switcher device. At least 5 myotubes were studied per dish. Maximal amplitudes of caffeine peaks after caffeine stimulation were measured using Clampfit software (Axon Instruments). Between 20 and 40 myotubes in total were studied for caffeine exposure experiments, from 4 different dishes. Thapsigargin (SERCA blocker) experiments (n = 16 tubes from two dishes) were conducted with an initial stimulation via a pulse of 20 mM caffeine; after Ca^{2+} concentration returned to baseline, the superfusate was switched to normal Tyrode or to Ca^{2+}-free Tyrode solution, and then to 300 nM thapsigargin (in the corresponding buffer, Ca^{2+}-free or normal Tyrode solution) for 3 minutes, after which two further 20 mM caffeine stimulations were recorded. Similar protocols were used when using tetracaine (n = 10 tubes from two dishes) and dantrolene (n = 15 tubes from two dishes) (50 μM and 10 μM respectively) to modify caffeine responses. To confirm that dantrolene had no direct effect on Indo-1 fluorescence, we compared the fluorescence emitted by Indo-1 pentapotassium salt, at a range of calcium concentrations (0 to 9 mM) in the presence and absence of dantrolene (10 μM).

Statistical analysis

Caffeine-response data at 2 and 3 weeks are expressed as mean ± S.E.M. Differences in data among groups were examined by 2 way repeated measurement ANOVA followed by Tukey's test for post hoc analysis. Differences were considered statistically significant when $p<0.05$.

Results

Caffeine responses in equine myotubes

To assess if calcium homeostasis of skin-derived myotubes is affected by differentiation time, we studied the response of the equine cultures to caffeine, after 2 or 3 weeks of differentiation. Figure 1 shows peak calcium release responses when cells were exposed to 5, 10 and 20 mM caffeine at each of the 2 time points. We observed significantly greater calcium release ($P<0.0001$) at 3 weeks compared to 2 weeks at two intermediate caffeine concentrations (5 and 10 mM) (Figure 1). As expected [49], we observed a dose-response in caffeine-induced calcium release (Figure 1), with a plateau (in 3 week differentiated cells) at around 10 mM caffeine. By 3 weeks of differentiation, caffeine responses were robust and reproducible: a functional excitation-calcium release-mechanism was indicated by the near maximal (in comparison with 20 mM caffeine) transients when cells were depolarised with 60 mM KCl (Figure 2). Within any one myotube, near maximal recovery to the KCl-induced response occurred after approximately 4 minutes (Figure 2). Cells remained responsive to sequential KCl-induced depolarisation or caffeine-induced calcium release as long as 30 minutes (when experiments were terminated); there was no apparent reduction in the amplitude of responses during this time (not shown).

Studies using calcium channel agonists/antagonists

To further characterize calcium homeostasis in our equine skin-derived cells, we used various agonists and antagonists of calcium regulatory proteins in calcium-containing and calcium-free solutions (Figures 3 and 4). Thapsigargin, a non-competitive antagonist of SERCA1 [55], almost completely abolished caffeine responses (Figure 3A). During treatment with thapsigargin there was an increase in Indo-1 basal fluorescence, revealing accumulation of cytoplasmic calcium when SERCA-1 activity is blocked. To ascertain whether this increase in calcium concentration was associated with sarcoplasmic Ca^{2+} leakage or to an influx of extracellular Ca^{2+}, we repeated the experiments using calcium-free bathing solutions. In absence of extracellular calcium, thapsigargin had the same effect: it induced a clear increase in Indo-1 fluorescence, indicative of a release of calcium from intracellular stores in skin-derived myotubes (Figure 3B). In order to determine whether this calcium leak was unique to skin-derived myotubes, we performed the same experiments in 15 day-old, primary equine myotubes derived from equine primary skeletal muscle cultures: our experiments revealed that these cells also had detectable SR leakage of calcium when SERCA was blocked (Figure 3C). Finally, we investigated whether this calcium leak occurred via RYR receptors: leakage through RYR can be blocked with tetracaine, an agent that inhibits spontaneous calcium release at low concentration [56]. In our model, tetracaine completely blocked the leak of sarcoplasmic calcium (Figure 3D), suggesting that calcium leakage occurs by way of the RYR receptor, and consistent with results observed in skeletal and cardiac muscle, which express RYR-1 and RYR-2 respectively [56,57].

As expected, dantrolene diminished the amplitude of the caffeine-induced calcium transient in skin-derived myotubes (Figures 4 A and B). We also detected a reduction in Indo1 fluorescence ratio (and hence cytoplasmic calcium concentration) in the presence of dantrolene (Figure 4): in order to confirm that this reduction was not an artefact associated with a direct effect of dantrolene on the Indo1 fluorescence ratio, we examined the influence of 10 μM dantrolene on the Indo1 fluorescence ratio at increasing predetermined calcium concentrations (0–9 mM): dantrolene had no effect on the Indo1 fluorescence signal (Figure 4C) confirming that dantrolene induced a reversible reduction in basal cytoplasmic calcium concentration in dermally-derived equine myotubes.

Discussion

There are several human and animal myopathies that involve disturbances in the regulation of skeletal muscle calcium homeostasis and hypersensitivity to agents that influence RYR1 channel opening, in particular, caffeine and halothane [16–18]. The precise nature of the perturbation can differ, even in patients with mutations in the same gene. For example, in some CCD-affected human patients, RYR1 mutations appear to induce an uncoupling between DHPR and RYR1, while in other patients with MH, the mutation makes the RYR1 channel leaky, leading to raised cytosolic calcium concentrations [58,59]. For many suspected RYR1 mutations however, the precise influence on muscle calcium homeostasis is unclear: when diagnosis largely depended on histological diagnosis following muscle biopsy, the IVCT was considered the gold standard test, but with the advent of direct next generation sequencing in patient diagnosis, there is likely reluctance to perform this more invasive procedure. In the human paediatric setting, or in valuable horses in full athletic training, use of muscle biopsy poses an additional diagnostic dilemma. A minimally-invasive method that can be used to investigate calcium homeostasis defects associated with known, or suspected myopathies is therefore especially attractive. Previously we revealed that an adenovirus expressing MyoD can convert both human and equine skin-derived fibroblasts to fusion competent myotubes, and further, that the cells respond similarly to primary myoblasts when exposed to incremental caffeine concentrations [49]. However, in order to understand the cellular model's potential for accurately defining defects in DHPR-RYR1 coupling, and in particular, RYR calcium leakage, it was important to evaluate in detail these

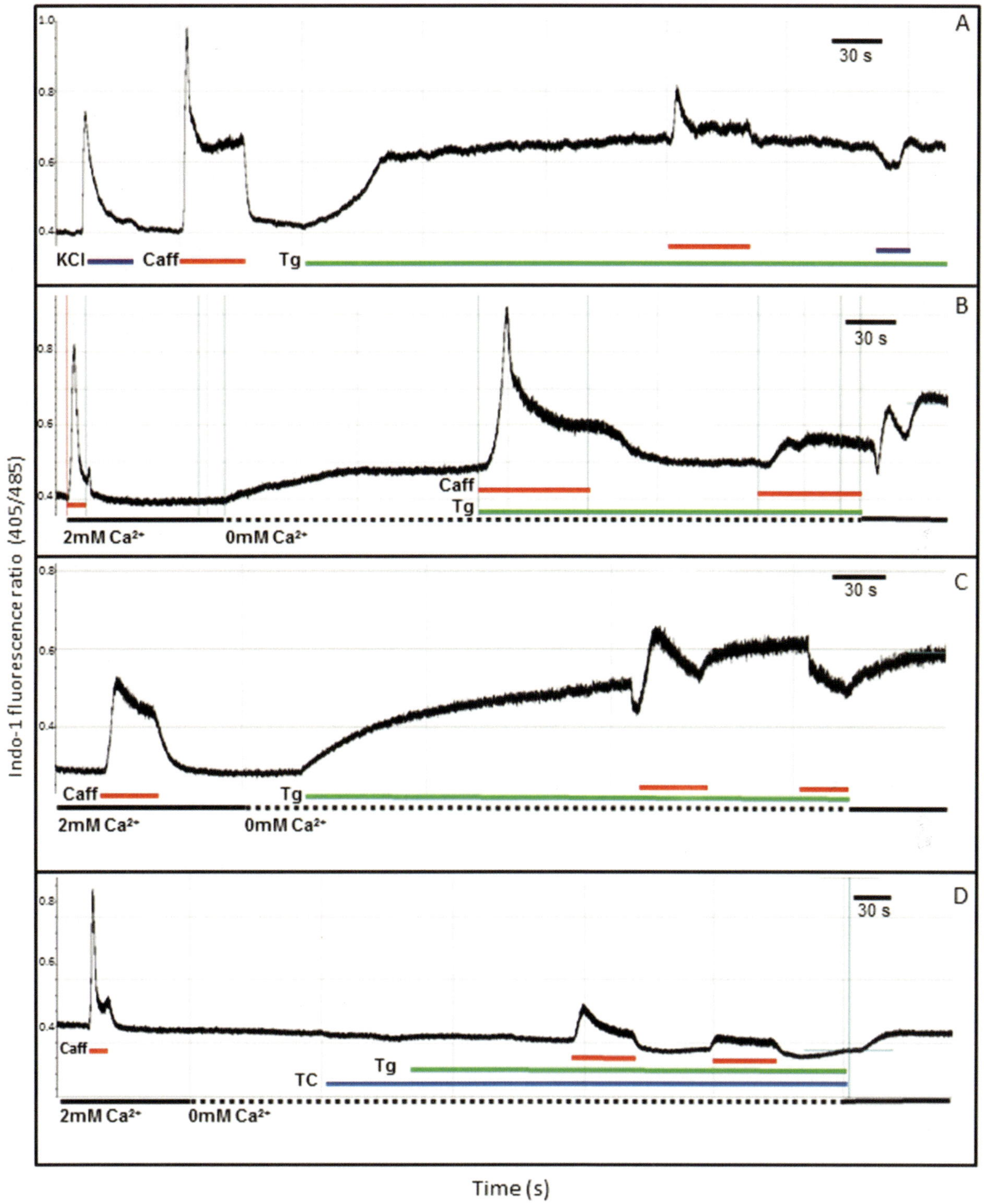

Figure 3. Calcium responses of skin-derived myotubes, treated with specific agonists and antagonists. A) Typical transients recorded following depolarisation with 60 mM KCl (blue line) and after exposure to 20 mM caffeine (red lines). The responses are almost abolished when the sarcoplasmic reticulum ATP-ase (SERCA-1) is blocked with thapsigargin (green line). Note that thapsigargin treatment induces an increase in Indo-1 fluorescence, that reveals leakage of SR calcium into the cytoplasm when SERCA-1 activity is blocked. B) Effect of thapsigargin on the response of skin-derived myotubes to caffeine, using calcium-free solution (dashed line). The increase in Ca^{2+} signal after the blockage of SERCA-1 supports the hypothesis of a leaky RYR-1 channel. C) Thapsigargin treatment was assayed on myotubes derived from primary, differentiated myoblasts, confirming that a similar leakage from the SR also occurs in these cells. D) When tetracaine is added to the perfusion system prior to the initiation of thapsigargin, the leakage is completely blocked, suggesting that RYR-1 is responsible for the leakage of SR calcium.

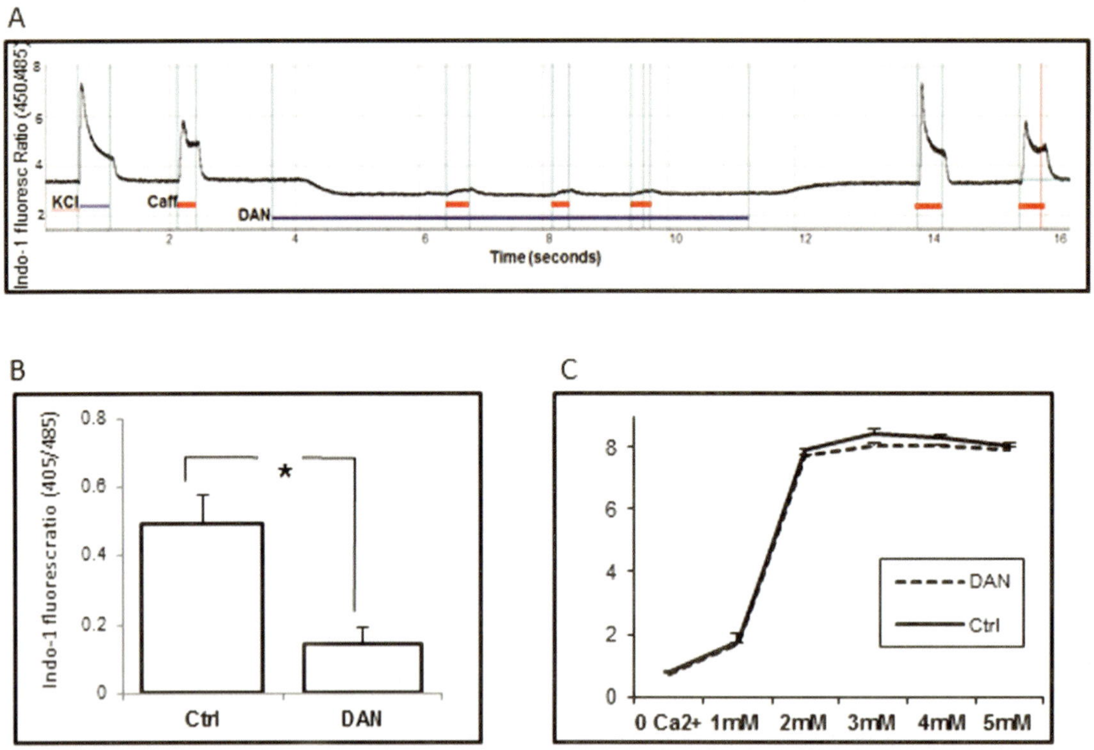

Figure 4. Effect of dantrolene on calcium transients. A) Depolarization with 60 mM KCl and 20 mM caffeine in normal buffer, followed by exposure to sequential exposures to caffeine in the presence of 10 μM dantrolene. B) The amplitude of the caffeine transient in the absence or presence of dantrolene. Note that dantrolene almost completely inhibits the ability of the myotubes to respond to caffeine ($p<0.05$) and lowers the cytoplasmic calcium concentration of resting myotubes. C) Indo-1 fluorescence at increasing calcium concentration, in the presence or absence of 10 μM dantrolene. Note that there was no direct effect of dantrolene on Indo-1 fluorescence.

aspects of the cells' physiology. The model's validation seems especially important given that similar techniques have been used previously to model calcium homeostasis defects in human patients [23].

In the current experiments, we conducted a detailed characterisation of calcium handling in dermally-derived myotubes using a range of agonists/antagonists of the main channels involved in EC-coupling. We detected the classical calcium release pathway mediated by RYR activation following cellular depolarisation and therefore revealed a functional coupling between DHPR and RYR proteins; however, in addition, our data supports the existence of a second, less well-defined and passive SR calcium efflux pathway, previously referred to as RYR calcium leak, which might occur through various proteins including RYR and translocons [58] [60,61]. We demonstrated these skin-derived myotubes' leak, by blocking SERCA-1 with thapsigargin and further, by showing that the rise in intracellular calcium occurred, even when the cells were maintained in calcium free buffer. We also revealed that the same response is seen in myotubes derived from primary myoblasts. Finally, we confirmed that this passive efflux of calcium was blocked by tetracaine, an RYR1 antagonist [60,61], revealing that the leak occurred via this receptor and was SR-derived [58,62,63].

The on-going recycling of calcium between SR and the cytoplasm mediated by this leak is overwhelmed by the massive release of SR that occurs during cell depolarisation or when cells are stimulated by caffeine. Interestingly, and as suggested previously [64] the extent of the leak appears to contribute to the basal cytoplasmic calcium concentration, since calcium concentration reduced when cells (in the resting state) were exposed to the RYR1 antagonist, dantrolene, thereby excluding excitation-coupled calcium entry [7,39]. In horses, dantrolene has been used both to treat [38] and prevent RER [65,66]. At higher doses, dantrolene can induce paresis in horses [37] presumably by limiting the extent of calcium release from the SR required for excitation-contraction coupling and as suggested by the diminished SR response to caffeine that we observed. However, our data suggest that the efficacy of dantrolene in equine RER and in MH, might relate to its lowering cytoplasmic calcium concentration in the cells' resting state (high cell calcium concentrations can stimulate cellular proteases and lead to rhabdomyolysis [67], [68]. Although further work is required, our data suggest that the drug might play a role in the treatment or management of additional RYR1-associated human or animal myopathies or other muscle disorders with primary or secondary defects in calcium homeostasis.

To date, there had been no "in depth" studies detailing the calcium handling of dermally-derived, virally-transduced cells. Our previous [48,49] and current work, reveals that these cells respond similarly to myotubes derived from primary muscle cultures. Whilst recognising the underlying cycling of calcium and the extent of SR calcium leakage that occurs in such cells, the system appears to offer a convenient, minimally-invasive model with which to test calcium homeostasis in patients that precludes any need for muscle biopsy. As such, the system might be more appropriate for evaluation of racehorses in training than intercostal muscle biopsy [69]; future work should be directed at comparison of responses detected in dermally-derived cells from horses and humans with known or suspected defects in cellular calcium homeostasis and controls.

Acknowledgments

The authors are grateful for the assistance provided by Mr Robert Pilsworth in collection of samples. This manuscript has been assigned the reference number CSS-00703 by the Royal Veterinary College's Research Office.

Author Contributions

Conceived and designed the experiments: RJP MF CMT. Performed the experiments: MF CMT PM GV. Analyzed the data: MF CMT RJP SCB. Contributed reagents/materials/analysis tools: CMT RJP PM GV. Wrote the paper: RJP MF.

References

1. Anderson K, Meissner G (1995) T-tubule depolarization-induced SR Ca2+ release is controlled by dihydropyridine receptor- and Ca(2+)-dependent mechanisms in cell homogenates from rabbit skeletal muscle. J Gen Physiol 105: 363–383.
2. Margreth A, Damiani E, Tobaldin G (1993) Ratio of dihydropyridine to ryanodine receptors in mammalian and frog twitch muscles in relation to the mechanical hypothesis of excitation-contraction coupling. Biochem Biophys Res Commun 197: 1303–1311.
3. Ma J, Anderson K, Shirokov R, Levis R, Gonzalez A, et al. (1993) Effects of perchlorate on the molecules of excitation-contraction coupling of skeletal and cardiac muscle. J Gen Physiol 102: 423–448.
4. Cherednichenko G, Hurne AM, Fessenden JD, Lee EH, Allen PD, et al. (2004) Conformational activation of Ca2+ entry by depolarization of skeletal myotubes. Proc Natl Acad Sci U S A 101: 15793–15798.
5. Huang J, van Breemen C, Kuo KH, Hove-Madsen L, Tibbits GF (2006) Store-operated Ca2+ entry modulates sarcoplasmic reticulum Ca2+ loading in neonatal rabbit cardiac ventricular myocytes. Am J Physiol Cell Physiol 290: C1572–1582.
6. Zhao X, Yoshida M, Brotto L, Takeshima H, Weisleder N, et al. (2005) Enhanced resistance to fatigue and altered calcium handling properties of sarcalumenin knockout mice. Physiol Genomics 23: 72–78.
7. Bannister RA, Pessah IN, Beam KG (2009) The skeletal L-type Ca(2+) current is a major contributor to excitation-coupled Ca(2+) entry. J Gen Physiol 133: 79–91.
8. Denborough MA, Forster JF, Lovell RR, Maplestone PA, Villiers JD (1962) Anaesthetic deaths in a family. Br J Anaesth 34: 395–396.
9. Healy JM, Lehane M, Heffron JJ, Farrell M, Johnson K, et al. (1990) Localization of the malignant hyperthermia susceptibility locus to human chromosome 19q12-q13.2. Biochem Soc Trans 18: 326.
10. Hull MJ, Webster WW, Gatz E (1971) The effects of pentobarbital on 2,4-dinitrophenol induced malignant hyperthermia during halothane general anesthesia in dogs. J Oral Surg 29: 640–648.
11. Roberts MC, Mickelson JR, Patterson EE, Nelson TE, Armstrong PJ, et al. (2001) Autosomal dominant canine malignant hyperthermia is caused by a mutation in the gene encoding the skeletal muscle calcium release channel (RYR1). Anesthesiology 95: 716–725.
12. Jurkat-Rott K, McCarthy T, Lehmann-Horn F (2000) Genetics and pathogenesis of malignant hyperthermia. Muscle Nerve 23: 4–17.
13. Aleman M, Riehl J, Aldridge BM, Lecouteur RA, Stott JL, et al. (2004) Association of a mutation in the ryanodine receptor 1 gene with equine malignant hyperthermia. Muscle Nerve 30: 356–365.
14. Fujii J, Otsu K, Zorzato F, de Leon S, Khanna VK, et al. (1991) Identification of a mutation in porcine ryanodine receptor associated with malignant hyperthermia. Science 253: 448–451.
15. Harrison GG (1972) Pale, soft exudative pork, porcine stress syndrome and malignant hyperpyrexia–an identity? J S Afr Vet Assoc 43: 57–63.
16. Mickelson JR, Louis CF (1996) Malignant hyperthermia: excitation-contraction coupling, Ca2+ release channel, and cell Ca2+ regulation defects. Physiol Rev 76: 537–592.
17. Lopez JR, Alamo L, Caputo C, Wikinski J, Ledezma D (1985) Intracellular ionized calcium concentration in muscles from humans with malignant hyperthermia. Muscle Nerve 8: 355–358.
18. Lopez JR, Alamo LA, Jones DE, Papp L, Allen PD, et al. (1986) [Ca2+]i in muscles of malignant hyperthermia susceptible pigs determined in vivo with Ca2+ selective microelectrodes. Muscle Nerve 9: 85–86.
19. Tilgen N, Zorzato F, Halliger-Keller B, Muntoni F, Sewry C, et al. (2001) Identification of four novel mutations in the C-terminal membrane spanning domain of the ryanodine receptor 1: association with central core disease and alteration of calcium homeostasis. Hum Mol Genet 10: 2879–2887.
20. Ducreux S, Zorzato F, Muller C, Sewry C, Muntoni F, et al. (2004) Effect of ryanodine receptor mutations on interleukin-6 release and intracellular calcium homeostasis in human myotubes from malignant hyperthermia-susceptible individuals and patients affected by central core disease. J Biol Chem 279: 43838–43846.
21. Ghassemi F, Vukcevic M, Xu L, Zhou H, Meissner G, et al. (2009) A recessive ryanodine receptor 1 mutation in a CCD patient increases channel activity. Cell Calcium 45: 192–197.
22. Zhou H, Brockington M, Jungbluth H, Monk D, Stanier P, et al. (2006) Epigenetic allele silencing unveils recessive RYR1 mutations in core myopathies. Am J Hum Genet 79: 859–868.
23. Zhou H, Yamaguchi N, Xu L, Wang Y, Sewry C, et al. (2006) Characterization of recessive RYR1 mutations in core myopathies. Hum Mol Genet 15: 2791–2803.
24. Zvaritch E, Kraeva N, Bombardier E, McCloy RA, Depreux F, et al. (2009) Ca2+ dysregulation in Ryr1(I4895T/wt) mice causes congenital myopathy with progressive formation of minicores, cores, and nemaline rods. Proc Natl Acad Sci U S A 106: 21813–21818.
25. Lynch PJ, Tong J, Lehane M, Mallet A, Giblin L, et al. (1999) A mutation in the transmembrane/luminal domain of the ryanodine receptor is associated with abnormal Ca2+ release channel function and severe central core disease. Proc Natl Acad Sci U S A 96: 4164–4169.
26. Avila G, O'Brien JJ, Dirksen RT (2001) Excitation–contraction uncoupling by a human central core disease mutation in the ryanodine receptor. Proc Natl Acad Sci U S A 98: 4215–4220.
27. Zhou H, Rokach O, Feng L, Munteanu I, Mamchaoui K, et al. (2013) RyR1 deficiency in congenital myopathies disrupts excitation-contraction coupling. Hum Mutat 34: 986–996.
28. Voermans NC, Laan AE, Oosterhof A, van Kuppevelt TH, Drost G, et al. (2012) Brody syndrome: a clinically heterogeneous entity distinct from Brody disease: a review of literature and a cross-sectional clinical study in 17 patients. Neuromuscul Disord 22: 944–954.
29. Hovnanian A (2007) SERCA pumps and human diseases. Subcell Biochem 45: 337–363.
30. Drogemuller C, Drogemuller M, Leeb T, Mascarello F, Testoni S, et al. (2008) Identification of a missense mutation in the bovine ATP2A1 gene in congenital pseudomyotonia of Chianina cattle: an animal model of human Brody disease. Genomics 92: 474–477.
31. McCarthy TV, Quane KA, Lynch PJ (2000) Ryanodine receptor mutations in malignant hyperthermia and central core disease. Hum Mutat 15: 410–417.
32. Cole FL, Mellor DJ, Hodgson DR, Reid SW (2004) Prevalence and demographic characteristics of exertional rhabdomyolysis in horses in Australia. Vet Rec 155: 625–630.
33. Upjohn MM, Archer RM, Christley RM, McGowan CM (2005) Incidence and risk factors associated with exertional rhabdomyolysis syndrome in National Hunt racehorses in Great Britain. Vet Rec 156: 763–766.
34. MacLeay JM, Sorum SA, Valberg SJ, Marsh WE, Sorum MD (1999) Epidemiologic analysis of factors influencing exertional rhabdomyolysis in Thoroughbreds. Am J Vet Res 60: 1562–1566.
35. Dranchak PK, Valberg SJ, Onan GW, Gallant EM, Binns MM, et al. (2006) Exclusion of linkage of the RYR1, CACNA1S, and ATP2A1 genes to recurrent exertional rhabdomyolysis in Thoroughbreds. Am J Vet Res 67: 1395–1400.
36. Isgren CM, Upjohn MM, Fernandez-Fuente M, Massey C, Pollott G, et al. (2010) Epidemiology of exertional rhabdomyolysis susceptibility in standardbred horses reveals associated risk factors and underlying enhanced performance. PLoS One 5: e11594.
37. Court MH, Engelking LR, Dodman NH, Anwer MS, Seeler DC, et al. (1987) Pharmacokinetics of dantrolene sodium in horses. J Vet Pharmacol Ther 10: 218–226.
38. McKenzie EC, Valberg SJ, Godden SM, Finno CJ, Murphy MJ (2004) Effect of oral administration of dantrolene sodium on serum creatine kinase activity after exercise in horses with recurrent exertional rhabdomyolysis. Am J Vet Res 65: 74–79.
39. Bannister RA (2013) Dantrolene-induced inhibition of skeletal L-type Ca2+ current requires RyR1 expression. Biomed Res Int 2013: 390493.
40. Klein A, Lillis S, Munteanu I, Scoto M, Zhou H, et al. (2012) Clinical and genetic findings in a large cohort of patients with ryanodine receptor 1 gene-associated myopathies. Hum Mutat 33: 981–988.
41. Dlamini N, Voermans NC, Lillis S, Stewart K, Kamsteeg EJ, et al. (2013) Mutations in RYR1 are a common cause of exertional myalgia and rhabdomyolysis. Neuromuscul Disord 23: 540–548.
42. Larach MG (1989) Standardization of the caffeine halothane muscle contracture test. North American Malignant Hyperthermia Group. Anesth Analg 69: 511–515.
43. Jungbluth H, Sewry CA, Muntoni F (2011) Core myopathies. Semin Pediatr Neurol 18: 239–249.
44. Burton NM, Vierck J, Krabbenhoft L, Bryne K, Dodson MV (2000) Methods for animal satellite cell culture under a variety of conditions. Methods Cell Sci 22: 51–61.
45. Yasin R, Van Beers G, Nurse KC, Al-Ani S, Landon DN, et al. (1977) A quantitative technique for growing human adult skeletal muscle in culture starting from mononucleated cells. J Neurol Sci 32: 347–360.
46. Lattanzi L, Salvatori G, Coletta M, Sonnino C, Cusella De Angelis MG, et al. (1998) High efficiency myogenic conversion of human fibroblasts by adenoviral vector-mediated MyoD gene transfer. An alternative strategy for ex vivo gene therapy of primary myopathies. J Clin Invest 101: 2119–2128.

47. Abe T, Takano K, Suzuki A, Shimada Y, Inagaki M, et al. (2004) Myocyte differentiation generates nuclear invaginations traversed by myofibrils associating with sarcomeric protein mRNAs. J Cell Sci 117: 6523–6534.
48. Fernandez-Fuente M, Ames EG, Wagner ML, Zhou H, Strom M, et al. (2008) Assessment of the transformation of equine skin-derived fibroblasts to multinucleated skeletal myotubes following lentiviral-induced expression of equine myogenic differentiation 1. Am J Vet Res 69: 1637–1645.
49. Fernandez-Fuente M, Martin-Duque P, Vassaux G, Brown SC, Muntoni F, et al. (2014) Adenovirus-mediated expression of Myogenic Differentiation Factor 1 (MyoD) in equine and human dermal fibroblasts enables their conversion to caffeine-sensitive myotubes. Neuromuscul Disord: 24(3): 250–8.
50. Choi J, Costa ML, Mermelstein CS, Chagas C, Holtzer S, et al. (1990) MyoD converts primary dermal fibroblasts, chondroblasts, smooth muscle, and retinal pigmented epithelial cells into striated mononucleated myoblasts and multinucleated myotubes. Proc Natl Acad Sci U S A 87: 7988–7992.
51. Weintraub H, Tapscott SJ, Davis RL, Thayer MJ, Adam MA, et al. (1989) Activation of muscle-specific genes in pigment, nerve, fat, liver, and fibroblast cell lines by forced expression of MyoD. Proc Natl Acad Sci U S A 86: 5434–5438.
52. Walmsley GL, Arechavala-Gomeza V, Fernandez-Fuente M, Burke MM, Nagel N, et al. (2010) A duchenne muscular dystrophy gene hot spot mutation in dystrophin-deficient cavalier king charles spaniels is amenable to exon 51 skipping. PLoS One 5: e8647.
53. Larsen J, Pettersson OJ, Jakobsen M, Thomsen R, Pedersen CB, et al. (2011) Myoblasts generated by lentiviral mediated MyoD transduction of myotonic dystrophy type 1 (DM1) fibroblasts can be used for assays of therapeutic molecules. BMC Res Notes 4: 490.
54. He TC, Zhou S, da Costa LT, Yu J, Kinzler KW, et al. (1998) A simplified system for generating recombinant adenoviruses. Proc Natl Acad Sci U S A 95: 2509–2514.
55. Rogers TB, Inesi G, Wade R, Lederer WJ (1995) Use of thapsigargin to study Ca2+ homeostasis in cardiac cells. Biosci Rep 15: 341–349.
56. Gyorke S, Lukyanenko V, Gyorke I (1997) Dual effects of tetracaine on spontaneous calcium release in rat ventricular myocytes. J Physiol 500 (Pt 2): 297–309.
57. Laver DR, van Helden DF (2011) Three independent mechanisms contribute to tetracaine inhibition of cardiac calcium release channels. J Mol Cell Cardiol 51: 357–369.
58. Yang T, Esteve E, Pessah IN, Molinski TF, Allen PD, et al. (2007) Elevated resting [Ca(2+)](i) in myotubes expressing malignant hyperthermia RyR1 cDNAs is partially restored by modulation of passive calcium leak from the SR. Am J Physiol Cell Physiol 292: C1591–1598.
59. Tong J, McCarthy TV, MacLennan DH (1999) Measurement of resting cytosolic Ca2+ concentrations and Ca2+ store size in HEK-293 cells transfected with malignant hyperthermia or central core disease mutant Ca2+ release channels. J Biol Chem 274: 693–702.
60. Csernoch L, Szentesi P, Sarkozi S, Szegedi C, Jona I, et al. (1999) Effects of tetracaine on sarcoplasmic calcium release in mammalian skeletal muscle fibres. J Physiol 515 (Pt 3): 843–857.
61. Garcia J, Avila-Sakar AJ, Stefani E (1991) Differential effects of ryanodine and tetracaine on charge movement and calcium transients in frog skeletal muscle. J Physiol 440: 403–417.
62. Hollingworth S, Chandler WK, Baylor SM (2006) Effects of tetracaine on voltage-activated calcium sparks in frog intact skeletal muscle fibers. J Gen Physiol 127: 291–307.
63. Eltit JM, Li H, Ward CW, Molinski T, Pessah IN, et al. (2011) Orthograde dihydropyridine receptor signal regulates ryanodine receptor passive leak. Proc Natl Acad Sci U S A 108: 7046–7051.
64. Eltit JM, Yang T, Li H, Molinski TF, Pessah IN, et al. (2010) RyR1-mediated Ca2+ leak and Ca2+ entry determine resting intracellular Ca2+ in skeletal myotubes. J Biol Chem 285: 13781–13787.
65. DiMaio Knych HK, Arthur RM, Taylor A, Moeller BC, Stanley SD (2011) Pharmacokinetics and metabolism of dantrolene in horses. J Vet Pharmacol Ther 34: 238–246.
66. McKenzie EC, Garrett RL, Payton ME, Riehl JH, Firshman AM, et al. (2010) Effect of feed restriction on plasma dantrolene concentrations in horses. Equine Vet J Suppl: 613–617.
67. Gissel H (2005) The role of Ca2+ in muscle cell damage. Ann N Y Acad Sci 1066: 166–180.
68. Glahn KP, Ellis FR, Halsall PJ, Muller CR, Snoeck MM, et al. (2010) Recognizing and managing a malignant hyperthermia crisis: guidelines from the European Malignant Hyperthermia Group. Br J Anaesth 105: 417–420.
69. Lentz LR, Valberg SJ, Mickelson JR, Gallant EM (1999) In vitro contractile responses and contracture testing of skeletal muscle from Quarter Horses with exertional rhabdomyolysis. Am J Vet Res 60: 684–688.

15

A Sensitive, Reproducible and Objective Immunofluorescence Analysis Method of Dystrophin in Individual Fibers in Samples from Patients with Duchenne Muscular Dystrophy

Chantal Beekman, Jessica A. Sipkens, Janwillem Testerink, Stavros Giannakopoulos, Dyonne Kreuger, Judith C. van Deutekom, Giles V. Campion, Sjef J. de Kimpe*, Afrodite Lourbakos

Prosensa Therapeutics BV, Leiden, the Netherlands

Abstract

Duchenne muscular dystrophy (DMD) is characterized by the absence or reduced levels of dystrophin expression on the inner surface of the sarcolemmal membrane of muscle fibers. Clinical development of therapeutic approaches aiming to increase dystrophin levels requires sensitive and reproducible measurement of differences in dystrophin expression in muscle biopsies of treated patients with DMD. This, however, poses a technical challenge due to intra- and inter-donor variance in the occurrence of revertant fibers and low trace dystrophin expression throughout the biopsies. We have developed an immunofluorescence and semi-automated image analysis method that measures the sarcolemmal dystrophin intensity per individual fiber for the entire fiber population in a muscle biopsy. Cross-sections of muscle co-stained for dystrophin and spectrin have been imaged by confocal microscopy, and image analysis was performed using Definiens software. Dystrophin intensity has been measured in the sarcolemmal mask of spectrin for each individual muscle fiber and multiple membrane intensity parameters (mean, maximum, quantiles per fiber) were calculated. A histogram can depict the distribution of dystrophin intensities for the fiber population in the biopsy. This method was tested by measuring dystrophin in DMD, Becker muscular dystrophy, and healthy muscle samples. Analysis of duplicate or quadruplicate sections of DMD biopsies on the same or multiple days, by different operators, or using different antibodies, was shown to be objective and reproducible (inter-assay precision, CV 2–17% and intra-assay precision, CV 2–10%). Moreover, the method was sufficiently sensitive to detect consistently small differences in dystrophin between two biopsies from a patient with DMD before and after treatment with an investigational compound.

Editor: James M. Ervasti, University of Minnesota, United States of America

Funding: Funding provided by Prosensa Therapeutics BV, Leiden, the Netherlands. The funder provided support in the form of salaries, equipment and facilities for all authors, but did not have any additional role in the study design, data collection and analysis, decision to publish, or preparation of the manuscript.

* Email: s.dekimpe@prosensa.nl

Introduction

Duchenne muscular dystrophy (DMD) is characterized by progressive muscle fiber degeneration as a result of a dystrophin deficiency at the muscle fiber sarcolemmal membranes. The underlying mutations in the *DMD* gene are typically deletions of one or more exons (in 63% of patients) interrupting the open-reading frame. RNA-modulating therapy is the most advanced and promising strategy for this severe childhood muscle disease [1]. Several antisense oligonucleotides (AONs) are currently in (pre)clinical development. AON-induced exon skipping can restore the open-reading frame and, although the deletion and additional removal of an extra (flanking) exon seems paradoxical, the protein itself clearly allows such modification, as demonstrated in patients with the typically milder phenotype, Becker muscular dystrophy (BMD). Mutations in these patients result in an internally shortened but in-frame transcript and a dystrophin protein that is functional, especially when the mutation is located in the central rod domain between exons 10 and 60.

In current clinical studies aiming to increase dystrophin expression in patients with DMD, the pharmacodynamic effect of treatment can be assessed at the RNA or protein level. Such data can provide support for the mechanism of action and dose selection. Dystrophin bioanalytical assays need to consider "trace" dystrophin expression and "revertant" fibers. The expression of very low levels of trace dystrophin in patients with DMD has been observed before [1,2], but emerging methodologies on imaging and quantification of expression levels have shown that trace dystrophin is expressed more commonly in nearly all fibers in the majority of DMD muscle biopsies [3–7]. The incidence of revertant fibers that express relatively high levels of dystrophin is generally low (<5%) and appears to be dependent on the deletion and can reach 14% [6,7]. Trace dystrophin and revertant fibers can be recognized and accounted for in immunofluorescence analysis (IFA) of muscle biopsy cross-sections. Similarly, the presence of fibrosis and adipose tissue in a biopsy can be identified and excluded from analysis of muscle biopsies in IFA. IFA has the advantage that it can detect the effect of treatment on dystrophin expression at the sarcolemma of the muscle fibers in a biopsy.

Historically, significant efforts have been made to objectively measure dystrophin intensities. One image analysis method determined the average dystrophin intensity from all fibers in an image that co-localized with a spectrin signal in a software-generated mask defining the sarcolemmal area [4]. Another method assessed dystrophin expression by manually placing circles on randomly selected areas of the sarcolemma of a selected number of fibers per biopsy and measured the maximum membrane intensity within that circle [5,6]. It has been reported that the intensity of dystrophin may vary between fibers in a healthy control muscle [4,5] and that this variability is even more pronounced in BMD and DMD muscle [2,3,5]. Therefore, it would be more informative to measure not only the average intensity of all sarcolemmal membranes in an image or the maximum intensity in a limited number of fibers, but to determine the complete dystrophin expression at the membrane of each individual fiber in a biopsy cross-section. Ideally, image analysis should be automated to allow for higher throughput and unbiased interpretation of expression in a fiber or an image.

Here, we present a standardized IFA method that is sensitive, operator-independent, and reproducible. It is based on imaging by confocal microscopy and semi-automated image analysis using computer software. Individual fibers are identified by spectrin co-staining and dystrophin intensity is measured at each fiber membrane to determine the distribution of dystrophin expression over individual fibers in the cross-section of a muscle biopsy. We demonstrate that the method is fit-for-purpose for the analysis and comparison of muscle samples from healthy controls and from patients with BMD and DMD.

Materials and Methods

Ethics Statement

Human control muscle tissues were obtained from a commercial tissue bank (Asterand, Hertfordshire, UK; http://asterand.com/Asterand/about/ethics.htm) and from the Vrije Universiteit Medical Center (VUMC, Amsterdam, the Netherlands). The use of post-mortem material was approved by the VUMC research committee (project 2011-67), where relatives have given explicit prior written consent that tissue taken at autopsy can be used for research, after completion of the diagnostic process and informed consents were approved by institutional review boards. BMD biopsies were kindly provided by the Leiden University Medical Center (LUMC, Leiden, the Netherlands) and approved by the LUMC medical ethics committee and after written informed consent was obtained from all subjects or legal representatives. DMD biopsies were obtained from patients participating in clinical studies (registered at clinicaltrials.gov; NCT01153932 and NCT01037309) after approval by the local medical ethics committees and after signed patient informed consent including the assessment of dystrophin. Please see our supporting information file for a full list of participating sites (Table S1).

Muscle Biopsies

The size of the muscle biopsies varied but was typically around 5×5×5 mm. The muscle biopsies were frozen in 2-methylbutane cooled in liquid nitrogen as described previously [8]. Muscle biopsies from the tibialis anterior were obtained from patients diagnosed with DMD or BMD. BMD biopsies (BMD 1–4) were kindly provided by Prof. dr. J.J. Verschuuren (LUMC). DMD biopsies were obtained from patients participating in clinical studies. The specific DMD mutation is for each donor indicated in Table 1. Samples DMD 1–3, 5, and 6 were naïve biopsies before treatment. DMD subject 5 participated in clinical study PRO044-CLIN-01 (Clinicaltrials.gov NCT01037309) and biopsies were taken before and after treatment with five weekly injections of 12 mg/kg antisense oligonucleotide PRO044, an investigational compound that can induce exon skipping to correct the reading frame of the mRNA.

Muscle samples from control donors were obtained post-mortem from individuals not suffering from DMD and kindly provided by Prof. dr. H.W. Niessen (VUMC, control 1 and 3, following storage of the body under cooled conditions (<5°C) for a maximum of 12 hours) and Asterand (control 2, following storage of the body for 7 hours). From healthy control 1, samples from six different muscle groups were obtained: tibialis anterior, quadriceps, gastrocnemius, biceps, triceps, and soleus. From control 3, only a quadriceps sample was obtained and from control 2, only a tibialis anterior sample.

Sectioning and Immunofluorescence Double-staining Procedure

Each experiment was performed by several operators and different operators were arbitrarily assigned to each of the subsequent processing steps (sectioning of muscle biopsies, staining of sections for dystrophin and spectrin, image acquisition by confocal microscopy, and software-assisted image analysis). Biopsy quality was assessed by hematoxylin and eosin staining and was routinely performed to evaluate freezing artefacts (biopsy handling, transport and storage) and relative amount of fibrotic and adipose tissue, and to ensure sufficient fibers for reliable IFA for dystrophin.

Using a cryotome (Thermo Fisher Scientific, Waltham, MA, USA), 8 μm muscle cross-sections were cut and placed on Superfrost Ultra Plus Microscope Slides (Thermo Fisher Scientific, VWR 631–0099). After drying at room temperature for 1 hour, the slides were placed in a −80°C freezer and used within 2 months. The staining procedure was performed at room temperature. Slides were removed from the freezer, air dried for 20 minutes, fixed with acetone for 1 minute, washed with PBS, blocked with PBS containing 0.05% Tween-20 and 5% horse serum for 1 hour, and subsequently washed with PBS. For each biopsy, two or four sections were stained. Double-staining for dystrophin and spectrin was performed with the following combination of antibodies: mouse monoclonal MANDYS106 rod-domain anti-dystrophin antibody [9,10] combined with a rabbit anti-spectrin antibody, or rabbit polyclonal ab15277 C-terminal anti-dystrophin antibody combined with a mouse anti-spectrin antibody (Table 2). Cross-reactivity to utrophin has been a concern for C-terminal anti-dystrophin antibodies, but is highly unlikely for ab15277 as it is raised to a peptide epitope unique to dystrophin and is affinity purified. Sections were incubated for 2 hours with anti-dystrophin or isotype antibody alone followed by a 1-hour incubation with anti-dystrophin and anti-spectrin antibodies combined, or isotype and anti-spectrin antibody combined. After the incubation with the primary antibodies, the sections were washed with PBS and then incubated with the appropriate secondary antibodies combined for 1 hour (Table 2). After washing again with PBS, the slides were mounted with Vectashield Mounting medium (Vector Laboratories, Burlingame, CA, USA; Brunschwig 6-H-1400) and imaged on the same day (Table 2).

Table 1. Control, BMD, and DMD muscle samples used.

Donor	Dystrophin mutation
Control 1	N/A
Control 2	N/A
Control 3	N/A
BMD 1	Deletion exon 45–47
BMD 3	Deletion exon 45–47
BMD 4	Deletion exon 03–07
BMD 2	Ex.19:c.2380+3A>C
DMD 1	Deletion exon 48–50
DMD 2	Deletion exon 45–50
DMD 3	Deletion exon 50
DMD 4	Deletion exon 45
DMD 5	Deletion exon 45
DMD 6	Deletion exon 43

BMD, Becker muscular dystrophy; DMD, Duchenne muscular dystrophy; N/A, not applicable.

Image Acquisition Procedure by Confocal Microscopy

Images were obtained using a Zeiss LSM 710 confocal microscope to enhance sharp membrane images. The standard imaging process captures 3-µm thick Z-slices. During development, we observed that the results were not influenced when using multiple Z-slices from the 8-µm section. From each muscle cross-section, five non-overlapping images at 25× magnification were acquired. Areas of the section containing very few muscle fibers or extensive fibrosis and adipose cells or sectioning artefacts were avoided. For the corresponding isotype staining for each biopsy, three non-overlapping images were obtained per section.

Pinhole size, image resolution, color depth, scan speed, and averaging (number of scans per image) were the same for all experiments. When imaging for an experiment that included healthy control and BMD/DMD biopsies, the microscope settings for laser intensity and detector gain for the dystrophin and spectrin channels were adjusted using the healthy control sample (with the highest signal intensity) so that only a few saturated pixels were present in the acquired images for the healthy control. When imaging for an experiment aiming to compare DMD samples, the imaging parameters for laser intensity and detector gain for the dystrophin channel were optimized for fluorescent beads (InSpeck Green [505/515] Microscope Image Intensity Calibration Kit; Invitrogen I-14785; 0.3% beads; Carlsbad, CA, USA), using higher laser intensity (DMD settings). Higher laser intensity makes better use of the 12-bit dynamic range (4095 arbitrary units) to detect differences at low expression levels. The spectrin settings were again optimized for the sample with the highest spectrin intensity, usually one of the DMD samples. In a single experiment, all images (control, DMD, or BMD) are taken at the same microscope, laser, and detector settings.

Image Analysis and Dystrophin Intensity Measurement Using Image Analysis Software

Image analysis was performed using Definiens Architect software (version 2.0) with a customized algorithm and application. Using the spectrin signal, the software identified the individual muscle fibers and determined within each fiber the sarcolemma and the cytoplasm. The software is able to distinguish between touching membranes of adjacent fibers using an algorithm based on maximum predicted membrane thickness and signal intensities from the individual fibers. On average, 400 fibers were analyzed per section (five images), for two or four sections per biopsy sample. Normally, at least 90% of the fibers in each image of a DMD patient-derived biopsy are sufficiently intact to be correctly identified (Figure 1B). The intensity of the dystrophin signal wass then determined. The dystrophin signal at the sarcolemma, as defined by spectrin, is considered to be dystrophin protein properly localized to the membrane. Images were processed automatically in batches, and identification of fibers was checked by operators. Mean intensity, minimum, maximum, and quantile dystrophin intensity values were determined per fiber. In addition, spectrin intensity per fiber was measured and morphology parameters calculated (such as cross sectional area of individual fibers and membrane thickness). The mean dystrophin membrane intensity (in arbitrary units [au]) is the average intensity of all pixels present in the spectrin surface area of an individual fiber. The quantile value of Q90 dystrophin intensity of a fiber, for instance, is the cut-off between 90% of pixels in the membrane with the lowest intensity and the 10% of pixels with the highest intensity. Generally, the "Q90–mean" of each fiber is used, which represents the mean intensity of the 10% of pixels with the highest intensity in the membrane of a fiber. The Q90-mean appears to represent what is observed by eye as the "brighter fluorescence" at the membrane and with high contrast to cytoplasm.

Table 2. Antibody reagents for immunofluorescence detection of dystrophin and spectrin.

Double-staining combination	Dystrophin primary antibody	Spectrin primary antibody	Secondary antibody antimouse	Secondary antibody antirabbit
MANDYS106 and spectrin	Mouse MANDYS106 [9][a]	Rabbit α-spectrin (Thermo Scientific PA1-46007)[c]	α-mouse AlexaFluor488 (Invitrogen A11029)[d]	α-rabbit AlexaFluor594 (Invitrogen A11037)[e]
Mouse isotype and spectrin	Mouse IgG2A (Sigma M5409)[b]	Rabbit α-spectrin (Thermo Scientific PA1-46007)[c]	α-mouse AlexaFluor488 (Invitrogen A11029)[d]	α-rabbit AlexaFluor594 (Invitrogen A11037)[e]
ab15277 and spectrin	Rabbit polyclonal (Abcam ab15277)[c]	Mouse α-spectrin (Novocastra NCL-SPEC1)[c]	α-mouse AlexaFluor594 (Invitrogen A11032)[e]	α-rabbit AlexaFluor488 (Invitrogen A11034)[d]
Rabbit isotype and spectrin	Rabbit polyclonal IgG (Abcam ab27478)[c]	Mouse α-spectrin (Novocastra NCL-SPEC1)[c]	α-mouse AlexaFluor594 (Invitrogen A11032)[e]	α-rabbit AlexaFluor488 (Invitrogen A11034)[d]

Dilution of primary antibodies in PBS containing 0.05% Tween, 5% FBS: [a]1:60, [b]1:300, [c]1:200.
Dilution of secondary antibodies in PBS containing 0.05% Tween: [d]1:250, [e]1:1000.
FBS, fetal bovine serum; Ig, immunoglobulin; PBS, phosphate-buffered saline.

The dystrophin intensity differs per fiber. The distribution of the dystrophin levels in a fiber population from a muscle biopsy can be assessed and depicted as a histogram (Figure 1C). The average for the mean dystrophin level per fiber can be calculated for the entire fiber population, but the range for the dystrophin level per fiber can vary considerably within a biopsy cross-section. In healthy (non-DMD) control muscle, the mean dystrophin expression in a fiber may vary by threefold (in the range of 500–1350 au mean intensity per fiber). Alternatively, this histogram can also be displayed as a plot of cumulative percentage of fibers, which results in an S-curve (Figure 1C). The heterogeneity of dystrophin expression in the fibers determines the slope of the S-curve and a steeper slope depicts a more homogeneous dystrophin expression between fibers of a biopsy. An increase in overall dystrophin levels will make the cumulative dystrophin curve shift to the right.

Statistical analysis

Reproducibility of the methodology has been assessed on the mean dystrophin intensity per fiber calculated for the biopsies.

Intra-assay precision: 2–4 replicate sections of a biopsy were analyzed in the same experiment and the percent coefficient of variation (CV) was calculated (CV% = standard deviation/ average dystrophin intensity * 100% for the different sections of the biopsy).

Inter-assay precision was assessed qualitatively by ranking and quantitatively by calculation of the CV%. For ranking, the same biopsies were analyzed in different experiments and the dystrophin intensity measured was used to rank order the biopsies. The ranking of the biopsies between the different experiments was compared. For the CV%, the dystrophin intensity result of the same biopsy analyzed for different experiments on different days were used for the calculation (CV% = standard deviation/ average dystrophin intensity * 100% for the different experiments on the biopsy).

To determine the statistical significance of the difference between pre- and post-treatment biopsy of subject DMD 4 analyzed in the same experiment, a linear mixed model was used. The dependent variable was log transformed in order to have a better normal distribution. Fixed term in the model was visit (before/after treatment) and random factors were sections within visits and images within sections.

Results

Method Optimization in Control Muscle Samples with Muscle and Donor Variability in Dystrophin Levels

In a series of experiments, the staining procedures for anti-dystrophin MANDYS106 and ab15277 antibodies, and image capture and analysis using Definiens architect software, were optimized using healthy control muscle samples from different muscle groups and donors. The method showed that dystrophin intensities vary widely between individual fibers within one cross-section and, therefore, comparison of samples should consider the distribution of membrane dystrophin intensities over individual fibers in a sample. In a representative experiment with MANDYS106 (Figure 2A), samples from six different muscle groups of one donor (control 1) were analyzed. The mean dystrophin membrane intensity and Q90 mean values per fiber varied between muscle groups. The highest dystrophin intensities were measured in the gastrocnemius muscle for the mean dystrophin per fiber (average = 764 au per fiber) and also for the mean of the 10% brightest pixels (average of the Q90-mean = 2041 au). The lowest dystrophin intensities were measured in the tibialis anterior muscle (mean of 590 au and Q90-mean of 1603 au per fiber) (Figure 2B). The distribution of dystrophin intensities in the entire fiber population differed between muscle groups (Figure 2C). The fiber dystrophin intensities in the tibialis anterior and quadriceps muscles were also analyzed for two different donors (control 2 and 3, respectively), and varied by up to 29% (quadriceps) between donors. The observation that dystrophin intensity varies between fibers within a healthy control muscle has been previously reported using epifluorescence and confocal microscopy [4–6]. Although the variance in dystrophin intensities between muscle groups and between donors, observed reproducibly in independent experiments using different cross-sections, is suggestive for differential dystrophin expression in muscle groups and donors, sample variation (site and timing of sampling) should also be taken into account.

Detection Range and Reproducibility in Control, BMD, and DMD Muscle Samples

The detection range and reproducibility of the method was assessed for two different anti-dystrophin antibodies, MANDYS106 and ab15277. Biopsies from the tibialis anterior muscle of donors with DMD (n = 2) or BMD (n = 4) were analyzed and compared to control 2. In a representative experiment (Figure 3A), MANDYS106 staining showed that the average mean dystrophin intensity per fiber was very low in the DMD biopsies (approximately 82 au) and intermediate in the BMD samples (ranging from 213 to 367 au) when compared to the 768 au in the control 2 sample (Figure 3B, Table 3). The intra-assay precision (CV%) ranged between 3 and 13% for replicate sections. The cumulative histogram plots of the control and BMD samples again highlight the typical variability in dystrophin expression between individual fibers in one cross-section but also show that the differences between patient biopsies apply across all fibers (Figure 3B). In addition, revertant fibers in the DMD samples had a higher dystrophin intensity, which was in the range of control muscle intensity (indicated by the asterisks in Figure 3B).

To evaluate the inter-assay precision of the method, two experiments were performed on different days with different operators for muscle biopsy staining, image acquisition, and processing. Muscle samples were ranked (1–7) based on their average dystrophin intensity. The ranking in the two experiments was very consistent (Table 3), except for two BMD samples (BMD 1 and 3) that expressed very similar dystrophin levels (7% and 11% difference between the 2 samples in 2 experiments). Using the dystrophin intensity arbitrary units measured for the same samples between experiments, the CV% was calculated to range between 4 and 13% for the control and BMD samples and between 24 and 43% for the DMD biopsies.

The consistency of dystrophin expression was also evaluated using the same control, BMD, and DMD samples but with staining with ab15277, a polyclonal rabbit antibody directed to the C-terminal end of the protein. Using ab15277, the lowest dystrophin intensity was measured in the DMD biopsies and higher levels in the BMD and control samples. The ab15277 antibody appears to be highly specific for dystrophin detection as indicated by the ability to detect also trace dystrophin and revertant fibers (Figure S1) and the very low staining observed in DMD biopsies is in agreement with previous work [4,11]. The same ranking of samples (1–7) was observed for two ab15277 experiments, and the MANDYS106 staining (Figure S1B). These results indicate that the IFA method using two different anti-dystrophin antibodies can reproducibly detect a wide range of dystrophin intensity levels. The resulting dystrophin intensity distribution plots are highly informative and reproducibly ranked

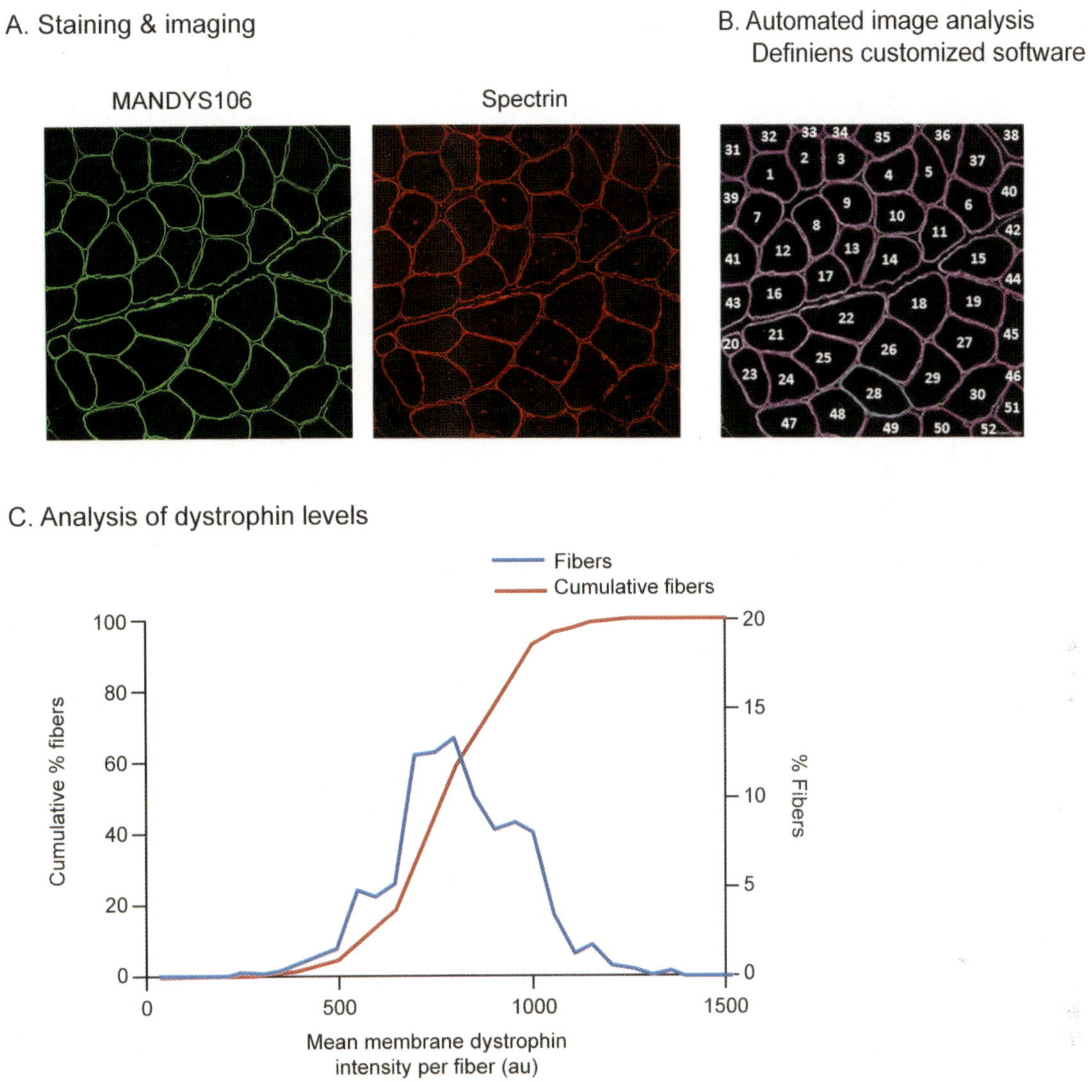

Figure 1. Immunofluorescence analysis of dystrophin intensities per fiber in a muscle fiber population. A. Cryosections of a healthy control muscle sample (control 3, quadriceps muscle) co-stained with anti-dystrophin antibody MANDYS106 and an anti-spectrin antibody. The sections were imaged using a confocal microscope, with the green channel (Alexa488) showing dystrophin and the red channel (Alexa594) showing spectrin. **B.** Images were analyzed using customized Definiens software, which automatically identifies individual muscle fiber membranes using their spectrin signal and measures the membrane dystrophin intensity per muscle fiber. **C.** Dystrophin intensity distribution in muscle fiber population analyzed, shown as a regular histogram (blue line) or a cumulative histogram (red line). (au: arbitrary units).

the different DMD and BMD muscle biopsies in an operator-independent manner.

Noteworthy are the mean spectrin intensities measured per fiber, which were typically higher in the DMD and BMD samples compared with the control sample (Figure S2). This was observed throughout all experiments (data not shown) and is in agreement with earlier reports describing qualitative assessments of immunofluorescence images for spectrin in fibers in diseased tissue [12,13].

Baseline Trace Dystrophin Intensities in DMD Muscle Biopsies

The inter-assay precision is lower for trace dystrophin levels in DMD biopsies and these can become indistinguishable at 1% laser intensity (Figure 3). To optimize imaging settings in this low range of detection, a 7% confocal laser intensity was used to be able to measure such subtle differences reproducibly. Fluorescent beads are used to determine the settings for the confocal microscopy and image acquisition and can also be used as a reference value between experiments. The number of fibers analyzed in a DMD muscle cross-section varied depending on the size of the muscle fibers and/or the disease state (i.e. the presence of connective and adipose tissue). Generally, each image contained an average of 80 fibers. With two sections analyzed per biopsy, between approximately 400 and 1350 fibers were included (average 800 fibers). With four sections per biopsy a maximum of ~3000 fibers was analyzed.

Using these optimized settings (7% laser intensity), variation in dystrophin expression per fiber within a DMD biopsy and between DMD biopsies also become apparent (Figure 4A). Whereas the dystrophin intensities vary between fibers, the spectrin intensities are generally similar and no correlation with the variability in dystrophin detection was observed. The intensity of trace dystrophin varied for individual fibers in a muscle biopsy

A.

C.

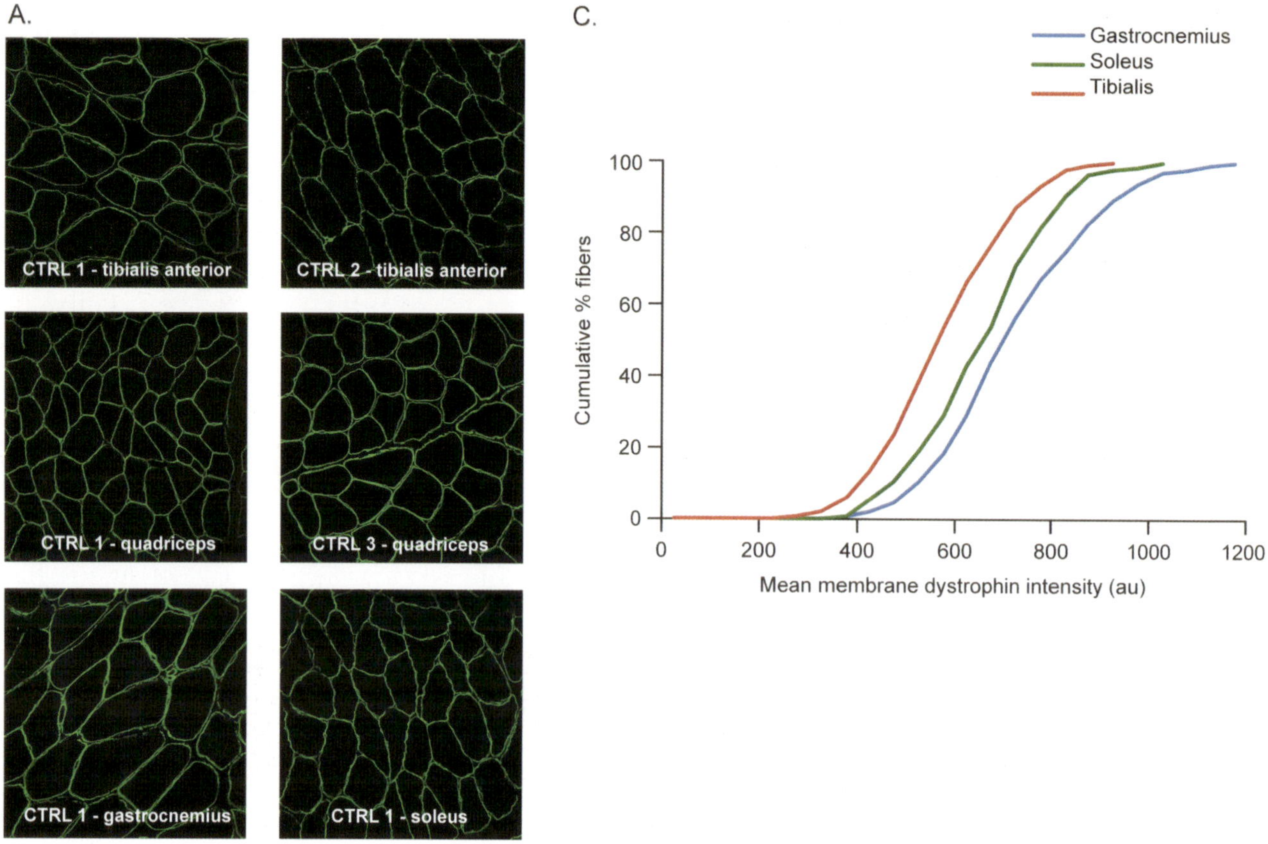

B.

Control donor	Muscle group	Number of fibers analyzed	Fiber surface area Mean ± SD (x10^3 µm^2)	Membrane thickness Mean ± SD (µm)	Spectrin intensity (au)	Dystrophin intensity MANDYS106 (au)		
						Mean (CV% 2 sections)	Q90 mean	Maximum
1	Gastrocnemius	305	7.7 ± 5.3	2.4 ± 0.4	793	764 (1)	2041	3660
1	Biceps	1010	2.8 ± 0.7	1.9 ± 0.3	781	637 (5)	1819	2884
1	Soleus	372	8.3 ± 3.3	1.9 ± 0.3	836	715 (4)	1939	3400
1	Triceps	728	4.4 ± 1.1	2.2 ± 0.4	734	607 (2)	1620	2951
1	Quadriceps	646	4.7 ± 1.4	2.0 ± 0.3	859	603 (5)	1628	2824
1	Tibialis	468	7.4 ± 2.9	2.2 ± 0.3	699	590 (5)	1603	2904
2	Tibialis	610	4.3 ± 1.7	1.8 ± 0.3	657	586 (8)	1787	3397
3	Quadriceps	510	6.3 ± 1.4	2.3 ± 0.4	862	777 (5)	2178	3468

Figure 2. Dystrophin expression in healthy (non-DMD) control muscle samples from different muscle groups and different donors using MANDYS106. Eight muscle samples were compared within one experiment: six muscle groups from one donor (control 1) and two muscle groups from two other donors (controls 2 and 3). Analysis was performed on two sections per sample; imaging was performed with microscope settings suitable for imaging control samples (1% laser intensity). A. Representative immunofluorescence images of different muscle groups from Controls 1–3. B. Summary of numbers of fibers analyzed per samples, morphology parameters (fiber cross-section surface area and membrane thickness), mean spectrin intensities and dystrophin intensity parameters (mean, Q90 mean and maximum) of all the samples analyzed. C. Dystrophin intensity distribution in the fiber populations (cumulative plots) of three different muscle groups analyzed for control 1. (au: arbitrary units; CV%: coefficient of variation of replicate sections; CTRL: control; DMD: Duchenne muscular dystrophy; SD: standard deviation).

A.

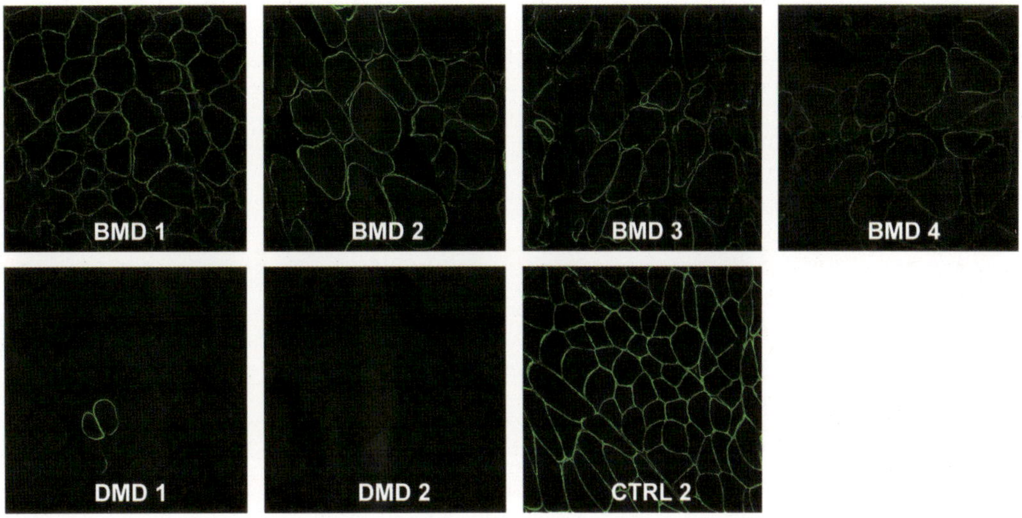

B.

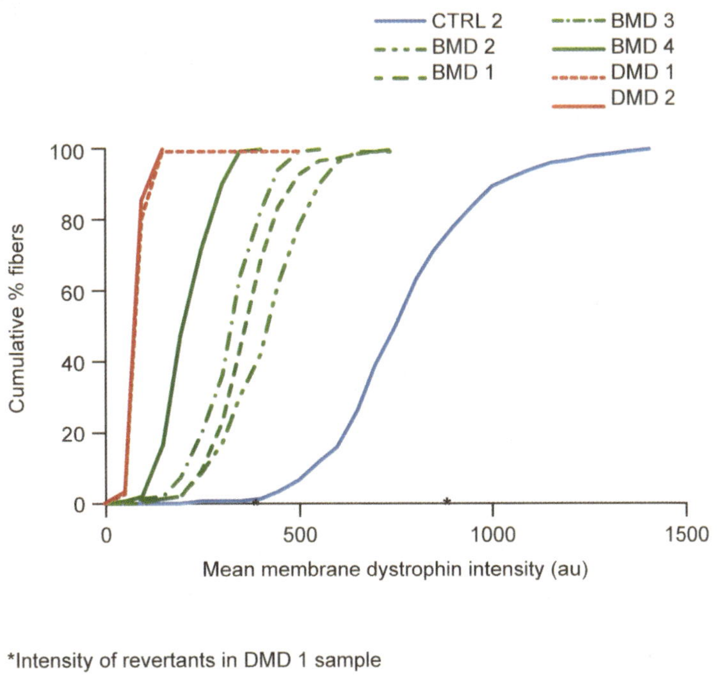

Figure 3. Dystrophin intensity in control muscle samples, and pre-treatment DMD and BMD muscle biopsies. A. Representative immunofluorescence images (1 of 10 images) from the tibialis anterior muscle samples (from one control subject (CTRL2), two patients with DMD and four patients with BMD. Analysis was performed in the same experiment using the MANDYS106 antibody and 'control' imaging settings (1% laser intensity). **B.** Corresponding dystrophin membrane intensity distribution in the fiber populations analyzed (cumulative graphs). (au: arbitrary units; BMD: Becker muscular dystrophy; CTRL: control; DMD: Duchenne muscular dystrophy).

population, typically between 200 and 800 au (eg, DMD example, Figure 4). For comparison, the intensity of the revertant fibers ranged from 800 to 2500 au.

The specificity of the detection of trace dystrophin in these DMD biopsies was confirmed by the increased signal intensity for the anti-dystrophin MANDYS106 antibody compared to the isotype control antibody control for aspecific binding (mouse IgG2a). Isotype staining for background is routinely applied in each experiment for each biopsy. The specificity of trace dystrophin was also confirmed by the DMD 6 biopsy, collected

Table 3. Reproducibility of detecting differences in dystrophin expression in muscle biopsies with a wide range of dystrophin levels from healthy controls to BMD and DMD samples by immunofluorescence using MANDYS106 antibody and Definiens intensity measurements (at 'control' microscope settings).

Sample	Experiment	Number of sections	Number of fibers analyzed	Cross sectional area of individual fibers; Mean ± SD ($x10^3$ μm^2)	Dystrophin membrane intensity MANDYS106 (au)					
					Mean	Intra-assay precision CV% sections	Inter-assay precision CV% experiments	Q90 mean	Maximum	Ranking
Control 2	1	2	625	4.4±1.8	929	13%	13%	2397	3609	1
	2	2	544	4.3±1.9	768	3%		2169	3640	1
BMD 1	1	2	262	4.8±2.7	415	3%	9%	1224	2425	2
	2	2	337	4.9±2.2	367	6%		1076	2195	3
BMD 3	1	2	173	7.2±3.6	387	13%	4%	1125	2366	3
	2	2	221	7.2±3.8	412	7%		1195	2439	2
BMD 4	1	2	250	5.8±3.9	359	4%	7%	1062	2152	4
	2	2	102	7.7±4.9	323	6%		993	2122	4
BMD 2	1	2	300	4.4±3.3	200	7%	4%	668	1553	5
	2	2	197	6.4±4.2	213	4%		689	1552	5
DMD 1	1	2	1102	2.3±1.1	58	6%	24%	154	341	6
	2	2	739	3.0±1.8	82	13%		198	399	6
DMD 2	1	2	937	2.6±1.5	44	10%	43%	115	243	7
	2	2	816	2.5±1.4	82	6%		184	334	7

The intra-assay precision (CV%) was calculated for the mean dystrophin intensity of multiple sections of a biopsy/sample analyzed in the same experiment. Inter-assay precision between experiments performed on different days was assessed in two ways by ranking of the samples based on the dystrophin intensity in each experiment and by calculating the CV% from the mean dystrophin intensity in each experiment (experiment 1 and 2 performed 102 days apart).

BMD, Becker muscular dystrophy; CV, coefficient of variation; DMD, Duchenne muscular dystrophy; SD, standard deviation.

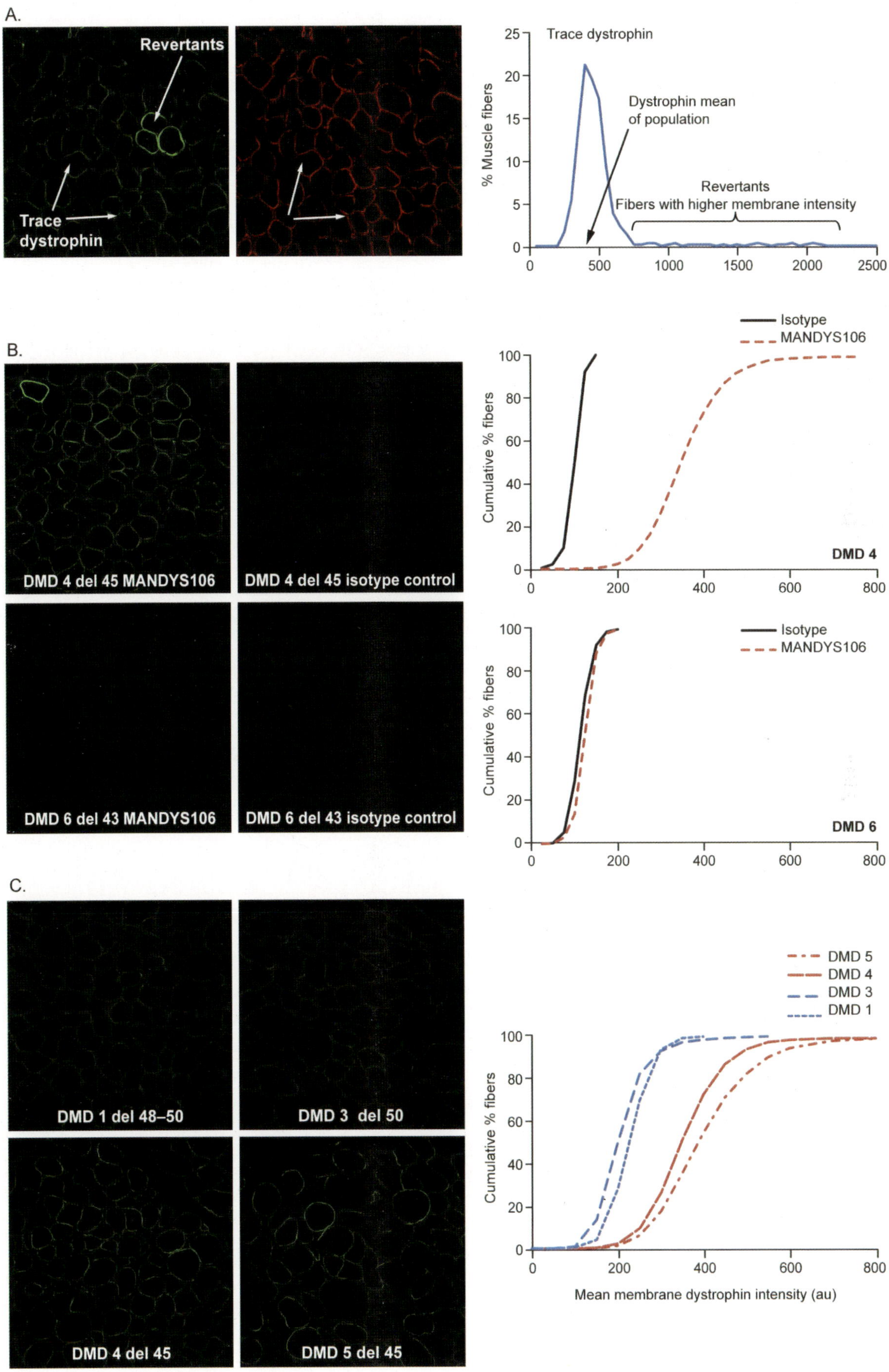
A.
Revertants
Trace dystrophin
Trace dystrophin
Dystrophin mean of population
Revertants
Fibers with higher membrane intensity
% Muscle fibers
B.
DMD 4 del 45 MANDYS106
DMD 4 del 45 isotype control
DMD 6 del 43 MANDYS106
DMD 6 del 43 isotype control
Isotype
MANDYS106
Cumulative % fibers
DMD 4
DMD 6
C.
DMD 1 del 48–50
DMD 3 del 50
DMD 4 del 45
DMD 5 del 45
DMD 5
DMD 4
DMD 3
DMD 1
Cumulative % fibers
Mean membrane dystrophin intensity (au)

Figure 4. Dystrophin signal specificity using MANDYS106. Immunofluorescence intensities measured in pre-treatment biopsies of different patients with DMD at microscope settings suitable for imaging DMD samples (7% laser intensity). **A.** (Left): Dystrophin staining (AlexaFluor488). All fibers exhibit varying intensities of dystrophin (trace dystrophin) and certain fibers termed "revertants" express higher levels of dystrophin. (Middle): Spectrin staining (AlexaFluor594): Fibers with equivalent spectrin intensities exhibited varying levels of dystrophin staining. (Right): Histogram of the mean dystrophin intensity in the fiber population depicting the fibers expressing trace dystrophin and revertant fibers. The mean dystrophin intensity of the fiber population expressing trace dystrophin is indicated by the arrow. **B.** Specificity of MANDYS106 antibody compared with isotype control for measuring dystrophin expression. Immunofluorescence images of MANDYS106 (left) or negative control isotype staining (right) of patients DMD 4 (deletion exon 45) and DMD 6 (deletion exon 43), and the corresponding histograms of mean dystrophin intensity (cumulative graphs). **C.** Dystrophin intensities in patients with DMD with different exon deletions (DMD patient 1: deletion exon 48–50; DMD patient 3: deletion exon 50; DMD patient 5: deletion exon 45; DMD patient 6: deletion exon 45). These samples were analyzed in the same experiment. (au: arbitrary units; del: deletion; DMD: Duchenne muscular dystrophy).

from a patient with DMD with a deletion of exon 43. As the epitope for the MANDYS106 antibody is encoded by this exon, no trace dystrophin expression was detected in this biopsy (Figure 4B). In contrast, in sample DMD 4 (deletion of exon 45), MANDYS106 staining exceeded isotype control staining (Figure 4B).

Trace dystrophin expression is typically much higher in patients with exon 44 flanking deletions (DMD 4 and 5) than in patients with exon 51 flanking deletions (DMD 1 and 3) (Figure 4C, Table 4). The cumulative distribution plots of the membrane dystrophin intensity per fiber show a clear shift of the whole fiber population to higher dystrophin intensities for exon 44 samples DMD 4 and DMD 5 compared with exon 51 samples DMD 1 and DMD 3. This is in accordance with the higher levels of spontaneous exon 44 skipping on the RNA level that we detected in multiple non-treated muscle cell cultures and baseline biopsies of patients with exon 44 flanking deletions (data not shown).

The reproducibility of dystrophin measurement in DMD samples was determined by comparing the dystrophin intensity of multiple sections of a DMD biopsy within one experiment (intra-assay precision) and between different experiments performed on separate days (inter-assay precision). The mean dystrophin intensity of four sections of the same DMD sample analyzed in the same experiment showed a CV% of between 2 and 10%. In experiments with two sections, CV% ranged from 4 to 10% (Table 4). The inter-assay precision was assessed in three independent experiments performed by different operators on three different days over the course of 1.5 years. Using the dystrophin intensity measured, the DMD samples were ranked and the order was consistent between the three experiments (Table 4). The CV% for the dystrophin intensity between experiments was calculated to range between 2 and 17% for the DMD biopsies. This indicates that, under these imaging conditions, the ranking and comparison of DMD samples is reproducible. A summary of the experiments performed is given (Table 5).

Dystrophin Intensities in Pre- and Post-Treatment DMD Muscle Biopsies

Using the optimized staining protocol, confocal image acquisition and Definiens analysis procedures, it is possible to accurately, objectively, and reproducibly assess differences in dystrophin levels in DMD between pre- and post-treatment muscle samples from clinical studies in DMD aiming to correct the open-reading frame and restore (internally truncated) dystrophin expression in patients with DMD. As an example, in a patient with DMD with an exon 44 flanking deletion treated for 5 weeks with 12 mg/kg PRO044 (by subcutaneous injections), the average dystrophin mean intensity in the fiber population was measured in the post and pre treatment biopsy. The % difference in dystrophin intensity between the post and pre-treatment biopsy was calculated (% dystrophin difference = ([dystrophin intensity post-treatment – dystrophin intensity pre-treatment]/dystrophin intensity pre-treatment ×100). The dystrophin intensity was higher in the post-treatment biopsy by 32% for MANDYS106 and 30% for ab15277, when compared with the pre-treatment biopsy (Figure 5). Also, the cumulative fiber plots for mean dystrophin intensities showed a clear shift to higher intensities for the post-treatment biopsies. Duplicate sections showed an intra-assay precision between 1 and 7%. To demonstrate reproducibility, the experiment with each antibody was repeated in a second experiment and the average membrane dystrophin mean intensity per fiber in the post-treatment biopsy was similarly higher by 30% using MANDYS106 and 19% using ab15277, compared to the pre-treatment biopsy. The difference between the pre- and post-treatment dystrophin levels was statistically significant ($P<0.05$) (Figure 5C). Hence, a difference in dystrophin intensity between two biopsies of the same DMD patient can be reproducibly demonstrated. Whether this is a treatment effect would require analysis of multiple biopsies, including placebo-treated control subjects.

Discussion

Dystrophin analysis in muscle biopsies is especially relevant for potential therapeutic approaches that aim to increase dystrophin expression in patients with DMD, such as recent efforts in gene replacement, read-through of stop codon mutations, or antisense-induced exon skipping. Measurement of dystrophin expression can provide proof-of-mechanism or support dose selection [8,14]. The occurrence of trace dystrophin levels in muscle fibers, and in addition the incidence of strong dystrophin-positive revertant fibers in patients with DMD, should be reported and taken into account in the interpretation of dystrophin assessments using tissue homogenates such as RT-PCR, Western blot, or mass-spectrometer analysis. Generally, Western Blot provides information on the total amount of dystrophin present and immunofluorescence gives insight on the functional dystrophin present at the sarcolemma of individual fibers and thus the methods are complementary. IFA of muscle cross-sections can be used to differentiate a potential drug effect from trace and revertant fiber dystrophin expression. IFA can also focus on the dystrophin levels in muscle fibers while avoiding fibrotic areas and fatty cells that increase with disease progression. Nevertheless, comparison of two biopsies remains best when both biopsies have been sampled from areas of similar relative muscle content. A disadvantage for IFA may be that image analysis of cross-sections requires relatively well preserved morphology of the biopsy and to obtain and preserve high quality samples without freeze artifacts may be a challenge in multicenter, international trials.

We present here an objective, sensitive, reproducible, and standardized IFA method to assess dystrophin intensity levels per individual fiber in an entire fiber population in a semi-automated manner. The current IFA method uses double-staining for dystrophin and spectrin and the results have shown that the assay

Table 4. Reproducibility of detecting differences in dystrophin expression in DMD muscle biopsies by immunofluorescence using MANDYS106 antibody and Definiens intensity measurements (at high laser settings).

Sample	Experiment	Day	Number of sections	Number of fibers	Dystrophin membrane intensity MANDYS106 (au)				
					Mean	Intra-assay precision CV% sections	Inter-assay precision CV% experiments	Q90 mean	Ranking
DMD 3	3	1	2	777	255	6%	10%	635	4
	4	17	2	803	241	3%		662	
	7	527	4	1849	208	10%		589	
DMD 1	3	1	2	976	286	8%	14%	701	3
	4	17	2	1075	298	2%		729	
	7	527	4	2103	228	3%		604	
DMD 4	5	142	2	572	306	4%	17%	843	2
	6	324	2	579	427	5%		1152	
	7	527	4	2012	354	2%		997	
DMD 5	5	142	2	583	406	4%	2%	1094	1
	7	527	4	1375	397	6%		1148	

The intra-assay precision (CV%) was calculated for the mean dystrophin intensity of multiple sections of a biopsy/sample analyzed in the same experiment. Inter-assay precision between experiments performed on different days was assessed in two ways by ranking of the samples based on the dystrophin intensity in each experiment and by calculating the CV% from the mean dystrophin intensity in each experiment (different experiments 3, 4, 5, 6, and 7 were performed over the course of 1.5 years with the day of experiment shown in the table).
CV, coefficient of variation; DMD, Duchenne muscular dystrophy.

Table 5. Summary of experiments: different operators performing the staining, imaging, and Definiens image processing.

Experiment	Intensity of control beads (% laser intensity)	Operators		
		Staining	Image acquisition	Definiens processing
7	2302 (7%)	1, 9	4, 8	8, 9, 4, 10
6	2137 (7%)	1, 3	2, 4	3, 6, 7
5	2076 (7%)	1, 2	3, 4	3, 4
4	1887 (7%)	2, 6	5, 7	1
3	2295 (7%)	5, 6	4, 3	3, 6, 1
2	340 (1%)	3, 5	1, 4	1, 3
1	N/D	3	3, 4	3, 4, 5

N/D, not determined.

is (i) specific, (ii) sensitive, (iii) reproducible, and (iv) operator-independent. Specificity was shown by comparing the dystrophin-specific antibody staining with isotype staining for aspecific binding and by including a genetic control lacking the dystrophin epitope for the MANDYS106 antibody. Sensitivity was demonstrated by the detection of even minor differences at a wide range of dystrophin signal intensities from high dystrophin expression levels in healthy control samples to intermediate levels for BMD and low levels for DMD samples. Reproducibility was shown by the low intra-assay precision with a CV% between different sections of a biopsy generally less than 10%. The inter-assay precision between separate experiments performed over long interval periods was calculated to have a CV% between 2 and 17% for the DMD samples measured. The ranking of different biopsies and the percentage difference between post- and pre-treatment biopsies remained highly similar between different experimental days and using two different antibodies binding to the rod domain (MANDYS106) or to the C terminus of the dystrophin protein (ab15277). A calibration curve or quality control standards are not available for dystrophin measurement by immunofluorescence and the staining and absolute fluorescence can differ somewhat between experimental days. Therefore, a paired comparison of biopsies provides the best sensitivity and reproducibility when analyzed within the same experiment. Finally, the method employs semi-automated fiber recognition software using the spectrin staining as a mask. Therefore, multiple samples can be assessed relatively quickly and independent of operator bias, which is a major advantage over methods based on visually counting cells or selecting random areas for measurement [4–6].

Spectrin was chosen as the membrane control protein to detect individual fibers and to define a mask for measurement of the dystrophin signal intensity, as it shows a better co-localization with dystrophin than laminin (data not shown). In a previous report, spectrin levels were assessed by averaging all fibers in an image, and no statistical difference between disease and healthy muscle samples was found [4]. We observed, however, typically higher spectrin intensities in the BMD and DMD samples than in control samples. This is in agreement with earlier reports describing qualitative assessments of immunofluorescence images for spectrin in diseased tissue from neuromuscular diseases including DMD [12] and in avian dystrophic muscle [13]. In the current method, spectrin is used only as a membrane identifier, not for normalization of the dystrophin signal, so any such potential disease pattern would not affect the outcome. We are currently gathering data to assess trends in spectrin and dystrophin in a large number of DMD samples.

Employing a method that takes individual fibers into account and uses software for semi-automated measurements to reduce operator bias appears especially important in DMD because baseline biopsy samples show levels of trace dystrophin in almost all fibers. Therefore, the distribution of dystrophin expression over the different muscle fibers and the positive shift to a higher dystrophin (staining) intensity for the entire fiber population become key differentiators to detect a dystrophin difference upon treatment. Interestingly, the method showed that dystrophin intensities vary widely between fibers within one biopsy, and two- to threefold between fibers with the lowest and highest mean dystrophin intensity per fiber. Also, differences in the average dystrophin intensity were observed between different muscle groups and between different donors, which is in agreement with up to 40% difference between 2 controls reported previously using both epifluorescence and confocal microscopy [4–6]. The difference in dystrophin expression between fibers, muscle groups, and donors may be correlated to transcript levels, but it may also be regulated post-transcriptionally by, for instance, non-coding RNAs. In addition to the lack of a standardized control, dilutions are not possible and, hence, dilution linearity and accuracy cannot be demonstrated by immunofluorescence analysis. Various recent studies, that have depicted dystrophin intensity as % of control by immunofluorescence analysis, have reported a wide variety of trace dystrophin levels for DMD patients between 0% and 25% when compared to healthy control dystrophin intensity and those extrapolated intensity levels also differed dependending on the antibody used [4,5,15,16]. The wide variability in results and dependency on antibody indicate that proportional extrapolation from control is likely inaccurate. Although Western Blot analysis is generally less sensitive compared to immunofluorescence analysis, it does allow for direct comparison with different dilutions of control sample and thereby improved accuracy. Taylor et al. (2012) [4] and Anthony et al. (2014) [15] detected higher % of control levels of dystrophin for immunofluorescence compared to Western blot analysis for the same DMD sample. All these points are highly relevant for clinical studies aiming to assess dystrophin levels in pre- and post-treatment muscle biopsies or express dystrophin levels in percentages of control. The choice of the muscle to obtain a biopsy, the consistent use of that muscle during a study for that patient, and, in case of normalization to control, the choice of the healthy donor tissue may directly affect the outcome. It is, therefore, difficult to compare results between

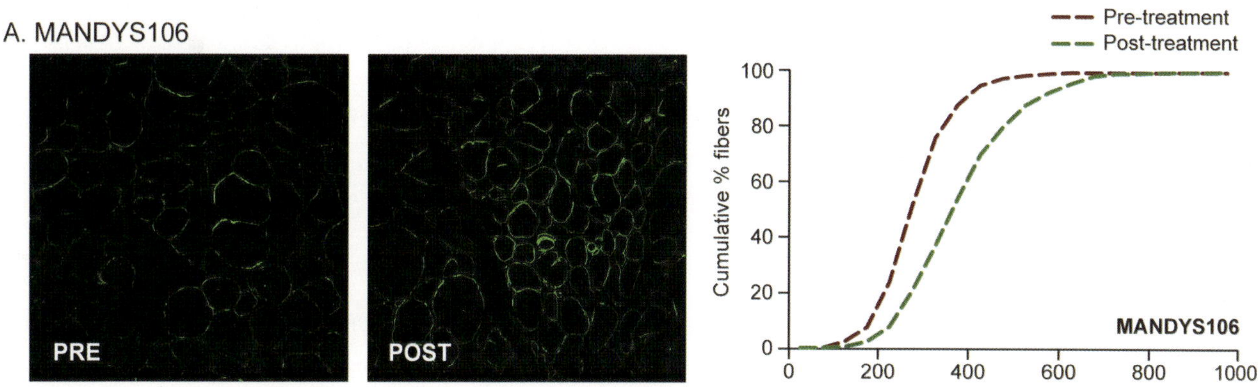

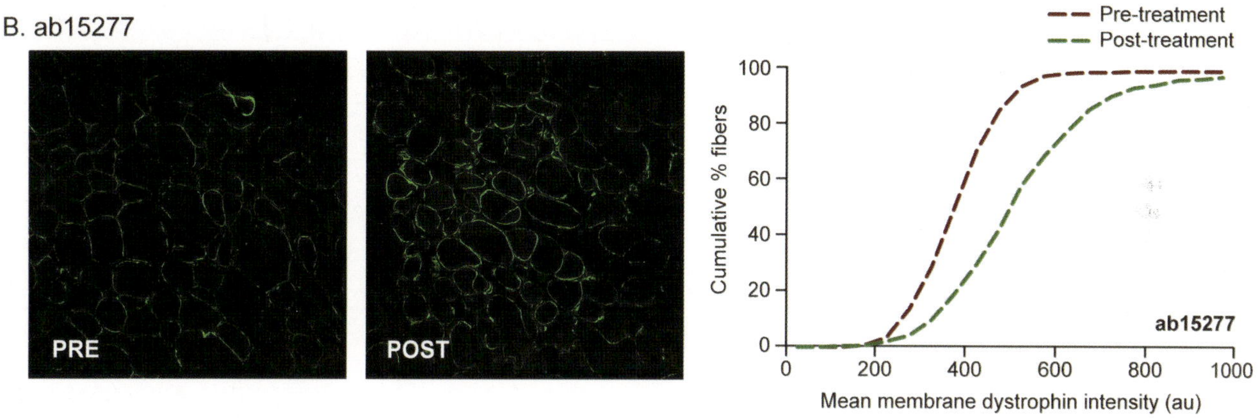

C.

Experiment MANDYS106	Operators			Intensity control beads 7% laser	Sample	Number of fibers analyzed	Spectrin membrane intensity (au)	Dystrophin membrane intensity MANDYS106 (au)		Dystrophin difference post- compared to pre-treatment		
	Staining	Imaging	Definiens processing					Mean (CV% 2 sections)	Q90 mean	Mean	Q90 mean	Significance (mean)
5	3, 5	2, 4	1, 4	2076	DMD 4 pre	572	1114	306 (4)	843	+32%	+34%	0.021
					DMD 4 post	741	1145	404 (1)	1131			
6	3, 1	3, 2, 4	6, 7	2137	DMD 4 pre	579	991	427 (5)	1152	+30%	+27%	0.000
					DMD 4 post	514	966	556 (2)	1460			

Experiment ab15277	Operators			Intensity control beads 7% laser	Sample	Number of fibers analyzed	Spectrin membrane intensity (au)	Dystrophin membrane intensity ab15277 (au)		Dystrophin difference post- compared to pre-treatment		
	Staining	Imaging	Definiens processing					Mean (CV% 2 sections)	Q90 mean	Mean	Q90 mean	Significance (mean)
8	1, 2	4, 3	3, 4	2299	DMD 4 pre	617	N/D	407 (2)	1030	+34%	+28%	0.000
					DMD 4 post	559	N/D	548 (2)	1314			
9	5, 2	3, 1, 4	3, 1	2116	DMD 4 pre	307	500	318 (6)	870	+19%	+17%	0.059
					DMD 4 post	604	390	378 (7)	1017			

Figure 5. Dystrophin intensities in pre- and post-treatment biopsies from DMD patient 4 (deletion exon 45) using two different anti-dystrophin antibodies. A. Representative immunofluorescence images (1 of 10) and dystrophin intensity measurements of the muscle fiber population of pre- and post-treatment biopsies using MANDYS106 (left) and the corresponding cumulative graphs (right). **B.** Representative immunofluorescence images (1 of 10) and dystrophin intensity measurements of the muscle fiber population of pre- and post-treatment biopsies using ab15277 (left) and the corresponding cumulative graphs (right). **C.** Reproducibility of the detection of dystrophin intensity difference between post-treatment and pre-treatment biopsies using MANDYS106 and ab15277. Percentage dystrophin difference = ([dystrophin intensity post-treatment – dystrophin intensity pre-treatment]/dystrophin intensity pre-treatment ×100). The statistical significance was calculated using a mixed model analysis taking into account the following covariance parameters: variance between images of one section, variance between sections, variance between slides. The mean difference was significant at the 0.05 level. No difference was observed for the spectrin staining. (au: arbitrary units; CV: coefficient of variation; N/D: not determined).

studies that have used different muscles and different reference muscle samples.

Hence, the presented immunofluorescence analysis provides in general high sensitivity and localization of dystrophin expression and in this study we have presented a methodology that provides a reproducible result with high precision when comparing biopsies. However, the absolute difference between two biopsies should be interpreted with care. In the presented example, a reproducible difference of 30% in dystrophin intensity has been measured, underlining that the assay can reliably detect small differences. In the DMD pre- and post-treatment biopsies, the dystrophin levels were quite low. Using Western blot analysis, biopsies for non-treated DMD patients with 44 flanking deletions showed levels in the range of 1–10% of control (data not shown). Interpretation of the result is beyond the scope of this report and more patients should be evaluated and compared to placebo treated patients to establish whether the difference is a change related to treatment. Furthermore, comparison of such result with clinical performance would be needed to establish whether a small difference of 30% from baseline would be sufficient or whether 2 or more fold change would be needed for clinical benefit.

In conclusion, we have developed a semi-automated, objective, and reproducible immunofluorescence method optimized for assessing dystrophin levels in muscle biopsies from BMD or DMD patients in natural history studies or clinical studies with compounds aiming to restore dystrophin expression. It is highly sensitive for small differences between samples with an intra-assay precision with a CV% lower than 10%, allowing careful relative-quantitative comparison of biopsies within one experiment. Such comparison of a pre- and post-treatment biopsy within one experiment was also shown to be reproducible on different experimental days and independent of operators. This method has been tested as part of an international consortium initiative, the Biochemical Outcome Measures study group, focusing on the optimization of dystrophin assays and the standardization between different laboratories and operators; the results of this initiative will be reported in a forthcoming publication by the study group. Using the assay, variability was noted between donors of (non-DMD) control samples and, also, different muscle groups appear to exhibit different expression levels. Therefore, the choice and consistent use of muscle samples should be taken into account in clinical studies when analyzing biopsies for dystrophin expression and interpreting the results.

Supporting Information

Figure S1 A. Representative immunofluorescence images (1 of 10 images) from the tibialis anterior muscle samples (from one control subject (CTRL2), two patients with DMD and four patients with BMD. Analysis was performed in the same experiment using the antibody ab15277 and 'control' imaging settings (1% laser intensity). **B.** Corresponding dystrophin membrane intensity distribution in the fiber populations analyzed (cumulative graphs). (au: arbitrary units; BMD: Becker muscular dystrophy; CTRL: control; DMD: Duchenne muscular dystrophy).

Figure S2 Spectrin and dystrophin intensity in the tibialis anterior muscle from control and pre-treatment DMD and BMD muscle samples assessed by immunofluorescence staining and Definiens analysis. In general, spectrin levels appear somewhat lower in control samples but no consistent differences between DMD and BMD samples were observed. **A.** Tibialis anterior muscle from healthy control 2 was compared with two patients with DMD with exon 51 flanking deletions (DMD 1: deletion exon 48–50, DMD 2: deletion exon 45–50) and four patients with BMD); Dystrophin levels (from a MANDYS106-double staining with an anti-spectrin antibody) are different between the DMD, BMD and control samples. **B.** Spectrin levels for these same samples, measured from the staining with isotype for MANDYS106 with an anti-spectrin antibody. **C.** Tibialis anterior muscle from healthy control 1 was compared with two patients with DMD with exon 51 flanking deletions (DMD 1: deletion exon 48–50 and DMD 2: deletion exon 45–50). **D.** Tibialis anterior muscle from healthy control 2 was compared with two patients with DMD with exon 44 flanking deletions (DMD 4: deletion exon 45; DMD 5: deletion exon 45) (au: arbitrary units; BMD: Becker muscular dystrophy; CTRL: control; DMD: Duchenne muscular dystrophy).

Table S1 Overview DMD114117 and PRO044 hospital committees.

Acknowledgments

Operators L. Brasz, E. Geers, G. van Haalem, S. van Wijngaarden, P. de Bruijn and R. Kuper for performing experiments. For supplying biopsy muscle material: Prof. dr. H.W. Niessen (Department of Pathology/Cardiac Surgery, VU University Medical Centre, Amsterdam, the Netherlands) and Prof. dr J.J. Verschuuren (Leiden University Medical Centre, Leiden, the Netherlands). T. Mrowiec (Definiens AG Germany) for development of rule set for dystrophin measurements using the Definiens software. For review and discussion: Dr. S. Hood and R. Geeske (GlaxoSmithKline, UK and USA). Dr G. Morris (Wolfson Centre for Inherited Neuromuscular Disease, RJAH Orthopaedic Hospital, UK) for providing MANDYS106. Prof. dr. T. Stijnen (Department of Medical Statistics and Bioinformatics, Leiden University Medical Center, the Netherlands) for statistical analysis. The authors take full responsibility for the content of the paper but thank Sarah Brown BSc (Hons) and Catherine Kidd PhD (Caudex Medical, Oxford, UK, supported by Prosensa Therapeutics BV) for editorial assistance.

Author Contributions

Conceived and designed the experiments: JAS AL SK CB SG. Performed the experiments: JT SG CB DK. Analyzed the data: JT SG CB DK JAS AL SK. Wrote the paper: SK JD CB AL GC.

References

1. van Deutekom JC, de Kimpe SJ, Campion GC (2013) Antisense oligonucleotides as personalized medicine for Duchenne muscular dystrophy. Drug Discov Today: Ther Strat: doi: 10.1016/j.ddstr.2013.04.001.
2. Nicholson LV, Johnson MA, Gardner-Medwin D, Bhattacharya S, Harris JB (1990) Heterogeneity of dystrophin expression in patients with Duchenne and Becker muscular dystrophy. Acta Neuropathol 80: 239–250.
3. Voit T, Stuettgen P, Cremer M, Goebel HH (1991) Dystrophin as a diagnostic marker in Duchenne and Becker muscular dystrophy. Correlation of immunofluorescence and western blot. Neuropediatrics 22: 152–162.
4. Taylor LE, Kaminoh YJ, Rodesch CK, Flanigan KM (2012) Quantification of dystrophin immunofluorescence in dystrophinopathy muscle specimens. Neuropathol Appl Neurobiol 38: 591–601.
5. Arechavala-Gomeza V, Kinali M, Feng L, Brown SC, Sewry C, et al. (2010) Immunohistological intensity measurements as a tool to assess sarcolemma associated protein expression. Neuropathol Appl Neurobiol 36: 265–274.
6. Arechavala-Gomeza V, Kinali M, Feng L, Guglieri M, Edge G, et al. (2010) Revertant fibres and dystrophin traces in Duchenne muscular dystrophy: implication for clinical trials. Neuromuscul Disord 20: 295–301.
7. Lourbakos A, Sipkens J, Beekman C, Kreuger D, Brasz L, et al. (2011) The incidence of revertant and trace dystrophin expression in muscle biopsies of Duchenne Muscular Dystrophy patients with different exon deletions [P1.6]. Neuromuscul Disord. 21: 643.
8. van Deutekom JC, Janson AA, Ginjaar IB, Frankhuizen WS, Aartsma-Rus A, et al. (2007) Local dystrophin restoration with antisense oligonucleotide PRO051. N Engl J Med 357: 2677–2686.
9. Nguyen TM, Cartwright AJ, Morris GE, Love DR, Bloomfield JF, et al. (1990) Monoclonal antibodies against defined regions of the muscular dystrophy protein, dystrophin. FEBS Lett 262: 237–240.
10. Nguyen TM, Morris GE (1993) Use of epitope libraries to identify exon-specific monoclonal antibodies for characterization of altered dystrophins in muscular dystrophy. Am J Hum Genet 52: 1
11. Hollinger K, Yang CX, Montz RE, Nonneman D, Ross JW, et al. (2014) Dystrophin insufficiency causes selective muscle histopathology and loss of dystrophin-glycoprotein complex assembly in pig skeletal muscle. FASEB J 28: 1600–1609.
12. Appleyard ST, Dunn MJ, Dubowitz V, Scott ML, Pittman SJ, et al. (1984) Monoclonal antibodies detect a spectrin-like protein in normal and dystrophic human skeletal muscle. Proc Natl Acad Sci U S A 81: 776–780.
13. Repasky EA, Pollina CM, Menold MM, Hudecki MS (1986) Increased concentration of spectrin is observed in avian dystrophic muscle. Proc Natl Acad Sci U S A 83: 802–806.
14. Kinali M, Arechavala-Gomeza V, Feng L, Cirak S, Hunt D, et al. (2009) Local restoration of dystrophin expression with the morpholino oligomer AVI-4658 in Duchenne muscular dystrophy: a single-blind, placebo-controlled, dose escalation, proof-of-concept study. Lancet Neurol 8: 918–928.
15. Anthony K, Arechavala-Gomeza V, Ricotti V, Torelli S, Feng L, et al. (2014) Biochemical characterization of patients with in-frame or out-of-frame DMD deletions pertinent to exon 44 or 45 skipping. JAMA Neurol 71: 32–40.
16. Cirak S, Arechavala-Gomeza V, Guglieri M, Feng L, Torelli S, et al. (2011) Exon skipping and dystrophin restoration in patients with Duchenne muscular dystrophy after systemic phosphorodiamidate morpholino oligomer treatment: an open-label, phase 2, dose-escalation study. Lancet 378(9791): 595–605.

Single Muscle Fiber Gene Expression with Run Taper

Kevin Murach, Ulrika Raue, Brittany Wilkerson, Kiril Minchev, Bozena Jemiolo, James Bagley, Nicholas Luden, Scott Trappe*

Human Performance Laboratory, Ball State University, Muncie, Indiana, United States of America

Abstract

This study evaluated gene expression changes in gastrocnemius slow-twitch myosin heavy chain I (MHC I) and fast-twitch (MHC IIa) muscle fibers of collegiate cross-country runners (n = 6, 20±1 y, VO_{2max} = 70±1 ml•kg^{-1}•min^{-1}) during two distinct training phases. In a controlled environment, runners performed identical 8 kilometer runs (30:18±0:30 min:s, 89±1% HR_{max}) while in heavy training (~72 km/wk) and following a 3 wk taper. Training volume during the taper leading into peak competition was reduced ~50% which resulted in improved race times and greater cross-section and improved function of MHC IIa fibers. Single muscle fibers were isolated from pre and 4 hour post run biopsies in heavily trained and tapered states to examine the dynamic acute exercise response of the growth-related genes Fibroblast growth factor-inducible 14 (*FN14*), Myostatin (*MSTN*), Heat shock protein 72 (*HSP72*), Muscle ring-finger protein-1 (*MURF1*), Myogenic factor 6 (*MRF4*), and Insulin-like growth factor 1 (*IGF1*) via qPCR. *FN14* increased 4.3-fold in MHC IIa fibers with exercise in the tapered state ($P<0.05$). *MSTN* was suppressed with exercise in both fiber types and training states ($P<0.05$) while *MURF1* and *HSP72* responded to running in MHC IIa and I fibers, respectively, regardless of training state ($P<0.05$). Robust induction of *FN14* (previously shown to strongly correlate with hypertrophy) and greater overall transcriptional flexibility with exercise in the tapered state provides an initial molecular basis for fast-twitch muscle fiber performance gains previously observed after taper in competitive endurance athletes.

Editor: Stephen E. Alway, West Virginia University School of Medicine, United States of America

Funding: Funding provided by National Institutes of Health (AG 038576). The funders had no role in study design, data collection and analysis, decision to publish, or preparation of the manuscript.

* Email: strappe@bsu.edu

Introduction

Athletes routinely reduce training volume prior to a major competition to help facilitate peak performance. A 3–4 week reduced training phase, known as taper, typically results in a 2–4% improvement in race performance [1–3]. In the last 30 years, taper research has identified increased power output at the whole muscle and single muscle fiber level as an important physiological basis for improved performance [1,2,4]. More specifically, tapering has been repeatedly shown to target fast-twitch muscle fibers by increasing their size [1–3] and power [1,2] with improvements in contractile performance largely accounted for by hypertrophy. However, little is known about molecular alterations that are contributing to performance gains in fast-twitch muscle fibers with tapering.

Recent methodological advances in our laboratory have established the ability to examine gene expression at the single muscle fiber level [5–7]. We sought to apply this novel approach with tapering to better understand potential molecular adaptations in fast-twitch muscle fibers. We were guided into these single muscle fiber gene studies by previous work in cross-country runners (for whom muscle biopsy samples were still available) that had an altered transcriptional response in mixed-muscle homogenate samples after identical 8 km running bouts in the heavily trained versus tapered state [2]. This alteration was intriguing since previous research has shown a blunted transcriptional response to exercise in well-conditioned skeletal muscle [6,8]. Thus, it appears that skeletal muscle of highly trained athletes may be more sensitive at the molecular level to various training phases than previously thought. Further support for conducting these single fiber gene studies was that the runners' MHC IIa fibers hypertrophied (+15%) and increased power output (+9%) with taper [2]. The combination of single muscle fiber gene measurements at strategically timed muscle biopsies after a heavily trained and tapered state 8 km run provided a unique opportunity to gauge the transcriptional flexibility of the MHC IIa fibers during these two training periods.

For the single muscle fiber gene experiments, we selected six genes that have been implicated in muscle size regulation and remodeling and included *FN14*, *MSTN*, *HSP72*, *MURF1*, *MRF4*, and *IGF1*. In developed human skeletal muscle, Fibroblast growth factor-inducible 14 (*FN14/TNFRSF12A*) was recently shown to strongly correlate with fast-twitch specific growth in response to exercise [6,9], the cytokines Myostatin (*MSTN/GDF8*) and Insulin-like growth factor 1 (*IGF1*) are components of major growth pathways [10], Myogenic factor 6 (*MRF4/MYF6*) is associated with exercise-induced remodeling [7], Muscle ring-finger protein-1 (*MURF1/TRIM63*) is a marker of ubiquitin-proteasome mediated myofibrillar breakdown [11], and Heat shock protein 72 (*HSP72/HSPA1A*) combats protein degradation [12]. We hypothesized that advantageous post exercise regulation of *HSP72*, *MURF1*, and *MRF4* previously observed in mixed-muscle with taper [2] would be more pronounced in MHC IIa fibers and that favorable *FN14*, *MSTN*, and *IGF1* expression would be targeted to the MHC IIa muscle fibers.

Materials and Methods

Subjects

Seven male runners from Taylor University's (Upland, Indiana) cross-country team volunteered to participate in a previous study [2]. Of these seven subjects, six were used for this investigation (age [y] 20±1, height [cm] 178±5, weight [kg] 66.1±5.1) (Table 1) as insufficient tissue at one time point for one subject negated molecular analysis. Details of the general study design and taper program are outlined in our previous investigation [2] and briefly profiled here (Figures 1 and 2). Subjects were competitive runners with 8 km lifetime best average performances of 26:32±0:32 (min:s). Prior to the investigation, subjects competitively participated in running for ~7 years (range: 4.5–10.0 y). Subjects were provided with written and oral information about experimental procedures and potential risks prior to providing written consent.

Ethics Statement

Support was granted by the coaching staff and all procedures were approved by the Ball State University and Taylor University Institutional Review Boards.

Experimental Design

A schematic of the study design is presented in Figure 3. Identical laboratory procedures were performed in the heavily trained (T1 and T2) and tapered (T3 and T4) conditions. Resting (heavily trained - T1, tapered - T3) and 4 h post exercise (heavily trained - T2, tapered - T4) gastrocnemius muscle biopsies were collected around an 8 km standardized indoor track run. MHC I and IIa fibers were individually isolated and pooled in order to conduct targeted fiber type specific gene expression analysis via reverse transcription quantitative real-time polymerase chain reaction (qPCR). The effect of taper was examined by conducting exercise response comparisons (T1:T2 and T3:T4) in both fiber types. Subjects were treadmill tested for aerobic capacity before and after the taper period.

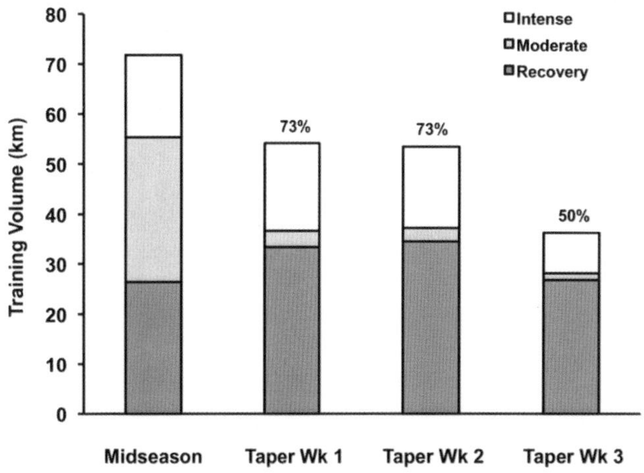

Figure 2. Summary of training volume and intensity during heavy training (11 wks) and each week of taper (3 wks), reproduced from Luden et al. [2] **with permission from the American Physiological Society.**

Training

Taylor University coaching staff prescribed the training performed throughout the 11 wk season (8 wks of midseason heavy training +3 wks of reduced-volume taper) based upon recommendations from our laboratory team. Training load was quantified using heart rate monitor data (Polar, Lake Success, NY) and self-reported running logs while mid-season training load (8 wks) was aggregated to represent one mean for heavy training. Average mid-season weekly running volume (6 d/wk) was approximately 72 km. During the 3 wk taper, weekly running volume in the moderate intensity range was progressively reduced

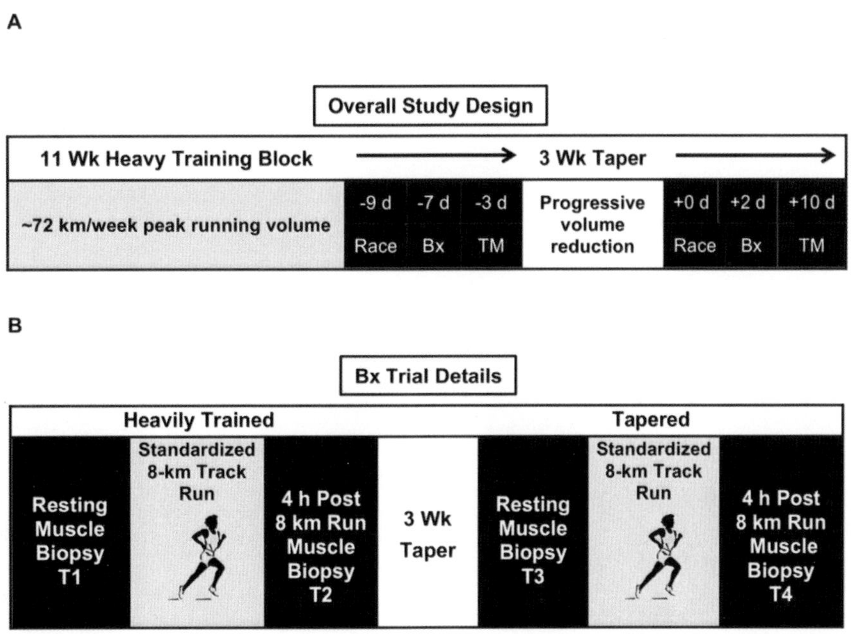

Figure 1. Overall study design (A), and Biopsy trial details (B). Bx = lateral gastrocnemius muscle biopsy, TM = Treadmill VO_{2max} testing.

Table 1. Subject characteristics and physiological data (n = 6).

	Heavily Trained	Tapered	% Δ
MHC IIa CSA (μm²)	5812±622	6631±758	+14%
MHC IIa Power (μN•FL⁻¹•s⁻¹)	58.7±6.4	63.5±7.3	+9%
VO_{2max} (ml•kg⁻¹•min⁻¹)	70.0±1.1	69.1±1.1	↔
X-Country Race Performance (min:s)	27:42±0:25	27:00±0:30	−3%

Data derived from Luden et al. [2] less one subject.

to 50% of mid-season training while high intensity training volume was maintained (Figure 2).

Standardized 8 km Indoor Track Run

Subjects were instructed to run 8 km on a 200 m indoor track between 15.2 and 16.0 km/h (~45–48 s/lap) depending on talent level (30:18±0:30 min:s, 89±1% HR_{max}). This pace was chosen because it corresponded to a training velocity commonly performed by this group. Lap times were verbalized throughout the run to ensure even pacing and each lap split was recorded manually. Subjects performed identical runs in the heavily trained and tapered state and were monitored by the investigative team.

Muscle Biopsy

Four muscle biopsies (T1, T2, T3, T4) were obtained from the lateral head of the gastrocnemius. The gastrocnemius was chosen based on its documented use during running [13] and the large amount of gastrocnemius research conducted in runners over the past 40 years. Subjects reported to Taylor University having refrained from physical activity for two days (~48 h). After 30 min of supine rest, a resting muscle biopsy was obtained (T1, T3) followed by a standardized 8 km run on a 200 m indoor track. Subjects then underwent 4 h of supine rest upon which a second biopsy was obtained from the opposite leg (T2, T4). The rationale for the 4 h post exercise biopsy time point was based on previous post exercise mRNA time course investigations from our laboratory [7,14]. From each biopsy, a muscle sample weighing ~15 mg was placed in 0.5 ml of RNA*later* (Ambion, Austin, TX), stored at 4°C overnight, and subsequently stored at −20°C until fiber separation and RNA extraction.

Muscle Fiber Separation and MHC Identification

See Figure 3 for a schematic representation of the method used for fiber type-specific isolation and fiber pooling for qPCR. Individual muscle fibers were isolated in RNAlater using fine tweezers under a light microscope at room temperature as previously described [5,11,15,16]. An average of 129 fibers were isolated from each of the 24 samples (6 subjects×4 biopsies) for a total of 3,096 fibers. Approximately one quarter of each fiber was clipped and placed into 40 μl sodium dodecyl sulfate (SDS) buffer (1% SDS, 6 mg/ml ethylenediaminetetraacetic acid [EDTA], 0.06 M Tris [pH 6.8], 2 mg/ml bromophenol blue, 15% glycerol, and 5% b-mercaptoethanol) for SDS-PAGE (sodium dodecyl sulfate polyacrylamide gel electrophoresis) MHC identification as previously described by our laboratory [5,11,15,16]. The remaining fiber segment was placed into an individual well of a number-labeled 96-well plate with 75 μl RNA*later* and stored at −20°C until MHC type was confirmed and before fiber type-specific pooling. Overall MHC fiber type distribution of each subject's lateral gastrocnemius was determined using all fibers extracted from each individual.

Fiber Pooling and RNA Extraction

Following MHC isoform identification, the corresponding MHC I and IIa fiber segments were located in the 96-well plate. Muscle fibers of each type (MHC I and IIa) at each time point (T1, T2, T3, T4) were extracted from their individual wells containing RNA*later* and combined in a tube containing 500 μl TRI Reagent (Molecular Research Center, Cincinnati OH) used for RNA extraction. RNA extraction was performed according to the manufacturers protocol (MRC) and total RNA concentration (4.07±0.15 ng/μl) was determined using the Quant-iT RNA assay kit (Invitrogen, Carlsbad, CA) in conjunction with the Qubit fluorometer (Invitrogen). Forty-eight samples (24 samples×2 fiber types) were ultimately generated containing 36±6 (range 23–54) fibers, an amount sufficient to yield an RNA concentration of > 1.5 ng/μl [6,7].

Reverse Transcription and qPCR

Oligo (dT) primed first-strand cDNA was synthesized (16.5 ng of total RNA) using SuperScript II RT (Invitrogen) and quantification of mRNA levels (in duplicate) was performed in a 72-well Rotor-Gene 3000 Centrifugal Real-Time Cycler (Corbett Research, Mortlake, NSW, Australia). Ribosomal protein, large, P0 (*RPLP0*) was used as a reference gene as we have previously described [17]. All primers used in this study were mRNA-specific (on different exons and crossing over an intron) and designed for qPCR (Vector NTI Advance 9 software, Invitrogen) using SYBR Green chemistry. The primer sequences for *FN14* were: Forward -ACTTCTGCCTGGGCTGCGCT and Reverse - TCTCCTGCGGCATCGTCTCC, Genbank number: NM_016639.2. Primer sequences and characteristics for *MSTN*, *HSP72*, *MURF1*, *MRF4*, and *IGF1* as well as qPCR parameters have been reported previously from our laboratory [2,5,7,14,18]. For each qPCR run, a melting curve analysis was generated to validate the presence of only one product and a serial dilution curve (cDNA made of 500 ng total RNA from human skeletal muscle; Ambion, Austin, TX) was generated to evaluate reaction efficiencies. The amplification calculated by the Rotor-Gene software was specific and highly efficient (efficiency = 1.03±0.02; R^2 = 0.99±0.00; slope = 3.24±0.04). The gene expression response to exercise (8 km run) was examined in the heavily trained and tapered state using the $2^{-\Delta\Delta C_T}$ (fold change) quantification method [14,19,20].

Statistics

Data were checked for normality and sphericity and original or log transformed data were used for statistical analyses. Within each fiber type, the gene expression response to exercise in the heavily trained and tapered state was evaluated using a repeated measures two-way ANOVA with factors of time (T1–T4) and training state (heavily trained and tapered). Due to the minimal number of hybrids (<8%) and no IIx fibers in these highly trained runners,

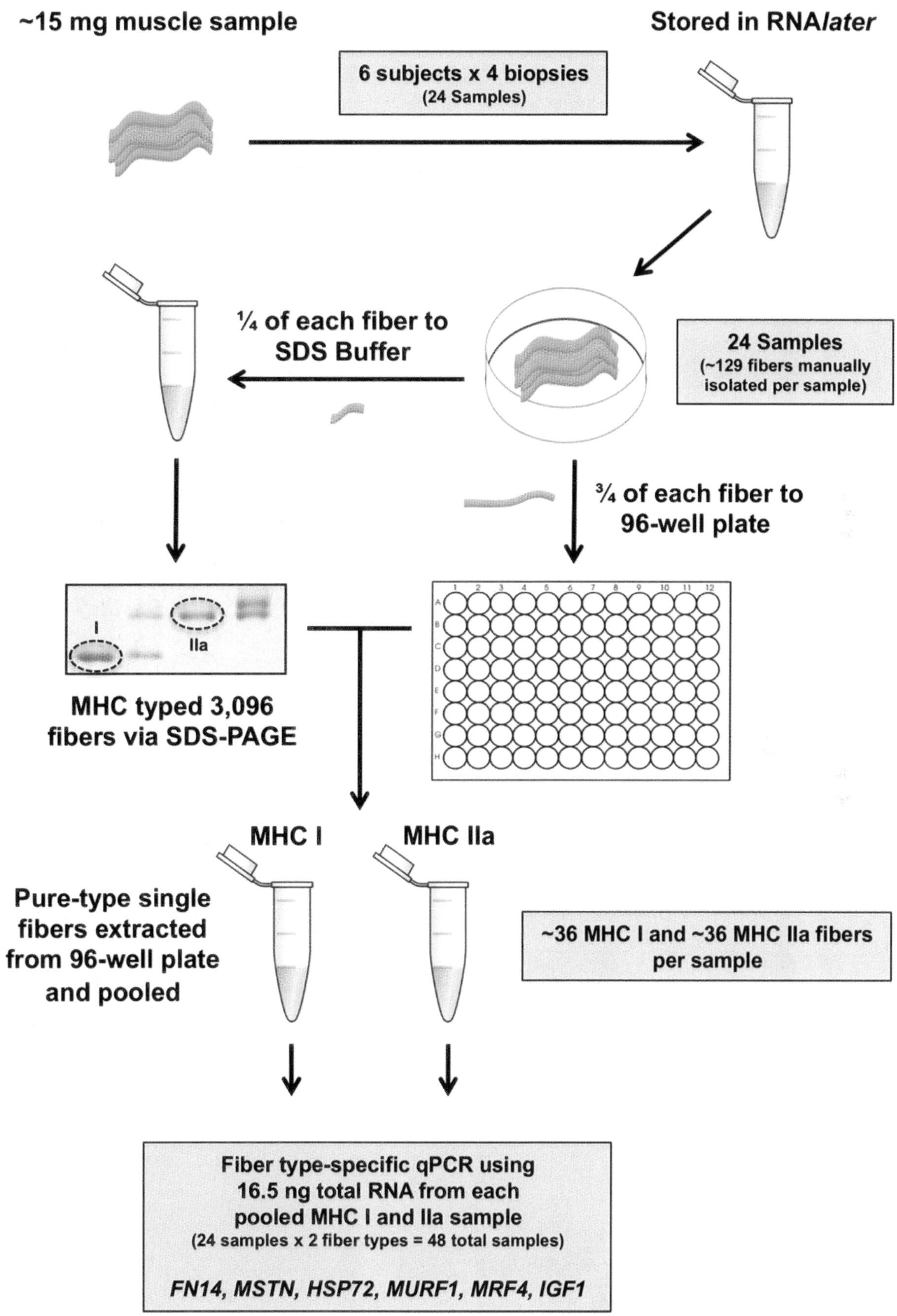

Figure 3. Schematic of method used to conduct fiber type-specific isolation of single muscle fibers for qPCR analysis.

gene expression analysis was limited to MHC I and MHC IIa fibers. All statistics were conducted in SPSS 17.0 for Windows, all data are presented as means ± SE, and significance was set at $P < 0.05$.

Results

Exercise-Induced (T1:T2 and T3:T4) Gene Expression in MHC IIa fibers

In the tapered state (T3:T4), *FN14* mRNA increased 4.3-fold (time and interaction effect, $P<0.05$, Figure 4) 4 h following the 8 km run. *MSTN* decreased 1.6-fold in the heavily trained state and 2.0-fold in the tapered state (time effect, $P<0.05$, Figure 5A). *MURF1* increased 2.7-fold in the heavily trained state and 4.0-fold in the tapered state (time effect, $P<0.05$, Figure 6). No changes were observed with exercise for *FN14* in the heavily trained state or *HSP72*, *MRF4*, or *IGF1* in the heavily trained or tapered state (Table 2).

Exercise-Induced (T1:T2 and T3:T4) Gene Expression in MHC I fibers

Exercise decreased *MSTN* 1.7-fold in the heavily trained state and 1.1-fold in the tapered state (time effect, $P<0.05$, Figure 5B). *HSP72* increased 1.7-fold in the heavily trained state and 2.0-fold in the tapered state (time effect, $P<0.05$, Figure 7). No changes occurred in *FN14*, *MURF1*, *MRF4*, or *IGF1* with exercise in the heavily trained or tapered state (Table 3).

Lateral Gastrocnemius Fiber Type

The average fiber type distribution (percentage) of the gastrocnemius in these runners was: 61.7±4.0% MHC I, 4.5±1.6% MHC I/IIa, 30.9±3.1% MHC IIa, 2.7±1.7% MHC IIa/IIx, and 0.2±0.1% MHC I/IIa/IIx. There were no MHC IIx fibers found in any subject. Fibers expressing multiple isoforms (MHC I/IIa, MHC IIa/IIx, and MHC I/IIa/IIx) comprised 7.4% of the total fiber population.

Discussion

The unique aspect of this investigation was the examination of MHC I and IIa gene responses in competitive collegiate runners after identical 8 km runs in the heavily trained versus tapered state. The 8 km running stimulus used in our study design reflects a typical weekly training run (~89% HR_{max}) these athletes performed throughout the competitive season. The post 4 h run time point coincides with anabolic and catabolic mRNA expression patterns following exercise [7,14] and captures elements of muscle remodeling. The main finding was that *FN14*, a gene strongly associated with fast-twitch hypertrophy [6,9], was robustly induced in MHC IIa fibers with exercise in the tapered state. Additionally, *MSTN* was suppressed with exercise in

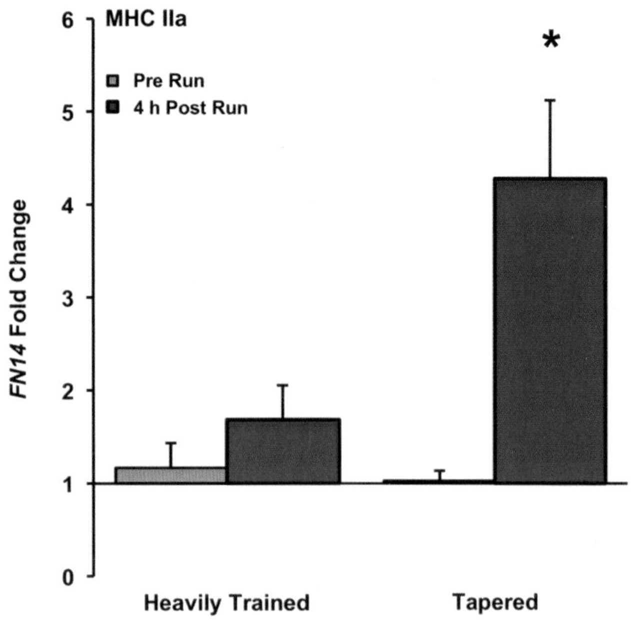

Figure 4. *FN14* gene expression response after an 8 km run in the heavily trained (T1:T2) and tapered (T3:T4) state in MHC IIa fibers, presented as fold change, *Time and interaction effect, P<0.05.

both fiber types and training states while *MURF1* and *HSP72* responded to running in MHC IIa and I fibers, respectively, regardless of training state. Contrary to the notion that exercise gene response [6,8,21,22] and adaptive potential [23] are attenuated as training status improves, these data indicate transcriptional flexibility in MHC I and IIa fibers of highly trained runners after an effective three week taper. The marked *FN14* response in MHC IIa fibers provides an initial molecular basis to support MHC IIa hypertrophy observed with taper, a stimulus that generally produces the highest calculated fast-twitch fiber growth rate in humans.

Tapered training of ≤3 weeks in aerobically fit runners [2], swimmers [1], and cyclists [3] can be calculated to confer MHC IIa growth rates of 5.0%, 8.0%, and 14.2% per week, respectively. By comparison, MHC IIa growth with progressive resistance training in young healthy individuals occurs at a maximum rate of 3.8% by 4 weeks [24] and approaches an asymptote by 12 weeks [25] as adaptation becomes more refined (see Table S1 for comprehensive review of fast-twitch growth with exercise). Despite being highly conditioned, fast-twitch muscle fibers of trained endurance athletes can rapidly change size in response to training adjustments which measurably affects whole muscle and single

Table 2. Genes not responsive to exercise in MHC IIa fibers in the heavily trained or tapered state.

	Heavily Trained		Tapered	
	T1	T2	T3	T4
HSP72	1.07±0.17	1.31±0.32	1.06±0.15	1.77±0.32
MRF4	1.03±0.12	0.84±0.09	1.15±0.28	0.9±0.11
IGF1	1.09±0.17	1.02±0.21	1.18±0.30	0.77±0.12

Presented as fold change, mean ± SE.

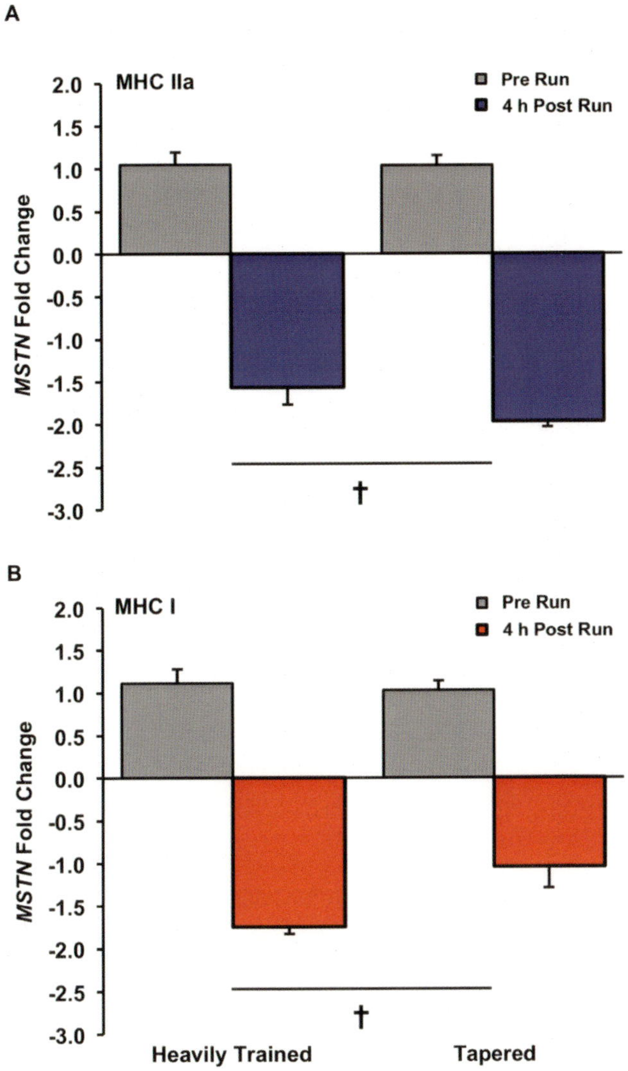

Figure 5. *MSTN* gene expression response after an 8 km run in the heavily trained (T1:T2) and tapered (T3:T4) state in MHC I (A) and IIa (B) fibers, presented as fold change, Main time effect for exercise, P<0.05.

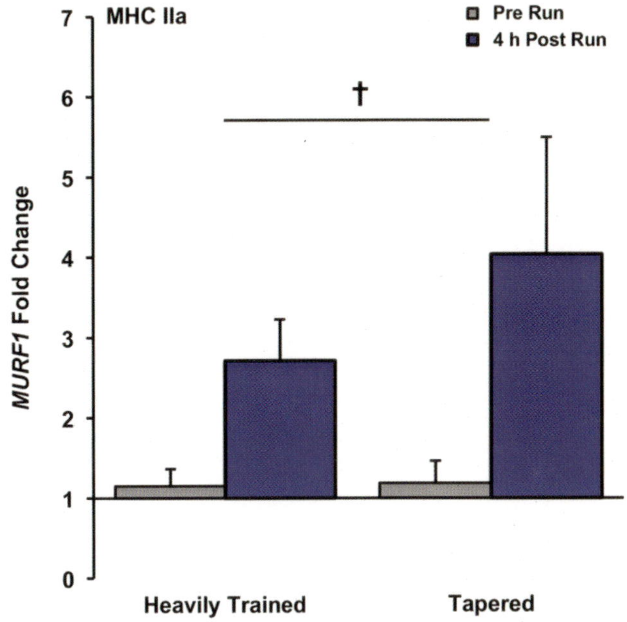

Figure 6. *MURF1* gene expression response after an 8 km run in the heavily trained (T1:T2) and tapered (T3:T4) state in MHC IIa fibers, presented as fold change, Main time effect for exercise, P<0.05.

fiber power [1,2,26,27]. However, the only transcript-level insight into mediators of fiber type-specific size regulation in humans has been in reference to resistance exercise. Acute resistance exercise elicits differential MHC I and IIa proteolytic mRNA responses [11] and activates a distinct MHC IIa transcriptome that precedes resistance training-induced increases in MHC IIa single fiber cross sectional area [6,9]. The current investigation reinforces the differential gene regulation concept, namely that *FN14* induction may augment the capacity of MHC IIa fibers to quickly grow and improve contractile function with taper.

The 4.3-fold *FN14* induction post run in tapered MHC IIa fibers aligns with our laboratory's recent finding that robust *FN14* expression after exercise is associated with isolated fast-twitch fiber size increases from resistance training [6,9]. A member of the TNFα superfamily, FN14 is a cell-surface receptor found on a variety of tissues including skeletal muscle [28] and appears to signal through the diverse NF-Kβ pathway [28,29]. While linked to atrophy in pathological conditions [30], FN14 also appears necessary for muscle proliferation, differentiation, and regeneration in mice and cell culture [31,32]. In this investigation, *FN14* gene induction after running in the tapered state was uniform (six of six subjects) and four responses were larger (≥4.4-fold) than the largest heavily trained response (2.8-fold). These occurrences highlight the magnitude of this fiber type-specific induction and further implicate *FN14* as an important component specific to the MHC IIa remodeling process in humans' response to exercise.

MSTN decreased post-run in both conditions and fiber types. Myostatin is a negative regulator of skeletal muscle mass that is blunted following a hypertrophic stimulus in humans [9,14,33–36]. Interestingly, Myostatin is also suppressed at the gene and protein level in humans after non-hypertrophic exercise [14,37,38]. This could signal a metabolic purpose for down-regulation [38,39] or Myostatin's supporting role in muscle remodeling and homeostasis after aerobic exercise [40]. It is worth noting, however, that the largest *MSTN* reduction observed here (2.0-fold) was in tapered MHC IIa fibers. Skeletal muscle reportedly has ~2–3 times the amount of Myostatin necessary to restrain growth [41] while animal [42–46] and human [47–49] fast-twitch muscle appears most sensitive to *MSTN* alterations. The 2.0-fold tapered state reduction in *MSTN* with running may have surpassed a physiologically significant threshold for Myostatin-mediated growth to occur and could have contributed to previously observed MHC IIa hypertrophy with taper [2].

MURF1 was responsive to run exercise in the heavily trained and tapered state in MHC IIa fibers. A marker of myofibrillar protein breakdown, *MURF1* increases after acute resistance [14,20,50] and endurance [14,51] exercise and is elevated concomitant with training-induced hypertrophy [52]. Increased *MURF1* with exercise may therefore represent a normal component of the MHC IIa remodeling process in healthy human muscle. *HSP72*, *MRF4*, and *IGF1* were not altered with exercise in MHC IIa fibers in either training state. In animals, heat shock protein is less constitutively expressed in fast-twitch than slow-twitch muscle [53–55] and is less responsive to exercise in human Type IIa fibers [56]. A lack of *HSP72* response to intense training

Table 3. Genes not responsive to exercise in MHC I fibers in the heavily trained or tapered state.

	Heavily Trained		**Tapered**	
	T1	**T2**	**T3**	**T4**
FN14	2.04±1.14	3.18±0.92	1.47±0.53	2.25±1.13
MURF1	1.12±0.19	3.94±1.88	1.17±0.29	1.04±0.27
MRF4	1.05±0.16	1.45±0.17	1.25±0.41	1.09±0.12
IGF1	1.09±0.19	1.03±0.13	1.06±0.17	0.77±0.06

Presented as fold change, mean ± SE.

and taper may therefore reflect a normal pattern of heat shock protein expression in MHC IIa fibers. *MRF4* induction after taper observed previously in mixed-muscle of these runners was relatively modest (1.4 fold) [2] and was abolished at the single fiber level in both fiber types. This discrepancy could result from a combinatorial effect of all fiber types yielding significant *MRF4* expression in mixed-muscle or the potential influence of satellite cells (express *MRF4* upon activation [57,58]). Common mRNA markers of quiescent satellite cells (*NCAM1, CD34, CDH15, CALCR*) are present in fibers mechanically dissected using the method described here [6] which suggests satellite cell presence but the extent of satellite cell adhesion has not yet been determined. IGF1 activates the Akt/mTOR pathway and is strongly implicated in exercise-induced muscle hypertrophy [10]. However, *IGF1* transcript is shown to not change appreciably in the early recovery from aerobic [18] or resistance exercise [18,59,60] which agrees with our findings.

HSP72 responded to exercise in MHC I fibers in both training states. This induction is consistent with greater HSP72 protein levels in Type I vs IIa fibers following 30 minutes of acute exercise [56]. In well-conditioned aerobic athletes, the greatest increase in basal HSP72 protein level occurs with intensified training but overall content peaks following a reduced training period [61]. While speculative, it is conceivable that improved translational efficiency in reaction to tapering along with a slightly more pronounced *HSP72* response to exercise in tapered MHC I fibers (Figure 7) of the trained runners studied here ultimately results in greater HSP72 protein levels after taper. This could be interpreted as a positive adjustment to the post run cellular environment that would aid in the localized stress tolerance of intense exercise performance [12] that coincides with peak level competition [1,2,4].

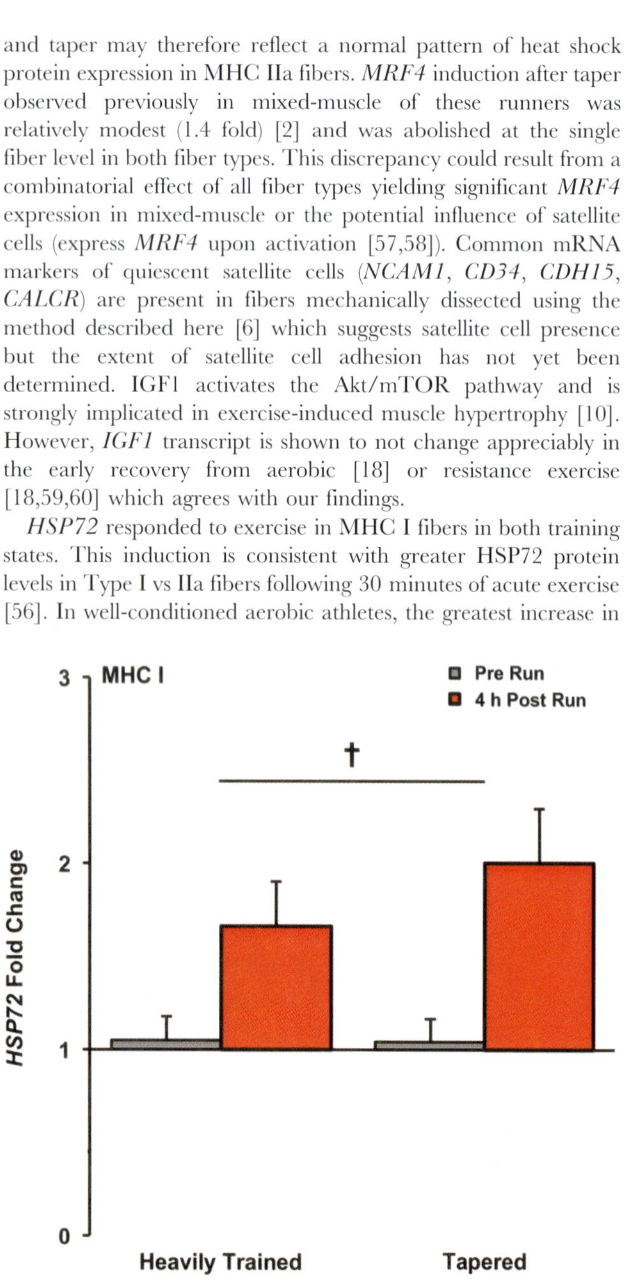

Figure 7. ***HSP72* gene expression response after an 8 km run in the heavily trained (T1:T2) and tapered (T3:T4) state in MHC I fibers, presented as fold change, Main time effect for exercise, P<0.05.**

A properly conducted taper program in athletes prior to peak competition improves performance that appears to be mediated, in part, by increased power at the whole muscle and single muscle fiber level. The single muscle fiber performance gains with taper are targeted to MHC IIa fibers and are primarily driven by hypertrophy [1,2]. The current study extends these MHC IIa-specific muscle fiber adaptations with taper to the molecular level and reports a sizeable *FN14* induction in the tapered state that may have contributed to rapid fast-twitch remodeling. A potentially meaningful *MSTN* suppression with tapered state exercise may also help support a favorable fast-twitch growth environment. We speculate that intense aerobic training periods reduce MHC IIa plasticity of growth-related gene targets and that taper reverses this process. To what extent the taper-induced MHC IIa adaptations are due to super-compensation from intense training or recovery to levels prior to the heavy training phase has not been established. The current study illustrates how tapering can promote transcriptional flexibility not previously thought possible in well-conditioned muscle [6,8]. These basic alterations at the molecular level provide a framework for expanded studies (i.e. transcriptome, protein quantification, epigenetics, etc.) to further our understanding of MHC IIa plasticity with exercise training paradigms.

Supporting Information

Table S1 Summary of literature on selective fast-twitch size alterations in young healthy individuals.

Acknowledgments

We would like to thank the Taylor University cross-country team, Ted Bowers (head coach), and the coaching staff for their enthusiastic participation in this research. Thank you to Dr. David Costill for his review and comments on the manuscript. We also wish to thank Drs. Erik Hayes, Andrew Galpin, Matt Harber, and Todd Trappe for their assistance with data collection during the taper project and Dr. Holmes Finch for his invaluable insight concerning statistics.

Author Contributions

Conceived and designed the experiments: ST K. Murach NL UR. Performed the experiments: K. Murach UR BW K. Minchev BJ JB. Analyzed the data: K. Murach UR BJ ST. Contributed reagents/materials/analysis tools: ST. Wrote the paper: K. Murach ST.

References

1. Trappe S, Costill D, Thomas R (2000) Effect of swim taper on whole muscle and single muscle fiber contractile properties. Med Sci Sports Exerc 32: 48–56.
2. Luden N, Hayes E, Galpin A, Minchev K, Jemiolo B, et al. (2010) Myocellular basis for tapering in competitive distance runners. J Appl Physiol 108: 1501–1509.
3. Neary JP, Martin TP, Quinney HA (2003) Effects of taper on endurance cycling capacity and single muscle fiber properties. Med Sci Sports Exerc 35: 1875–1881.
4. Costill D, King D, Thomas R, Hagreaves M (1985) Effects of Reduced Training on Muscular Power in Swimmers. The Physician and Sports Medicine 13: 94–101.
5. Jemiolo B, Trappe S (2004) Single muscle fiber gene expression in human skeletal muscle: validation of internal control with exercise. Biochem Biophys Res Commun 320: 1043–1050.
6. Raue U, Trappe TA, Estrem ST, Qian HR, Helvering LM, et al. (2012) Transcriptome signature of resistance exercise adaptations: mixed muscle and fiber type specific profiles in young and old adults. J Appl Physiol 112: 1625–1636.
7. Yang Y, Creer A, Jemiolo B, Trappe S (2005) Time course of myogenic and metabolic gene expression in response to acute exercise in human skeletal muscle. J Appl Physiol 98: 1745–1752.
8. Schmutz S, Dapp C, Wittwer M, Vogt M, Hoppeler H, et al. (2006) Endurance training modulates the muscular transcriptome response to acute exercise. Pflugers Arch 451: 678–687.
9. Raue U, Slivka D, Minchev K, Trappe S (2009) Improvements in whole muscle and myocellular function are limited with high-intensity resistance training in octogenarian women. J Appl Physiol 106: 1611–1617.
10. Harridge SD (2007) Plasticity of human skeletal muscle: gene expression to in vivo function. Exp Physiol 92: 783–797.
11. Yang Y, Jemiolo B, Trappe S (2006) Proteolytic mRNA expression in response to acute resistance exercise in human single skeletal muscle fibers. J Appl Physiol 101: 1442–1450.
12. Yamada P, Amorim F, Moseley P, Schneider S (2008) Heat shock protein 72 response to exercise in humans. Sports Med 38: 715–733.
13. Costill DL, Sparks K, Gregor R, Turner C (1971) Muscle glycogen utilization during exhaustive running. J Appl Physiol 31: 353–356.
14. Louis E, Raue U, Yang Y, Jemiolo B, Trappe S (2007) Time course of proteolytic, cytokine, and myostatin gene expression after acute exercise in human skeletal muscle. J Appl Physiol 103: 1744–1751.
15. Dickinson JM, Lee JD, Sullivan BE, Harber MP, Trappe SW, et al. (2010) A new method to study in vivo protein synthesis in slow- and fast-twitch muscle fibers and initial measurements in humans. J Appl Physiol 108: 1410–1416.
16. Galpin AJ, Raue U, Jemiolo B, Trappe TA, Harber MP, et al. (2012) Human skeletal muscle fiber type specific protein content. Anal Biochem 425: 175–182.
17. Trappe TA, Carroll CC, Jemiolo B, Trappe SW, Dossing S, et al. (2008) Cyclooxygenase mRNA expression in human patellar tendon at rest and after exercise. Am J Physiol Regul Integr Comp Physiol 294: R192–199.
18. Coffey VG, Jemiolo B, Edge J, Garnham AP, Trappe SW, et al. (2009) Effect of consecutive repeated sprint and resistance exercise bouts on acute adaptive responses in human skeletal muscle. Am J Physiol Regul Integr Comp Physiol 297: R1441–1451.
19. Livak KJ, Schmittgen TD (2001) Analysis of relative gene expression data using real-time quantitative PCR and the 2(-Delta Delta C(T)) Method. Methods 25: 402–408.
20. Raue U, Slivka D, Jemiolo B, Hollon C, Trappe S (2007) Proteolytic gene expression differs at rest and after resistance exercise between young and old women. J Gerontol A Biol Sci Med Sci 62: 1407–1412.
21. Egan B, O'Connor PL, Zierath JR, O'Gorman DJ (2013) Time course analysis reveals gene-specific transcript and protein kinetics of adaptation to short-term aerobic exercise training in human skeletal muscle. PLoS One 8: e74098.
22. Perry CG, Lally J, Holloway GP, Heigenhauser GJ, Bonen A, et al. (2010) Repeated transient mRNA bursts precede increases in transcriptional and mitochondrial proteins during training in human skeletal muscle. J Physiol 588: 4795–4810.
23. Saltin B, Henriksson J, Nygaard E, Andersen P, Jansson E (1977) Fiber types and metabolic potentials of skeletal muscles in sedentary man and endurance runners. Ann N Y Acad Sci 301: 3–29.
24. Woolstenhulme MT, Conlee RK, Drummond MJ, Stites AW, Parcell AC (2006) Temporal response of desmin and dystrophin proteins to progressive resistance exercise in human skeletal muscle. J Appl Physiol (1985) 100: 1876–1882.
25. Hakkinen K, Alen M, Komi PV (1985) Changes in isometric force- and relaxation-time, electromyographic and muscle fibre characteristics of human skeletal muscle during strength training and detraining. Acta Physiol Scand 125: 573–585.
26. Fitts RH, Costill DL, Gardetto PR (1989) Effect of swim exercise training on human muscle fiber function. J Appl Physiol 66: 465–475.
27. Kohn TA, Essen-Gustavsson B, Myburgh KH (2011) Specific muscle adaptations in type II fibers after high-intensity interval training of well-trained runners. Scand J Med Sci Sports 21: 765–772.
28. Winkles JA (2008) The TWEAK-Fn14 cytokine-receptor axis: discovery, biology and therapeutic targeting. Nat Rev Drug Discov 7: 411–425.
29. Burkly LC, Michaelson JS, Zheng TS (2011) TWEAK/Fn14 pathway: an immunological switch for shaping tissue responses. Immunol Rev 244: 99–114.
30. Mittal A, Bhatnagar S, Kumar A, Lach-Trifilieff E, Wauters S, et al. (2010) The TWEAK-Fn14 system is a critical regulator of denervation-induced skeletal muscle atrophy in mice. J Cell Biol 188: 833–849.
31. Dogra C, Hall SL, Wedhas N, Linkhart TA, Kumar A (2007) Fibroblast growth factor inducible 14 (Fn14) is required for the expression of myogenic regulatory factors and differentiation of myoblasts into myotubes. Evidence for TWEAK-independent functions of Fn14 during myogenesis. J Biol Chem 282: 15000–15010.
32. Girgenrath M, Weng S, Kostek CA, Browning B, Wang M, et al. (2006) TWEAK, via its receptor Fn14, is a novel regulator of mesenchymal progenitor cells and skeletal muscle regeneration. EMBO J 25: 5826–5839.
33. Costa A, Dalloul H, Hegyesi H, Apor P, Csende Z, et al. (2007) Impact of repeated bouts of eccentric exercise on myogenic gene expression. Eur J Appl Physiol 101: 427–436.
34. Kim JS, Petrella JK, Cross JM, Bamman MM (2007) Load-mediated downregulation of myostatin mRNA is not sufficient to promote myofiber hypertrophy in humans: a cluster analysis. J Appl Physiol 103: 1488–1495.
35. Raue U, Slivka D, Jemiolo B, Hollon C, Trappe S (2006) Myogenic gene expression at rest and after a bout of resistance exercise in young (18–30 yr) and old (80–89 yr) women. J Appl Physiol 101: 53–59.
36. Roth SM, Martel GF, Ferrell RE, Metter EJ, Hurley BF, et al. (2003) Myostatin gene expression is reduced in humans with heavy-resistance strength training: a brief communication. Exp Biol Med (Maywood) 228: 706–709.
37. Harber MP, Crane JD, Dickinson JM, Jemiolo B, Raue U, et al. (2009) Protein synthesis and the expression of growth-related genes are altered by running in human vastus lateralis and soleus muscles. Am J Physiol Regul Integr Comp Physiol 296: R708–714.
38. Hittel DS, Axelson M, Sarna N, Shearer J, Huffman KM, et al. (2010) Myostatin decreases with aerobic exercise and associates with insulin resistance. Med Sci Sports Exerc 42: 2023–2029.
39. Chen Y, Ye J, Cao L, Zhang Y, Xia W, et al. (2010) Myostatin regulates glucose metabolism via the AMP-activated protein kinase pathway in skeletal muscle cells. Int J Biochem Cell Biol 42: 2072–2081.
40. Matsakas A, Friedel A, Hertrampf T, Diel P (2005) Short-term endurance training results in a muscle-specific decrease of myostatin mRNA content in the rat. Acta Physiol Scand 183: 299–307.
41. Welle S, Burgess K, Thornton CA, Tawil R (2009) Relation between extent of myostatin depletion and muscle growth in mature mice. Am J Physiol Endocrinol Metab 297: E935–940.
42. Arounleut P, Bialek P, Liang LF, Upadhyay S, Fulzele S, et al. (2013) A myostatin inhibitor (propeptide-Fc) increases muscle mass and muscle fiber size in aged mice but does not increase bone density or bone strength. Exp Gerontol 48: 898–904.
43. Carlson CJ, Booth FW, Gordon SE (1999) Skeletal muscle myostatin mRNA expression is fiber-type specific and increases during hindlimb unloading. Am J Physiol 277: R601–606.
44. Liu CM, Yang Z, Liu CW, Wang R, Tien P, et al. (2008) Myostatin antisense RNA-mediated muscle growth in normal and cancer cachexia mice. Gene Ther 15: 155–160.
45. Magee TR, Artaza JN, Ferrini MG, Vernet D, Zuniga FI, et al. (2006) Myostatin short interfering hairpin RNA gene transfer increases skeletal muscle mass. J Gene Med 8: 1171–1181.
46. Wehling M, Cai B, Tidball JG (2000) Modulation of myostatin expression during modified muscle use. FASEB J 14: 103–110.
47. Jespersen JG, Nedergaard A, Andersen LL, Schjerling P, Andersen JL (2011) Myostatin expression during human muscle hypertrophy and subsequent atrophy: increased myostatin with detraining. Scand J Med Sci Sports 21: 215–223.
48. Reardon KA, Davis J, Kapsa RM, Choong P, Byrne E (2001) Myostatin, insulin-like growth factor-1, and leukemia inhibitory factor mRNAs are upregulated in chronic human disuse muscle atrophy. Muscle Nerve 24: 893–899.
49. Wojcik S, Nogalska A, Engel WK, Askanas V (2008) Myostatin and its precursor protein are increased in the skeletal muscle of patients with Type-II muscle fibre atrophy. Folia Morphol (Warsz) 67: 6–12.
50. Nedergaard A, Vissing K, Overgaard K, Kjaer M, Schjerling P (2007) Expression patterns of atrogenic and ubiquitin proteasome component genes with exercise: effect of different loading patterns and repeated exercise bouts. J Appl Physiol (1985) 103: 1513–1522.

51. Harber MP, Konopka AR, Jemiolo B, Trappe SW, Trappe TA, et al. (2010) Muscle protein synthesis and gene expression during recovery from aerobic exercise in the fasted and fed states. Am J Physiol Regul Integr Comp Physiol 299: R1254–1262.
52. Leger B, Cartoni R, Praz M, Lamon S, Deriaz O, et al. (2006) Akt signalling through GSK-3beta, mTOR and Foxo1 is involved in human skeletal muscle hypertrophy and atrophy. J Physiol 576: 923–933.
53. Hernando R, Manso R (1997) Muscle fibre stress in response to exercise: synthesis, accumulation and isoform transitions of 70-kDa heat-shock proteins. Eur J Biochem 243: 460–467.
54. Larkins NT, Murphy RM, Lamb GD (2012) Absolute amounts and diffusibility of HSP72, HSP25, and alphaB-crystallin in fast- and slow-twitch skeletal muscle fibers of rat. Am J Physiol Cell Physiol 302: C228–239.
55. Locke M, Noble EG, Atkinson BG (1991) Inducible isoform of HSP70 is constitutively expressed in a muscle fiber type specific pattern. Am J Physiol 261: C774–779.
56. Tupling AR, Bombardier E, Stewart RD, Vigna C, Aqui AE (2007) Muscle fiber type-specific response of Hsp70 expression in human quadriceps following acute isometric exercise. J Appl Physiol (1985) 103: 2105–2111.
57. Cornelison DD, Wold BJ (1997) Single-cell analysis of regulatory gene expression in quiescent and activated mouse skeletal muscle satellite cells. Dev Biol 191: 270–283.
58. Yablonka-Reuveni Z, Rivera AJ (1994) Temporal expression of regulatory and structural muscle proteins during myogenesis of satellite cells on isolated adult rat fibers. Dev Biol 164: 588–603.
59. Hameed M, Orrell RW, Cobbold M, Goldspink G, Harridge SD (2003) Expression of IGF-I splice variants in young and old human skeletal muscle after high resistance exercise. J Physiol 547: 247–254.
60. Psilander N, Damsgaard R, Pilegaard H (2003) Resistance exercise alters MRF and IGF-I mRNA content in human skeletal muscle. J Appl Physiol 95: 1038–1044.
61. Liu Y, Mayr S, Opitz-Gress A, Zeller C, Lormes W, et al. (1999) Human skeletal muscle HSP70 response to training in highly trained rowers. J Appl Physiol 86: 101–104.

17

Redox State and Mitochondrial Respiratory Chain Function in Skeletal Muscle of LGMD2A Patients

Mats I. Nilsson, Lauren G. Macneil, Yu Kitaoka, Fatimah Alqarni, Rahul Suri, Mahmood Akhtar, Maria E. Haikalis, Pavneet Dhaliwal, Munim Saeed, Mark A. Tarnopolsky*

Department of Pediatrics and Medicine, Neuromuscular Clinic, McMaster University Hospital, Hamilton, Ontario, Canada

Abstract

Background: Calpain-3 deficiency causes oxidative and nitrosative stress-induced damage in skeletal muscle of LGMD2A patients, but mitochondrial respiratory chain function and anti-oxidant levels have not been systematically assessed in this clinical population previously.

Methods: We identified 14 patients with phenotypes consistent with LGMD2A and performed *CAPN3* gene sequencing, CAPN3 expression/autolysis measurements, and *in silico* predictions of pathogenicity. Oxidative damage, anti-oxidant capacity, and mitochondrial enzyme activities were determined in a subset of muscle biopsies.

Results: Twenty-one disease-causing variants were detected along the entire *CAPN3* gene, five of which were novel (c.338 T>C, c.500 T>C, c.1525-1 G>T, c.2115+4 T>G, c.2366 T>A). Protein- and mRNA-based tests confirmed *in silico* predictions and the clinical diagnosis in 75% of patients. Reductions in antioxidant defense mechanisms (SOD-1 and NRF-2, but not SOD-2), coupled with increased lipid peroxidation and protein ubiquitination, were observed in calpain-3 deficient muscle, indicating a redox imbalance primarily affecting non-mitochondrial compartments. Although ATP synthase levels were significantly lower in LGMD2A patients, citrate synthase, cytochrome *c* oxidase, and complex I+III activities were not different from controls.

Conclusions: Despite significant oxidative damage and redox imbalance in cytosolic/myofibrillar compartments, mitochondrial respiratory chain function is largely maintained in skeletal muscle of LGMD2A patients.

Editor: Jianhua Zhang, University of alabama at birmingham, United States of America

Funding: Work was supported with private donations from Jessica Heikoop and family and Jay's Drive Fore MD Golf Tournament. The funders had no role in study design, data collection and analysis, decision to publish, or preparation of the manuscript.

* Email: tarnopol@mcmaster.ca

Introduction

Limb-girdle muscular dystrophy (LGMD) are a heterogeneous group of genetic disorders and characterized by progressive weakness and wasting of the proximal limb girdle muscles and dystrophic muscle pathology. To date, 24 forms of LGMD have been identified with either autosomal dominant (1A-1H) or recessive (2A-2Q) inheritance patterns. Primary calpainopathy (LGMD2A, OMIM 253600), caused by mutations in the 40-kb *CAPN3* gene (OMIM 114240, mapped to 15q15.1-q21.1), is the most frequent form of recessive LGMD, with a prevalence of 1:15,000–1:150,000 depending on the population [1]. Disease onset generally occurs in early childhood to the second decade of life and is distinguished by an increase in serum creatine kinase (CK), symmetrical involvement of shoulder/pelvic girdles, and a dystrophic muscle pathology [2], ultimately causing loss of ambulation and wheel-chair dependence in adulthood [3].

The *CAPN3* gene contains 24 exons encoding for the 94-kDa Na^+/Ca^{2+}-dependent cysteine protease calpain-3 (CAPN3) [4,5], which serves both structural and proteolytic roles within sarcomeres of skeletal muscle [6,7,8], interacting mainly with α-actinin and titin to regulate myofibrillar disassembly, protein turnover, and mechanotransduction [9,10,11]. Muscle-specific CAPN3 consists of four domains (I–IV [Fig. S1]) and has three unique insertions sequences NS, IS1 (autolytic sites) and IS2 (titin-binding and nuclear translocation signal). Deficiency of CAPN3 is associated with build-up of toxic debris, oxidative damage, degeneration, and necrosis in LGMD2 patients, proving that it is indispensable for the maintenance and function of skeletal muscle. While the majority of the reported ~480 pathological *CAPN3* mutations impair autolysis and enzyme activity of calpain-3 (www.dmd.nl), titin-anchorage and substrate binding may also be affected [3], which is exemplified by the fact that 20–30% of LGMD2A patients exhibit normal calpain-3 protein levels and no loss in autolytic activity [12,13,14,15]. As such, the assessment of protein expression and Ca^{2+}-dependent autolysis of calpain-3 may be a cost-effective diagnostic approach (particularly in the absence of substrate-specific enzyme activity assays); however, *CAPN3* gene sequencing is essential for assigning a specific diagnosis in a significant portion of LGMD2A patients and remains the gold standard. Gene sequencing allows the practitioner to differentiate between primary and secondary calpainopathies and to perform genotype-phenotype correlations. Furthermore, the discovery of novel mutations improves our current understanding of molecular pathology, protein function, and may uncover previously unknown cellular roles of calpain-3.

Among the recently elucidated roles of CAPN3 is stabilization of the ryanodine receptor (RyR) and regulation of Ca^{2+} release during excitation-contraction coupling in the skeletal muscle triads. RyR expression, Ca^{2+} release, and CAMKII signaling are significantly reduced in CAPN3 knock-out (KO) mice, causing a decreased sensitivity to exercise stimuli, abnormal morphology and organization of mitochondria, decreased ATP production, and preferential involvement of slow-twitch muscle fibers [6,7,8,16]. Although proteomic studies support the notion that CAPN3 is an important regulator of mitochondrial function [16,17], and slow-twitch muscle fibers (↑ mitochondrial abundance in slow vs. fast) are predominately affected in LGMD2A patients [7,18,19], expression and activities of rate-limiting enzymes in the Kreb's cycle and mitochondrial respiratory chain (MRC) have not been assessed in calpain-3 deficient humans to date. Furthermore, the effect of calpainopathy on mitochondrial anti-oxidants are unknown despite the fact that oxidative damage is a hallmark of LGMD2A and mitochondria are postulated to generate the majority of cellular free radicals [20]. To this end, we measured oxidative damage, anti-oxidant capacity, protein ubiquitination, and expression/activities of rate-limiting mitochondrial enzymes in skeletal muscle of genetically confirmed LGMD2A patients. From our cohort of 14 subjects, we identified 21 mutations of the *CAPN3* gene, including five previously unreported sequence variants, and present biochemical data and *in silico* predictions of pathogenicity to strengthen genotype-phenotype correlations.

Methods

Clinical diagnosis, muscle biopsy and blood collection

All experiments were conducted according to the principles expressed in the Declaration of Helsinki. Written informed consent for muscle biopsies and approval for the use of archived patient samples were given by all subjects and the research ethics board at Hamilton Health Sciences (HIREB project # 10-327-T).

Fourteen out of 272 patients with confirmed or suspected muscular dystrophy in the Neuromuscular Disease Clinic at McMaster University Hospital exhibited clinical features consistent with LGMD2A. Major diagnostic criteria included absence of an autosomal dominant or X-linked inheritance pattern, atrophy and progressive weakness of shoulder/hip girdles, preferential posterior involvement of thighs/calves, sparing of facial, oculomotor, and cardiac muscles, and CK levels 5–80 times above normal [2,21,22]. Additional clinical features seen in some patients were waddling gate, winging scapulae, loss of ambulation, and wheelchair dependence. Upon review of clinical records, patients were further classified into Erb phenotype (scapulohumeral), early pelvifemoral phenotype ($\leq$12 y), classical pelvifemoral phenotype (Leyden-Möbius;13–29 y), late onset pelvifemoral phenotype ($\geq$30 y), or asymptomatic phenotype (hyperCKemia) if possible [13,21]. To confirm clinical diagnosis, whole blood from antecubital vein (N = 14) and/or a skeletal muscle biopsy from *vastus lateralis* (N = 12) were obtained and sent for *CAPN3* mutational testing and electron/light microscopy. Upon receiving genetic and pathology results, a sub-set of biopsies, previously snap-frozen in liquid nitrogen and stored at −80°C, were used for mitochondrial and CAPN3 mRNA/protein expression studies (WB and RT-PCR), oxidative damage/autolytic activity tests, and immunohistochemistry. For diagnostic purposes, those patients with one identified *CAPN3* sequence variant were prioritized for biochemical analyses and compared to subjects with proven pathology and age/gender-matched controls. Control muscles were obtained from our biopsy bank, which contains specimens from healthy subjects that have previously consented to the use of their tissues in our research. Bioinformatic software tools were used to predict pathogenicity of all mutations and strengthen genotype-phenotype correlations. Molecular tests and/or gene sequencing were done to rule out Duchenne/Becker muscular dystrophy (DMD/BMD), facioscapulohumeral muscular dystrophy (FSHD), Emery Dreifuss muscular dystrophy, LGMD2B (*DYSF*), LGMD2C-F (sarcoglycanopathies), and LGMD2I (*FKRP*) in select patients.

CAPN3 mutation and *in silico* analyses

Whole blood samples from patients were sent to PreventionGenetics (Marshfield, WI) and Athena Diagnostics (Worcester, MA) for *CAPN3* DNA sequence testing as previously described [23,24]. PreventionGenetics extracted genomic DNA using a Gentra PUREGENE kit and used PCR to amplify the full coding region (24 exons, 2466 basepairs) as well as ~50 bases of flanking intronic or other non-coding sequences. After cleaning of PCR products, cycle sequencing was carried out using the ABI Big Dye Terminator v.3.0 kit. Products were resolved by electrophoresis on an ABI 3130×l capillary sequencer and compared with reference sequences. Sequencing was performed separately in both forward and reverse directions. Similarly, Athena Diagnostics isolated highly purified genomic DNA, followed by automated unidirectional DNA sequencing of the coding region and 20 bases surrounding each exon. All abnormal variants were confirmed bidirectionally and detectable at an overall sensitivity approaching 99%. All test results were reviewed, interpreted, and reported by ABMG certified clinical molecular geneticists.

Pathogenicity of identified mutations was predicted using bioinformatics software as previously described by our laboratory [23,25]. Missense mutations were assessed by SIFT (sift.jcvi.org, SIFT sequence, UniProt-TrEMBL 2009 Mar) and PolyPhen2 (http://genetics.bwh.harvard.edu/pph2/) whereas intronic sequence variants were evaluated by the Human Splicing Finder program, version 2.4.1 (http://www.umd.be/HSF/). NetGene2 and BDGP Splite Site Prediction were used to verify the results obtained from HSF. Evolutionary conservation analysis of non-mutated nucleotides/amino acids was carried out using the UCSC Genome Browser (http://genome.ucsc.edu/cgi-bin/hgGateway). Mutations that alter highly conserved nucleotides/amino acids are likely to be deleterious, as these nucleotides/amino acids may be vital to mRNA/protein structure or function. As such, evolutionary conservation analysis was carried out with the UCSC Genome Browser using the "Feb.2009 (GRCH37/hg19)" assembly. Conservation of non-mutated nucleotides/amino acids across 46 species from the subphylum *Vertebrata* was assessed, including 36 mammalian species (*Mammalia;* 33 eutharians with chorioallontoic placenta, two metatherians with choriovitelline/yolk placenta, and one egg-laying prototherian), five species of bony fish (*Osteichthyes*), one jawless fish (*Agnatha*), two birds (*Aves*), one frog (*Amphibia*), and one lizard (*Reptilia*). Among these vertebrates were chimp, orangutan, rhesus, mouse, rat, guinea pig, rabbit, dolphin, cow, dog, elephant, opossum, lizard, *Xenopus tropicalis*, tetraodon, fugu, zebrafish, and lampreys. Mutation nomenclature adheres to the guidelines from the Human Genome Variation Society and nucleotide accession # NM000070.2 and protein accession # NP000061.1.

RNA isolation and quantitative real-time PCR (RT-PCR)

Total RNA isolation, first strand cDNA synthesis, and PCR amplification were performed as previously described with minor modifications [23]. Total RNA was extracted from approximately 25 mg of quadriceps muscle that was homogenized in 1 mL TRIzol® reagent (Invitrogen, Burlington, ON, Canada). Following homogenization, 0.2 mL of chloroform was added to each sample and the clear aqueous phase was transferred to RNeasy spin columns, followed by RNA isolation as per manufacturer's instructions (Qiagen, Germantown, Maryland, USA). The samples were DNase treated on the spin columns to prevent contamination with genomic DNA (Qiagen) and the absorbances at 230 nm (OD_{230}), 260 nm (OD_{260}), and 280 nm (OD_{280}) were determined using an ultraviolet spectrophotometer (NanoDrop 1000; Thermo Scientific). Measurements were repeated twice with a coefficient of variation of <7.5% and $OD_{260/280}$ and $OD_{260/230}$ ratios >1.5. Reverse transcription was performed on 150 ng of total RNA primed with random hexamers on a gradient thermocycler (MyCycler, Biorad, Hercules, CA, USA) as per manufacturer's instructions (Applied Biosystems, Foster City, CA, USA). Real-time polymerase chain reaction (RT-PCR) was performed with the 7300 Real-time PCR system (Applied Biosystems, Foster City, CA, USA) using SYBR® Green chemistry (PerfeCTa SYBR® Green Supermix with ROX, Quanta Biosciences, Gaithersburg, MD, USA) with standard thermocycling conditions. Primers, based on human gene sequences from GenBank (http://www.ncbi.nlm.nih.gov/genbank/), were designed for CAPN3 (NM_000070; F: 5′-atgactcggaggtgatttgc-3′, R: 3′-tttgggaacctcgtagatgg-5′) and β2-microglobulin (NM_004048.2; F: 5′-ggctatccagcgtactccaa-3′; R: 3′-gatgaaacccagacacatagca-5′) using Primer3 software (http://biotools.umassmed.edu/bioapps/primer3_www.cgi). Melt curve analysis was performed on all primers to ensure the validity of amplification. Tm for forward and reverse CAPN3 primers was 60.08°C and 59.93°C, respectively. CAPN3 mRNA expression was thereafter quantified using the $2^{-\Delta Ct}$ method and normalized to β2-microglobulin.

Western blotting

In order to minimize CAPN3 Ca^{2+} autolysis, whole quadriceps muscle was homogenized in 1:10 wt/vol in 0.4 M Tris hydrochloride, 25 mM EGTA ($[Ca^{2+}]$ <10 nM), 4% SDS, and protease inhibitor mixture (Complete Tablets, Roche) (pH 6.8) as previously described with minor modifications [11,26]. Immediately following homogenization, samples were heated to 95°C in SDS loading buffer for 10 min (0.125 M Tris hydrochloride, 10% glycerol, 4% SDS, 4 M urea, 10% mercaptoethanol, and 0.0001% bromophenol blue, pH 6.8) and stored at −80°C. A small aliquot of muscle homogenate, obtained prior to denaturation, was analyzed for protein concentration by a standard colorimetric assay [27].

The samples were loaded in equal amounts on 4–15% SDS polyacrylamide gels (10–20 µg), electrophoresed for one hour at 25 mA, and wet-transferred in Otter buffer (49.6 mM Tris, 384 mM glycine, 20% methanol, and 0.01% SDS) for 50 min at 400 mA onto 0.45 µM nitrocellulose membranes (Amersham Hybond-ECL, GE Healthcare). Following a 1-hr block step, membranes were incubated at 1:1000 (unless otherwise noted) with primary antibodies from Novacastra (CAPN 3*, NL-CALP-12A2, 1:100), Abcam (4-HNE#, ab48506, 1:3000; SOD1*, ab16831; SOD2*, ab13534), MitoSciences (total OXPHOS*, MS601), and Santa Cruz (Ub*, sc-8017; NRF-2*, C-20/sc-722; Keap-1*, sc15246) at 1:1000 overnight at 4°C. Standard HRP-linked secondary antibodies from GE Healthcare (NA931V [anti-mouse]; NA934V [anti-rabbit]) and Bio-Rad (anti-goat) diluted 1:5000 were used to detect primary IgGs, and reacted with Immobilon Western Chemiluminescent HRP Substrate from Millipore. Lastly, the membranes were developed in a dark room with Amersham Hyperfilm (GE Healthcare), and relative intensities of specific antigen bands or entire lanes (ubiquitin and 4-HNE) were quantified digitally with ImageJ 1.37v software. Blocking was performed in 1% milk* (m) or 5% m# (1×TBS), primary incubations in 1% m* or 5% BSA# (1×TBS), and secondary incubations in 1% m* or 5% m# (1×TBS). All incubation steps were followed by 3×5 min washes in TBS. CAPN3 blots were repeated twice with homogenates prepared from two separate pieces of muscle. Equal loading was verified by Ponceau S stain following wet transfer, which in our hands is a more consistent way of normalizing WB data compared to the use of single house-keeping proteins. Select membranes were probed for actin to confirm accuracy of Ponceau S.

Mitochondrial enzyme assays

Cytochrome *c* oxidase (COX; EC 1.9.3.1), complex I+III, and citrate synthase (CS; EC 2.3.3.1) activities were measured in quadriceps homogenates as previously described by our group [28,29,30]. All samples were analyzed in duplicate on a Cary 300 Bio UV–visible spectrophotometer (Varion, Inc., Palo Alto, CA) and the intra-assay coefficient of variation for all samples was less than 5%.

For COX activity, oxidized cytochrome *c* (Sigma C7752) was reduced by sodium ascorbate in 0.05 M potassium phosphate buffer (KH_2PO_4, pH 7.4). Fifteen microliters of muscle homogenate were added to 955 µL of 0.05 M potassium phosphate buffer and 15 µL of reduced cytochrome *c* in a 1.5 mL cuvette. The rate of oxidation of reduced cytochrome *c* was measured at 550 nm for 3 min at 37°C. COX activity was expressed in nmol/min/mg protein.

Complex I+III activity (NADH-cytochrome *c* oxidoreductase) was assessed by adding 15 µL of oxidized cytochrome *c* (40 mg/ml) to 1 mL of reaction buffer (0.1 M potassium phosphate and 1 mM sodium azide, pH~7.0, 37.5°C) in two 1.5 mL cuvettes. Following mixing, five µL of 1 mM rotenone (Sigma R8875) was added to a "rotenone-sensitive" cuvette (back) and 20 µl of muscle homogenate (~50–150 µg total protein) were added to both (front and back). A blank reading was done after 1 min equilibration and 5 µL of NADH was added to the front cuvette only at the start of the measurement. The reduction of oxidized cytochrome *c* was measured over two minutes at 550 nm. Activity was expressed in µmol cytochrome *c* reduced · min^{-1}· mg $protein^{-1}$.

CS activity was determined by measuring the formation of thionitrobenzoate anion. Fifteen microliters of muscle homogenate were added to 810 µL buffer (0.1 M Tris–HCl buffer, pH 8.0) along with 10 µL of acetyl CoA (7.5 mM in 0.1 M Tris-HCL buffer, pH 8.0) and 100 µL of 0.1 mM dithionitrobenzoic acid. The reaction was started by adding 50 µL of 9.0 mM oxaloacetate. Absorbance was measured at 412 nm for 2 min at 37°C. CS activity was expressed in nmol·min^{-1}·mg of $protein^{-1}$.

Calpain 3 autolytic activity immunoblots

The autolytic activity assay is based on the observation that full-length CAPN3 (94-kDa) undergoes gradual degradation into lower molecular weight products (56-, 58-, and 60-kDA [NL-CALP-12A2]) when incubated in a calcium-enriched saline solution for ≥ 5 min [14,15,31]. Cellular Ca^{2+} concentrations are ~100 nM at rest and increase to ~250 nM for 24 hrs following eccentric exercise, which is enough to activate CAPN3 autolysis [11]. As such, muscle was homogenized in 1:10 wt/vol saline solution (0.9% NaCl) with 5 mM $CaCl_2$ and incubated at room

Table 1. LGMD2A phenotypes, CAPN3 sequence variants, and *in silico* predictions.

ID / Sex	[A]Age / [B]Pheno	Mutation	[C]Ex/In	Nucleotide	Amino Acid	[D]Dom	[E]Zyg	[F]Nov	[G]Bioinformatics (missense/deletion) SIFT	Poly2	Cons
*P1	37/31/14	Transition	10	c.1250 C>T	p.Thr417Met	III	Het	N	Y	Y	42
M	Classical	Transition	4	c.500 T>C	p.Phe167Ser	II	Het	Y	Y	Y	44
*P2	39/38/34	Transversion	22	c.2338 G>C	p.Asp780His	IV	Het	N	Y	Y	42
M	Late	Transversion	22	c.2366 T>A	p.Leu789Gln	IV	Het	Y	Y	Y	43
*P3	39/36/36	Deletion	13	c.1573_1575 del	p. Phe525del	III	Het	N	–	–	37
F	Asympt.	Transition	20	c.2120 A>G	p.Asp707Gly	IV	Het	N	Y	Y	41
*P4	[†]56/53/18	Transversion	19i	IVS19+4 T>G	Cryptic splice site[$]	IV	Hom	Y	–	–	–
M	Classical	(intronic)		(c.2115+4 T>G)							
P5	w28/23/14	Transversion	4i	IVS4+1 G>C	Donor splice site[#]	II	Hom	N	–	–	–
M	Classical	(intronic)		(c.632+1 G>C)							
P6	w39/32/4	Deletion	4	c.550 del A	p.Thr184ArgfsX36	II	Hom	N	–	–	–
F	Early	(Frameshift)									
P7	54/50/39	Transition	11	c.1477 C>T	p.Arg493Trp	III	Het	N	Y	Y	40
F	Late	Deletion (Frameshift)	4	c.550 del A	p.Thr184ArgfsX36	II	Het	N	–	–	–
P8	w37/33/15	Deletion	3	c.483 del G	p.Ile162SerfsX17	II	Hom	N	–	–	–
M	Classical	(Frameshift)									
P9	15/14/13	Transition	9	c.1162 C>T	p.Gln388Stop	II	Het	N	–	–	–
M	Classical	Transition	11	c.1465 C>T	p.Arg489Trp	III	Het	N	Y	Y	38
*P10	54/50/c	Transition	13	c.1621 C>T	p.Arg541Trp	III	Het	N	Y	Y	38
M	Early	Transition	2	c.338 T >C	p.Ile113Thr	II	Het	Y	Y	N	33
*P11	40/33/30	Transversion	10	c.1257 T>G	p.Asp419Glu	III	Het	N	Y	Y	43
M	Late										
*P12	39/32/27	Transversion	11i	IVS11–1 G>T	Acceptor splice	III	Het	Y	–	–	–
F	Unspecified	(intronic)		(c.1525–1 G>T)	site[‡]						
*P13	45/45/38	Transition	1	c.224 A>G	p.Tyr75Cys	I	Het	N	Y	Y	35
M	Late	Transition	8	c.1099 G>A	p.Gly367Ser	II	Het	N	Y	Y	43
P14	30/28/15	Transition	4	c.527 T>C	p.Val176Ala	II	Het	N	Y	Y	43
M	Classical	Deletion	5	c.759_761 del	p. Lys254 del	II	Het	N	–	–	41

[A]Current age/age at biopsy (or genetic confirmation)/first symptoms noted, [†] = deceased, w = wheelchair, c = childhood;
[B]Phenotypic classification into Erb (scapulohumeral), early pelvifemoral (≤12 y), classical pelvifemoral (Leyden-Möbius;13–29 y), late onset pelvifemoral (≥30 y), or asymptomatic phenotype (hyperCKemia);
[C]*CAPN3* exon/intron;
[D]CAPN3 domains;
[E]Zygosity;
[F]Novelty;

Table 1. Cont.

ᴳ*In silico* predictions of pathogenicity of missense mutations with SIFT (Uni-Prot TrEMBL 2009 Mar) and PolyPhen-2 (v2.2.2r398). Y = pathological; N = benign. Conservation of exchanged/deleted amino acids with UCSC genome browser (Human Feb. 2009 [GRCh37/hg19] Assembly) across 46 species. Effects of intronic mutations on pre-mRNA splicing with Human Splicing Finder program (version 2.4.1).
§Mutation in 5′ end of intron 19 creates a cryptic splice site that is used instead of the regular site.
#Mutation in 5′ end of intron 4 destroys donor splice site.
‡Mutation in 3′ end of intron 11 destroys the acceptor splice site.
*Selected for further biochemical testing.

temperature for 5 min to ensure partial autolysis. The reaction was blocked by adding 1:1 vol/vol loading buffer containing Ca^{2+}-chelating EDTA (0.05 DTT, 0.1 M EDTA, 0.125 M Tris hydrochloride, 4% SDS, 10% glycerol, and 0.005% bromophenol blue, pH 8.0), followed by immediate heating at 95°C for 10 min and storage at −80°C. Protein concentration and CAPN3 expression were measured as previously described for the conventional Western blot. CAPN3 autolytic tests were repeated twice with homogenates prepared from two separate pieces of muscle. Equal loading was verified with Ponceau S stain as previously described.

Calpain 3 immunohistochemistry

Quadriceps muscle (1.5 mm^3) was embedded in Optimal Cutting Temperature compound (OCT) and immersed in liquid nitrogen-cooled isopentane, followed by cryosectioning of 8 µm slices that were mounted on polylysine-coated slides and stored at −80°C. The slides were brought to room temperature, fixed in acetone for 10 min, rinsed 2×2 min, and stained according to manufacturer's protocol using the Vector Elite ABC detection system (Vector Laboratories, Burlingame, CA) [32]. Briefly, slides were incubated with 1:50 CAPN3 (NL-CALP-12A2) for 60 min, followed by quenching of endogenous peroxidase activity with 0.3% H_2O_2 and washing 3×2 min. A secondary biotinylated anti-mouse antibody was applied at a 1:500 dilution for 60 min and samples washed for 3×5 min. Slides were then incubated with Vectastain ABC reagent for 30 min, washed 1×5 min, and exposed to peroxidase substrate (3,3′-diaminobenzidine; DAB) for 5 min. Following a rinse in tap-water, the sections were counterstained with hematoxylin for nuclear detail, dehydrated in ascending concentrations of ethanol, and cleared in xylene to increase tissue transparency and improve focus of internal structures. Sections were cover-slipped with Permount and visualized using bright-field microscopy at 400× total magnification as previously described [29]. Antibody incubations and wash steps were done in 0.25% BSA/0.025% Triton X100/TBS solution and TBS, respectively.

Statistical analysis

Data analysis was performed using independent t-tests (Sigma Stat®, ver. 3.5). Statistical significance was set at $P \leq 0.05$. To increase reproducibility, assays were repeated twice for each patient and presented as means ± standard error.

Results

Clinical findings

We studied 14 patients (10 males and 4 females [Table 1]) that fulfilled the diagnostic criteria for LGMD2A proposed by the European Neuromuscular Centre Workshop [22], including atrophy and progressive weakness of shoulder/hip girdles, elevated CK levels, and muscle biopsies consistent with a dystrophic/myopathic process. The age at onset ranged from 4 to 39 y and the majority of patients presented with pelvic girdle weakness or asymptomatic hyperCKemia (92.9%). In this cohort we identified two subjects with early onset (14.3%), six with the classical Leyden Mbius phenotype (42.9%), four with late onset (28.6%), one asymptomatic (7.1%), and one unspecified (7.1%). Surprisingly, no patients exhibited primary shoulder-girdle involvement/onset (Erb phenotype). At the time of the investigation three subjects were wheelchair-bound (P5, P6, and P8) and one (P4) had passed away.

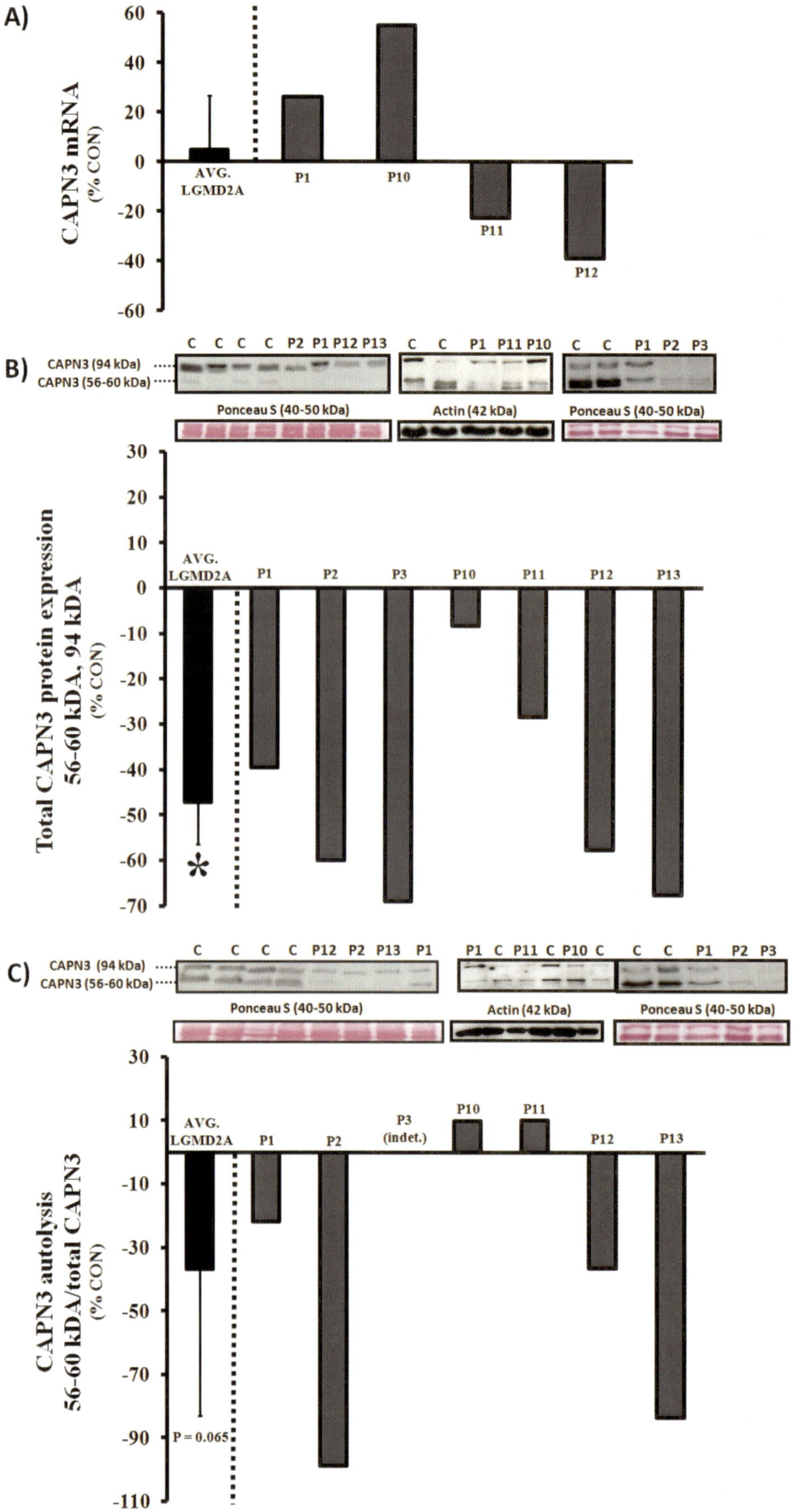
A)
CAPN3 mRNA
(% CON)
60
40
20
0
-20
-40
-60
AVG.
LGMD2A
P1
P10
P11
P12
B)
C C C C P2 P1 P12 P13
C C P1 P11 P10
C C P1 P2 P3
CAPN3 (94 kDa)
CAPN3 (56-60 kDa)
Ponceau S (40-50 kDa)
Actin (42 kDa)
Ponceau S (40-50 kDa)
Total CAPN3 protein expression
56-60 kDA, 94 kDA
(% CON)
30
20
10
0
-10
-20
-30
-40
-50
-60
-70
AVG.
LGMD2A
P1
P2
P3
P10
P11
P12
P13
*
C)
C C C C P12 P2 P13 P1
P1 C P11 C P10 C
C C P1 P2 P3
CAPN3 (94 kDa)
CAPN3 (56-60 kDa)
Ponceau S (40-50 kDa)
Actin (42 kDa)
Ponceau S (40-50 kDa)
CAPN3 autolysis
56-60 kDA/total CAPN3
(% CON)
30
10
-10
-30
-50
-70
-90
-110
AVG.
LGMD2A
P1
P2
P3
(indet.)
P10
P11
P12
P13
P = 0.065

Figure 1. Expression and autolysis of CAPN3 in quadriceps muscle of LGMD2A patients. A) CAPN3 mRNA expression (RT-PCR); B) CAPN3 protein (Western blot); C) Ca^{2+}-induced autolytic activity of CAPN3 (Western blot). Calpain-3 autolytic activity is presented as a ratio between autolyzed fragments and total CAPN3 (representing *relative autolytic capacity* of protein present), but the results should also be interpreted in the context of total protein expression from regular Western blots. Logically, a reduction in total CAPN3, obtained from Ca^{2+}-free homogenates, equates to a decrease in *total autolytic capacity.* All CAPN3 data were normalized to a suitable housekeeping gene (β2-microglobulin), protein (actin), or total proteins levels (Ponceau S stain) and graphed as % age/gender-matched healthy controls. Representative images of CAPN3 blots (56–60 kDa, 94 kDa), Ponceau S stain (40–50 kDa), or actin (42 kDa) are shown in B–C. For total protein expression and autolytic activity, N = 7 (LGMD2A) and N = 8 (control), while N = 4 (LGMD2A) and N = 6 (control) for mRNA. Bars to the far left represent the average of all LGMD2A patients (AVG. LGMD2A). INDT: Indeterminate. *Significantly lower compared to controls (P≤0.05).

Pathological findings

Biopsies and/or blood were collected and used for *CAPN3* mutational analysis and muscle histopathology as described in the methods section (mean age 35.6±2.9 y, range 14–53 y) [Table 1, Figs. S1–S2]. For further diagnostic and biochemical testing, a sub-set of patients were selected (N = 8; mean age 39.8±3.0 y, range 31–50 y) and compared to age- and gender-matched controls (N = 7; mean age 36.6±3.7 y, range 25–50 y) or as noted in the figure legends. Muscle histopathology (electron microscopy and IHC) ranged from mild to moderate to acute dystrophic processes and consisted of internalized nuclei, variation in fiber size, necrosis, degeneration/regeneration, and fiber splitting. Three patients (P1, P10, and P11) were randomly chosen for fiber-type quantification and revealed selective type 1 atrophy (−16% avg. diameter vs. CON) and type II dominance in P11 (83% fast/17% slow vs. 61%/39% in CON) [Fig. S2]. PAS, Oil-Red-O, succinate dehydrogense, cytochrome *c* oxidase, and NADH dehydrogenaze stains generally showed normal triglyceride abundance, glycogen content, and activity/distribution of mitochondria in all patients. Intra-mitochondrial crystalloid inclusions were present in electron micrographs of P4, but no other mitochondrial abnormalities were observed. Unless otherwise noted, immunohistochemistry showed normal reactivity towards dystrophin, spectrin, merosin, sarcoglycans (α,β,γ,δ), beta dystroglycan, caveolin III, desmin, and dysferlin in all subjects.

Genotype-phenotype correlations

Gene sequencing of the *CAPN3* gene revealed 21 sequence variants in our cohort of 14 patients, including 13 missense mutations, 1 nonsense mutation, 4 deletions (frameshifts/premature stop), and 3 intronic mutations (Table 1). Consistent with idea of mutation clustering in specific exons of the *CAPN3* gene (i.e. 1, 4, 5, 8, 10, 11, 21), ~60% of identified variants in this study occurred in aforementioned exons (Fig. S1). The majority of patients were compound heterozygotes with the exception of four homozygous individuals (P4, P5, P6, and P8) and two subjects with one mutation identified but with a clinical and/or biochemical phenotype consistent with LGMD2A (P11 and P12). All mutations were predicted to be pathogenic with bioinformatic software programs, exchanging highly conserved amino acids in the enzyme or nucleotides indispensable for splicing of the pre-mRNA. Five of these pathological sequence variants were novel and had not been reported in the Leiden database previously. Biochemical analyses were a priority in those patients exhibiting novel mutations (P1, P2, P4, P10, and P12) and/or one pathological sequence variant (P10 and P11), which were compared to subjects with proven pathology (P3 and P13) and age/gender-matched controls. Collectively, we confirmed the *in silico* predictions in75% of patients using WB or IHC for CAPN3 levels/autolytic activity and RT-PCR for mRNA expression, including subject P12, but not in P4 or P10 (Fig. 1A–C; Table S1; Fig. S2). Immunoblotting was the most robust test in this study, while RT-PCR and IHC were less useful for diagnostic purposes. Gene sequencing was necessary for specific diagnosis in P4 and P10. Mutations predicted to be pathogenic are presented in Table 1 and novel variants are also described in the text.

Proband 1 is of European Canadian decent and diagnosed with classical pelvifemoral LGMD2A (Leyden-Möbius). *CAPN3* sequencing revealed a unique combination of missense mutations [c.1250 C>T (p.Thr417Met) and c.500 T>C (p.Phe167Ser)]. Upon biochemical analyses, moderate reductions in protein expression and autolytic activity of calpain-3 were noted, but no defects in mRNA abundance. The former sequence variant exchanges a highly conserved threonine for a methione in domain III and results in an absence of CAPN3 protein when combined with c.2362_2363delinsTCATCT [33]. The second mutation in proband 1 is novel and exchanges a highly conserved phenylalanine (nonpolar, neutral, and hydrophobic) for a serine (polar, neutral, and hydrophilic) in domain II, which contains the catalytic module of CAPN3. Because there is no biochemical data on either mutation in the homozygous state, individual contributions of each sequence variant to the phenotype are difficult to determine.

Proband 2 is of South-East Asian heritage and exhibited two compound heterozygous missense mutations [c.2338 G>C (p. Asp780His) and c.2366 T>A (p.Leu789Gln)] causing late-onset pelvifemoral LGMD2A. Protein expression and autolytic activity, but not mRNA levels, were significantly reduced and the biochemical phenotype was more severe than P1 despite the late-onset form. Both sequence variants exchange evolutionary conserved amino acids in domain IV of CAPN3 (exon 22), which may affect Ca^{2+}-binding with downstream effects on autolytic activity. Interestingly, c.2338 G>C was inherited from his mother and is a recently recognized founder mutation originating from northern India in the Agarwal community, whose clan members practice intra-communal exogamy and are postulated to be descendants of King Agrasen [34]. This mutation was previously shown to cause pelvifemoral LGMD2A in the homozygous state and in combination with c.2099-1 G>T or c.1106 G>A, but effects on CAPN3 expression were inconclusive (protein non-significantly reduced vs. absent) [34,35]. We speculate that the novel sequence variant c.2366 T>A has deleterious effects on protein expression and autolysis of CAPN3, although verification in a homozygous patient or through site-directed mutagenesis is preferred.

Proband 4 was born in Pakistan and died at 56 years of age due to respiratory insufficiency. The patient exhibited a classical pelvifemoral LGMD2A phenotype with an onset in his late teens and he was wheelchair-bound at the time of his death. We identified a novel homozygous transversion (c.2115+4 T>G) in intron 19, which is predicted to create a cryptic splice site that is used instead of the regular site. Activation of a previously dormant cryptic splice may result in exon skipping or intron retention, and considering that CAPN3 reactivity appeared largely normal on IHC in this patient, we surmise that the gene product is stable but that the protein is truncated or otherwise dysfunctional.

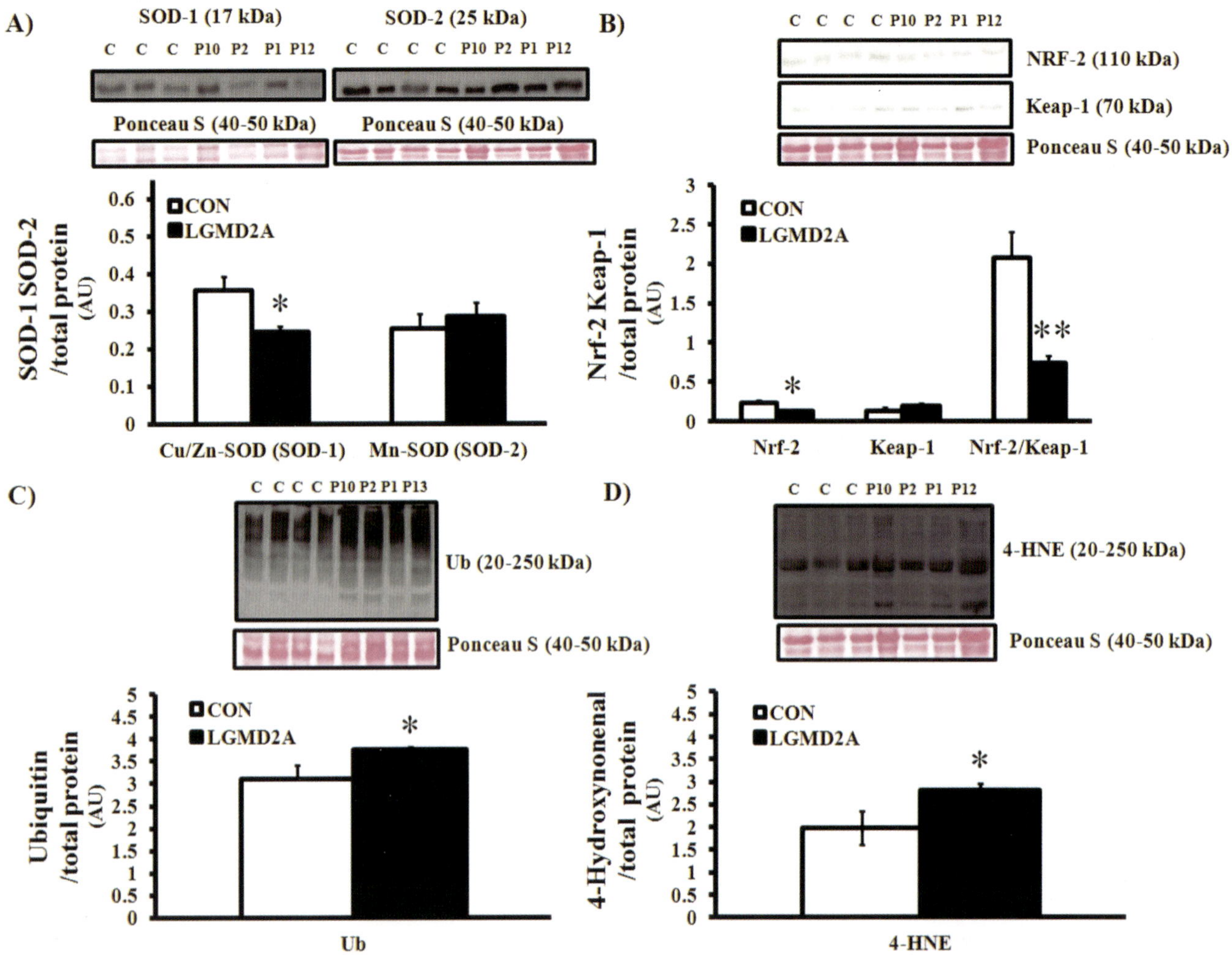

Figure 2. Western blot analyses of anti-oxidant capacity (SOD-1, SOD-2, NRF-2/Keap-1), oxidative damage (lipid peroxidation; 4-HNE), and ubiquitination (Ub) in LGMD2A patients. *P≤0.05 vs. control. **P≤0.01 vs. control. All data were normalized to total protein levels (Ponceau S stain) and represent averages of age/gender-matched controls (N = 3–4; white bars) and LGMD2A patients (N = 4; black bars). Representative images of blots and Ponceau S stain (40–50 kDa) are shown.

Proband 10 is of Irish decent and was clinically diagnosed with early onset pelvifemoral LGMD2A. The patient was found to be compound heterozygous for two missense mutations [c.1621 C>T (p.Arg541Trp) and c.338 T>C (p.Ile113Thr)], affecting conserved amino acids and predicted to be pathological by SIFT analysis. While the muscle biopsy showed a definite dystrophic pattern, we did not detect CAPN3 deficiency using the standard RT-PCR, WB, or IHC tests, possibly indicating that other functions, such as substrate recognition/binding or proteolytic activity, are impaired. c.1621 C>T has previously been reported in LGMD2A patients in the compound heterozygous and homozygous states and is associated with a reduction in CAPN3 expression in both Erb and Leyden-Möbius phenotypes [13,36]. c.338 T>C is a novel mutation exchanging isoleucine (nonpolar, neutral, and hydrophobic) for threonine (polar, neutral and hydrophilic), and is predicted by SIFT to be pathogenic and may impair proteolytic activity in domain II of CAPN3.

Proband 12 is of Iranian heritage and exhibited the major diagnostic criteria for primary calpainopathy, but clinical records were insufficient to pinpoint a specific LGMD2A phenotype. The mutational screen revealed a novel transversion in intron 11 (c.1525-1 G>T) that was predicted to destroy an acceptor splice site, but a second sequence variant was not identified. Canonical mutations of conserved nucleotides in positions −2, −1, +1, and +2 will significantly affect splicing (minus/plus signs indicate upstream/downstream from 5′ and 3′ ends of the exon, respectively) and may cause exon skipping or intron retention [37], ultimately affecting the mRNA stability and/or protein structure. CAPN3 protein levels, mRNA abundance, and autolytic activity were significantly reduced in P12, which strongly suggests that the mutation is pathogenic and confirms the clinical diagnosis.

Redox balance and mitochondrial function

Although structural and distributional abnormalities of mitochondria, oxidative damage, and markers of degradation may be hallmarks of the dystrophic process in calpain-3 deficient skeletal muscle [18,20,38], mitochondrial enzyme function and anti-oxidant defense have not been assessed in LGMD2A patients to date. As such, we measured the expression of CuZn-SOD (SOD-1), Mn-SOD (SOD-2), Nrf-2/Keap-1 and assessed the degree of oxidative damage, protein ubiquitinylation, and mitochondrial function in a sub-set of patient biopsies. Interestingly, SOD-1 and the Nrf-2/Keap-1 ratio were significantly lower in LGMD2A tissue, while SOD-2 levels were normal (Fig. 2A–B). As expected,

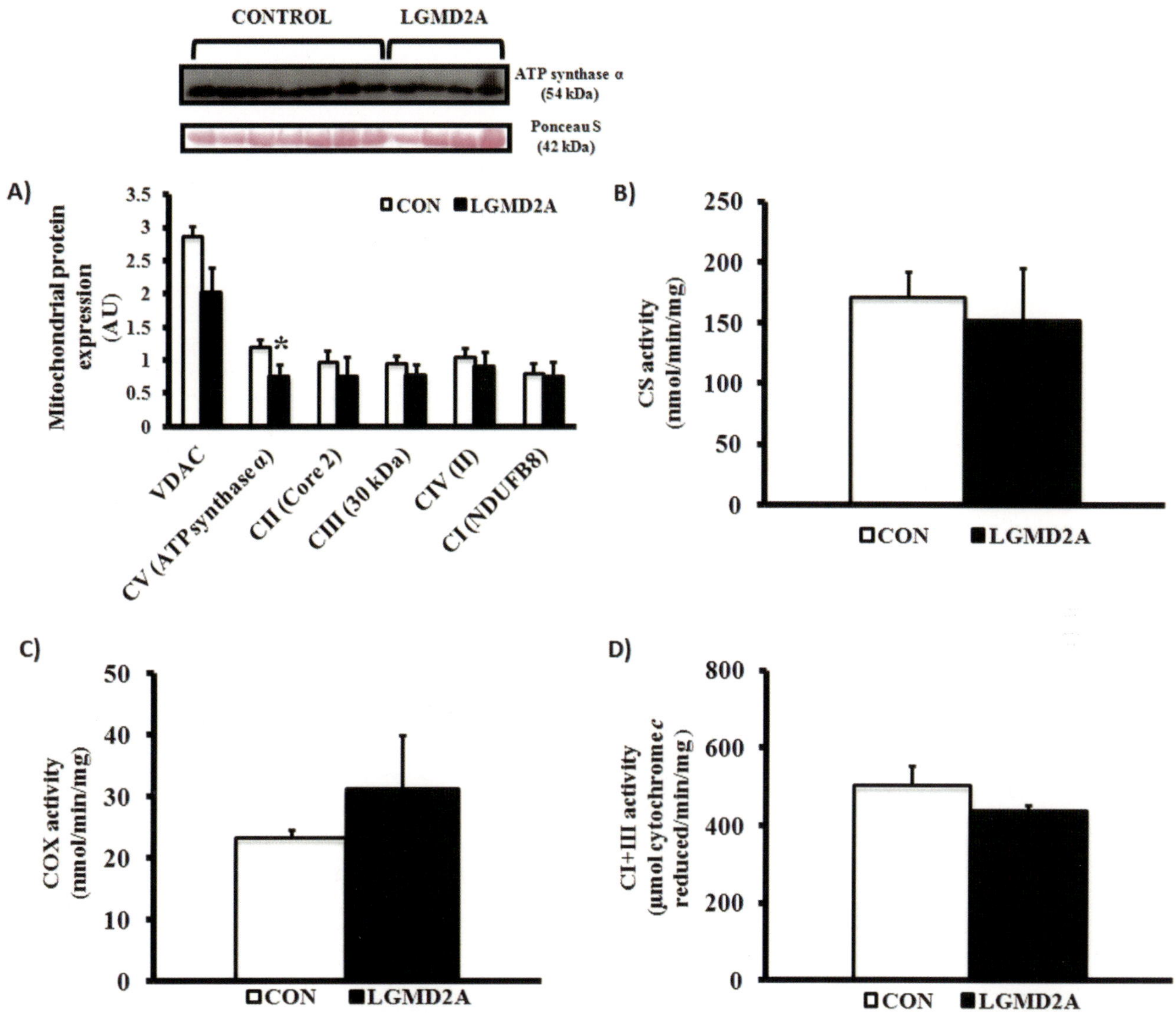

Figure 3. Western blot analyses of OXPHOS expression (complex I–V) and ETC enzyme activities (CS, COX, and complex I+III) in LGMD2A patients. *Significantly lower ATP synthase expression in calpain-3 deficient muscle ($P \leq 0.05$). All Western blot data were normalized to total protein levels (Ponceau S stain) and represent averages of age/gender-matched controls (N = 7 for OXPHOS and enzyme assays; N = 5 for VDAC) and LGMD2A patients (N = 5 for OXPHOS and VDAC; N = 2–3 for enzyme assays). Representative images of OXPHOS blots and Ponceau S stain (42 kDa) are shown.

lipid peroxidation (4-HNE) and total ubiquitin expression were elevated in calpain-3 deficient muscle (Fig. 2C–D). Activities of citrate synthase, COX, and complex I+III were not different from age/gender-matched controls, although a moderate reduction of complex V (ATP synthase) was detected on immunoblots (Fig. 3A–D).

Discussion

Herein we present five novel sequence variants that add to the mutational spectrum of LGMD2A and provide further insights into the cellular mechanisms underlying pathology in this patient population. Our results support the contention that gel-based tests (protein expression and autolytic activity) are the most important diagnostic tools next to *CAPN3* gene sequencing, while microscopy-based methods may be less useful for genotype-phenotype correlations and confirmation of clinical diagnosis.

In addition to our mutational data, we assessed oxidative damage, key anti-oxidant markers, and mitochondrial enzyme function in a subset of patient biopsies. Although the limited sample size prohibits us from making generalized statements, our findings leave open the possibility of mitochondrial enzyme dysfunction not being a universal feature of calpainopathy in humans, which appears to be the case in CAPN3 KO mice [16]. We found that the activities of rate-limiting enzymes in the Kreb's cycle (citrate synthase), mitochondrial respiratory chain (cytochrome *c* oxidase and NADH-cytochrome *c* oxidoreductase), and expression of OXPHOS proteins were largely normal in LGMD2A patients. In support of these observations, SOD-2 levels were comparable to age- and gender-matched controls, suggesting a preserved ability of mitochondria to catalyze highly reactive superoxide anions from complex I and III into hydrogen peroxide. Conversely, Nrf-2, Nrf-2/Keap1 ratio, and CuZn-SOD (SOD-1) were significantly suppressed in calpain-3 deficient skeletal muscle, collectively indicating a primary cytosolic/myofibrillar redox imbalance. Considering that Nrf-2 dissociates from its cytosolic inhibitor Keap1 and moves to the nucleus to regulate the transcription of anti-oxidant genes under stress conditions, aberrant regulation of Nrf-2 is generally synonymous with a reduction in cytoprotection, as previously shown by our group [39]. Given the results of the current study, and others [20,40,41], cellular redox imbalance appears to be compartment-specific and induces the ubiquitin-proteasome pathway, which in turn orchestrates protein degradation and muscle wasting in LGMD2A.

Calpain-3 associates with the ryanodine receptor and regulates Ca^{2+} release at the muscle triads, and calpain-3 deficiency impairs Ca^{2+} transport, RyR expression, and CAMKII signaling in CAPN3 KO mice [6,7,8]. Calcium kinetics play an important role in loading-induced muscle adaptations and maintenance of slow fiber phenotype in humans, and LGMD2A patients may exhibit lower RyR levels and a preferential involvement of slow muscle fibers [7]. Although the connection between calpain-3 and mitochondrial function remains unclear, two reports have demonstrated mitochondrial abnormalities in Japanese LGMD2A patients [18,38]. In partial agreement with aforementioned studies, ATP synthase levels were suppressed and type 1 fibers preferentially affected in our patient cohort, but we did not find general deficits in mitochondrial enzyme function, protein expression, or ultra-structure. Interestingly, ATP production is impaired in CAPN3 KO mice [16], but neither ATP synthase activity or energy status were assessed in our study. Because Ca^{2+} modulates the phosphorylation of subunit *c* of F_0F_1 ATPase and increased Ca^{2+} levels activates a number of nuclear genes encoding mitochondrial proteins (including ATP synthase) [42,43], calpainopathy may impair transcription of ATP synthase and/or its function. Selective type 1 fiber atrophy conceivably lowers the total amount of mitochondria in CAPN3-deficient skeletal muscle, and in light of our finding that VDAC was symmetrically reduced (albeit not significantly) compared to F_0F_1 ATPase, further research is necessary to delineate potential complex-specific deficiencies in isolated mitochondrial fractions.

In summary, we confirmed pathogenicity of *CAPN3* mutations in 75% of LGMD2A patients selected for biochemical analyses, which stresses the importance of gene sequencing in the diagnostic process. Assessment of total CAPN3 expression and autolysis by immunoblotting were the most reliable diagnostic tools (compared to RT-PCR and IHC) in the absence of substrate-specific enzymatic activity assays. We confirmed that oxidative damage is a hallmark of LGMD2A and expanded on previous studies by showing that calpain-3 deficiency is associated with cytosolic redox imbalance and a mild reduction in ATP synthase levels. Given the fact that CAPN3 regulates calcium release and Ca^{2+} is necessary for transcription and function of ATP synthase, future studies elucidating potential deficits in ATP production and F_0F_1 ATPase activity in LGMD2A patients may be warranted.

Supporting Information

Figure S1 Localization and distribution of 21 *CAPN3* sequence variants from our cohort of 14 LGMD2A patients along pre-mRNA (top), mRNA (middle), and protein (bottom). Mutational data adhere to the guidelines proposed by the Human Genome Variation Society (www.hgvs.org/mutnomen) and nucleotide numbering reflects the cDNA sequence with +1 corresponding to the A of the ATG translation initiation codon in the reference sequence. Exons 4, 11, 13, and 22 show the highest number of mutations, affecting protein domains II (3 mutations), III (4 mutations), and IV (2 mutations). Intronic mutations mainly affect domains III and IV. Domain I has regulatory role, domain II is the proteolytic module, domain III has a C2-like domain, and domain IV binds Ca^{2+} ions. NS, IS1, and IS2 are calpain-3 specific insertions.

Figure S2 Hematoxylin and eosin stain, immunohistochemical determination of fiber-type, and CAPN3 reactivity on flat sections in a sub-set of LGMD2A patients (total magnification 200×–400×). Top panel: Red circles show markedly increased abundance of internalized nuclei in calpain-deficient muscle. Middle panel: Primarily slow-twitch fiber atrophy and increased variation in fiber size/shape in LGMD2A patients. Note fast-twitch fiber dominance in P11. Lower panel: Normal CAPN3 reactivity in all subjects despite pathological mutations.

Table S1 [a]Clinical diagnosis: Phenotype consistent with major criteria of LGMD2A (see methods); [b]CAPN3 mRNA expression by RT-PCR (Fig. 1A); [c]Total CAPN3 protein expression on Western blot (Fig. 1B); [d]Ca^{2+}-induced CAPN3 autolytic activity assessed on immunoblot (Fig. 1C); [e]CAPN3 reactivity on 8 μm frozen sections (Fig. S2); ND: Not done; INDT: Indeterminate.

Acknowledgments

We gratefully acknowledge the patients and the volunteers in the Neuromuscular and Neurometabolic Clinic at McMaster University Hospital.

Author Contributions

Conceived and designed the experiments: MN MT. Performed the experiments: MN FA LM MH YK MA RS PD MS. Analyzed the data: MN FA LM MH YK MA RS PD MS. Contributed reagents/materials/analysis tools: MT. Contributed to the writing of the manuscript: MN MT.

References

1. Duguez S, Bartoli M, Richard I (2006) Calpain 3: a key regulator of the sarcomere? FEBS Journal 273: 3427–3436.
2. Saeenz A, Leturcq F, Cobo AM, Poza JJ, Ferrer X, et al. (2005) LGMD2A: genotype-phenotype correlations based on a large mutational survey on the calpain 3 gene. Brain 128: 732–742.
3. Kramerova I, Beckmann JS, Spencer MJ (2007) Molecular and cellular basis of calpainopathy (limb girdle muscular dystrophy type 2A). Biochimica et Biophysica Acta (BBA) - Molecular Basis of Disease 1772: 128–144.
4. Ono Y, Ojima K, Torii F, Takaya E, Doi N, et al. (2010) Skeletal muscle-specific calpain is an intracellular Na+-dependent protease. Journal of Biological Chemistry 285: 22986–22998.
5. Richard I, Broux O, Allamand Ve, Fougerousse Fo, Chiannilkulchai N, et al. (1995) Mutations in the proteolytic enzyme calpain 3 cause limb-girdle muscular dystrophy type 2A. Cell 81: 27–40.
6. Ojima K, Ono Y, Ottenheijm C, Hata S, Suzuki H, et al. (2011) Non-proteolytic functions of calpain-3 in sarcoplasmic reticulum in skeletal muscles. Journal of Molecular Biology 407: 439–449.
7. Kramerova I, Kudryashova E, Ermolova N, Saenz A, Jaka O, et al. (2012) Impaired calcium calmodulin kinase signaling and muscle adaptation response in the absence of calpain 3. Human Molecular Genetics 21: 3193–3204.
8. Kramerova I, Kudryashova E, Wu B, Ottenheijm C, Granzier H, et al. (2008) Novel role of calpain-3 in the triad-associated protein complex regulating calcium release in skeletal muscle. Human Molecular Genetics 17: 3271–3280.
9. Ojima K, Kawabata Y, Nakao H, Nakao K, Doi N, et al. (2012) Dynamic distribution of muscle-specific calpain in mice has a key role in physical-stress adaptation and is impaired in muscular dystrophy. The Journal of Clinical Investigation 120: 2672–2683.

10. Ojima K, Ono Y, Doi N, Yoshioka K, Kawabata Y, et al. (2007) Myogenic stage, sarcomere length, and protease activity modulate localization of muscle-specific calpain. Journal of Biological Chemistry 282: 14493–14504.
11. Murphy RM, Goodman CA, McKenna MJ, Bennie J, Leikis M, et al. (2007) Calpain-3 is autolyzed and hence activated in human skeletal muscle 24 h following a single bout of eccentric exercise. Journal of Applied Physiology 103: 926–931.
12. Milic A, Daniele N, Lochmuller H, Mora M, Comi GP, et al. (2007) A third of LGMD2A biopsies have normal calpain 3 proteolytic activity as determined by an in vitro assay. Neuromuscular Disorders 17: 148–156.
13. Fanin M, Fulizio L, Nascimbeni AC, Spinazzi M, Piluso G, et al. (2004) Molecular diagnosis in LGMD2A: Mutation analysis or protein testing? Human Mutation 24: 52–62.
14. Fanin M, Nascimbeni AC, Angelini C (2007) Screening of calpain-3 autolytic activity in LGMD muscle: a functional map of CAPN3 gene mutations. Journal of Medical Genetics 44: 38–43.
15. Fanin M, Nascimbeni AC, Fulizio L, Trevisan CP, Meznaric-Petrusa M, et al. (2003) Loss of calpain-3 autocatalytic activity in LGMD2A patients with normal protein expression. The American Journal of Pathology 163: 1929–1936.
16. Kramerova I, Kudryashova E, Wu B, Germain S, Vandenborne K, et al. (2009) Mitochondrial abnormalities, energy deficit and oxidative stress are features of calpain 3 deficiency in skeletal muscle. Human Molecular Genetics 18: 3194–3205.
17. Cohen N, Kudryashova E, Kramerova I, Anderson LVB, Beckmann JS, et al. (2006) Identification of putative in vivo substrates of calpain 3 by comparative proteomics of overexpressing transgenic and nontransgenic mice. Proteomics 6: 6075–6084.
18. Chae J, Minami N, Jin Y, Nakagawa M, Murayama K, et al. (2001) Calpain 3 gene mutations: genetic and clinico-pathologic findings in limb-girdle muscular dystrophy. Neuromuscular Disorders 11: 547–555.
19. Fardeau M, Eymard B, Mignard C, Tome FMS, Richard I, et al. (1996) Chromosome 15-linked limb-girdle muscular dystrophy: Clinical phenotypes in Reunion Island and French metropolitan communities. Neuromuscular Disorders 6: 447–453.
20. Rajakumar D, Alexander M, Oommen A (2013) Oxidative stress, NF-KB and the ubiquitin proteasomal pathway in the pathology of calpainopathy. Neurochemical Research: 1–10.
21. Angelini C, Fanin M (2005) Calpainopathy. In: Pagon R, Adam M, Bird T, editors. GeneReviews^{TM}. Seattle (WA): University of Washington.
22. Beckmann J, Bushby K (1996) Advances in the molecular genetics of the limb-girdle type of autosomal recessive progressive muscular dystrophy. Curr Opin Neurol (5): 389–393.
23. Nilsson MI, Laureano ML, Saeed M, Tarnopolsky MA (2013) Dysferlin aggregation in limb-girdle muscular dystrophy type 2B/Miyoshi myopathy necessitates mutational screen for diagnosis. Muscle & Nerve 47: 740–747.
24. Wu Y, Weber JL, Vladutiu GD, Tarnopolsky MA (2011) Six novel mutations in the myophosphorylase gene in patients with McArdle disease and a family with pseudo-dominant inheritance pattern. Molecular Genetics and Metabolism 104: 587–591.
25. Nilsson MI, Kroos MA, Reuser AJ, Hatcher E, Akhtar M, et al. (2014) Novel GAA sequence variant c.1211 A>G reduces enzyme activity but not protein expression in infantile and adult onset Pompe disease. Gene 537: 41–45.
26. Murphy RM, Snow RJ, Lamb GD (2006) u-Calpain and calpain-3 are not autolyzed with exhaustive exercise in humans. American Journal of Physiology - Cell Physiology 290: C116–C122.
27. Smith PK, Krohn RI, Hermanson GT, Mallia AK, Gartner FH, et al. (1985) Measurement of protein using bicinchoninic acid. Anal Biochem 150: 76–85.
28. McKenzie S, Phillips SM, Carter SL, Lowther S, Gibala MJ, et al. (2000) Endurance exercise training attenuates leucine oxidation and BCOAD activation during exercise in humans. American Journal of Physiology - Endocrinology and Metabolism 278: E580–E587.
29. Nilsson MI, Samjoo IA, Hettinga BP, Koeberl DD, Zhang H, et al. (2012) Aerobic training as an adjunctive therapy to enzyme replacement in Pompe disease. Molecular Genetics and Metabolism 107: 469–479.
30. Safdar A, Hamadeh MJ, Kaczor JJ, Raha S, deBeer J, et al. (2010) Aberrant mitochondrial homeostasis in the skeletal muscle of sedentary older adults. PLoS ONE 5: e10778.
31. Fanin M, Nascimbeni AC, Tasca E, Angelini C (2008) How to tackle the diagnosis of limb-girdle muscular dystrophy 2A. Eur J Hum Genet 17: 598–603.
32. Kolski HK, Hawkins C, Zatz M, De Paula F, Biggar D, et al. (2008) Diagnosis of limb-girdle muscular dystrophy 2A by immunohistochemical techniques. Neuropathology 28: 264–268.
33. Krahn M, Bernard R, Pécheux C, Hammouda EH, Eymard B, et al. (2006) Screening of the CAPN3 gene in patients with possible LGMD2A. Clinical Genetics 69: 444–449.
34. Ankala A, Kohn JN, Dastur R, Gaitonde P, Khadilkar SV, et al. (2013) Ancestral founder mutations in calpain-3 in the Indian Agarwal community: Historical, clinical, and molecular perspective. Muscle & Nerve 47: 931–937.
35. Todorova A, Kress W, Mueller C (2005) Novel mutations in the calpain 3 gene in Germany. Clinical Genetics 67: 356–358.
36. Piluso G, Politano L, Aurino S, Fanin M, Ricci E, et al. (2005) Extensive scanning of the calpain-3 gene broadens the spectrum of LGMD2A phenotypes. Journal of Medical Genetics 42: 686–693.
37. Desmet F-O, Hamroun D, Lalande M, Collod-Beroud G, Claustres M, et al. (2009) Human Splicing Finder: an online bioinformatics tool to predict splicing signals. Nucleic Acids Research 37: e67.
38. Kawai H, Akaike M, Kunishige M, Inui T, Adachi K, et al. (1998) Clinical, pathological, and genetic features of limb-girdle muscular dystrophy type 2A with new calpain 3 gene mutations in seven patients from three Japanese families. Muscle & Nerve 21: 1493–1501.
39. Kitaoka Y, Ogborn DI, Nilsson MI, Mocellin NJ, MacNeil LG, et al. (2013) Oxidative stress and Nrf2 signaling in McArdle disease. Mol Genet Metab 110: 297–302.
40. Fanin M, Nascimbeni AC, Angelini C (2013) Muscle atrophy in Limb Girdle Muscular Dystrophy 2A: a morphometric and molecular study. Neuropathology and Applied Neurobiology 39: 762–771.
41. Whitehead NP, Yeung EW, Froehner SC, Allen DG (2010) Skeletal muscle NADPH oxidase is increased and triggers stretch-induced damage in the mdx mouse. PLoS ONE 5: e15354.
42. Hood DA (2001) Invited Review: Contractile activity-induced mitochondrial biogenesis in skeletal muscle. Journal of Applied Physiology 90: 1137–1157.
43. Grover GJ, Marone PA, Koetzner L, Seto-Young D (2008) Energetic signalling in the control of mitochondrial F1F0 ATP synthase activity in health and disease. The International Journal of Biochemistry & Cell Biology 40: 2698–2701.

18

Effects of Intermittent Training on Anaerobic Performance and MCT Transporters in Athletes

Grégoire Millet[1,2], David J. Bentley[3], Belle Roels[4], Lars R. Mc Naughton[5]*, Jacques Mercier[6], David Cameron-Smith[7,8]

1 ISSUL Institute of Sport Sciences University of Lausanne, Lausanne, Switzerland, **2** Department of Physiology, University of Lausanne, Lausanne, Switzerland, **3** Faculty of Health Science, University of Adelaide, Adelaide, South Australia, Australia, **4** ORION, Clinical Services Ltd, London, England, **5** Department of Sport and Physical Activity, Edge Hill University, Ormskirk, Lancashire, England, **6** Laboratoire de physiologie des Interactions EA 701, Institut de Biologie, Montpellier, France, **7** School of Nutrition and Exercise Sciences, Deakin University, Melbourne, Victoria, Australia, **8** Liggins Institute, University of Auckland, Auckland, New Zealand

Abstract

This study examined the effects of intermittent hypoxic training (IHT) on skeletal muscle monocarboxylate lactate transporter (MCT) expression and anaerobic performance in trained athletes. Cyclists were assigned to two interventions, either normoxic (N; n = 8; 150 mmHg P_IO_2) or hypoxic (H; n = 10; ~3000 m, 100 mmHg P_IO_2) over a three week training (5×1 h-1h30.week^{-1}) period. Prior to and after training, an incremental exercise test to exhaustion (EXT) was performed in normoxia together with a 2 min time trial (TT). Biopsy samples from the *vastus lateralis* were analyzed for MCT1 and MCT4 using immuno-blotting techniques. The peak power output (PPO) increased ($p<0.05$) after training (7.2% and 6.6% for N and H, respectively), but VO_2max showed no significant change. The average power output in the TT improved significantly (7.3% and 6.4% for N and H, respectively). No differences were found in MCT1 and MCT4 protein content, before and after the training in either the N or H group. These results indicate there are no additional benefits of IHT when compared to similar normoxic training. Hence, the addition of the hypoxic stimulus on anaerobic performance or MCT expression after a three-week training period is ineffective.

Editor: Jonathan A. Coles, Glasgow University, United Kingdom

Funding: The International Olympic Committee (http://www.olympic.org/ioc) and the French Ministry of Sport (http://www.sports.gouv.fr/) supported this study. Additional funding was provided by the Molecular and Medical Research Strategic Research Cluster, Deakin University (www.deakin.edu.au), Melbourne, Australia. The funders had no role in study design, data collection and analysis, decision to publish, or preparation of the manuscript.

* E-mail: lars.mcnaughton@edgehill.ac.uk

Introduction

Traditionally the effects of intermittent hypoxic exposure or altitude training have been investigated on prolonged endurance performance. The proposed benefits of altitude training are an increase in red blood cell mass and haemoglobin concentration, which have the potential to enhance oxygen (O_2) transport capacity and therefore endurance performance upon return to sea-level [17,36,42]. There is now considerable debate on the use of the different high-intensity hypoxic training methods as intermittent hypoxic training (IHT), which is frequent training of a higher intensity in hypoxia, or repeated sprints training in hypoxia (RSH) to improve endurance performance or repeated sprint ability in normoxia/at sea-level [8,18,25,34,35]. A variety of individual and team sports comprise a considerable anaerobic component [37]. The scientific rationale supporting the use of altitude training for anaerobic performance improvement is less compelling than that for the use of altitude training for the enhancement of endurance performance. However there is some evidence that altitude training can benefit sprinting or other short-term high-intensity performance that requires a substantial anaerobic metabolic contribution [2,7,9,]. However only few scientific studies have examined the effects of IHT on anaerobic performance [27].

One important physiological adaptation that may occur as a result of altitude training is an improvement in the capacity to buffer the exercise-induced increase in the concentration of hydrogen ions (H^+) in skeletal muscle. Few studies have reported increase in buffering capacity following spring training in normoxia [17] as well with "living high – training high" [26] or "living high training low" [9] altitude methods. However, to date little is known about the effects of intermittent hypoxic stimulus on anaerobic performance.

The transport of lactate across the sarcolemma of skeletal muscle is mediated by proton-linked monocarboxylate transporters (MCT1 and MCT4) [12,13,16,21,30,31,43]. Due to the 1:1 ratio between the lactate transport and the H^+ transport, an increase in MCT1 and MCT4 could reduce the intracellular pH perturbations [13]. The MCT1 is expressed in the mitochondria [4] and facilitates the lactate influx into the muscle [13]. The MCT4 however, facilitates the removal of lactic acid and is mainly expressed in glycolytic fibers [13]. An increase in MCT1 and MCT4 protein expression is likely to decrease intracellular pH perturbations due to the coupled H^+ transport [13]. Exercise training above VO_2max in normoxic conditions is known to induce increases in both MCT1 and MCT4 content [2,29].

However, there are limited studies investigating the effects of hypoxia on MCT expression in human skeletal muscle [5,41]. In one study the authors concluded that 20 consecutive nights (9–10 h $night^{-1}$) of hypoxic exposure (N_2 enriched altitude house with simulated altitude at 2650 m, F_IO_2 = 16.3%), a 'live high-train low' (LHTL) scenario, decreased lactate production (as measured by stable isotope methodology) during intense exercise in well-trained athletes [5]. However, there was no effect of hypoxic exposure on MCT1 and MCT4 protein expression [5]. Aside from this investigation, there is little information concerning the effects of IHT on MCT expression in human skeletal muscle. The effects of IHT at high intensity on anaerobic performance in normoxia have also not been clearly established in trained athletes. The present study was therefore designed to evaluate the effects of acute intermittent hypoxic training on anaerobic performance and MCT expression, in human skeletal muscle. We tested the hypothesis that IHT would not provide larger MCT expression or anaerobic performance enhancement, when compared to the same similar training in normoxia.

Methods

Subjects

Eighteen male cyclists voluntarily participated in the study after giving written informed consent. The experimental procedures were approved by the institutional ethics committee (CPP Sud Méditerranée III, Faculty of Medicine, Nimes, France). All subjects were familiarized with the testing protocols and equipment used in the experiment. In addition, all the subjects were sea-level residents with no history of recent travel to altitude. After recruitment, the subjects were randomly allocated into two training groups, a Hypoxic group (H; n = 10) and a Normoxic group (N, n = 8). The subject characteristics for each group are presented in Table 1. The experiment took place in the pre-season prior to the main competition phase of the season.

Experimental design

During the course of the experimental period (W1–W3), the subjects performed two interval-training and three continuous sessions per week in conjunction with their regular endurance training. Each training session included a 15 min warm-up and 15 min cool-down. The continuous training session consisted of 60 min at 60% of VO_{2max}. The interval-training required the subjects to perform two sets of three repetitions each two min in duration and at an intensity of 100% Peak Power Output (PPO) [33]. Two min of rest was allowed between each repetition with 6 min rest between each set. Each session was performed at the same relative intensity specific to each condition (e.g. 100% PPO and 60% of VO_{2max} measured in normoxia or hypoxia for N or H, respectively) to ensure an equivalent training stimulus. The subjects trained on their own bicycle fixed on an electromagnetic resistant home-trainer (Elite Travel, Milan, Italy). Each session was meticulously controlled by the same researcher.

Training sessions were performed either in normoxic (P_IO_2 of 150 mmHg) or hypoxic (P_IO_2 of 100 mmHg, simulated altitude of ~3000 m) environment for N and the H group, respectively. The average duration of the hypoxic stimulus per week during the training period was 382±8 min. No supplementary interval training was performed outside the supervised interval-training sessions.

Pre (W0) and post-training period (W4), a medical examination and determination of physical characteristics were completed (Table 1) and muscle biopsy samples were taken. The subjects performed an incremental exercise test to exhaustion in normoxic conditions. An identical incremental test to exhaustion under hypoxic conditions (P_IO_2 ~100 mmHg) on a separate visit to the laboratory was also performed by the H group. An all-out exercise trial (~2 min) was also performed under normoxic conditions by both groups to determine anaerobic performance. All the tests were randomized for both groups. A physician was in attendance at all times and was responsible for the safety of the subjects during the study. The weekly training that took place outside the experimental training was controlled.

Environmental stimulus

The hypoxic environment (equivalent to ~3000 m) was induced by the continued delivery of a hypoxic gas mixture by a system that modifying nitrogen content and therefore decreased the inspired O_2 fraction (Altitrainer 200, SMTEC, Geneva, Switzerland). This device allows the production of large quantities of hypoxic gas mixture, up to 200 $L{\cdot}min^{-1}$, with an easily adjustable O_2 fraction over a large range and with a short response time. Air inhaled from outside the machine is controlled with a fixed quantity of nitrogen from a bottle which is then mechanically mixed prior to being stocked in a buffer tank of 30 L. The first safety check is ensured by the mixer's mechanical limit, which cannot exceed a certain nitrogen fraction (F_IO_2 = 9.7%). The user inhales the mixture contained in the tank through a Hans Rudolph two-way respiratory valve. An O_2 probe, a second safety check, plunged in the buffer tank, measures the PO_2. This probe, with aid of a microprocessor, allows the PO_2 of the inhaled mixture, or the equivalent altitude to be displayed and cannot decrease less than 66 mmHg (5500 m). If necessary, the user can constantly modify the composition of the air which they breathe and thus change the simulated altitude. A breath-by-breath analyser was attached to the system in order to measure respiratory exchange.

Performance Tests

The subjects completed two different performance tests before (W0) and after (W4) the training.

1) Incremental test to exhaustion. The subjects performed an incremental test to exhaustion to determine the maximal oxygen uptake (VO_{2max}; $ml{\cdot}kg^{-1}{\cdot}min^{-1}$), the peak power output (PPO; W), maximal heart rate (HR_{max}; bpm), and maximal

Table 1. The subjects' physical characteristics of Normoxic (N: n = 8) and Hypoxic (H: n = 10) groups.

	W0		W4	
	N	H	N	H
Age (years)	24.2±0.4	24.4±0.3		
Height (cm)	181.6±0.03	180.1±0.5		
Weight (kg)	71.3±0.8	73.2±0.8	72.0±0.8	72.6±0.8

Mean ± SE; W0: pre-; W4: post-training.

ventilation (VE; $l \cdot min^{-1}$). The test began with a three min stage at an initial power output of 60 W and than the workload progressively increased by 30 W every minute until exhaustion. Exhaustion was reached when two out of three of the following criteria were obtained: 1) heart rate (HR) approaching an age predicted maximum value (220 - age); 2) a plateau in VO_2 despite an increase in exercise intensity; and 3) a RER >1.1. PPO was defined as the highest mechanical power maintained during one min.

In addition, only the H group performed the same test also under hypoxic conditions on a separated laboratory visit and prior the start of the training protocol and biopsy (data not presented in this paper). This test was necessary to provide data to determine the workloads (100% PPO and 60% of VO_{2max}) under hypoxic conditions for the training sessions for the H group.

2) All-out exercise test. The all-out exercise test consisted of cycling at the highest power output to exhaustion, approximately 2 min, in normoxic conditions. This test is a reliable measurement for anaerobic performance [22]. This test assessed the subject's anaerobic capacity expressed as maximal accumulated oxygen deficit (MAOD) [23], the peak oxygen consumption (VO_{2peak}, $ml \cdot kg^{-1} \cdot min^{-1}$), average power output (P_{aver}, W) and maximal lactate (La_{max}; $mmol \cdot L^{-1}$) accumulation were measured.

Physiological parameters

Respiratory gas exchange was measured pre and post intervention using a $K4^{b2}$ (Cosmed, Rome, Italy). Prior to each test, the system was calibrated according to manufacturer's recommendations. Breath-by-breath data were reduced to 30 s averages and $VO_{2max/peak}$ was determined as the highest 30 s VO_2 average. Heart rate (HR) was constantly recorded by the means of a HR monitor (S810, Polar, Kempele, Finland) integrated to the Cosmed system.

The accumulated oxygen (AO_2) deficit was calculated as the difference between the AO_2 demand and the AO_2 uptake measured during the all-out exercise test [23]. The AO_2 demand was taken as the product of the O_2 demand and the duration of the exercise, assuming that the O_2 demand was constant throughout the whole exercise period. The AO_2 deficit calculated was reported as the "maximal AO_2 deficit" (MAOD) for cycling [22,23]. Changes in MAOD determined after the training period were reported as the percentage increase, calculated from the pre-test values (W0).

All the tests were performed on a bicycle equipped with an SRM road professional powermeter (Schoberer Rad Messtechnik, Jülich, Welldorf, Germany). The saddle height on the cycle ergometer was kept identical for all the tests. Power output and pedalling cadence were recorded every second and 30-s averaged values were stored. The calibration procedure and technical aspects concerning SRM crank system have previously been described in detail. The SRM road professional powermeter is constructed with four strain gauges and shown to have a high accuracy in power measurement. The 95% limits of agreement is 2.1 W which is equivalent to 1.8% [11]. After each test the rate of perceived exertion (RPE) was recorded.

Training outside experimental design

The training completed outside the experimental design was recorded daily using a computerized training diary during the three weeks of training period. The type of activity, *i.e.* cycling, swimming, running, and the intensity were recorded, with training intensity divided into five intensity levels [28]. All training sessions outside the protocol were individually timed and each exercise categorized according to the five intensity levels. The performed training duration was multiplied by its corresponding multiplying factor, *i.e.* 2, 4, 6, 10, and 16, respectively and the sum was then divided by the overall duration of the session to calculate the average intensity of each training session. It was deemed not valid to compare hourly volume as the subjects performed exercise training in different modes (swimming, running).

Muscle biopsy

One week after all cycling sessions, muscle samples were obtained from the *vastus lateralis* using the percutaneous needle biopsy technique after administration of local anesthesia (xylocaine) as previously described and performed in our laboratory [38,39]. The biopsies were taken by the same researcher from the same site, *i.e.* in the middle of the line between *spina iliaca* anterior superior and the upper outer corner of the *patella* at a depth of 1.5 - 2.0 cm from the fascia in all the subjects. The muscle samples were immediately frozen in liquid nitrogen and stored at −80°C until further analysis.

Western Blotting

Whole muscle protein was isolated from each sample by a method previously described and previously used in our laboratory [6,39]. Muscle protein concentration was determined in duplicate by bicinchoninic acid assay (Pierce, Interchim, Montluçon, France) with the use of BSA as a standard.

Affinity polyclonal antibodies directed against the carboxy terminus of human MCT1 and MCT4 were produced with the synthetic peptide C-Ahx-KDTEGGPKEEESPV-OH for MCT1 and C-AHX-GEVVHTPETSV-OH for MCT4, like the sequence used in other research work [4,5,7,18]. Western Blotting was probed with these antibodies and Chemicon International antibodies (Temecula, California, USA. Rabbit anti-MCT1: AB3538P and rabbit anti-MCT4: AB3316P). Polyclonal antibodies yielded a single band on a Western blot that corresponded to 43 kD, consistent with the molecular mass reported earlier [21]. Antibody specificities were confirmed in preliminary experiments in which the peptides blocked the detection of MCT1 and MCT4. Samples of muscle homogenates (12 μg protein) and pre-stained molecular mass markers (Bio-Rad), were separated on 10% Bis-Tris-acrylamide gels (200 V for ~60 min) with the Novex system (Invitrogen, Groningen, The Netherlands). Proteins were then transferred from the gels to polyvinylidene difluoride (PVDF) membranes (30 V, 180 min), and the membranes were incubated on a shaker overnight at 4°C temperature in buffer D (20 $mmol.l^{-1}$ Tris base, 137 $mmol.l^{-1}$ NaCl, 0.1 $mol.l^{-1}$ HCl, adjusted to pH 7.5, 0.1% [vol/vol] Tween 20, and 5% [wt/vol] non-fat dried milk). The membranes were then incubated with diluted carboxy-terminal of either MCT1 antibody (1:90 000) or MCT4 (1:90 000) in buffer D for 2 hours at room temperature, followed by 4 washes (4×5 min washes) in buffer E, *i.e.*, buffer D without dried milk and then incubated for 50 min with goat anti-rabbit immunoglobulin G horse-radish peroxidase-conjugated secondary antibody (1:10 000, BI2407, BioSys, Compiègne, France) in buffer E. Membranes were washed as previously described and MCT1 or MCT4 expression was detected by ECL (Biomax MR films, Kodak, Reuil-Malmaison, France). The identified bands were developed and fixed using a Hyperprocessor (RNP 1700, Amersham, Les Ulis, France). MCT1 and MCT4 protein band densities determined by scanning the blots on a scanner (AGFA Duo Scan T1200, New York, USA) and Scion Image software (Scion Corp, Frederick, MD). Results were expressed in arbitrary optical density (OD) units (a.u.) as previously [6,38,39].

Table 2. Averaged percentage (Mean ± SE) of target power output (target PO), *i.e.* 100% PPO for interval sessions and 60% of VO_{2max} and the averaged absolute power output ($W_{absolute}$; W) for continuous training sessions, of Normoxic (N, n = 8) and Hypoxic (H; n = 10) groups.

	Continuous		Interval	
	% of target PO	$W_{absolute}$	% of target PO	$W_{absolute}$
N	91.7±0.6	185.0±7.5	91.0±0.7	310.9±4.5
H	91.8±1.6	130.0±0.3	91.8±1.0	259.4±0.3

mRNA analysis

Total cellular RNA was extracted as previously described [40]. The RT-PCR was performed using the Applied Biosystems 7500 Real Time PCR Machine (Applied Biosystems, Foster City, CA). PCR was performed in duplicate with reaction volumes of 20 µl, containing SYBR Green 1 (Applied Biosystems, Foster City, CA), forward and reverse primers and cDNA template (diluted 1:20). Data were analyzed using a comparative critical threshold (Ct) method where the amount of target normalized to the amount of endogenous control relative to control value is given by $2^{-\Delta\Delta Ct}$. The efficacy of *cyclophilin* as an endogenous control was examined using the equation $2^{-\Delta Ct}$. It was considered an appropriate control for this study when no changes in the expression of the gene were observed (data not shown) [19]. Primers were designed using Primer Express software package version 3.0 (Applied Biosystems, Foster City, CA) from gene sequences obtained from GenBank. Primers were designed spanning intron-exon boundaries to prevent amplification of the target region for any contaminating DNA. Primer sequence specificity was also confirmed using BLAST. A melting point dissociation curve was generated by the PCR instrument for all PCR products to confirm the presence of a single amplified product.

Statistical analysis

All values are reported as mean ± standard error (SE). A power calculation was conducted for the primary outcome measure of average power in the time trial for the initial 20 subjects (10 per group) recruited. The calculation (using PASS 11) was based upon unpublished test-retest reliability data from our laboratory to produce an effect size of 0.72 and a power of 86% [10]. Since we had two subjects withdraw, a re-calculation of power indicated that, eight subjects in the control group and 10 in the experimental group gave 81% power to detect a standardised effect size of 0.72 for the condition-by-time interaction.

After analysis of the normality and the homogeneity of variance of the tested samples, the influence of the two training methods on the measured variables was analyzed using a two-way (training group × time) analysis of variance (ANOVA) with repeated measures on the second factor. A student Newman-Keuls post-hoc test was used to analyze significant effects. All analyses were undertaken using SigmaStat 2.3 (Jandel Corporation, San Rafael, CA). Statistical significance was accepted at $P<0.05$.

Table 3. Mean (± SE) intensity of additional training outside the experimental design of each training week for Normoxic (N; n = 8) and Hypoxic (H; n = 10) groups.

	W1	W2	W3
N	3.1±0.05	3.1±0.06	3.2±0.1
H	2.9±0.09	3.0±0.05	3.0±0.07

W1: first week; W2: second week; W3: third week of training protocol.

Results

Table 2 presents the workloads of each group averaged over the three weeks for the interval training and continuous workload sessions. No significant differences in (relative) training workloads in- and outside the training sessions were observed between the groups (Table 3). No significant differences were observed in PPO or VO_2max obtained during the incremental exercise test or performance during the 2 min all-out trial values before the training period between the two training groups (Table 4). PPO significantly ($p<0.01$) increased with training but this increase was not different between training groups (7.2% and 6.6% for N and H, respectively). No significant improvement was found for VO_2max in the two training groups. Both groups significantly ($p<0.01$) improved performance (P_{aver}) during the 2 min all-out exercise trial (7.3 and 6.4% for N and H group, respectively). The H group showed a significant decrease ($P = 0.006$) of −5.1% in VO_2peak measured during the 2 min all-out test between W0 and W4 (Table 5). The N group showed no significant difference in VO_{2peak} (−2.4%) between W0 and W4 (Table 5). No statistical differences were found in muscle MCT1 and MCT4 protein and mRNA content after each training intervention (Figure 1 and 2). Furthermore, we did not find any relationship between MCT content and anaerobic performance.

Discussion

This study was conducted to examine the effects of IHT (compared to conventional interval-training in normoxia) on anaerobic performance and MCT expression in human skeletal muscle. The key findings of the study were that PPO at sea-level increased with training regardless of whether this was performed in hypoxia or normoxia. Furthermore, anaerobic exercise performance at sea-level increased to a similar extent after the hypoxic and normoxic training period. In addition, neither the hypoxic nor normoxic training had any effect on MCT1 and MCT4 protein content. Hence, these results indicate there are no additional effect of the hypoxic stimulus on anaerobic performance after a three-week training period.

The PPO and all-out exercise performance improved after three weeks of training. This suggests that three weeks of training consisting of two interval training sessions and three steady work training sessions are sufficient to obtain significant improvements in sea-level aerobic and anaerobic performance. Meanwhile, neither VO_{2max} nor VO_{2peak} enhanced after the training period in well-trained athletes. The present results are in accordance with a previous study where the authors evaluated a lower intensity hypoxic training of 105 min of cycling training at 60 to 70% of HR reserve a day during 10 consecutive days at 2500 m in eight triathletes [24]. After the training protocol, VO_{2max} was unchanged in both groups indicating that performance can be improved without complimentary changes in VO_2max. However, PPO significantly increased with 6% and also significant improvements in anaerobic power (5%) and anaerobic capacity (4%) measured during a 30-s Wingate test were observed in the IHT group. The authors concluded that 10 days of ~2 hours a day of IHT did not induce changes in VO_{2max} of elite triathletes, but did enhance anaerobic power and capacity [24]. An enhanced

Table 4. Mean (± SE) values of the incremental test to exhaustion of Normoxic (N; n = 8) and Hypoxic (H; n = 10) groups.

	N		H	
	W0	**W4**	**W0**	**W4**
VO_{2max}(ml·kg^{1}.min^{-1})	58.1±0.8	61.0±1.2	58.5±0.7	58.3±0.6
PPO (W)	341.7±3.5	366.3±3.2*	339.0±0.5	361.5±4.4*
HR_{max} (bpm)	190.1±1.1	188.3±1.5	189.7±1.1	189.4±1.0
VE_{max} (L·min^{-1})	159.9±2.6	174.3±2.5	154.2±1.4	155.0±1.7
RPE_{max}	17.9±0.2	17.9±0.1	16.4±0.2§	16.9±0.2

W0: pre-; W4: post-training; VO_{2max}: highest value of the oxygen consumption averaged over 30 s; PPO: peak power output; VE_{max}: highest value of ventilation averaged over 30 s; RPE: rate of perceived exertion.
*P<0.05 for the differences within a group versus W0; §P<0.05 for the differences between groups at a matched time point.

H^+-buffering capacity has been shown to be associated with the improvement in anaerobic/sprint performance following spring training in normobaric conditions. It has been reported in Danish national team cross-country skiers who lived at 2100 m and trained at 2700 m for 14 days, a significant 29% increase in maximal oxygen deficit, as well as a significant 6% increase in the buffering capacity of the *gastrocnemius* muscle [26]. However, as there was no sea-level control group data in this study, it is therefore difficult to draw definitive conclusions regarding the findings. Others [9]found a significant 18% increase in *in-vitro* muscle buffer capacity (βm) of the *vastus lateralis* in male athletes after 23 days of living high-training low at a simulated altitude of 3000 m. These authors [9] suggested therefore that the chronic hypoxic stimulus per se increased the βm.

The observed increase in the aerobic and anaerobic performance without any changes in VO_{2max} and VO_{2peak} could also be explained by a decrease in the rates of lactate appearance (R_a) and disappearance (R_d). Whilst lactate kinetics during exercise were not measured during this study, others [5] have investigated the effect of 20 nights of 9–10 h of LHTL at a simulated altitude of 2650 m, and found an decrease in whole body R_a during 30 min exercise, at 85% VO_{2peak}, in well-trained athletes. Meanwhile, these authors [5] investigated the effect of hypoxia during rest and/or sleeping in contrast with the present study where training rather than rest and/or sleeping was performed under hypoxic conditions. Moreover, the buffering capacity and pH regulation did not show any changes after the 20 nights of LHTL [5]. Therefore, the observed increase in PPO and anaerobic exercise performance are likely due to mechanisms independent of lactate metabolism, *i.e.* buffer capacity and MCTs.

The present work is one of the first studies to examine change in anaerobic performance with IHT. The results show that whilst IHT can be beneficial for performance of 2 min of all-out exercise, the effect does not have any additional benefits than conventional training in normoxia. Whilst these results suggest that IHT should only be reserved for athletes aiming to improve performance in events with a considerable aerobic component, it should be considered that performance at altitude could be improved. A previous study showed that work performance in hypoxia was improved after a period of training in hypoxic conditions [33]. Moreover, there were no differences between or within both groups for citrate synthase and hydroxyacyl-CoA-dehydrogenase activity [33]. Since anaerobic performance is strongly associated to high lactate transport/oxidation, it is of interest that we did not observe any significant changes in the MCT protein expression. In other words, three weeks of IHT does not result in an up-regulation of MCT protein, and is in accordance with previous findings [5]. These authors did not observe an effect of hypoxic exposure, *i.e.* 20 nights of LHTL on MCT1 and MCT4 protein density. Similarly, other authors found no changes in MCT1 and MCT4 content in the *vastus lateralis* muscles after eight weeks at natural altitude of 4100 m [14]. In contrast, other researchers [20] observed that in female Wistar rats, after eight weeks in a hypobaric hypoxic environment (4300 m), a similar decrease of

Table 5. Mean (± SE) values of the 2-min all-out exercise of Normoxic (N; n = 8) and Hypoxic (H; n = 10) groups.

	N (n = 8)		H (n = 10)	
	W0	**W4**	**W0**	**W4**
P_{aver} (W)	377.6±3.4	405.3±2.5*	345.5±5.3	367.6±5.3*
VO_{2peak} (ml·min^{-1}·kg^{-1})	57.5±0.6	56.1±0.7	56.7±0.6	53.8±0.6*
HR_{max} (bpm)	178.7±1.4	178.0±1.2	186.6±1.0	181.8±0.9
VE_{max} (L·min^{-1})	156.8±2.0	177.2±3.0	150.9±1.8	144.3±1.4§
RPE_{max}	17.7±0.3	18.4±0.2	16.8±0.2	16.3±0.2§
La_{max} (mmol·L^{-1})	15.1±0.2	16.6±0.3	14.8±0.3	14.6±0.3
MAOD (ml·kg^{-1})	32.7±1.0	35.4±1.1	31.8±1.0	34.3±0.1

W0: pre-; W4: post-training; P_{aver}: average power output; VO_{2peak}: highest 30 s VO_2 average; HR: highest value of heart rate averaged over 30 s; VE_{max}: highest value of ventilation averaged over 30 s; RPE: rate of perceived exertion; La_{max}: maximal lactate; MAOD: maximal accumulated oxygen deficit.
*P<0.05 for the differences within a group versus W0; §P<0.05 for the differences between groups at a matched time point.

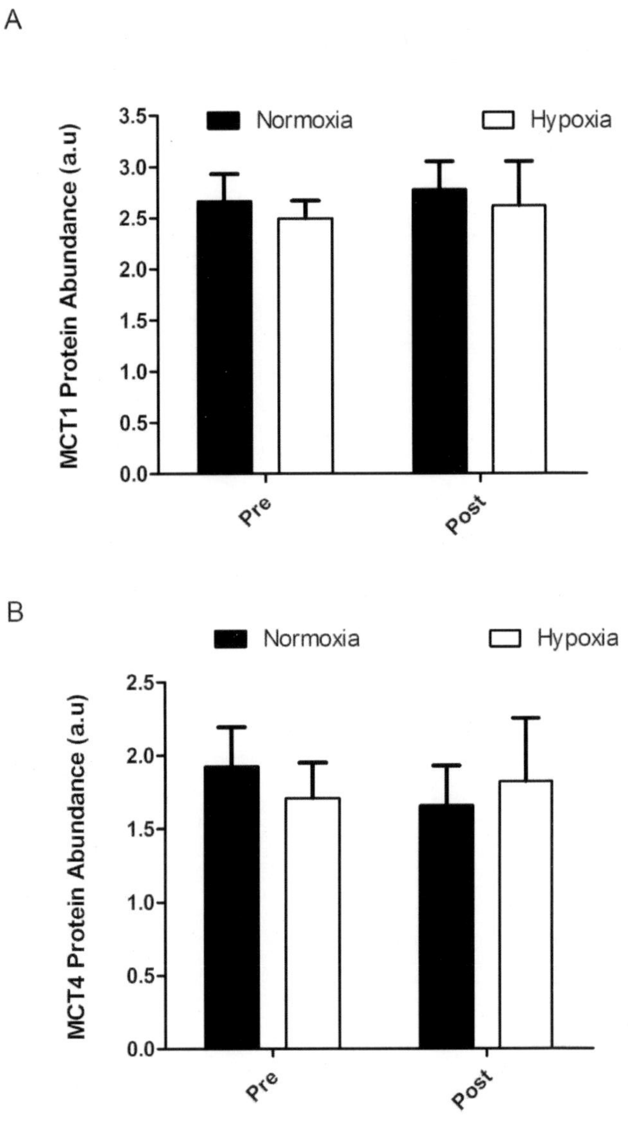

Figure 1. The MCT1 (A) andMCT4 (B) protein content for the normoxic (N; n = 8) and hypoxic (H; n = 10) groups, pre (W0) and post (W4) the 3 wk IHT period.

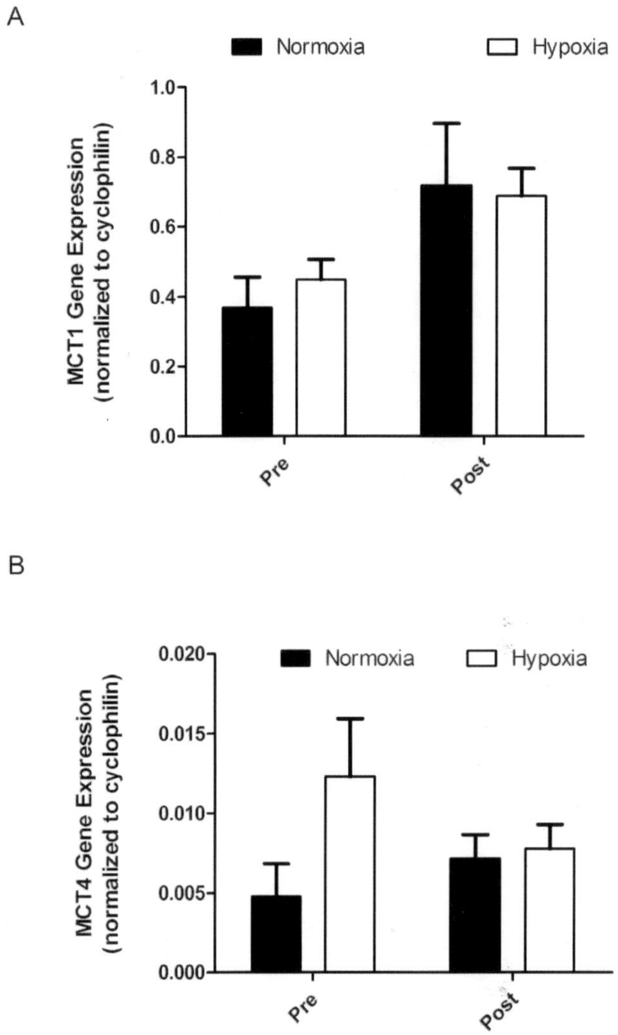

Figure 2. The MCT1 (A) and, MCT4 (B) mRNA for the normoxic (N; n = 6) and hypoxic (H; n = 8) groups, pre (W0) and post (W4) the 3 wk IHT period.

47% in MCT1 and MCT4 of in the *plantaris* muscle. Moreover, these authors found also a tissue-specific effect of hypoxic training on the protein expression [20]. Therefore, as suggested, human muscle could also experience similar fibre-type-dependent changes which in the *vastus lateralis* muscle - as analyzed in the present study - due to its mixed fibre-type composition, could have been overwritten [15].

The lack of any change in MCT1 and MCT4 expression could be due to the training intensity in the present study not of a sufficient magnitude to induce changes in MCT protein content. Indeed, some authors have suggested that the changes in MCT protein expression are related to the training intensity [3]. These authors suggested that MCT1 and MCT4 protein content might increase after an intense anaerobic exercise training, as has been previously observed [30] and that only MCT1 protein content might increase after an aerobic training as they observed [3]. After three weeks of chronic muscle stimulation of 24 h/day in red *tibialis anterior* muscle, MCT1 protein content was significantly increased by 78%, whereas MCT4 protein expression was not altered [3]. However, after eight weeks of one-legged knee-extensor high-intensity exercise training in healthy male subjects, the MCT1 and MCT4 protein content had increased significantly by 76 and 32% respectively [30]. In addition, it has been shown that after seven to eight weeks of one-legged knee-extensor exercise training at an intensity of 150% of thigh VO_{2max}, the MCT1 protein content increased with 115% ($P < 0.05$), whereas no significant difference was observed for the MCT4 protein content (+111%, $P > 0.05$) [14]. Whilst this study demonstrates supramaximal exercise training may evoke large increases in MCT1 and MCT4 expression, some precaution should be taken when interpreting these results, as the study design involved single-leg knee-extensor exercise training which might not induce the same physiological adaptations compared to the present study where "whole body" cycling exercise training was incorporated. Even if a strong point of the present study was that the relative exercise intensity (e.g. 91–92% of PPO – Table 2) during interval-training was similar in normoxia and in hypoxia, this intensity and the duration of the work-interval (e.g. 2-min) were likely not optimal for inducing a high lactate production. It was reported that the increase in lactate/H+ transport capacity is more likely in response to the high-intensity training than the hypoxic condition per se [16]. Therefore, one may assume that the present training intensity was not enough 'glycolytic' for inducing an increase in MCTs in any group. In addition, MCT4 was reported more sensitive than MCT1 to hypoxia since after chronic hypobaric hypoxia exposure [32] or extreme hypoxic conditions [41], only MCT4 protein or mRNA levels increased. In the present study, the low hypoxic dose (combination of a total exposure <20 h and a moderate normobaric hypoxia level; e.g. simulated altitude of 3000 m) explains probably why neither MCT4 nor MCT1 were increased.

In conclusion, three weeks of intermittent hypoxic training increased incremental exercise performance at sea-level. At the same time, anaerobic performance was enhanced without altering the expression of MCT1 and MCT4 protein content. However, no additional benefits of training in hypoxia were observed when compared to similar high-intensity training in normoxia. Therefore, IHT at intensity at or close to PPO as a technique to further improve anaerobic performance at sea-level is questionable.

Impact and Perspective

Scientists, coaches and athletes should have a better understanding of the role that hypoxia plays in training for anaerobic exercise or indeed training for such intermittent high intensity performance. No additional adaptations or anaerobic performance enhancement should be expected above that which athletes can accomplish at sea-level.

Author Contributions

Conceived and designed the experiments: GM BR JM DCS. Performed the experiments: GM BR JM. Analyzed the data: GM DCS LM JM. Contributed reagents/materials/analysis tools: GM BR JM LM DB DCS. Wrote the paper: GM BR JM LM DB. Re-wrote several drafts of the manuscript: LM GM DB DCS.

References

1. Bell GJ, Wenger HA (1988) The effect of one-legged sprint training on intramuscular pH and non bicarbonate buffering capacity. Eur J Appl Physiol Occup Physiol, 58: 158–164
2. Bickham DC, Bentley DJ, Le Rossignol PF, Cameron-Smith D (2006) The effects of short-term sprint training on MCT expression in moderately endurance-trained runners. European Journal of Applied Physiology & Occupational Physiology, 96: 636–643
3. Bonen A, Tonouchi M, Miskovic D, Heddle C, Heikkila JJ, et al. (2000) Isoform-specific regulation of the lactate transporters MCT1 and MCT4 by contractile activity. Am J Physiol Endocrinol Metab, 279: E1131–1138
4. Brooks GA, Brown MA, Butz CE, Sicurello JP, Dubouchaud H (2004) Cardiac and skeletal muscle mitochondria have a monocarboxylate transporter MCT1. Journal of Applied Physiology, 1999, 87: 1713–1718
5. Clark SA, Aughey RJ, Gore CJ, Hahn AG, Townsend NE, et al. (2004) Effects of live high, train low hypoxic exposure on lactate metabolism in trained humans. Journal of Applied Physiology, 96: 517–525
6. Eydoux N, Dubouchaud H, Py G, Granier P, Prefaut C, et al. (2000) Lactate transport in rat sarcolemmal vesicles after a single bout of submaximal exercise. International Journal of Sports Medicine, 21: 393–399
7. Faiss R, Leger B, Vesin JM, Fournier PE, Eggel Y, et al. (2013) Significant molecular and systemic adaptations after repeated sprint training in hypoxia. PLoS ONE 8: e56522
8. Faiss R, Girard O, Millet GP (2013) Advancing hypoxic training in team sports: from intermittent hypoxic training to repeated sprint training in hypoxia. Br J Sports Med 47 Suppl 1: i45–i50
9. Gore CJ, Hahn AG, Aughey RJ, Martin DT, Ashenden MJ, et al.(2001) Live high:train low increases muscle buffer capacity and submaximal cycling efficiency. Acta Physiol Scand, 173: 275–286
10. Hintze J (2011) using PASS 11, LLC. Kaysville, Utah, USA. Available: www.ncss.com.
11. Jones SM, Passfield L (1998) The dynamic calibration of bicycle power measuring cranks. In: Haake SJ (ed) The Engineering of Sport Blackwell Science, Oxford, pp. 265–274
12. Juel C (1996) Lactate/proton co-transport in skeletal muscle: regulation and importance for pH homeostasis. Acta Physiol Scand, 156: 369–374
13. Juel C, Halestrap AP (1999) Lactate transport in skeletal muscle - role and regulation of the monocarboxylate transporter. J Physiol, 517 (Pt 3). 633–642
14. Juel C, Klarskov C, Nielsen JJ, Krustrup P, Mohr M, et al. (2004) Effect of high-intensity intermittent training on lactate and H+ release from human skeletal muscle. Am J Physiol Endocrinol Metab, 286: E245–251
15. Juel C, Lundby C, Sander M, Calbet JA, Hall G (2003) Human skeletal muscle and erythrocyte proteins involved in acid-base homeostasis: adaptations to chronic hypoxia. Journal of Physiology, 548: 639–648
16. Juel C, Pilegaard H. (1998) Lactate/H+ transport kinetics in rat skeletal muscle related to fibre type and changes in transport capacity. Pflugers Archiv, 436(4): 560–564
17. Levine BD (2002) Intermittent hypoxic training: fact and fancy. High Alt Med Biol, 3: 177–193
18. Lundby C, Millet GP, Calbet JA, Bartsch P, Subudhi AW (2012) Does 'altitude training' increase exercise performance in elite athletes? Br J Sports Med 46: 792–795
19. Mahoney DJ, Carey K, Fu MH, Snow R, Cameron-Smith D, et al. (2004) Real-time RT-PCR analysis of housekeeping genes in human skeletal muscle following acute exercise. Physiol Genomics, 18: 226–231
20. McClelland GB, Brooks GA (2002) Changes in MCT 1, MCT 4, and LDH expression are tissue specific in rats after long-term hypobaric hypoxia. Journal of Applied Physiology, 92: 1573–1584
21. McCullagh KJ, Poole RC, Halestrap AP, O'Brien M, Bonen A (1996) Role of the lactate transporter (MCT1) in skeletal muscles. Am J Physiol, 271: E143–150
22. Medbo JI, Jebens E (2002) Leg gas exchange, release of glycerol, and uptake of fats after two minutes bicycling to exhaustion. Scandinavian journal of clinical and laboratory investigation 62: 211–221
23. Medbo JI, Mohn AC, Tabata I, Bahr R, Vaage O, et al. (1988) Anaerobic capacity determined by maximal accumulated O2 deficit. Journal of Applied Physiology, 64: 50–60
24. Meeuwsen T, Hendriksen IJ, Holewijn M (2001) Training-induced increases in sea-level performance are enhanced by acute intermittent hypobaric hypoxia. European Journal of Applied Physiology and Occupational Physiology, 84: 283–290.
25. Millet GP, Faiss R, Brocherie F, Girard O (2013) Hypoxic training and team sports: a challenge to traditional methods? Br J Sports Med 47 Suppl 1: i6–i7
26. Mizuno M, Juel C, Bro-Rasmussen T, Mygind E, Schibye B, et al. (1990) Limb skeletal muscle adaptation in athletes after training at altitude. Journal of Applied Physiology, 68: 496–502
27. Morton JP, Cable NT (2005) Effects of intermittent hypoxic training on aerobic and anaerobic performance. Ergonomics, 48: 1535–1546
28. Mujika I, Busso T, Lacoste L, Barale F, Geyssant A, et al. (1996) Modelled Responses to Training and Taper in Competitive Swimmers. Medicine and Science in Sports and Exercise, 28: 251–258
29. Perry CG, Heigenhauser GJ, Bonen A, Spriet LL (2008) High-intensity aerobic interval training increases fat and carbohydrate metabolic capacities in human skeletal muscle. Appl Physiol Nutr Metab, 33: 1112–1123
30. Pilegaard H, Domino K, Noland T, Juel C, Hellsten Y, et al. (1999) Effect of high-intensity exercise training on lactate/H+ transport capacity in human skeletal muscle. Am J Physiol, 276: E255–261
31. Pilegaard H, Terzis G, Halestrap A, Juel C (1999) Distribution of the lactate/H+ transporter isoforms MCT1 and MCT4 in human skeletal muscle. Am J Physiol, 276: E843–848
32. Py G, Eydoux N, Lambert K, Chapot R, Koulmann N, et al. (2005) Role of hypoxia-induced anorexia and right ventricular hypertrophy on lactate transport and MCT expression in rat muscle. Metabolism, 54(5):634–644
33. Roels B, Bentley DJ, Coste O, Mercier J, Millet GP (2007) Effects of intermittent hypoxic training on cycling performance in well-trained athletes. European Journal of Applied Physiology and Occupational Physiology, 101: 359–368
34. Roels B, Millet GP, Marcoux CJ, Coste O, Bentley DJ, et al. (2005) Effects of hypoxic interval training on cycling performance. Medicine and Science in Sports and Exercise, 37: 138–146
35. Roels B, Thomas C, Bentley DJ, Mercier J, Hayot M, et al. (2007) Effects of intermittent hypoxic training on amino and fatty acid oxidative combustion in human permeabilized muscle fibers. Journal of Applied Physiology, 102(1): 79–86
36. Rusko HR (1996) New aspects of altitude training. Am J Sports Med, 24: S48–52
37. Stolen T, Chamari K, Castagna C, Wisloff U (2005) Physiology of soccer: an update. Sports Medicine, 35: 501–536
38. Thomas C, Perrey S, Lambert K, Hugon G, Mornet D, et al. (2005) Monocarboxylate transporters, blood lactate removal after supramaximal exercise, and fatigue indexes in humans. Journal of Applied Physiology, 98: 804–809
39. Thomas C, Sirvent P, Perrey S, Raynaud E, Mercier J (2004) Relationships between maximal muscle oxidative capacity and blood lactate removal after supramaximal exercise and fatigue indexes in humans. Journal of Applied Physiology, 97: 2132–2138

40. Trenerry MK, Carey KA, Ward AC, Cameron-Smith D (2007) STAT3 signalling is activated in human skeletal muscle following acute resistance exercise. Journal of Applied Physiology, 102: 1483–1489
41. Ullah MS, Davies AJ, Halestrap AP (2006) The plasma membrane lactate transporter MCT4, but not MCT1, is up-regulated by hypoxia through a HIF-1alpha-dependent mechanism. Journal of Biological Chemistry, 281(14): 9030–9037
42. Wilber RL (2001) Current trends in altitude training. Sports Medicine, 31: 249–265.
43. Wilson MC, Jackson VN, Heddle C, Price NT, Pilegaard H, et al. (1998) Lactic acid efflux from white skeletal muscle is catalyzed by the monocarboxylate transporter isoform MCT3. J Biol Chem, 273: 15920–15926

19

Muscle MR Imaging in Tubular Aggregate Myopathy

Valeria Beltrame[1], Paolo Ortolan[1], Alessandro Coran[1], Riccardo Zanato[1], Matteo Gazzola[1], Annachiara Frigo[2], Luca Bello[3], Elena Pegoraro[3], Roberto Stramare[1]*

1 Department of Medicine, Section of Radiology, University of Padova, Padova, Italy, **2** Department of Cardiac, Thoracic and Vascular Sciences, University of Padova, Padova, Italy, **3** Department of Neurosciences, University of Padova, Padova. Italy

Abstract

Purpose: To evaluate with Magnetic Resonance (MR) the degree of fatty replacement and edematous involvement in skeletal muscles in patients with Tubular Aggregate Myopathy (TAM). To asses the inter-observer agreement in evaluating muscle involvement and the symmetry index of fatty replacement.

Materials and Methods: 13 patients were evaluated by MR to ascertain the degree of fatty replacement (T1W sequences) according to Mercuri's scale, and edema score (STIR sequences) according to extent and site.

Results: Fatty replacement mainly affects the posterior superficial compartment of the leg; the anterior compartment is generally spared. Edema was generally poor and almost only in the superficial compartment of the leg. The inter-observer agreement is very good with a Krippendorff's coefficient >0.9. Data show a total symmetry in the muscular replacement (McNemar-Bowker test with $p = 1$).

Conclusions: MR reveals characteristic muscular involvement, and is a reproducible technique for evaluation of TAM. There may also be a characteristic involvement of the long and short heads of the biceps femoris. It is useful for aimed biopsies, diagnostic hypotheses and evaluation of disease progression.

Editor: Barry J. Byrne, Earl and Christy Powell University, United States of America

Funding: The authors have no support or funding to report.

* E-mail: roberto.stramare@unipd.it

Introduction

Tubular Aggregate Myopathy (TAM) is a congenital myopathy characterized by progressive loss of strength, mainly proximal, and frequent cramps and muscle pains induced by exercise. Histologically, it is characterized by tubular aggregates in muscle fibers. According to available data, tubular aggregates are believed to form as a consequence of genetic and/or functional variations, which mainly affect the mechanisms involved in muscle excitation or calcium regulation [1].

To date, no gene responsible for the pathology has been identified: as no specific genetic test is available, clinical and histological examinations, immunohistochemical and histoenzymatic analyses of muscle biopsies, electron microscopy and electromyography are performed for diagnosis.

Evaluation of myopathies/dystrophies by Magnetic Resonance imaging (MR) has always mainly focused on primary and secondary inflammatory skeletal muscle diseases. Several studies report that imaging can also assess the degree of muscle atrophy and the severity of the pathology with high accuracy and sometimes with greater sensitivity than clinical assessment [2]. The different distribution patterns shown by variations in the intensity and severity of muscle involvement may help to achieve differential diagnosis, to identify asymptomatic subjects and to follow up myopathic patients [2–7].

This study aimed at evaluating the extent and distribution of fatty replacement and extracellular edema by MR in subjects with TAM, together with assessment of inter-observer agreement, index of symmetry (left and right hemibodies) and a search for the typical signs of the pathologies which MR can provide.

Materials and Methods

After the review board of the University of Padova had approved this prospective study, our Neurophysiology Center selected 13 patients with TAM (M/F: 8/5, average age 40.4, range 17–67), according to the following criteria:

- clinical condition characterized by progressive loss of strength and/or muscle pains, with cramps and increased hematic CK;
- muscle biopsy revealing tubular aggregates defined as basophilic material in H&E, reddish in color with modified Gomori trichrome stain, intensely reactive to NADH-TR and with negative reaction to SDH; in some cases, diagnosis of TAM was confirmed by electron microscopy;
- absence of other neuromuscular disorders involving loss of strength and tubular aggregates (e.g., limb girdle myasthenia, alcoholic myopathy).

All patients gave their written consent to all tests and to treatment of their data.

MR assessment

Patients underwent MR assessment (1.5 T, Avanto, Siemens, Erlangen, Germany) with T1-weighted axial scans and Short Tau Inversion Recovery (STIR) sequences (8 mm slice thickness, 150° flip angle) according to the following acquisition parameters: pelvic girdle (FOV: 400, 30 slices, TR: 478 ms, TE: 8.8 msec) and STIR (FOV: 400, 30 slices, TR: 4160 msec, TE: 72 msec) and lower limb (FOV: 400, 32 slices, TR: 596 msec, TE: 8.7 msec) and STIR (FOV: 400, 32 slices,TR: 4160 msec, TE: 72 msec). Images were acquired with a body coil and a simultaneous scan of both sides. 32 slices were acquired in the mid of the thighs and legs, because at this level, the images are more representative of the whole muscle features. Moreover, where the muscle bulk is greater, the muscle involvement could be more clearly analyzed.

Tests generally lasted about 30 minutes.

The skeletal muscles assessed were the following: pelvic girdle (gluteus maximus, medius and minimus, tensor of fascia lata and iliopsoas), anterior compartment of thigh (vastus lateralis, intermedius and medialis, rectus femoris), posterior compartment of thigh (sartorius, gracilis, adductor, semimembranosus, semitendinosus, long and short heads of biceps femoris), anterior compartment of leg (anterior tibial, peroneal, extensor digitorum and extensor hallucis), deep posterior leg compartment (posterior tibial, flexor digitorum and hallucis) and superficial posterior leg compartment (gastrocnemius and soleus).

Areas of signal hyperintensity in T1W sequences were interpreted as areas of fatty infiltration. The extent of fatty replacement and its distribution in muscles were evaluated by staging, specific scores being assigned (modified Mercuri scale) [8][9] (Fig. 1): normal appearance (score 0); early moth-eaten appearance, with small scattered areas of increased intensity of T1 signal (score 1); late moth-eaten appearance with many discrete areas of increased signal intensity with initial confluence, comprising less than 30% of the volume of the single individual muscle (score 2); late moth-eaten appearance with many quite extended areas of increased intensity of T1, comprising 30–60% of the volume of each individual muscle (score 3); faded, confused appearance, produced by confluent areas of increased signal intensity (score 4); last-stage appearance, with muscle replaced with adipose and connective tissue with increased signal intensity, only a thin muscle fascia preserved, and neuromuscular structures still distinguishable (score 5).

Short Tau Inversion Recovery sequences (STIR) can identify injury in muscles which appear normal in T1 and can clarify the nature of the signal abnormalities common to several muscular disorders caused by various genetic or protein defects[10]. Hyperintense signals in STIR sequences were used to assess the degree of edema, divided into 3 levels (absent, mild, moderate). The distribution of edema was also classified as interfascicular (fluid in interfascicular space) or intrafascicular (fluid in space between individual myofibers). Edema was defined as segmented if it affected less than half of the acquired muscle sections, and comprehensive if it affected more than half of the axial acquisitions. A specific edema score was also used: absent (score 0); mild, intrafascicular (1); mild, intrafascicular, segmented (2); mild, intrafascicular, global (3), moderate intrafascicular, segmented (4); moderate intrafascicular, global (5).

The images of the 13 patients were analysed in a blind study by three doctors with at least two years of experience in musculoskeletal MRI assessment. Each observer evaluated the 26 muscles of patients' lower limbs (total 1014 ratings). Each of the investigated muscles was analyzed separately and, when a different score was assigned to the proximal and distal images, the average score was used.

Statistical evaluation

In view of the ordinal nature of our data, Krippendorff's coefficient ("alpha") [11] was used to quantify inter-observer agreement, and 95% confidence limits were calculated by bootstrap sampling [12], in order to take the small sample size into account. The closer the alpha coefficient to 1, the greater the agreement (alpha 0.00–0.20: minimum agreement; 0.21–0.40: intermediate; 0.41–0.60: moderate; 0.61–0.80; substantial: 0.81–1.00, almost perfect) [11].

For symmetry evaluation of left and right (hemibodies), the McNemar-Bowker statistical test [13] was employed (test for dependent samples).

Results

13 patients were examined for TAM (Tab. 1). Their average age at the onset of symptoms was 17.1 years (minimum 3 years, maximum 66) with an average disease duration of 22.7 years. Most of the patients (9 out of 13) showed autosomal dominant inheritance; the remaining 4 were sporadic cases. Symptoms at onset were variable.

Analysis of the degree of fatty muscle replacement, according to anatomical area, showed that the superficial posterior leg compartment was the most frequently involved, with an average Mercuri score of 2–2.2. The anterior leg compartment was the least affected (Fig. 2).

Analysis of each muscle (Fig. 3) showed that those most affected by fatty involution were the medial gastrocnemius, semimembranosus, gastrocnemius lateralis, semitendinosus, long head of the biceps femoris, vastus lateralis and soleus. Less affected muscles were the iliopsoas, peroneal, flexor digitorum longus and hallucis, posterior tibial, extensors of fingers and hallux, and tibialis anterior (Tab. 2).

As regards the degree of edema, the most afflicted muscle area was the superficial posterior leg compartment, with an average edema score of 0.9.

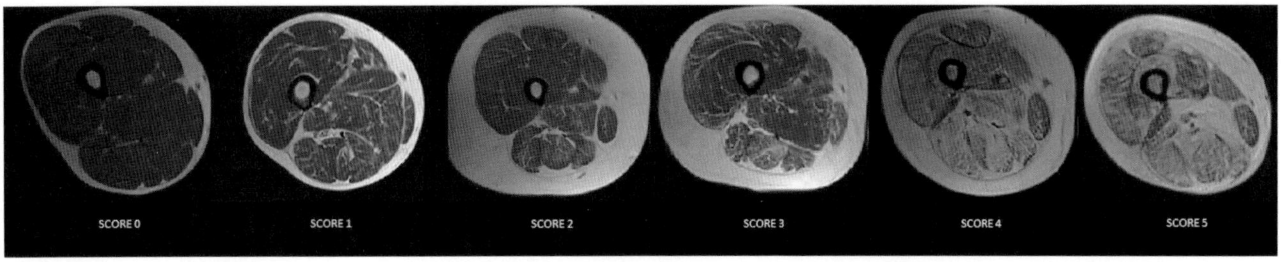

Figure 1. Modified Mercuri's scores, showing progressive grades of muscular fatty replacement.

Table 1. Clinical features of patients with Tubular Aggregate Myopathy.

Patient	Age/gender	Age at onset of symptoms (yrs)	Duration of illness (yrs)	Presenting symptom	Transmission	CK (U/L)
1.	20/F	6	14	weakness lower limbs	AD	4500
2.	38/F	7	31	weakness lower limbs	AD	1200
3.	46/F	6	40	difficulties in running	AD	2500
4.	43/M	6	37	weakness lower limbs	AD	N/A
5.	34/M	21	13	increased CPK	AD	2000
6.	64/F	6	58	difficulties in running	AD	N/A
7.	17/F	7	10	weakness lower limbs	AD	N/A
8.	41/M	7	34	weakness lower limbs	AD	N/A
9.	28/M	3	25	difficulties in running	S	240
10.	28/M	3	25	difficulties in running	S	130
11.	56/M	46	10	exercise intolerance	AD	1000
12.	43/M	38	5	cramps	S	800
13.	67/M	66	1	weakness of extensor muscles of neck	S	Normal

Most muscles appeared to be only slightly affected by edema; in others, it appeared to be completely absent.

Inter-observer agreement was assessed according to each observer's scores with respect to the parameter "fatty replacement", as the extent of edema was too small to reach statistical significance. Inter-observer agreement was calculated according to Krippendorff's coefficient. Agreement in all areas was "almost perfect", the coefficient always being >0.9.

As regards individual muscle assessment, most muscles (21/26) showed "nearly perfect" concordance; 3/26 had "substantial" agreement. Inter-observer agreement was "fair" (alpha <0.35) (Tab. 2) only for the flexor hallucis longus and flexor digitorum longus.

The left and right (hemibodies) overlapped almost perfectly, as confirmed by the McNemar-Bowker test ($p = 1$).

Four out of ten patients showed a different degree of fatty replacement in the short and long heads of the biceps femoris. In particular, the long rather than the short head was more involuted (Fig. 4), as confirmed by Fisher's exact test ($p = 0.0004$).

The difference in involution between the long and short heads of the biceps femoris increased with greater fatty replacement.

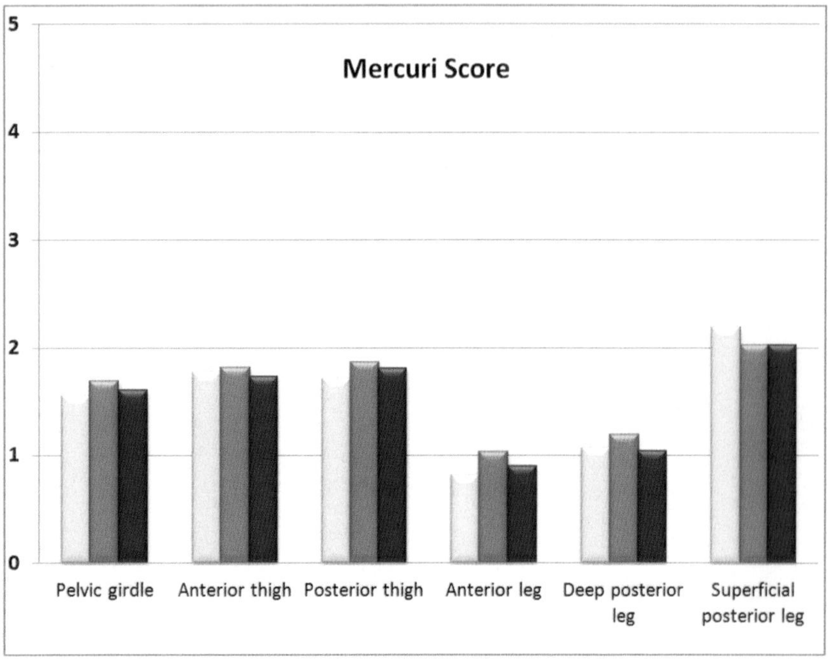

Figure 2. Mercuri scores of muscles divided into areas (three observers).

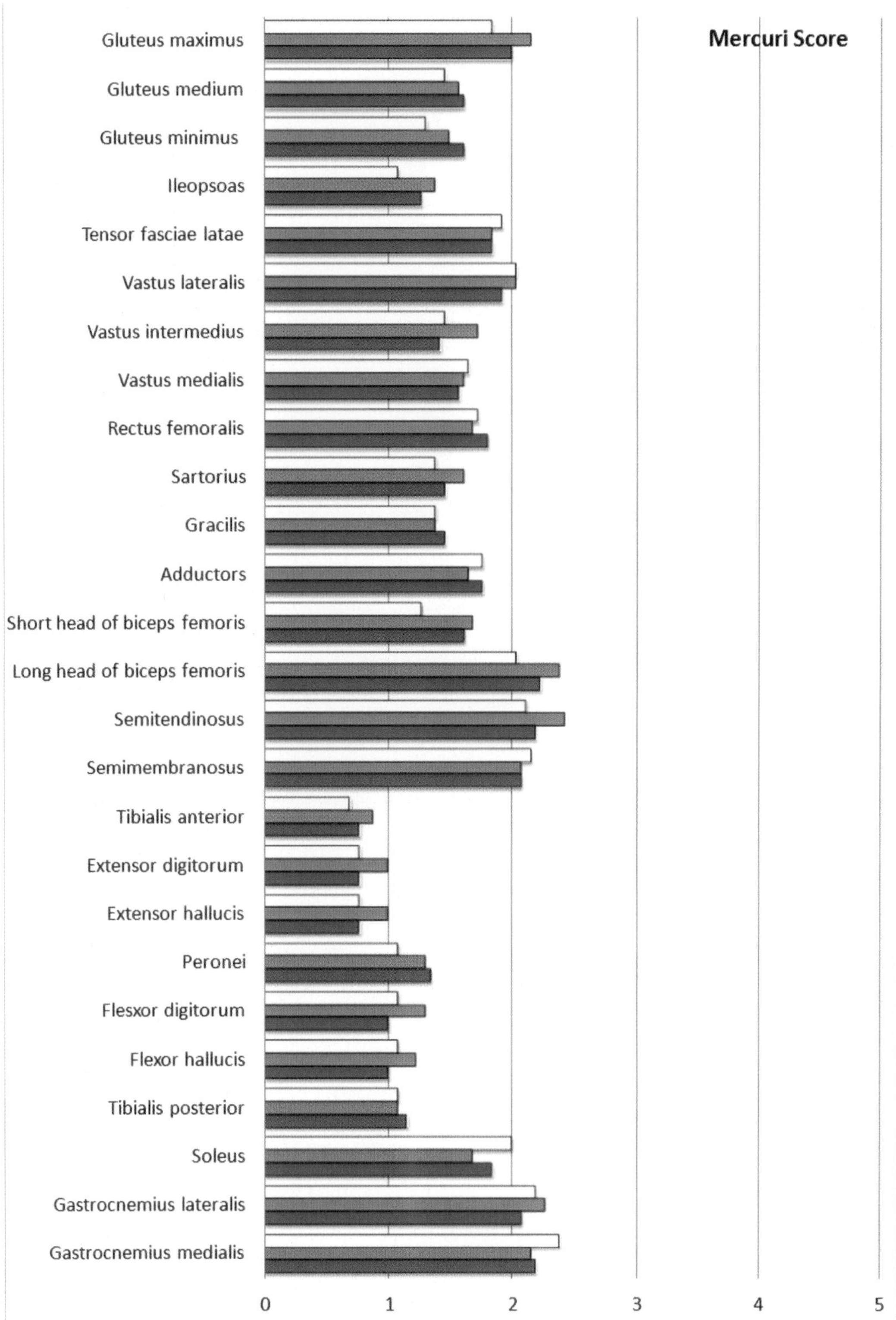

Figure 3. Mercuri scores of individual muscles (three observers).

In patients with a higher average replacement rate of the lower limb, the long head appeared proportionally much more affected than the short head: this difference increased with the greater severity of the illness (Fig. 5).

Discussion

Tubular aggregates were described for the first time by Engel in 1966 in the muscle fibers of patients suffering from periodic paralysis and congenital myotonia [10]. These aggregates are

Table 2. Inter-observer agreement: values of Krippendorf's alpha coefficient of individual muscles with 95% confidence limits.

Muscle	Krippendorff's alpha	LL95CI	UL95CI
Gluteus maximus	0.7517	0.4951	0.9404
Gluteus medius	0.8165	0.6199	0.9616
Gluteus minimus	0.7543	0.5588	0.9152
Iliopsoas	0.8866	0.7968	0.9616
Tensor of fascia lata	0.9870	0.9767	0.9957
Vastus lateralis	0.9649	0.9453	0.9828
Vastus intermedius	0.8975	0.8001	0.9729
Vastus medialis	0.9047	0.8433	0.9562
Rectus femoris	0.9726	0.9531	0.9894
Sartorius	0.9031	0.8486	0.9506
Gracilis	0.9018	0.8382	0.9566
Adductors	0.9060	0.8670	0.9428
Biceps femoris, short head	0.7484	0.6058	0.8779
Biceps femoris, long head	0.9124	0.8399	0.9716
Semitendinosus	0.9167	0.8409	0.9773
Semimembranosus	0.9883	0.9762	0.9979
Anterior tibial	0.8589	0.6409	0.9990
Extensor digitorum	0.9260	0.8409	0.9893
Extensor hallucis	0.9260	0.8424	0.9898
Peroneus	0.9040	0.8112	0.9752
Flexor digitorum brevis	0.3391	−0.0324	0.6544
Flexor hallucis longus	0.3475	−0.0192	0.6659
Posterior tibial	0.9409	0.8815	0.9855
Soleus	0.9000	0.8602	0.9392
Gastrocnemius lateralis	0.9573	0.9192	0.9855
Medial gastrocnemius	0.9667	0.9483	0.9846

predominantly subsarcolemmal inclusions of densly packed membranous tubules, originating from the sarcoplasmic reticulum [1] and associated with various pathologies, both congenital and acquired [11–15], such as hypo- or hypercalcemia, periodic paralysis, congenital myotonia, malignant hyperthermia, inflammatory myopathy, alcoholic myopathy and Whipple's disease [16]. It has been proved that tubular aggregates affect calcium homeostasis at subsarcolemmal level and that the sarcoplasmic reticulum is involved in their formation [1]. In the case of TAM, they represent the main histological feature.

Imaging in myopathic patients is useful in clarifying both evolutionary and presymptomatic aspects [2]. MR applications in the study of muscular dystrophies were first employed after experience with CT, which had already made a significant contribution. Cupler's study (1998) of Miyoshi myopathy highlighted the presence of extracellular edema in STIR in the posterior leg compartment at the onset of the disease [17].

Thanks to high definition of anatomical details, T1W sequences can visualize and quantify the extent of fatty muscle replacement which characterizes muscle pathologies and which worsens

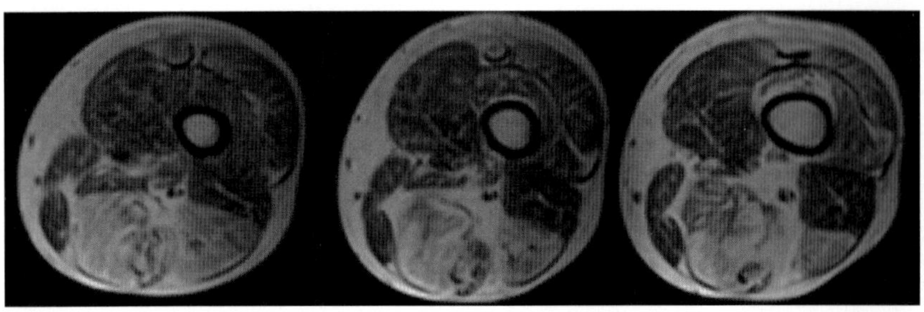

Figure 4. T1W sequence of thigh of same patient in cranio-caudal progression. Different fatty replacement between long head (black arrow) and short head (white arrow) of biceps femoris. Hyperintense appearance, due to fat replacement of long head of biceps femoris, is similar to that of semimembranosus and semitendinosus muscles.

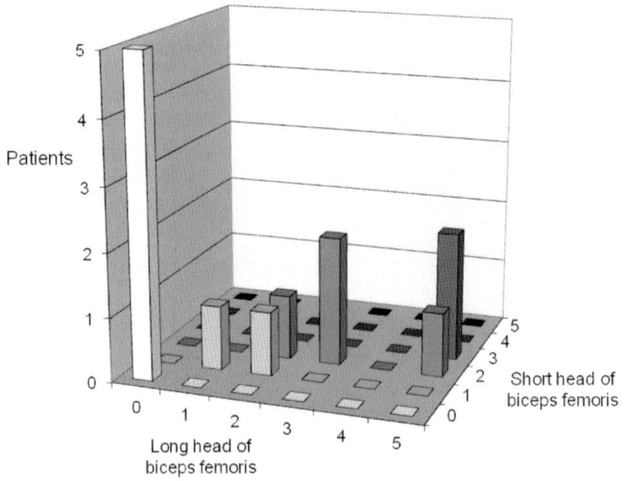

Figure 5. Comparison between degree of fatty replacement (modified Mercuri scale) of long and short heads of biceps femoris in 13 patients. A degree of fatty replacement of long head corresponds to a degree of replacement equal to or less than that of short head. Note in particular how difference between two heads increases with increasing degree of replacement of long head.

progressively. Signal hyperintensity in T1W sequences is an expression of muscle fatty replacement. STIR sequences can detect edema in tissues (such as signal hyperintensity), a sign of inflammatory reaction.

In our 13 TAM patients, 41% of the muscles examined did not show any pathological involvement; 17% of them were classified according to a Mercuri score of 1, 14% with a score of 2, 13% with 3, and 8% with 4. Only 7% of the muscles appeared to be completely replaced.

As described in the past for other muscle diseases, the superficial posterior compartment was the worst affected and the anterior compartment the least [18–20].

Among individual muscles, the most affected were the gastrocnemius, semimembranosus and semitendinosus, and the tibialis anterior, extensor hallucis longus and extensor digitorum longus the least.

This may indicate that, in myopathies, the process of fatty involution and myofiber degeneration affects the most commonly used muscles, as myocells show greater inability to respond to stress.

Unlike fatty replacement, muscle edema was hardly ever found in the areas analysed. The most affected area was the superficial posterior leg compartment. Other muscle compartments were virtually free of edema. In the case of myositis and also of many dystrophies, the MR aspect differs.

As regards assessment of inter-observer agreement, our data showed good agreement in fatty replacement scores according to the modified Mercuri scale. Only the flexor digitorum longus and flexor hallucis longus in the deep posterior leg compartment showed poor agreement. This was very probably due partly to the difficulty of identifying and isolating these muscles in anatomical MR images, especially in patients who do not display particularly trophic activity, and partly to the small number of patients and low scores found by the three observers.

The literature contains few works identifying MR characteristics typical of some muscle pathologies. Works on type 1 myotonic dystrophy, hyaline body myopathy and girdle dystrophy are rare [18–20].

The literature does not contain any records of MR analysis of patients with TAM. In our records, the different replacement level between the long and short heads of the biceps femoris seems peculiar:

Studies have reported that long head of the biceps femoris is more severely affected in Duchenne muscular dystrophy than the short head of the biceps femoris. Akima et al. [21], showed that in Duchenne muscular dystrophy the long head of the biceps femoris was composed of 33% of non-contractile tissue versus 10% in the short head of the biceps femoris.

This pattern has not been described so far in patients with myopathyes. Although limited to 13 patients, this study reports higher progressive fatty replacement of the long head of the biceps femoris compared with the short head, reaching statistical significance. In particular, the short head never reaches a score higher than 3, whereas the long head in three of our patients scored 5. The long head usually has a fatty replacement level similar to that of the semitendinosus muscle, with which it originates at the level of the ischial tuberosity (Fig. 4). The long head, together with the semitendinosus and semimembranosus, makes up the hamstring muscle group which, in addition to extraflexion and rotation of the thigh (like the short head of the biceps femoris), extends the pelvis and aids external rotation of the hip.

As in Duchenne dystrophy, in patients with TAM, the different bio-mechanic of the two biceps femoris heads are probably emphasized.

Conclusions

MR has several roles to play in the approach to TAM, because it can assess the extent of muscle damage (staging), guide biopsies and assess disease progression.

If confirmed by other studies, the particular finding of more progressive fatty replacement of the long head of the biceps femoris than in the short head may become a feature of TAM muscle involvement.

Author Contributions

Conceived and designed the experiments: RS EP. Performed the experiments: VB LB. Analyzed the data: PO AC RZ MG. Contributed reagents/materials/analysis tools: AF. Wrote the paper: VB PO AC RZ MG.

References

1. Salviati G, Pierobon-Bormioli S, Betto R, Damiani E, Angelini C, et al. (1985) Tubular aggregates: sarcoplasmic reticulum origin, calcium storage ability, and functional implications. Muscle Nerve 8(4):299–306.
2. Schedel H, Reimers CD, Nagele M, Witt TN, Pongratz DE, et al. (1992) Imaging techniques in myotonic dystrophy. A comparative study of ultrasound, computed tomography and magnetic resonance imaging of skeletal muscles. Eur J Radiol 15(3):230–8.
3. Schreiber A, Smith WL, Ionasescu V, Zellweger H, Franken EA, et al. (1987) Magnetic resonance imaging of children with Duchenne muscular dystrophy. Pediatr Radiol 17(6):495–7.
4. Messineo D, Cremona A, Trinci M, Francia A, Marini A (1998) MRI in the study of distal primary myopathopies and of muscular alterations due to peripheral neuropathies: possible diagnostic capacities of MR equipment with low intensity field (0.2 T) dedicated to peripheral limbs. Magn Reson Imaging 16(7):731–41.
5. Lamminen AE (1990) Magnetic resonance imaging of primary skeletal muscle diseases: patterns of distribution and severity of involvement. Br J Radiol 63(756):946–50.
6. Castillo J, Pumar JM, Rodriguez JR, Prieto JM, Arrojo L, et al. (1993) Magnetic resonance imaging of muscles in myotonic dystrophy. Eur J Radiol 17(3):141–4.

7. May DA, Disler DG, Jones EA, Balkissoon AA, Manaster BJ (2000)Abnormal signal intensity in skeletal muscle at MR imaging: patterns, pearls, and pitfalls. Radiographics 20 Spec No S295–315.
8. Martin JJ, Ceuterick C, Van Goethem G (1997) On a dominantly inherited myopathy with tubular aggregates. Neuromuscul Disord 7(8):512–20.
9. Muller HD, Vielhaber S, Brunn A, Schroder JM (2001) Dominantly inherited myopathy with novel tubular aggregates containing 1–21 tubulofilamentous structures. Acta Neuropathol 102(1):27–35.
10. Engel AG (1966) Electron microscopic observations in primary hypokalemic and thyrotoxic periodic paralyses. Mayo Clin Proc 41(11):797–808.
11. Hayes AF, Krippendorff K (2007) Answering the call for a standard reliability measure for coding data. Communication Methods and Measures 1(1):77–89.
12. Efron B, Tibshirani RJ (1986) Bootstrap measures for standard errors, confidence intervals, and other measures of statistical accuracy. Statistical Science 1:54–77.
13. Bowker AH (1948) A test for symmetry in contingency tables. J Am Stat Assoc 43(244):572–4.
14. Chui LA, Neustein H, Munsat TL (1975) Tubular aggregates in subclinical alcoholic myopathy. Neurology 25(5):405–12.
15. Engel WK, Bishop DW, Cunningham GG (1970) Tubular aggregates in type II muscle fibers: ultrastructural and histochemical correlation. J Ultrastruct Res 31(5–6):507–25.
16. Morgan-Hughes JA (1998) Tubular aggregates in skeletal muscle: their functional significance and mechanisms of pathogenesis. Curr Opin Neurol 11(5):439–42.
17. Cupler EJ, Bohlega S, Hessler R, McLean D, Stigsby B, et al. (1998) Miyoshi myopathy in Saudi Arabia: clinical, electrophysiological, histopathological and radiological features. Neuromuscul Disord 8(5):321–6.
18. Stramare R, Beltrame V, Dal Borgo R, Gallimberti L, Frigo AC, et al. (2010) MRI in the assessment of muscular pathology: a comparison between limb-girdle muscular dystrophies, hyaline body myopathies and myotonic dystrophies. Radiol Med 115(4):585–99.
19. Wattjes MP, Kley RA, Fischer D (2010) Neuromuscular imaging in inherited muscle diseases. Eur Radiol 20(10):2447–60.
20. Mercuri E, Pichiecchio A, Allsop J, Messina S, Pane M, et al. (2007) Muscle MRI in inherited neuromuscular disorders: past, present, and future. J Magn Reson Imaging 25(2):433–40.
21. Akima H, Lott D, Senesac C, Deol J, Germain S, et al. (2012) Relationships of thigh muscle contractile and non-contractile tissue with function, strength, and age in boys with Duchenne muscular dystrophy. Neuromuscul Disord. 22(1): 16–25.

20

PECAM1$^+$/Sca1$^+$/CD38$^+$ Vascular Cells Transform into Myofibroblast-Like Cells in Skin Wound Repair

Julia Etich[1], Vera Bergmeier[1], Christian Frie[1], Sandra Kreft[1], Lena Bengestrate[1], Sabine Eming[2,3], Cornelia Mauch[3], Beate Eckes[3], Hikmet Ulus[4], Frances E. Lund[5], Gunter Rappl[2,6], Hinrich Abken[2,6], Mats Paulsson[1,2,7], Bent Brachvogel[1,2]*

1 Center for Biochemistry, Medical Faculty, University of Cologne, Cologne, North Rhine-Westphalia, Germany, **2** Center for Molecular Medicine Cologne (CMMC), Medical Faculty, University of Cologne, Cologne, North Rhine-Westphalia, Germany, **3** Department of Dermatology, University of Cologne, Cologne, North Rhine-Westphalia, Germany, **4** Clinic for Paediatric Surgery, Cologne, North Rhine-Westphalia, Germany, **5** Department of Medicine, University of Rochester Medical Center, Rochester, New York, United States of America, **6** Tumorgenetics, Department I of Internal Medicine, Medical Faculty, University of Cologne, Cologne, North Rhine-Westphalia, Germany, **7** Cologne Excellence Cluster on Cellular Stress Responses in Aging - Associated Diseases (CECAD), Cologne, North Rhine-Westphalia, Germany

Abstract

Skin injury induces the formation of new blood vessels by activating the vasculature in order to restore tissue homeostasis. Vascular cells may also differentiate into matrix-secreting contractile myofibroblasts to promote wound closure. Here, we characterize a PECAM1$^+$/Sca1$^+$ vascular cell population in mouse skin, which is highly enriched in wounds at the peak of neoangiogenesis and myofibroblast formation. These cells express endothelial and perivascular markers and present the receptor CD38 on their surface. PECAM1$^+$/Sca1$^+$/CD38$^+$ cells proliferate upon wounding and could give rise to α-SMA$^+$ myofibroblast-like cells. CD38 stimulation in immunodeficient mice reduced the wound size at the peak of neoangiogenesis and myofibroblast formation. In humans a corresponding cell population was identified, which was enriched in sprouting vessels of basal cell carcinoma biopsies. The results indicate that PECAM1$^+$/Sca1$^+$/CD38$^+$ vascular cells could proliferate and differentiate into myofibroblast-like cells in wound repair. Moreover, CD38 signaling modulates PECAM1$^+$/Sca1$^+$/CD38$^+$ cell activation in the healing process implying CD38 as a target for anti-angiogenic therapies in human basal cell carcinoma.

Editor: Richard L. Eckert, University of Maryland School of Medicine, United States of America

Funding: This project was supported by the DFG (SFB829-B04), BMBF (01-GN-0823); Wilhelm Sander-Stiftung and the Deutsche Krebshilfe to H.A. The funders had no role in study design, data collection and analysis, decision to publish, or preparation of the manuscript.

* E-mail: bent.brachvogel@uni-koeln.de

Introduction

The interaction of fibroblasts and vascular cells with the microenvironment is crucial to restore tissue integrity in skin wound healing. Resident fibroblasts are activated upon tissue injury to repopulate the wounded area and reconstruct the connective tissue. Therefore, fibroblasts undergo significant phenotypic changes into migrating and extracellular matrix-secreting myofibroblasts. Changes in the wound environment also initiate an angiogenic response during wound repair. Lining endothelial and perivascular cells migrate into the wound and form a new vascular bed to facilitate an adequate oxygen and nutrient supply. Both cell types may also transform into myofibroblast-like cells to promote non-vessel tissue repair [1]. Previous experiments indicated that PECAM1$^+$ endothelial cells can adapt a myofibroblast-like phenotype by forming α-smooth muscle actin (α-SMA)-containing stress fibers in corneal wounds [2] and give rise to fibroblast-like cells [3]. Perivascular cells (PVCs) are assumed to be activated during skin wound healing to migrate to the perivascular space and transform into myofibroblast-like cells [4,5]. Moreover, PVCs display mesenchymal stem cell-like properties [6,7] and are thought to contribute to the fibrotic reactions in spinal cord scar tissue formation [8]. Hence, endothelial cells and perivascular cells could represent a source for mesenchymal cells upon tissue repair [9,10]. Sca1 is often used to identify subpopulation of endothelial progenitor cells in the bone marrow or in the circulation [11,12]. We have previously detected Sca1 at the cell surface of a perivascular cell population in the vasculature of adult brain meninges [7,13] that can differentiate into various mesenchymal cell types.

In this work, we have used the expression of Sca1 and PECAM1 to analyze the contribution of the vasculature to myofibroblast formation and wound repair in the skin [9,10]. We identified a vascular PECAM1$^+$/Sca1$^+$ cell subpopulation, which was highly enriched in the granulation tissue of skin wounds and in neoangiogenic areas of human basal cell carcinoma. Surprisingly, cells expressed perivascular cell-specific genes like *Desmin*, *Pdgfrb* and *Angp1* and the endothelial cell-specific genes *Angpt2* and *Tie2*. In addition, the PECAM1 receptor *CD38* was found exclusively in PECAM1$^+$/Sca1$^+$ cells. PECAM1$^+$/Sca1$^+$/CD38$^+$ cells entered the cell cycle upon wounding and sorted cells could give rise to myofibroblast-like cells. Gain-of-function experiments in mice indicated a relevance of the CD38 receptor signaling for the activation of PECAM1$^+$/Sca1$^+$ cells in skin repair. Since CD38 can regulate cell activation, adhesion and migration events and its expression is restricted to PECAM1$^+$/Sca1$^+$ cells in the wound we propose that PECAM1$^+$/Sca1$^+$ cells can be activated by CD38 to transform into myofibroblast-like cells during wound repair. Data

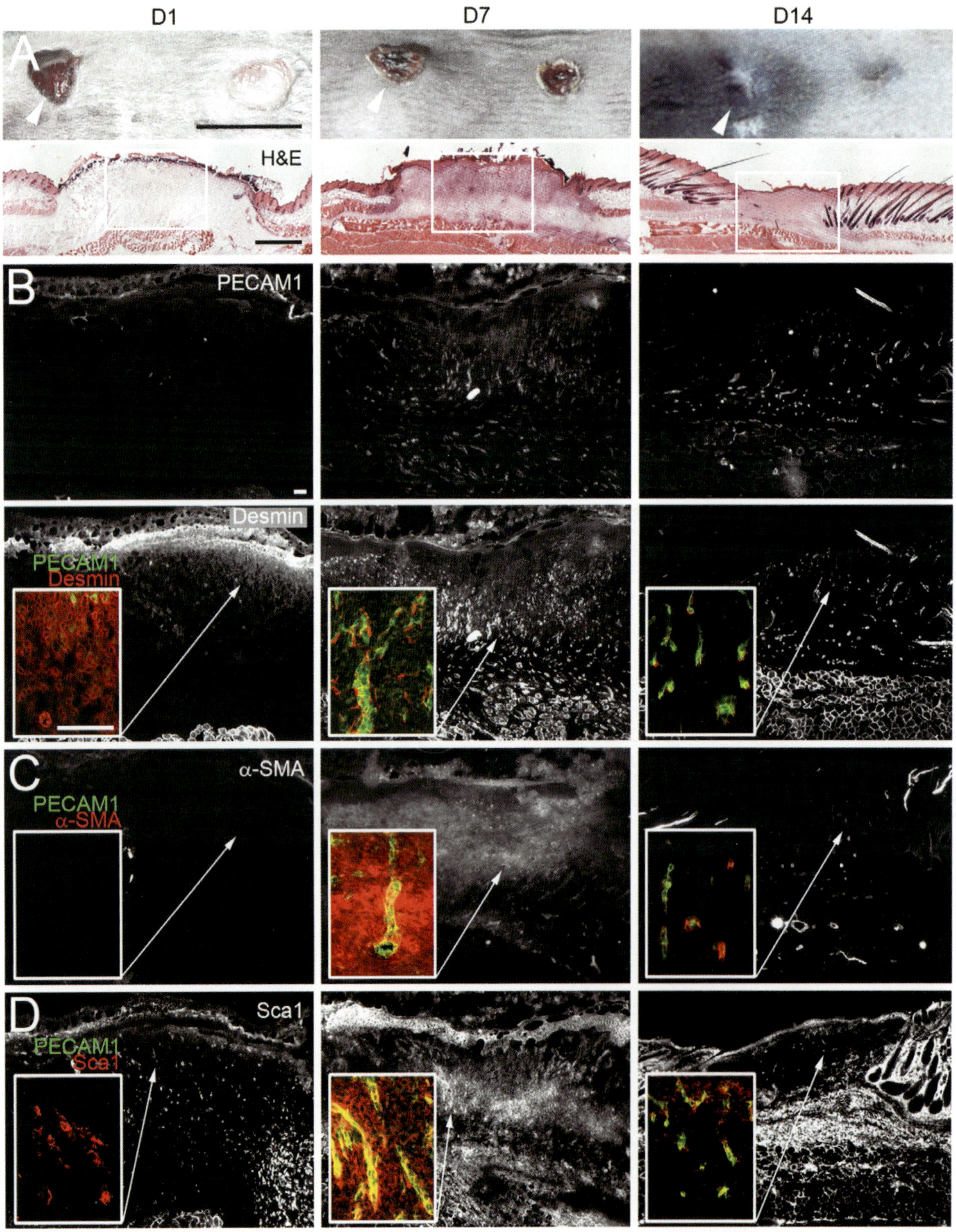

Figure 1. Expression of perivascular and endothelial cell-specific markers in wound repair. Analysis of PECAM1, desmin, α-SMA and Sca1 expression in the wounded skin. (A) Dorsal view of full thickness wounds on the back skin of mice one (D1), seven (D7) and 14 (D14) days post injury. Representative H&E-stained cryosections of selected wounds (arrowhead) during inflammation (D1), granulation (D7) and remodeling (D14) are shown. (B-D) Immunostaining of (B) PECAM1/desmin, (C) PECAM1/α-SMA or (D) PECAM1/Sca1 expression at the different stages of wound healing. The individual monochrome signals for PECAM1, desmin, α-SMA and Sca1 are shown in overviews. Squares within the images represent closeups of overlays for the PECAM1/desmin, PECAM1/α-SMA PECAM1/Sca1 stainings (B-D). Bars 1 cm (A, top), 1 mm (A, lower panel), 100 μm (B).

moreover imply CD38 as a target for anti-angiogenic therapy of human basal cell carcinoma.

Materials and Methods

Ethics Statement, Mice, Biopsies

Animal experiments were performed with C57BL/6N or C.129S6(B6)-Rag2tm1FwaN12 mice on BALB/c background in accordance with the animal ethics guidelines of the German law. Institutional review board: "Landesamt für Natur, Umwelt- und Verbraucherschutz NRW", (ethic approval no. 31.08.261, 20.11.057). Human foreskin samples and basal cell carcinoma biopsies were provided by the SFB829-core facilities. Institutional review board:" Ethik-Kommission der Medizinischen Fakultät der Universität zu Köln" (Ethic approval no. 08-144). Written informed consent was obtained from the patients.

Histology and Immunohistochemistry

Cryosections were used for histological and immunohistochemical analysis. For morphological assessment sections were stained for nuclei (hematoxylin) and cytoplasm (eosin) according to standard procedures. For immunofluorescence studies monoclonal rat anti-CD31 (BD), mouse anti- α-SMA (Sigma), mouse anti-desmin (Progen), rat anti-Sca1 (BD), rat anti-CD38 (Biolegend), rat anti-Tie2 (BD), rat anti-CD34 (BD) antibodies were used on paraformaldehyde-fixed sections. Corresponding secondary antibodies coupled to Alexa Fluor 488 (Molecular Probes) or Cy3 (Jackson Immuno Research) and DAPI (Invitrogen) were applied. Images were taken and analyzed by immunofluorescence (Nikon Eclipse TE2000-U Microscope) and confocal microscopy (LeicaTCS-SP5).

Wound Healing Experiments

Mice were anesthetized by i.p. injection of Ketavet/Rompun (Bayer) and full thickness wounds of 6 mm diameter were inflicted at the back. For antibody treatments 75 µg/150 µl of rat anti-CD38 or isotype control antibody (SouthernBiotech) were injected on day two, four and six post wounding into the retro-orbital venous sinus. Wounds were embedded in tissue tek (Sakura Finetek) and serial sections from the central portion of the wound (Leica Cryotome, CM3050) were stained with hematoxylin and eosin (H&E). Morphometric parameters [14] were determined using ImageJ software [15].

Fluorescence Activated Cell Sorting and Cell Culture

Isolated skin or wounds were digested with 0.5% (w/v) Dispase® II (Roche) in PBS at 4°C overnight. Subcutaneous tissue and epidermis were removed, dermis incubated in 0.2% (w/v) collagenase type 1 (Worthington) in DMEM-F12, 10% FCS for 1 ½ h at 37°C, washed with 5% FCS/PBS and passed through a 40 µm cell strainer (BD). $\sim 6 \times 10^5$ cells were recovered from skin or wound of a mouse. Cells were incubated for 15 min on ice in 5% FCS/PBS with mouse-Fc-Block (BD), and then stained for 15 min on ice with primary conjugated monoclonal antibodies specific for CD31, CD34, CD38, CD45, Sca1 or Tie2. Cells were washed, costained with 7-actinomycin (7AAD) followed by flow cytometry (FACSCantoII, BD) or cell sorting (FACSAriaIII, BD). To detect intracellular α-SMA, cells were fixed and permeabilized in IntraSure solution (BD) prior staining. For cell cycle analysis cells were labeled with antibodies, fixed and permeabilized in IntraSure solution (BD) and costained with propidium iodide (BD). Cells were analyzed by flow cytometry. The Watson algorithm [16] of the Flow Jo software (Tree Star, Inc) was used for data processing. For cell culture experiments 5000 sorted cells were cultured in VascuLife SMC medium (LifeLine Technology) containing 5 ng/ml FGF, EGF, insulin, 50 ng/ml ascorbic acid and 5% FCS at 37°C with 5% CO_2.

Semiquantitative RT-PCR

RNA from sorted cells was isolated using NucleoSpin-RNA-XS Kit (Macherey&Nagel) and quality was assessed by capillary electrophoresis according to the manufacturer's specifications (Agilent2100Bioanalyzer). RNA samples were reversely transcribed into cDNA using the SuperscriptIII 1°-strand Synthesis Kit (Invitrogen). Semiquantitative RT-PCRs were performed for *Desmin*, *Pdgfrb*, *Angpt1*, *Angpt2*, *Tie2*, *Pecam1*, *Sca1*, *CD34*, *CD38* and *Gapdh* according to standard procedures and band intensities of the electrophoretic gels were processed and quantified using Image J software [15]. Primer sequences will be provided on request.

Results

The Vasculature is Reorganized During Skin Repair

To study the distribution of the vasculature in skin repair, wounds were inflicted at the back of eight weeks old C57BL/6N mice (Fig. 1A) and vascular marker expression was analyzed. In the early phase of inflammation hardly any PECAM1$^+$ endothelial or desmin$^+$ perivascular cells were seen in the wound (Fig. 1B). At seven days post wounding PECAM1$^+$ endothelial and desmin$^+$ perivascular cells had invaded the wound and desmin$^+$ perivascular cells formed cytoplasmic protrusions along the PECAM1$^+$ vessels. With vessel regression the number of PECAM1$^+$/desmin$^+$ cells decreased. α-SMA$^+$ myofibroblasts were mainly detected in the granulation tissue seven days post injury (Fig. 1C). Stem cell antigen 1 (Sca1), known to be expressed in isolated perivascular cells from brain meninges [13], was hardly detected in the wound at one day post injury (Fig. 1D). After seven days the numbers of Sca1$^+$ cells transiently increased in the stroma and vasculature of the granulation tissue, while in 14 days old wounds Sca1 expression was primarily detected in PECAM1$^+$ vessels of the wound. Thus, the distribution of Sca1$^+$ cells partially resembled that of desmin$^+$ perivascular cells, PECAM1$^+$ endothelial cells and α-SMA$^+$ myofibroblasts.

PECAM1$^+$/Sca1$^+$ Vascular Cells are Enriched During Wound Repair

To define the origin of Sca1$^+$ cells we analyzed cell suspensions from dermis and wounds at various times points using flow cytometry. Cells were stained for 7AAD and the cell surface markers CD45, Sca1 and PECAM1. In the newborn dermis Sca1$^+$ cells represented 7.5% of the 7AAD$^-$ viable CD45$^-$ non-hematopoietic cell population, which increased to 43% and 49% in the juvenile and adult dermis, respectively (Fig. 2A, $n \geq 10$ mice). Approximately 1% of the newborn and up to 6.2% of the juvenile and adult dermal cells expressed PECAM1. In addition, 0.8% of the cells in newborn dermis and 2.3% in the juvenile and adult dermis expressed both proteins. In wounds no significant changes were seen for Sca1$^+$ cells at the analyzed time points, whereas the proportion of PECAM1$^+$ cells decreased from 5.6% in the unwounded control to 0.5% within the first three days after tissue injury (Fig. 2B, $n \geq 4$ mice). Later the proportion of PECAM1$^+$ cells increased to 2.4% of the cells. The percentage of PECAM1$^+$/Sca1$^+$cells increased from 2.7% in the unwounded skin to 11% at seven days post wounding. Thereafter the fraction of PECAM1$^+$/Sca1$^+$cells declined to 4.8% in 14 days old wounds. Hence, PECAM1$^+$/Sca1$^+$ cells were enriched at the peak of neoangiogenesis, matrix secretion and myofibroblast appearance.

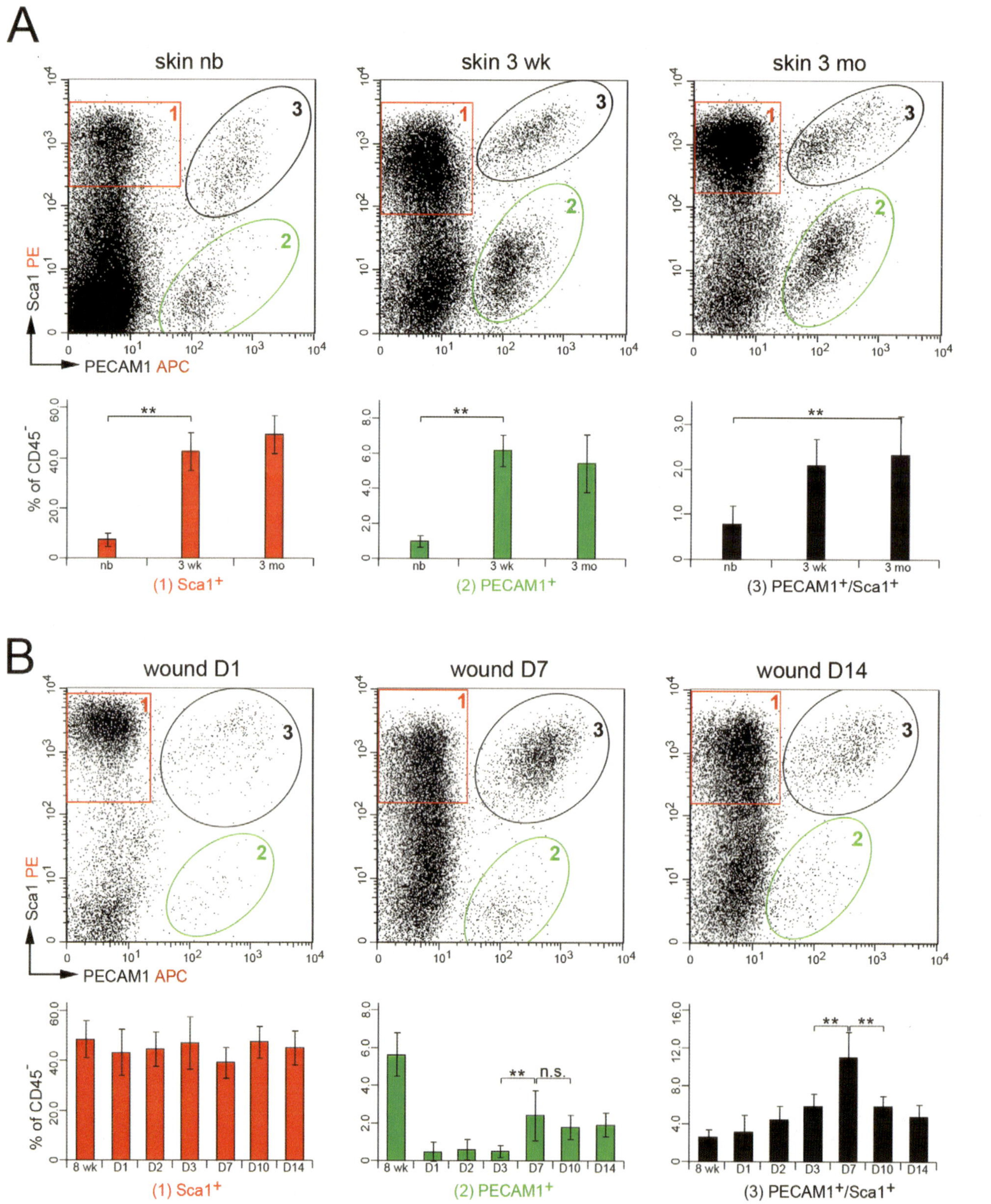

Figure 2. Distribution of PECAM1 and Sca1 protein on skin- and wound-derived cells. (A) Flow cytometry analysis of Sca1 and PECAM1 expression in CD45$^-$ non-hematopoietic cells isolated from newborn (nb), three weeks (3 wk) and three months (3 mo) old dermis. Sca1$^+$ (1, red box), PECAM1$^+$ (2, green ellipse) and PECAM1$^+$/Sca1$^+$ (3, black ellipse) cell populations are highlighted. (B) Dot plots of Sca1 and PECAM1 expression in cell suspensions isolated from full thickness wounds one (D1), seven (D7) and 14 days (D14) post injury of eight weeks old mice. Percentage of positive cell populations at the different time points of flow cytometry analysis (lower panel) is given with standard deviation and significant changes were determined using the unpaired two-tailed student's T-test (n≥3, **p≤0.01, n.s = not significant).

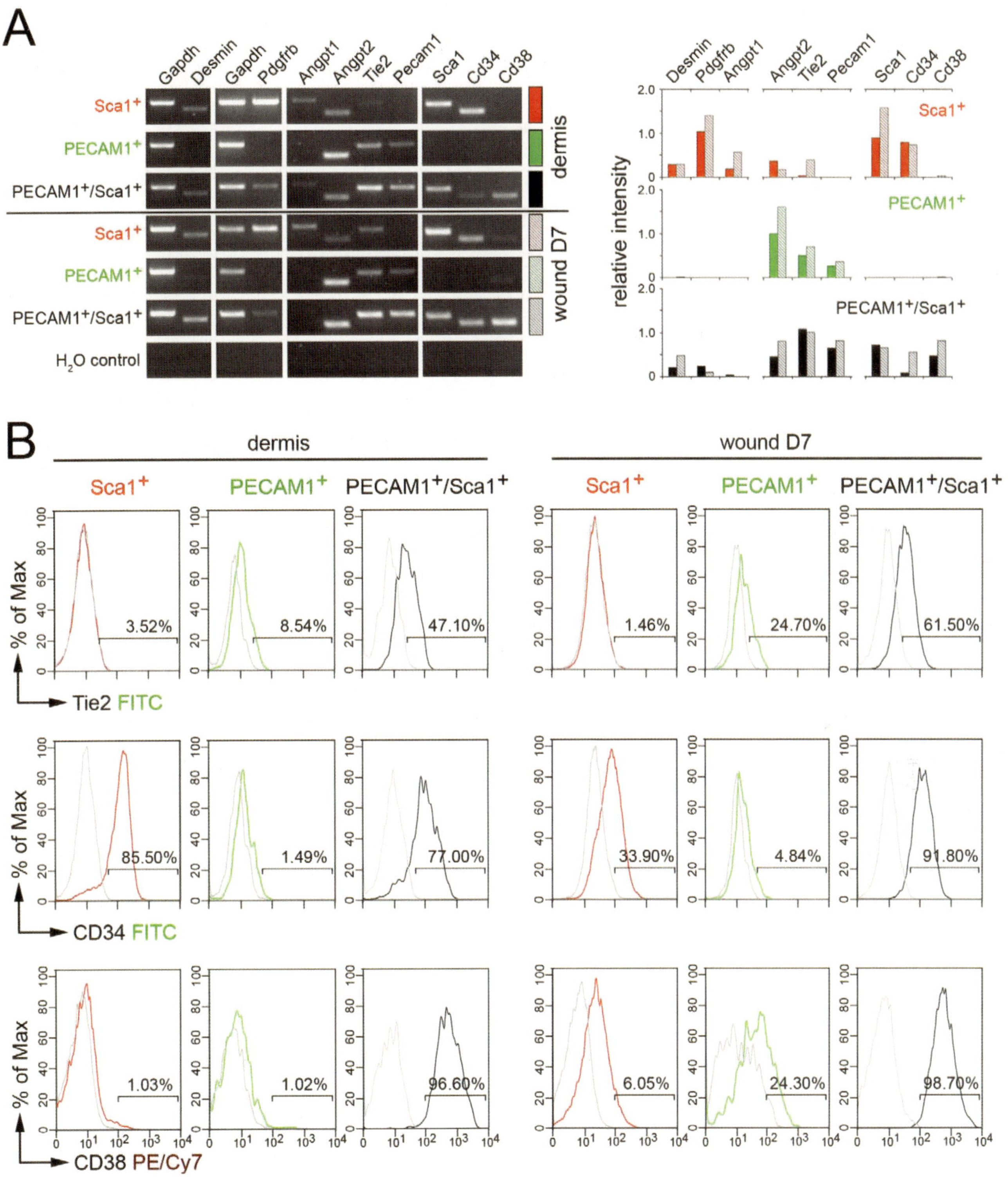

Figure 3. Expression profile of isolated Sca1^{+}, PECAM1^{+} and PECAM1^{+}/Sca1^{+} cells. Marker expression in the sorted cell populations isolated from dermis or wounds seven days post injury. (A) Relative mRNA expression levels of perivascular (*Desmin, Pdgfrb, Angpt1*), endothelial (*Angpt2, Tie2, Pecam1*), progenitor cell-specific markers (*Sca1, Cd34*) and of the CD38 receptor (*Cd38*) were determined by semiquantitative RT-PCR in non-hematopoietic Sca1^{+}, PECAM1^{+} and PECAM1^{+}/Sca1^{+} cell populations. The band intensities of the electrophoretic gels were processed and quantified using Image J software. The relative expression intensity of the individual genes compared to *Gapdh* is given. The lack of Sca1 or Pecam1 expression in sorted PECAM1^{+} or Sca1^{+} cells demonstrated the purity of the cell fractions. (B) Flow cytometric detection of TIE2, CD34, CD38 expression at the cell surface of Sca1^{+} (red), PECAM1^{+} (green) and PECAM1^{+}/Sca1^{+} (black) cells isolated from dermis or full thickness wounds seven days post injury.

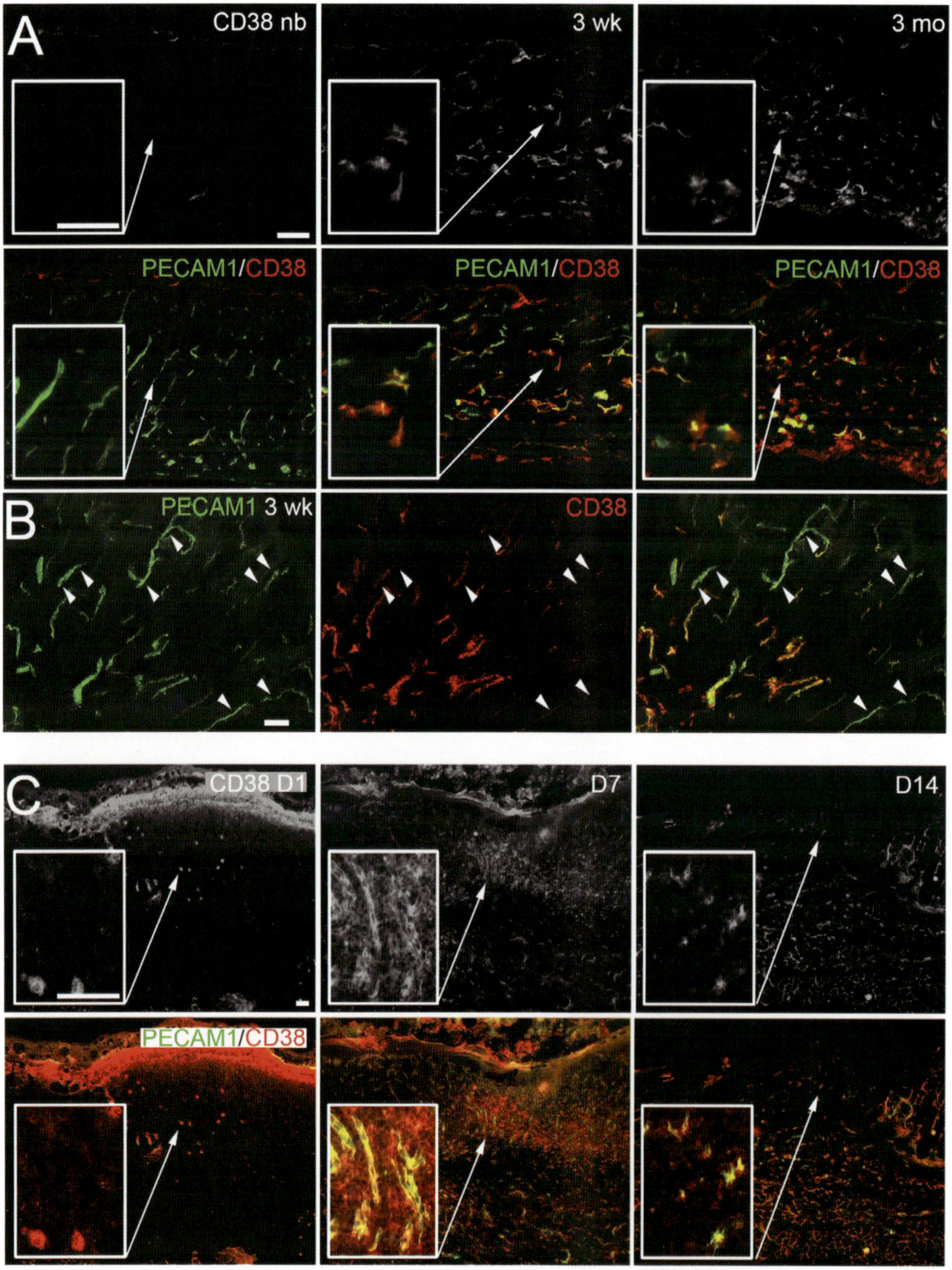

Figure 4. ***In situ*** **detection of the CD38 receptor in the maturing skin and wound.** (A) Expression of PECAM1 and CD38 in cryosections of newborn (nb), three weeks (3 wk) and three months (3 mo) old skin was detected by immunofluorescence microscopy. The fluorescence signal for CD38 (top row) and the overlay with PECAM1 is shown. (B) Confocal microscopy analysis of PECAM1/CD38 expression in three weeks old skin. PECAM1^{+} vessels lacking CD38 expression are indicated (arrowheads). (C) Localization of PECAM1 and CD38 expression in cryosections of wounds one (D1), seven (D7) and 14 days (D14) post injury. The fluorescence signal for CD38 (top row), the overlay with PECAM1 and higher magnifications of the wounded area are shown (A, C, squares). Bars 100 μm (A, C), 50 μm (B).

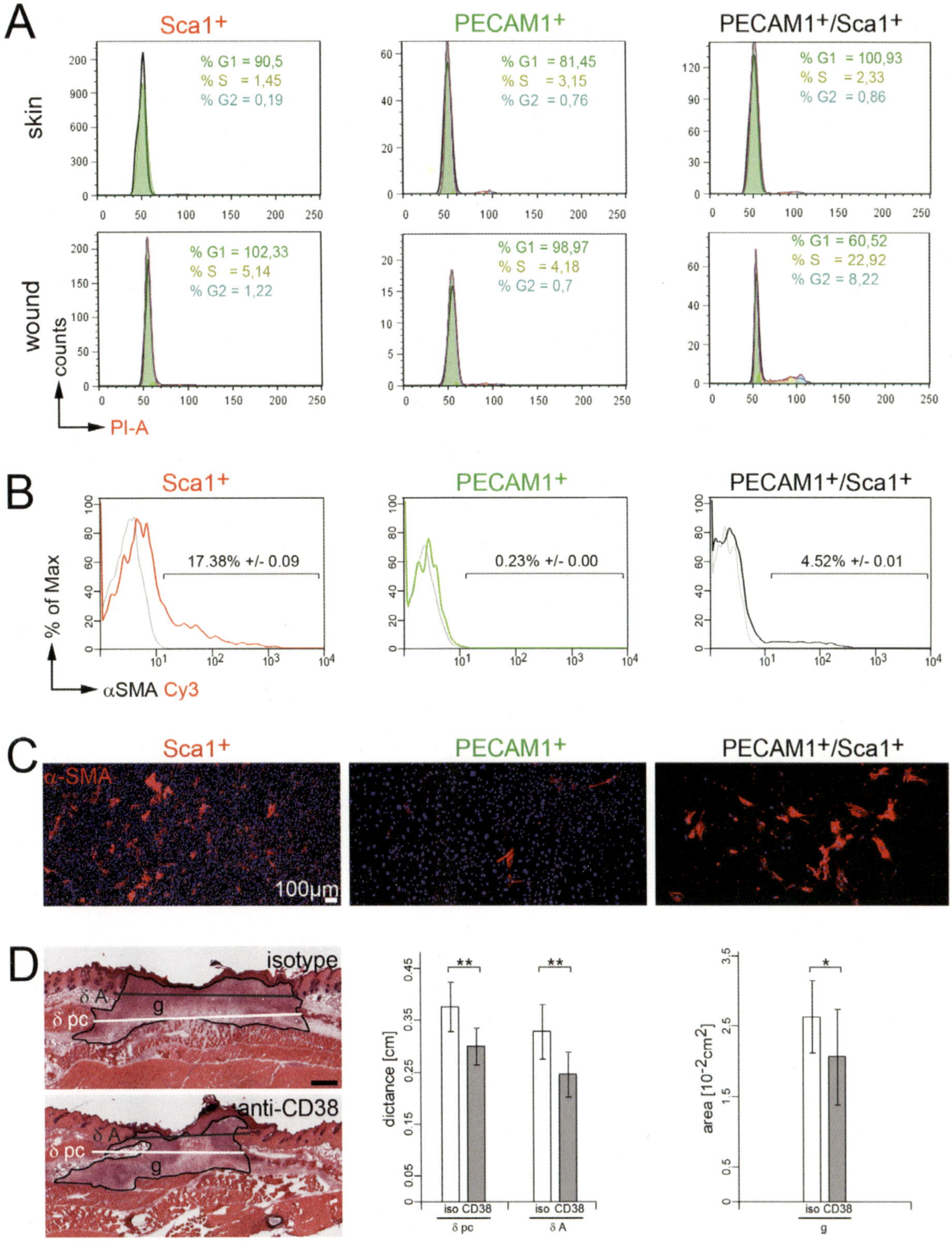

Figure 5. Myofibroblast-like cell formation and modulation of CD38 receptor activity. (A) Representative cell cycle analysis of skin- and wound-derived Sca1$^+$, PECAM1$^+$ and PECAM1$^+$/Sca1$^+$ cells seven days post injury using propidium iodide (PI) stain in flow cytometry analysis (see figure S1). The relative percentage of cells in G1 (green), S (ochre) and G2 (blue) are highlighted. (B) Flow cytometric detection of α-SMA in wound-derived Sca1$^+$, PECAM1$^+$/Sca1$^+$ and PECAM1$^+$ cells seven days post injury (n = 7 mice). (C) Immunofluorescence analysis of α-SMA expression in cultured wound-derived Sca1$^+$, PECAM1$^+$ and PECAM1$^+$/Sca1$^+$ cells. Nucleoli were detected using DAPI stain. (D) Morphometric analysis of wounds in immunodeficient mice stimulated with rat anti-CD38 or isotype matched antibodies (n = 4). Distances between edges of the panniculus carnosus (δ pc), hair follicles (δ A) and the area of the granulation tissue (g) were determined. Statistics: unpaired two-tailed student's T-test (*$p \leq 0.05$, **$p \leq 0.01$). Bars 100 µm (C), 500 µm (D).

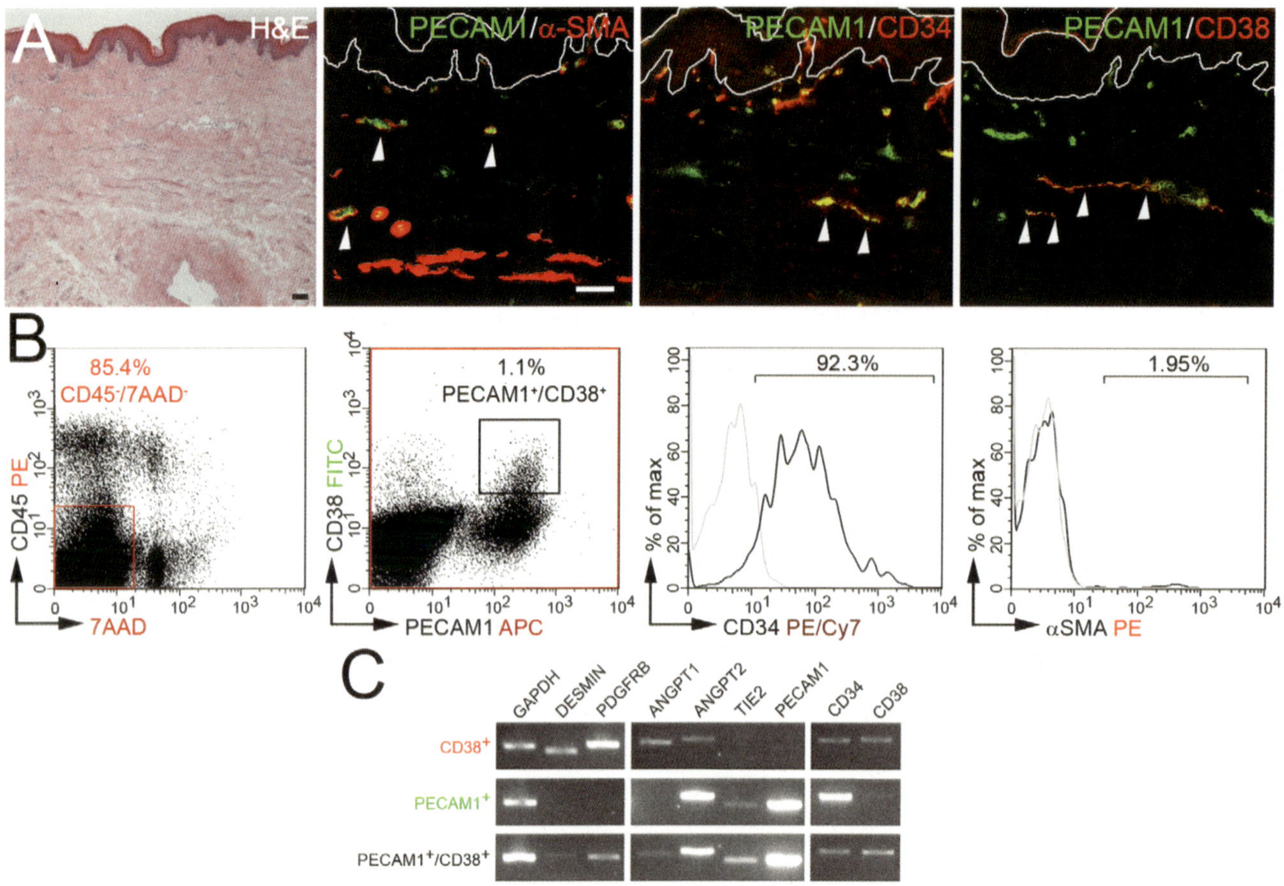

Figure 6. Identification of PECAM1⁺/CD38⁺ cells in human foreskin. (A) Expression of PECAM1, α-SMA, CD34 and CD38 in cryosections of 12 years old foreskin is detected by immunofluorescence microscopy. (B) Flow cytometry analysis of CD38 and PECAM1 expression. The proportion of CD34 and α-SMA expressing cells within the PECAM1⁺/CD38⁺ cell population was determined (histograms). (C) Expression profile of sorted non-hematopoietic CD38⁺, PECAM1⁺ and PECAM1⁺/CD38⁺ cell populations. Bars 100 μm.

PECAM1⁺/Sca1⁺ Vascular Cells Express CD38

The expression profile of sorted Sca1⁺, PECAM1⁺ and PECAM1⁺/Sca1⁺ cell populations from dermis and wounds seven days post injury were assayed by semiquantitative PCR to define the origin of PECAM1⁺/Sca1⁺ cells (Fig. 3A). Genes expressed in perivascular cells like *Desmin*, *Pdgfrb* and *Angpt1* were upregulated in dermis-derived Sca1⁺ cells, but were hardly detected in PECAM1⁺ cells. These cells mainly expressed endothelial cell-specific genes *Angpt2* and *Tie2*. Surprisingly, perivascular and endothelial cell-specific genes were expressed in PECAM1⁺/Sca1⁺ cells. The progenitor marker *CD34* was detected in Sca1⁺ cells and PECAM1⁺/Sca1⁺ cells and the PECAM1 receptor *CD38* was found exclusively in PECAM1⁺/Sca1⁺ cells. Similar expression profiles were seen in wound-derived cell populations. Flow cytometry confirmed the presence of TIE2, CD34 and CD38 proteins on the cell surface of the distinct cell populations (Fig. 3B). TIE2 protein was missing in Sca1⁺ cells but detected in 9% of PECAM1⁺ and 47% of PECAM1⁺/Sca1⁺ cells of the dermis. Wound-derived Sca1⁺ cells did not express TIE2 protein. The proportion of TIE2-expressing cells increased to 25% for PECAM1⁺ and 62% for PECAM1⁺/Sca1⁺ cells. CD34 was mainly detected on the cell surface of Sca1⁺ and PECAM1⁺/Sca1⁺ cells isolated from dermis or wounds. CD38 protein was found on all dermis-derived PECAM1⁺/Sca1⁺ cells but was not detected on Sca1⁺ and PECAM1⁺ single positive cells. In wounds CD38 expression was maintained on all PECAM1⁺/Sca1⁺ cells and 6% of the Sca1⁺ and 24% of the PECAM1⁺ cells started to express the CD38 receptor. These results indicated that PECAM1⁺/Sca1⁺ cells express CD34 and CD38 protein and activated Sca1⁺ or PECAM1⁺ cells gain CD38 expression upon injury.

The CD38 receptor mediates cell survival and migration signals [17] and may also activate PECAM1⁺/Sca1⁺ cells in the wound. We therefore studied the localization of CD38⁺ cells in the maturing skin and wounds by immunofluorescence analysis (Fig. 4). In newborn skin no signal for CD38 was seen, although PECAM1⁺ vessels were present throughout the dermis. In contrast, in skin at three weeks and three months a strong signal for CD38 was detected in a subpopulation of PECAM1⁺ vessels of the reticular dermis (Fig. 4A, B). In the early phase of the healing progress (D1) only a few CD38⁺ cells were present in the wound (Fig. 4C), whereas at later stages CD38⁺ cells were found in the intervascular space and in PECAM1⁺ vessels of the granulation tissue (D7). Upon remodeling CD38⁺ cells were mainly associated with PECAM1⁺ vessels (D14). The intervascular distribution of CD38⁺ cells pointed to a role of PECAM1⁺/Sca1⁺/CD38⁺ cells for non-vessel tissue repair.

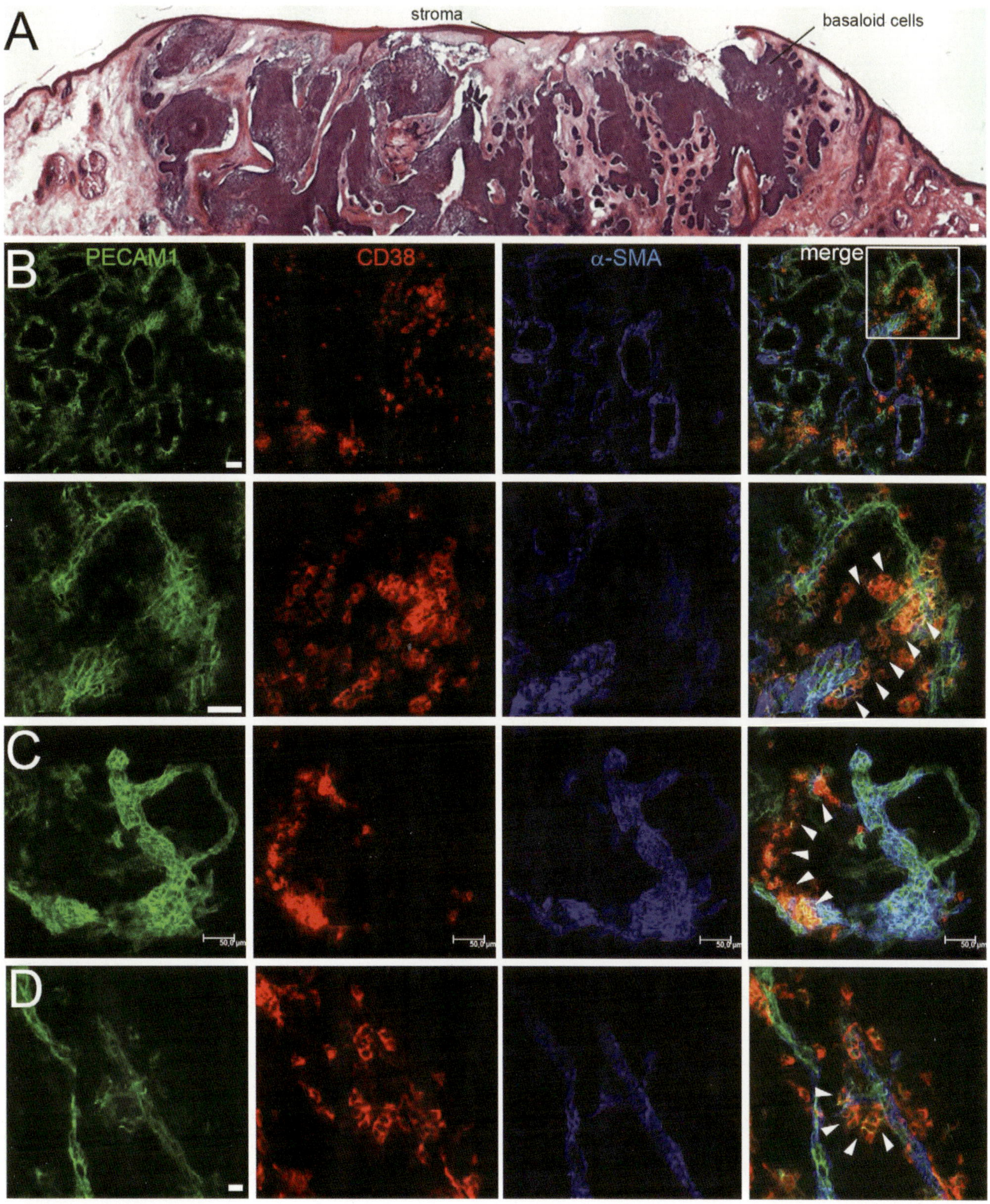

Figure 7. Identification of PECAM1⁺/CD38⁺ cells in human basal cell carcinomas (BCC). (A) H&E-stained cryosection of a BCC. (B–D) Confocal microscopy analysis of PECAM1, CD38 and α-SMA expression in two BCC biopsies (B–C, D). (B) Overview (top row) of the highly vascularized PECAM1^{+} stroma. Squares within the merged image indicate the magnified region (lower row). PECAM1^{low}/CD38^{+} cells are marked (arrowheads). Bars 100 µm (A), 50 µm (B, C), 10 µm (D).

PECAM1$^+$/Sca1$^+$/CD38$^+$ Vascular Cells form Myofibroblast-like Cells

We speculated that PECAM1$^+$/Sca1$^+$/CD38$^+$ can proliferate and differentiate into myofibroblast-like cells and therefore studied the cell-cycle status and the expression of the myofibroblast marker α-SMA in PECAM1$^+$/Sca1$^+$/CD38$^+$ cells at seven days post wounding (Fig. 5). For cell cycle analysis collagenase-digested skin or wound cell suspensions were stained with Sca1, Pecam1 and the DNA stain propidium iodide and then analyzed by flow cytometry. No proliferation was seen in skin-derived Sca1$^+$, PECAM1$^+$ or PECAM1$^+$/Sca1$^+$/CD38$^+$ cells. In wounds, most of the Sca1$^+$ and PECAM1$^+$ were still found in the G_0/G_1 phase of the cell cycle, whereas 23% of the PECAM1$^+$/Sca1$^+$/CD38$^+$ cells were found in the S-phase and 8% in the G2 phase of the cell cycle (Fig. 5A, Fig. S1). Hence, only PECAM1$^+$/Sca1$^+$/CD38$^+$ cells proliferate upon wounding at the peak of myofibroblast appearance. In addition, cells of skin and wounds were analyzed for α-SMA expression by flow cytometry analysis. In unwounded skin single PECAM1$^+$, Sca1$^+$ or PECAM1$^+$/Sca1$^+$/CD38$^+$ cells lack the expression α-SMA (Fig. S2C). This is in line with the immunofluorescence analysis of α-SMA expression in the newborn, 3 weeks and 3 months old skin, where α-SMA could only be found in the glassy membrane of the hair follicles and in the arrector pili muscle muscle tissue, but was nearly absent in the vasculature of the dermis (Fig. S2A). In the wound α-SMA was detected in 17% of Sca1$^+$ cells and 4.5% of PECAM1$^+$/Sca1$^+$ cells (Fig. 5B), whereas PECAM1$^+$ cells lack the expression of α-SMA.

In parallel sorted cells were cultured for five days on glass under conditions of mechanical tension and then assessed by immunofluorescence analysis for α-SMA expression. The presence of numerous intact DAPI$^+$ nuclei indicated that most cells of the Sca1$^+$ or PECAM1$^+$ cell population survived the isolation procedure (Fig. 5C), whereas number of PECAM1$^+$/Sca1$^+$/CD38$^+$ cells were significantly reduced. In cultures of Sca1$^+$ cells some α-SMA expressing cells emerged, while hardly any α-SMA$^+$ cells were present in PECAM1$^+$ cell cultures. In contrast, most of the cultured PECAM1$^+$/Sca1$^+$/CD38$^+$ cells expressed α-SMA, displayed a flattened morphology and formed a network of α-SMA$^+$ stress fibers. The results indicate that PECAM1$^+$/Sca1$^+$/CD38$^+$ cells can differentiate into α-SMA$^+$ myofibroblast-like cells.

To determine the function of CD38 for this differentiation process *in vivo* we triggered the CD38 receptor activity by intravenous injection of a CD38 antibody into wounded mice (n = 4). In order to avoid stimulatory effects of the injected antibody on CD38$^+$ lymphoid B- and T-cells, Rag2-deficient mice were used, which have no mature B- or T-cells [18]. Four wounds were inflicted on the back of the mice and the healing progress was studied seven days post injury. Wounds were isolated, sectioned and stained with hematoxylin and eosin (H&E). Morphometric assessment showed a significant reduction in wound size for anti-CD38 antibody-treated mice (Fig. 5D). The distances between the edges of the panniculus carnosus and the hair follicles were shortened by 20% and 25%, respectively, and the granulation tissue was reduced by 21%. These data indicate that CD38 receptor signaling in PECAM1$^+$/Sca1$^+$ cells promotes vessel-derived myofibroblast formation to support the healing progress.

PECAM1$^+$/CD38$^+$ Vascular Cells can be Identified in Human Foreskin and in Vascular Sprouts of Basal Cell Carcinomas

To identify a human orthologue vascular cell population we determined the distribution of CD38, PECAM1 and α-SMA by immunofluorescence analysis of human foreskin sections (Fig. 6A). Sca1 was not considered for analysis due to the lack of a human orthologue. PECAM1$^+$ endothelial cells were detected throughout the foreskin, whereas only a subpopulation of PECAM1$^+$ vessels expressed the CD34 or CD38 receptors. Flow cytometry analysis demonstrated that 1.1% of the viable non-hematopoietic cell population represent PECAM1$^+$/CD38$^+$ cells and within this population 92% of the cells expressed CD34. Approximately 2% of the PECAM1$^+$/CD38$^+$ cells contained α-SMA protein as shown by intracellular α-SMA staining (Fig. 6B). In a subsequent semiquantitative PCR study genes preferentially expressed in perivascular cells like *DESMIN*, *PDGFRB* and *ANGPT1* were detected in sorted CD38$^+$ cells, whereas endothelial cell-specific genes like *ANGPT2* and *TIE2* were mainly found in sorted PECAM1$^+$ cells (Fig. 6C). Both perivascular and endothelial cell-specific genes were expressed in sorted PECAM1$^+$/CD38$^+$ cells. Hence, a human counterpart for the murine PECAM1$^+$/Sca1$^+$/CD38$^+$ cell population was identified.

The vasculature may contribute to fibrotic tissue formation and pathological neoangiogenesis in humans. Therefore, the distribution of CD38 was studied on cryosections of biopsies from fibrotic scleroderma and neovascularised human basal cell carcinoma (BCC) patients. In four biopsies from patients with late fibrosis no signal for CD38 was detected in immunofluorescent analysis. In contrast, five out of seven BCC biopsies showed a staining for CD38 (Fig. S3). To define CD38$^+$ cells sections of two biopsies were costained with antibodies detecting PECAM1, CD38 and α-SMA and analyzed by confocal microscopy. A high density of vessels with strong PECAM1 expression (PECAM1^{high}) was found throughout the stroma of the first analyzed biopsy (Fig. 7B). CD38$^+$ cells were detected only in areas of low PECAM1 expression (PECAM1^{low}) in the outermost PECAM1$^+$ cell layer of sprouting vessels. CD38-expressing cells also originated from a dilated vessel to form a PECAM^{low}/CD38$^+$ loop-like structure (Fig. 7C), whereas the larger PECAM1^{high}/α-SMA$^+$ vessel and the smaller PECAM1^{high} vessel loop did not contain any CD38$^+$ cells. A similar distribution of CD38$^+$ cells was seen in the second tumor within a vascular outgrowth from a pre-existing small vessel. CD38 expression was detected in the PECAM1^{low} cells at the vascular tip (Fig. 7D, arrowheads), which seemed to migrate towards the nearby vessel to form a vascular bridge. In summary, CD38$^+$ cells are found in neoangiogenic PECAM1^{low} areas of the stromal vasculature in BCC biopsies.

Discussion

Sca1 and PECAM1 expression is commonly used to identify vascular progenitor cells in various tissues and previous studies suggested that tissue-resident Sca1$^+$ [11,19] or PECAM1$^+$/Sca1$^+$ [20] precursor cells may exist in the microvasculature to promote neoangiogenesis and tissue repair. In this study PECAM1 and Sca1 expression were used to define the vascular cell populations that are activated during skin repair.

The detection of both markers showed that non-hematopoietic Sca1$^+$ and PECAM1$^+$/Sca1$^+$ are present in the dermis of the skin. Sca1$^+$ cells expressed perivascular cell-specific marker genes such as *Pdgfrb* and *Desmin*, but some of the perivascular cell-specific genes may also be expressed by fibroblasts [5]. In contrast, a low proportion of PECAM1$^+$/Sca1$^+$ cells is found in the skin, which was transiently enriched in the granulation tissue of wounds seven days post injury coinciding temporally with neoangiogenesis and myofibroblast formation. These cells are capable of responding to environmental changes in the wound to enter the cell cycle upon injury and express endothelial and perivascular cell-specific genes as well as the progenitor cell marker CD34. The concomitant expression of endothelial and perivascular cell-specific genes may suggest that endothelial cells transiently undergo endothelial-to-mesenchyme transition in the vasculature of wounded skin. It is remarkable that all cells within the PECAM1$^+$/Sca1$^+$ population express CD34 and CD38, whereas PECAM1$^+$ or Sca1$^+$ cells fail to do so. Therefore, the purified cells represent a homogeneous population in a unique localization within the vasculature of the skin. CD34 expression has been reported for bone marrow-derived circulating endothelial progenitors [21]. PECAM1$^+$/Sca1$^+$/CD38$^+$ cells may originate from these CD34$^+$ bone marrow-derived precursors but the lack of the hematopoietic CD45 marker expression renders this scenario rather unlikely.

In order to promote non-vessel tissue repair PECAM1$^+$/Sca1$^+$/CD38$^+$ cells have to transform into mesenchymal cells. Myofibroblast-like cells in the intervascular stroma of wounds seven days post injury appear to emerge from pre-existing PECAM1$^+$/Sca1$^+$/CD38$^+$ vessels (see Fig. 1D and Fig. S2B). Mechanical challenge is an important trigger to induce myofibroblast formation from a variety of progenitors [1] and gain of α-SMA expression is a hallmark of this differentiation process. We detected intracellular α-SMA in 4% of the wound-derived PECAM1$^+$/Sca1$^+$/CD38$^+$ cells, which form extended α-SMA containing stress fibres *in vitro*, whereas PECAM1$^+$ single positive cells fail to do. Moreover, in cell suspensions from intact skin no intracellular α-SMA was detected in these cell populations. Therefore, it is likely that a proportion of PECAM1$^+$/Sca1$^+$/CD38$^+$ cells can undergo significant phenotypic changes upon wounding to transform into migrating, proliferating and matrix-secreting myofibroblast-like cells to contribute to the pool of myofibroblasts as it was previously described for endothelial cells in cardiac fibrosis [3].

In order to get activated PECAM1$^+$/Sca1$^+$/CD38$^+$ cells need to react to changes in the local environment. CD38 can interact with hyaluronan of the extracellular matrix [22], which is upregulated in skin wounds of mice. Elevated levels of hyaluronan are associated with faster closure, increased tensile strength, and less dermal scarring [23]. We showed that CD38 expression is restricted to the cell surface of PECAM1$^+$/Sca1$^+$/CD38$^+$ cells in the intact and repairing skin. PECAM1$^+$/Sca1$^+$/CD38$^+$ cells in the vasculature may therefore sense changes in the extracellular hyaluronan concentration via the CD38 receptor to become activated.

When stimulating the CD38 receptor by injection of CD38 antibody [24] a pronounced effect on wound healing progression was seen. In these mice the size of the wound was reduced by 20% and although the deposited antibodies hampered the analysis of the distribution of the vasculature we speculate that the stimulation of the PECAM1$^+$/Sca1$^+$ cell population via the CD38 receptor caused this size reduction. First, CD38 expression is exclusively expressed by PECAM1$^+$/Sca1$^+$/CD38$^+$ cells throughout the healing process (see Fig. 4) and second, effects of anti-CD38 antibodies on CD38$^+$ T- or B-cells can be excluded due to the usage of Rag2$^{-/-}$ mice, which fail to produce mature B- or T-lymphocytes [18]. Hence, PECAM1$^+$/Sca1$^+$/CD38$^+$ cells are the most likely target for the crosslinking CD38 antibodies in wounds. Therefore, the reduced wound size could be caused by the altered activation of the CD38 receptor on PECAM1$^+$/Sca1$^+$ cells, which is accompanied by changes in neoangiogenesis or myofibroblast formation. Interestingly, in human basal cell carcinoma (BCC) PECAM1^{low}/CD38$^+$ cells are mainly found in the highly vascularized tumor stroma in regions of newly formed vascular sprouts, whereas most of the mature PECAM1^{high} vessels lack CD38 expression. The availability of monoclonal CD38 antibodies [25] and the rather restricted expression upon pathological neoangiogenesis in the human BCCs makes the CD38 receptor also an attractive immunotherapeutic target to prevent new vessel formation and thereby tumor growth.

Supporting Information

Figure S1 Characterization of the cell proliferation in skin and wound. Cell cycle analysis of skin- and wound-derived Sca1$^+$, PECAM1$^+$ and PECAM1$^+$/Sca1$^+$cells seven days post injury using propidium iodide stain in flow cytometry analysis. The histograms of four individual mice are shown (mouse 1–4).

Figure S2 Myofibroblast-like cell formation. (A) Immunostaining of PECAM1/desmin and PECAM1/α-SMA expression at newborn stage (nb), three weeks (3 wk) and three months (3 mo). Squares within the images represent closeups of overlays for the PECAM1/desmin or PECAM1/α-SMA staining. Asterix depict the *arrector pili* muscle and arrows point to the glassy membrane of hair follicles. Only few of the large vessels are surrounded by α-SMA$^+$ cells and are highlighted by arrowheads. (B) Immunostaining of PECAM1/α-SMA expression at seven days post injury. The individual monochrome signals for PECAM1 and α-SMA are shown as well as the overlay for the PECAM1/α-SMA staining including the nuclear DAPI staining. PECAM1$^+$/α-SMA$^+$ cells around PECAM1$^+$ vessels are indicated by arrowheads. (C) Flow cytometric detection of α-SMA in Sca1$^+$, PECAM1$^+$/Sca1$^+$ and PECAM1$^+$ cells from unwounded skin ($n = 7$ mice). Bars 100 μm (A), 50 μm (B).

Figure S3 Identification of PECAM1$^+$/CD38$^+$ cells in vascular sprouts of human basal cell carcinomas. (A) Expression of PECAM1 and CD38 was defined by confocal microscopy analysis of five individual basal cell carcinoma biopsies (patient 1–5). (B) PECAM1 and isotype control (for CD38) staining. Bar 100 μm.

Author Contributions

Conceived and designed the experiments: JE SE BB. Performed the experiments: JE VB CF SK LB GR. Analyzed the data: JE LB SE CM BB. Contributed reagents/materials/analysis tools: CM BE HU FL HA MP. Wrote the paper: JE BB.

References

1. Hinz B (2007) Formation and function of the myofibroblast during tissue repair. J Invest Dermatol 127: 526–537.
2. Petroll WM, Barry-Lane PA, Cavanagh HD, Jester JV (1997) ZO-1 reorganization and myofibroblast transformation of corneal endothelial cells after freeze injury in the cat. Exp Eye Res 64: 257–267.
3. Zeisberg EM, Tarnavski O, Zeisberg M, Dorfman AL, McMullen JR, et al. (2007) Endothelial-to-mesenchymal transition contributes to cardiac fibrosis. Nat Med 13: 952–961.
4. Rajkumar VS, Shiwen X, Bostrom M, Leoni P, Muddle J, et al. (2006) Platelet-derived growth factor-beta receptor activation is essential for fibroblast and pericyte recruitment during cutaneous wound healing. Am J Pathol 169: 2254–2265.
5. Eming SA, Brachvogel B, Odorisio T, Koch M (2007) Regulation of angiogenesis: Wound healing as a model. Prog Histochem Cytochem 42: 115–170.
6. Sundberg C, Ivarsson M, Gerdin B, Rubin K (1996) Pericytes as collagen-producing cells in excessive dermal scarring. Lab Invest 74: 452–466.
7. Brachvogel B, Moch H, Pausch F, Schlotzer-Schrehardt U, Hofmann C, et al. (2005) Perivascular cells expressing annexin A5 define a novel mesenchymal stem cell-like population with the capacity to differentiate into multiple mesenchymal lineages. Development 132: 2657–2668.

8. Goritz C, Dias DO, Tomilin N, Barbacid M, Shupliakov O, et al. (2011) A pericyte origin of spinal cord scar tissue. Science 333: 238–242.
9. Torsney E, Xu Q (2011) Resident vascular progenitor cells. J Mol Cell Cardiol 50: 304–311.
10. Hoofnagle MH, Wamhoff BR, Owens GK (2004) Lost in transdifferentiation. J Clin Invest 113: 1249–1251.
11. Grenier G, Scime A, Le Grand F, Asakura A, Perez-Iratxeta C, et al. (2007) Resident endothelial precursors in muscle, adipose, and dermis contribute to postnatal vasculogenesis. Stem Cells 25: 3101–3110.
12. Luna G, Paez J, Cardier JE (2004) Expression of the hematopoietic stem cell antigen Sca-1 (LY-6A/E) in liver sinusoidal endothelial cells: possible function of Sca-1 in endothelial cells. Stem Cells Dev 13: 528–535.
13. Brachvogel B, Pausch F, Farlie P, Gaipl U, Etich J, et al. (2007) Isolated Anxa5(+)/Sca-1(+) perivascular cells from mouse meningeal vasculature retain their perivascular phenotype in vitro and in vivo. Exp Cell Res 313: 2730–2743.
14. Gerharz M, Baranowsky A, Siebolts U, Eming S, Nischt R, et al. (2007) Morphometric analysis of murine skin wound healing: standardization of experimental procedures and impact of an advanced multitissue array technique. Wound Repair Regen 15: 105–112.
15. Rasband W (1997–2011) ImageJ. U S National Institutes of Health, Bethesda, Maryland, USA.
16. Watson JV, Chambers SH, Smith PJ (1987) A pragmatic approach to the analysis of DNA histograms with a definable G1 peak. Cytometry 8: 1–8.
17. Deaglio S, Aydin S, Grand MM, Vaisitti T, Bergui L, et al. (2010) CD38/CD31 interactions activate genetic pathways leading to proliferation and migration in chronic lymphocytic leukemia cells. Mol Med 16: 87–91.
18. Shinkai Y, Rathbun G, Lam KP, Oltz EM, Stewart V, et al. (1992) RAG-2-deficient mice lack mature lymphocytes owing to inability to initiate V(D)J rearrangement. Cell 68: 855–867.
19. McQualter JL, Brouard N, Williams B, Baird BN, Sims-Lucas S, et al. (2009) Endogenous fibroblastic progenitor cells in the adult mouse lung are highly enriched in the sca-1 positive cell fraction. Stem Cells 27: 623–633.
20. Tsuchiya A, Heike T, Baba S, Fujino H, Umeda K, et al. (2008) Sca-1+ endothelial cells (SPECs) reside in the portal area of the liver and contribute to rapid recovery from acute liver disease. Biochem Biophys Res Commun 365: 595–601.
21. Peichev M, Naiyer AJ, Pereira D, Zhu Z, Lane WJ, et al. (2000) Expression of VEGFR-2 and AC133 by circulating human CD34(+) cells identifies a population of functional endothelial precursors. Blood 95: 952–958.
22. Nishina H, Inageda K, Takahashi K, Hoshino S, Ikeda K, et al. (1994) Cell surface antigen CD38 identified as ecto-enzyme of NAD glycohydrolase has hyaluronate-binding activity. Biochem Biophys Res Commun 203: 1318–1323.
23. Mack JA, Abramson SR, Ben Y, Coffin JC, Rothrock JK, et al. (2003) Hoxb13 knockout adult skin exhibits high levels of hyaluronan and enhanced wound healing. Faseb J 17: 1352–1354.
24. Hara-Yokoyama M, Kimura T, Kaku H, Wakiyama M, Kaitsu Y, et al. (2008) Alteration of enzymatic properties of cell-surface antigen CD38 by agonistic anti-CD38 antibodies that prolong B cell survival and induce activation. Int Immunopharmacol 8: 59–70.
25. de Weers M, Tai YT, van der Veer MS, Bakker JM, Vink T, et al. (2011) Daratumumab, a novel therapeutic human CD38 monoclonal antibody, induces killing of multiple myeloma and other hematological tumors. J Immunol 186: 1840–1848.

21

Insights from Computational Modeling in Inflammation and Acute Rejection in Limb Transplantation

Dolores Wolfram[1]*, Ravi Starzl[2], Hubert Hackl[3], Derek Barclay[4], Theresa Hautz[5], Bettina Zelger[6], Gerald Brandacher[7], W. P. Andrew Lee[7], Nadine Eberhart[1], Yoram Vodovotz[4], Johann Pratschke[5], Gerhard Pierer[1], Stefan Schneeberger[5,7]

1 Department of Plastic, Reconstructive and Aesthetic Surgery, Innsbruck Medical University, Innsbruck, Austria, **2** Language Technologies Institute, Carnegie Mellon University, Pittsburgh, Pennsylvania, United States of America, **3** Division of Bioinformatics, Biocenter, Innsbruck Medical University, Innsbruck, Austria, **4** Department of Immunology, University of Pittsburgh, Pittsburgh, Pennsylvania, United States of America, **5** Department of Visceral, Transplant and Thoracic Surgery, Innsbruck Medical University, Innsbruck, Austria, **6** Department of Pathology, Innsbruck Medical University, Innsbruck, Austria, **7** Department of Plastic and Reconstructive Surgery, Johns Hopkins University School of Medicine, Baltimore, Maryland, United States of America

Abstract

Acute skin rejection in vascularized composite allotransplantation (VCA) is the major obstacle for wider adoption in clinical practice. This study utilized computational modeling to identify biomarkers for diagnosis and targets for treatment of skin rejection. Protein levels of 14 inflammatory mediators in skin and muscle biopsies from syngeneic grafts [n = 10], allogeneic transplants without immunosuppression [n = 10] and allografts treated with tacrolimus [n = 10] were assessed by multiplexed analysis technology. Hierarchical Clustering Analysis, Principal Component Analysis, Random Forest Classification and Multinomial Logistic Regression models were used to segregate experimental groups. Based on Random Forest Classification, Multinomial Logistic Regression and Hierarchical Clustering Analysis models, IL-4, TNF-α and IL-12p70 were the best predictors of skin rejection and identified rejection well in advance of histopathological alterations. TNF-α and IL-12p70 were the best predictors of muscle rejection and also preceded histopathological alterations. Principal Component Analysis identified IL-1α, IL-18, IL-1β, and IL-4 as principal drivers of transplant rejection. Thus, inflammatory patterns associated with rejection are specific for the individual tissue and may be superior for early detection and targeted treatment of rejection.

Editor: Valquiria Bueno, UNIFESP Federal University of São Paulo, Brazil

Funding: Funding for this work was provided by the Armed Forces Institute for Advanced Regenerative Medicine Program (TATRC, DOD) Program, Department of Defense grant WX81XWH-07-1-0415, the Austrian Research Fund (Erwin Schrödinger Stipendium), the Austrian Society of Plastic and Reconstructive Surgery and the and the Pennsylvania Department of Health Commonwealth Universal Research Enhancement (CURE) program. The funders had no role in study design, data collection and analysis, decision to publish, or preparation of the manuscript.

* E-mail: dolores.wolfram@i-med.ac.at

Introduction

Rejection in Vascular Composite Allotransplantation (VCA) is characterized by an inflammatory cell-mediated cytotoxic process, which progressively harms the epidermis and the junction between dermis and epidermis, unless reversed or prevented by immunosuppression. Understanding the immune signaling patterns of skin rejection would enable the development of targeted and local therapy with fewer side effects.

The current gold standard for the diagnosis of rejection is histological evaluation of tissue biopsies according to the BANFF 2007 working classification [1]. Assessing rejection by histology suffers from latency between initiation of tissue damage and diagnosis. Often, histological signs of skin rejection have been found in protocol biopsies despite absence of clinical signs of rejection. As stated previously by our group and others, the histopathological alterations associated with rejection are not specific, but rather similar to several common inflammatory dermatoses [2,3] or the result of an inflammatory trigger [4]. The differential diagnosis between skin rejection, infection and unspecific inflammation can be challenging in hand- and especially face transplantation. The conditions are similar in their appearance and may interfere with or trigger each other [5].

Traditional methods are of limited value for elucidation of how the immune/inflammatory response in the skin affects VCA through intricate signaling patterns and context-dependent behaviors. Advanced computational methods such as language technologies and machine learning offer significant advances in deciphering complex processes from other areas of science [6,7].

We hypothesized that mechanisms of rejection in VCA are tissue specific and can be detected in advance of gross histological damage by assessing leukocyte expression patterns with advanced computational tools. Based on our findings, promising diagnostic markers for skin and muscle rejection as well as possible targets for new therapeutic interventions in VCA have been identified.

Methods

Experimental design

All animal procedures, care, and housing were reviewed and approved by the Institutional Animal Care and Use Committee

(IACUC) of the University of Pittsburgh (protocol number: 0808858B-2), and followed the National Institutes of Health guidelines for the care and use of laboratory animals. A summary of the cohorts and the conditions they represent are presented in Table 1. Limb transplantations including skin, muscle, bone and vessels, were performed as per a standardized technique between eight- to ten-week-old male Brown-Norway (BN) and Lewis rats (LEW) weighing 200–250 g with (group 3) or without (group 1) immunosuppression and compared with untreated isografts (group 2) [8]. Animals were anesthetized with a combination of xylazine (Xylasol, 5 mg/kg) and ketamine (Ketavet, 100 mg/kg), injected intramuscularly.

Assessment of rejection

Animals were inspected daily for signs of rejection. Skin rejection was classified per appearance: Grade 0 – no signs of rejection; Grade I – erythema of the transplanted leg, Grade II – erythema and edema, Grade III – epidermolysis of the transplanted skin, Grade IV – mummification of the leg (limb necrosis). In untreated animals (allografts, ATC), rejection occurs after 3-4 days (Grade I rejection) and progresses to Grade IV rejection between day 9 and 11. Samples from allograft skin and muscle were collected at postoperative days (POD) 3, 5, 7, 9 and 11 in all three groups in a staggered fashion. To out rule an impact of the trauma an the readout of subsequent tissue samples, biopsies were taken from sites distant to another on days 3, 5, 7 and 11, or days 5, 9 and 11 (see Table 2). Since all animals showed mummification of the graft on POD 11 with super infection in some, samples from this time point were excluded from the study.

The size of each tissue biopsy per chosen time point was approximately 25×10 mm. This tissue sample was divided into 3 identical parts for further analyses. One biopsy part (piece) was fixed in 10% buffered formalin and processed routinely for hematoxilyn and eosin (H&E) staining. Sections were evaluated for lymphocytic infiltration, dermal/epidermal interphase reaction, dermal-epidermal separation and necrosis by a pathologist in a blinded fashion. The other biopsy parts were preserved in RNALater for protein analysis and RNA isolation.

Protein isolation and protein expression analysis

Proteins from skin and muscle samples were isolated using a disperser (T10, basic ULTRA-TURRAX, IKA, Germany) with 1 ml 1 x Cell Lysis Buffer (Cell Signaling, Danvers, USA) per sample on ice. Proteins were quantified after homogenizing using the BCA Protein Assay Kit according to the manufacturer's protocol.

Inflammatory mediator expression at the protein levels was measured using the Luminex inflammatory mediator bead set (RCYTO-80K-PMX-14-plex Milliplex Map Kit from Millipore, Billerica, MA) that included interferon (IFN)-γ, IL-1α, IL-1β, IL-2, IL-4, IL-5, IL-6, IL-10, IL-12p70, IL-18, monocyte chemotactic protein (MCP-1), GRO/KC, TNF-α, and granulocyte-macrophage colony stimulating factor (GM-CSF) in a Luminex 100 IS (Luminex Corporation, USA) and analyzed by xPonent 3.1 Rev.2 Software (Luminex Corporation, USA). Results for each of the 14 analytes were read in pg/ml and subsequently normalized to total mass of sample protein (pg inflammatory mediator/mg protein) by multiplying with 0.025 ml standard sample volume and dividing with 0.1 mg added total protein for each sample. Any analytes indicating a concentration above 20,000 pg/μl were excluded from analysis (NA) as being outside the linear range of the Luminex assay.

Table 1. Study groups and design.

Group (Name)	Animals per group	Donor	Recipient	Treatment	Samples per time point (POD 3,5,7,9)	Samples per animal	Tissue
1 (ATC)	10	BN	LEW	none	5	3	Skin & Muscle
2 (ISO)	10	LEW	LEW	none	5	3	Skin & Muscle
3 (TAC)	10	BN	LEW	Tacrolimus*	5	3	Skin & Muscle

* 1 mg/kg/day (for 11 days).

Table 2. Appearance (Grading for skin rejection: I–IV) of each allograft on POD 1–11.

Animals ID	POD (Postoperative Day)										
	1	2	3	4	5	6	7	8	9	10	11
ATC 1	0	0	0	I	**I**	II	II	III	**III**	IV	**IV**
ATC 2	0	0	0	I	**II**	II	III	III	**IV**	IV	**IV**
ATC 3	0	0	**0**	0	**I**	II	**III**	III	IV	IV	**IV**
ATC 4	0	0	**0**	0	**I**	II	**II**	III	IV	IV	**IV**
ATC 5*	0	0	**0**								
ATC 6	0	0	**0**	0	I	II	**II**	III	**III**	IV	**IV**
ATC 7	0	0	**0**	I	II	II	**III**	III	**IV**	IV	**IV**
ATC 8	0	0	0	I	**II**	II	**II**	III	IV	IV	**IV**
ATC 9	0	0	0	I	**II**	II	II	III	**IV**	IV	IV
ATC 10	0	0	**0**	I	I	II	**II**	III	III	IV	IV
ATC 11	0	0	0	I	**II**	II	II	III	**III**	IV	**IV**

*This animal died on POD 3 during the anesthesia. Bold numbers mark biopsy timepoints (skin and muscle) for each animal.

Statistical and computational analysis

Analyses were performed with the statistical framework R 2.13.1 using packages including *stats, nnet, multtest, MASS, beeswarm, randomForest.* The non-parametric Kruskal-Wallis test was used to compare mediator abundance among groups 1-3 (ATC, ISO, TAC) at POD 3/POD 5. The Wilcoxon rank-sum test was used to identify the tissue levels of those mediators whose levels varied significantly between animals exhibiting rejection (ATC) and animals treated with tacrolimus to prevent rejection (TAC) in the early postoperative phase (POD 3/POD 5), as well for selected inflammatory mediators at POD 3. All p-values were adjusted for multiple hypothesis testing based on the false discovery rate (FDR) [9].

The multivariate extension of the one-way analysis of variance (MANOVA) or the discriminant function analysis (based on the same formulation as MANOVA with inflammatory mediators as independent variables and the rejection group as dependent variable in the latter case) are used to determine the coefficients of the two orthogonal discriminant vectors (DV), which enable maximal separation of the groups. As a measure of contribution to these vectors for each mediator, the sum of the absolute values of the respective coefficients (loadings) were used and related to the overall sum. Pillai's trace statistic was used to test for the differences in the vectors of means. The mediators showing significant differences among the 3 groups and with >2.5% contribution to the DVs in both skin and muscle were subjected to multinomial (logistic) regression analyses. A model for skin and one model for muscle were selected based on minimal Akaike information criterion [AIC]. Classifier performance was assessed using a 8-fold cross validation procedure and visualized using confusion tables. Accuracy was defined as 1- misclassification rate and Welch's test was used to test the differences between the mean of the number of true predicted and the mean of the sum of the respective number of false predicted.

To assess similarity of inflammatory mediator levels among different time points and tissue types, complete-linkage hierarchical clustering was performed and visualized as heat map using Genesis [10] based on mean-centered log2-transformed profiles. For this analysis, the mean value for each group and mediator was used.

A Random Forest (RF) [11] approach was used for classification of the rejection group (ATC, ISO, TAC) including all time points. This method was also used to identify those mediators most important for classification or diagnosis. Classifier performances were assessed by confusion tables and the out-of-bag (OOB) error rate. Principal Component Analysis (PCA) was used to rank most variable (important) mediators and potential therapeutic target candidates [12]. PCA reduces a multidimensional dataset to a few principal components, which account for the most variability in the dataset. The underlying hypothesis is that a mediator which changes during a process is important to that process [12,13]. In this analysis, the data were combined from skin and muscle, mean centered, and variance scaled. Components sufficient to capture at least 70% of total data variance observed were included.

Results

Progression of rejection

Appearance. On postoperative day (POD) 3, none of the allografts (n = 10) showed signs of rejection, on POD 5, 50% of the allografts displayed Grade I rejection and 5 animals (50%) II rejection. On postoperative day 7, rejection Grade II was present in 7 animals (70%) and rejection Grade III in 3 animals (30%). On day 9, 4 animals displayed Grade III rejection and 6 animals

Grade IV. None of the syngeneic controls or tacrolimus treated animals showed any signs of skin rejection/inflammation (Table 2).

Histological evaluation of skin biopsies. Histological evaluation of allograft skin biopsies on day 3 showed no or minimal inflammatory infiltrates (Grade 0) in six animals and a mild perivascular infiltrate (Grade I) in one biopsy. No tacrolimus-treated animals showed any signs of rejection while a mild perivascular infiltration was seen in one of the syngeneic control animal. On POD 5, biopsies from allogeneic transplants displayed Grade I rejection in three animals, as well as a moderate to severe perivascular inflammation with or without mild epidermal and/or adnexal epidermal dyskeratosis or apoptosis (Grade II) in three animals. One biopsy taken from the allogeneic group showed a severe skin rejection (Grade III), with dense inflammation and epidermal involvement with epithelial apoptosis, dyskeratosis and keratinolysis on POD 5. No inflammatory response was observed in isografts on POD 5, but two out of five biopsies in the tacrolimus treated animals did show an inflammatory infiltrate. On POD 7, allogeneic animals showed Grade III rejection and, one skin biopsy taken from the isograft group and one from the tacrolimus group displayed a moderate inflammation corresponding with Grade I/II rejection. At the endpoint, all samples from allografts showed rejection Grade III and one biopsy ($n = 5$) taken from the isografts displayed the characteristics of Grade I rejection. Two out of five biopsies in the tacrolimus group showed a mild rejection (Grade I) and one biopsy was classified as Grade II rejection (Table 3 and Figure 1).

Histological evaluation of muscle biopsies. H&E stains from allograft muscle samples showed no or rare inflammatory cells on POD 3 in four biopsies and Grade I rejection in two biopsies. Muscle biopsies from syngeneic controls showed a mild infiltration in two biopsies, severe inflammation similar to rejection Grade II in one graft, and no inflammatory response at this time point in two animals. On POD 5, two biopsies from the allogeneic transplants were classified as Grade 0 rejection, three samples as Grade I and one muscle biopsy as Grade II rejection, four biopsies from the isografts showed no or rare inflammation and only one sample a mild inflammation.

On POD 7, all biopsies ($n = 5$) from allografts displayed Grade I rejection and only one biopsy from an isografts showed a mild muscle inflammation on both day 7 and 9. Allograft muscle biopsies on day 9 showed rejection Grade I ($n = 1$, Grade II ($n = 2$) or Grade III ($n = 2$). Tacrolimus treated animals did not show any signs of rejection except for one animal displaying mild inflammation in the muscle on POD 9 (Table 4 and Figure 1).

Significant differences of inflammatory mediator levels at early postoperative time points among the different transplant models

We examined the levels of 14 inflammatory analytes in skin and muscle biopsies of allogeneic, syngeneic and immunosuppressed hind limb transplants at different postoperative days (POD 3, 5, 7, and 9) with a focus on the early postoperative phase where no histological alterations were observed (POD 3 and 5, Figure 2 and Figure S2). Non-parametric univariate analysis of the inflammatory mediators from skin and muscle were performed. Five inflammatory mediators (GM-CSF, IL1-α, IL-4, IL-12p70, IL-5, TNF-α) were significantly different at least in one group (adjusted $p<0.05$; Kruskal-Wallis test [KW]) in both skin and muscle. IL-12p70 and TNF-α were highly significantly different in the allograft versus the tacrolimus-treated animals (adjusted $p<0.005$; Wilcoxon-rank sum test [WR]; Table 5).

In Figure 2, the levels of the concentrations of these inflammatory mediators at POD 3 of all three groups within skin

Table 3. Histological evaluation of skin biopsies from postoperative (POD) 3 to 9.

SKIN	POD 3				POD 5				POD 7				POD 9			
GRADE	0	I	II	III	0	I	II	III	0	I	II	III	0	I	II	III
ATC	6	1				3	3	1				6				5
ISO	3	1			4				4		1		4	1		
TAC	5				3	2			4	1			2	2	1	

Number of biopsies taken on each postoperative day (POD 3,5,7,9) in skin according to their histological grading (Grad 0-III) based on H&E staining.

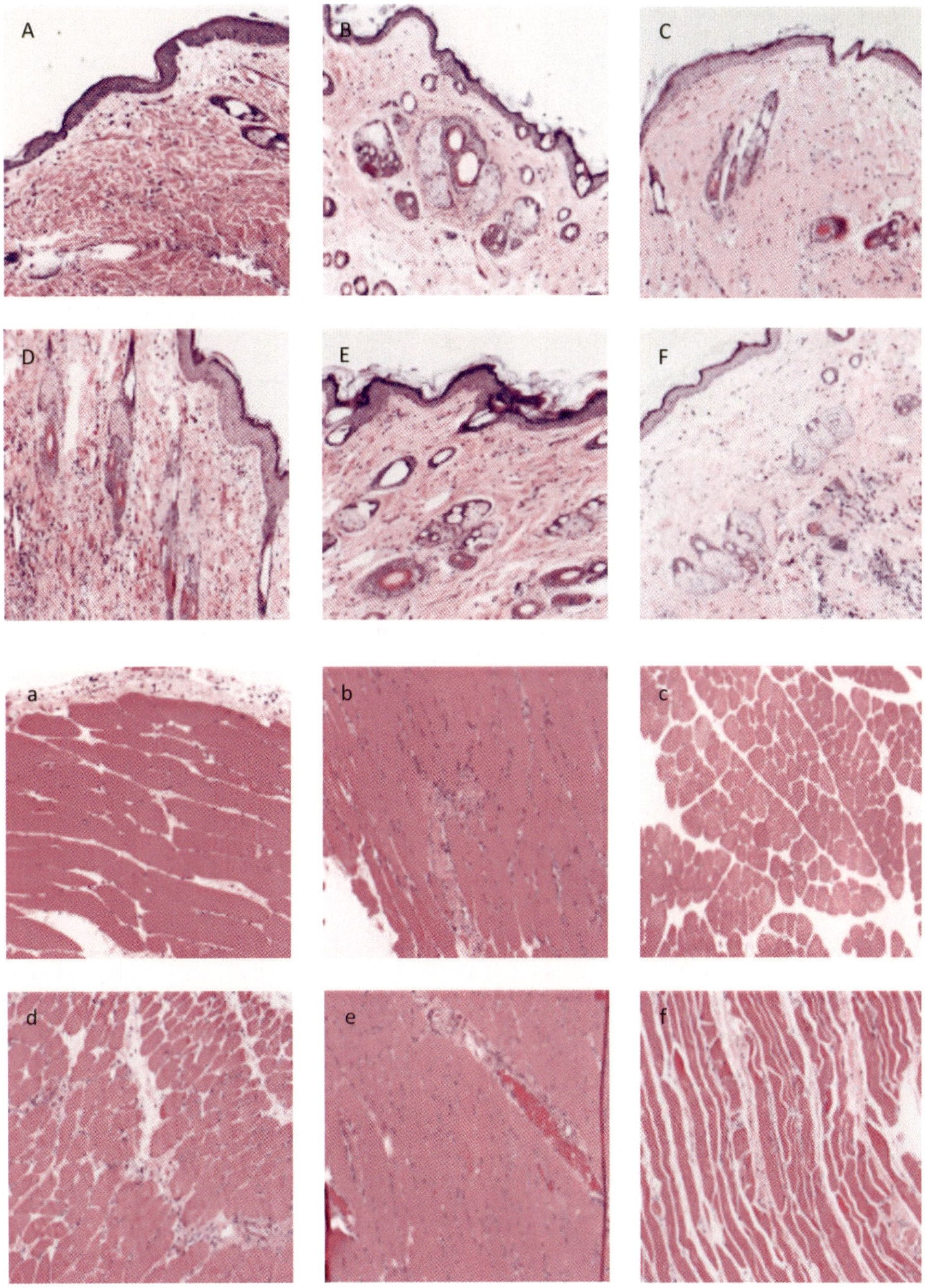

Figure 1. Histological evaluation of skin and muscle rejection in the early postoperative phase (POD 3 and 5). (A–C) Skin sample taken on POD 3 from an allograft without immunosuppression (A), from an isograft (B) and an allograft under TAC (C) showing no/rare inflammatory response (Grade 0 rejection). (D–F) Skin biopsies taken on POD 5 from a rejecting animal (D) displaying Grade 1 rejection, from an isograft (E) showing no/rare inflammatory response and a TAC treated allograft (F) characterized by a mild inflammatory response (Grade 0-I) in the deep dermis. (a–c) Muscle sample taken on POD 3 from an allograft without immunosuppression (a), from an isograft (b) and an allograft under TAC (c) showing no/rare inflammatory response (Grade 0 rejection). (d–f) Skin biopsies taken on POD 5 from a rejecting animal (d) displaying a mild inflammatory response (Grad 0-I rejection), from an isograft (E) and a TAC treated allograft (f) showing no/rare inflammatory response.

and muscle are depicted. Significantly higher concentrations of IL-12p70 in the skin from the allograft animals compared to the tacrolimus-treated animals (adjusted $p = 0.026$) as well as lower abundance of TNF-α in the allogeneic compared to the immunosuppressed transplants (adjusted $p = 0.026$) were detected. In muscle, numerical differences did not reach statistical significance (adjusted $p = 0.056$ in both cases).

For identification of inflammatory mediators with the highest predicting value, at early time points, multivariate analyses were performed. We fitted multivariate analysis of variance (MANOVA) models which resulted in $p = 8.9 \times 10^{-10}$ for skin and $p = 3.4 \times 10^{-5}$ for muscle from Pillai's trace statistic. Using these models, a functional discriminant analysis was performed. Mediators with the greatest absolute coefficients in the two resulting discriminant vectors might contribute most to the separation of groups (Table 5). The partition to the discrimination vectors for GM-CSF, IL-4, IL-12p70, IL-5, and TNF-α were > 2.5% in both tissues. We selected these inflammatory mediators as promising biomarkers candidates for further analyses.

Inflammatory mediators at early time points discern the procedure to which animals were subjected

A major goal of this study was to determine markers for early and accurate diagnosis of skin rejection in advance of major histological alterations. We applied several multivariate multinomial logistic regression models in skin and muscle samples for the classification of the three study groups at early postoperative time points (POD 3 and POD 5) using a combination of the selected inflammatory mediators (GM-CSF, IL-4, IL-12p70, IL-5, and TNF-α) as independent variables and study group as outcome. Based on the Akaike information criterion (AIC), which is a measure of the trade-off between the complexity of the model, i.e. number of variables, and the goodness of fit, optimal models for differentiation of the study groups could be found in skin rejection (based on IL-4, IL-12p70, and TNF-α: AIC = 16.0; residual deviance = 1.7×10^{-4}) and in muscle (based on IL-12p70 and TNF-α: AIC = 12.0; residual variance = 1.6×10^{-4}). The coefficients of the inflammatory mediators in the logistic regression models and classifier performance as assessed by 8-fold cross validation are detailed in Table 5. The prediction accuracy within skin was 87.1% and in muscle 100%, as derived from classification tables. A pairwise multivariate logistic regression analysis between the study groups (ATC vs. TAC, TAC vs. ISO, ISO vs. ATC) and applying a leave-one-out cross validation strategy resulted in an area under curve (AUC) from receiver operating characteristics (ROC) for skin of 0.5, 0.69, and 0.86 and for muscle of 1.0, 1.0, and 1.0, indicating a substantially better discrimination than by chance (AUC = 0.5) (Table 6).

Inflammatory mediator profiles are similar within each group

Hierarchical clustering was performed for all inflammatory mediators in the three experimental groups. Each row of the data matrix corresponds with one of the 14 inflammatory mediators, and each column corresponds with a group. The $\log_2$-transformed and mean-centered values (mean concentrations from each condition) are visualized as a heat map, with color codes shown in the color bar (Figure 3). The dendrogram on the x-axis shows the similarities among the samples. As expected, the rejection group (ATC skin and muscle samples), especially samples from later time points with pronounced histological changes, exhibit a completely different mediator clustering pattern vs. the control groups, with high abundance of IL-5, IL-18, IL-1β, MCP-1, IL-6, GRO-KC, and TNF-α. In TAC-treated animals, only IL-1α and TNF-α were highly abundant, whereas the expression of all other mediators assessed appeared suppressed.

The separation of the tacrolimus-treated group was also evident from the cluster analysis. Within sample cluster A (17 samples), 5.9% were from the tacrolimus and 94.1% were from study group ISO/ATC. In contrast, in cluster B (7 samples), 100% were from tacrolimus and 0% from the ISO/ATC groups. A Fisher's exact test ($p = 2.3\times10^{-5}$) suggested that the distribution between clusters A and B was not random. Profiles of MCP-1, IL-4, IL-1β, and IL-6 characterize rejecting grafts, whereas GM-CSF and IL-4 characterize isografts. This was also indicated by an absolute value of point-biserial correlation coefficient >0.6 comparing each group with the other groups. Interestingly, there appeared to be an

Table 4. Histological evaluation of muscle biopsies from postoperative (POD) 3 to 9.

MUSCLE	POD 3				POD 5				POD 7				POD 9			
GRADE	0	I	II	III	0	I	II	III	0	I	II	III	0	I	II	III
ATC	4	2			2	3	1			5				1	2	2
ISO	2	2	1		4	1			4	1			4	1		
TAC	5				5				5				4	1		

Number of biopsies taken on each postoperative day (POD 3,5,7,9) in muscle according to their histological grading (Grad 0-III) based on H&E grading. The first biopsy was taken from the lateral proximal part of the thigh, the second one from the lateral distal thigh, the third one from the ventral thigh and the last one from the medial part of the thigh.

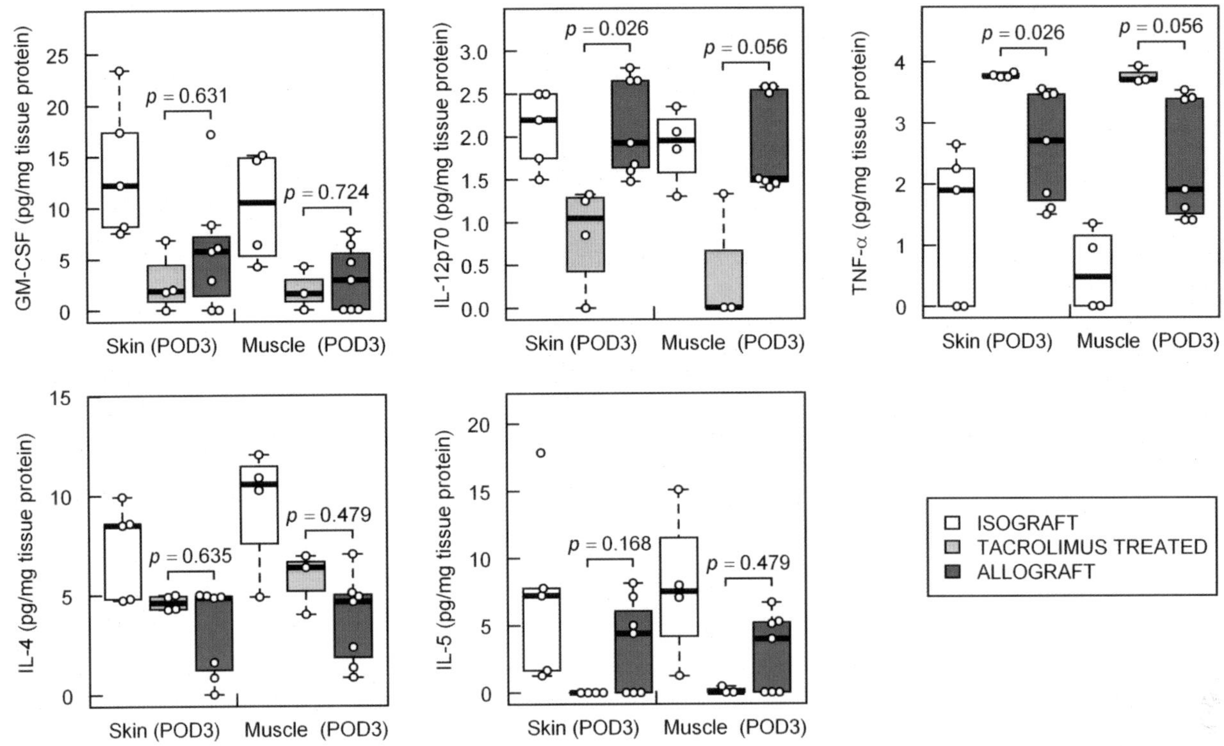

Figure 2. Distribution of inflammatory mediator levels at the earliest postoperative measurements (POD 3) in rat limb transplantation models. Adjusted p-values from Wilcoxon rank-sum test between the rejection group (ATC) vs. Tacrolimus treated group (TAC) for selected inflammatory mediators, which were tested to be included in a prediction model by multinomial logistic regression analysis, are presented.

Table 5. Statistical analysis for all 14 inflammatory mediator levels in skin and in muscle at early postoperative time points (combined group of POD 3 and POD 5).

	Skin POD 3/5			**Muscle POD 3/5**		
	p_{KW}	p_{WR}	**Partition on DVs [%]**	p_{KW}	p_{WR}	**Partition on DVs [%]**
GM-CSF	**0.0018**	0.3260	**4.26**	**0.0083**	0.6178	**2.60**
IL-1α	**0.0244**	1.0000	0.01	**0.0105**	0.0773	0.01
MCP-1	**0.0011**	**0.0026**	0.72	**0.0466**	0.3673	0.79
IL-4	**0.0040**	0.3421	**24.21**	**0.0194**	0.5312	**18.68**
IL-1β	0.2042	0.1577	0.10	0.8251	0.7577	0.09
IL-2	0.2042	0.2868	0.83	0.1779	0.5312	0.29
IL-6	0.1322	0.2824	0.27	0.5127	0.6178	0.29
IL-10	0.2777	0.2805	0.55	0.8251	0.8657	0.39
IL-12p70	**0.0019**	**0.0013**	**15.65**	**0.0030**	**0.0025**	**31.59**
IL-5	**0.0022**	**0.0123**	**4.85**	**0.0010**	0.2112	**5.03**
IFN-γ	0.2956	0.3729	**5.67**	0.2562	0.3619	1.90
IL-18	0.3462	0.2868	0.03	**0.0425**	0.7498	0.03
GRO-KC	**0.0040**	**0.0021**	0.27	0.5127	0.5312	0.11
TNF-α	$\mathbf{1.7 \times 10^{-4}}$	**0.0013**	**42.59**	**0.0001**	**0.0025**	**38.21**

Most promising inflammatory mediators for classification of rejection, based on early identification before histological manifestation of rejection is evident, are selected (p_{KW}<0.05 and *Partition on DVs* >1%, symbols in bold) and subjected to multinomial logistic regression analyses. For all measured inflammatory mediators adjusted p-values from Kruskal-Wallis test (KW) of overall equality between all 3 cohorts (ISO, TAC, ATC) and Wilcoxon rank-sum test (WR) for comparison between the rejection group (ATC) and the Tacrolimus treated group (TAC) as well as partition of each inflammatory mediator on the two discriminant vectors (DVs), which maximizes the separation between the 3 rejection groups, resulting from discriminant function analysis, are given.

Table 6. Results for multinomial logistic regression models in skin and muscle for classification of the rejection groups based inflammatory mediator/chemokine levels at early postoperative time points (POD 3/5) in rat transplantation models.

	Skin POD3/5			Muscle POD3/5		
ln(p(*TAC*)/p(*ATC*))	**-6.7-2.6*_IL4_-61.3*_IL12p70_+25.6*_TNFa_**			**-6.9-18.8*_IL12p70_+11.3*_TNFa_**		
ln(p(*ISO*)/p(*ATC*))	**-1094.8+112.6*_IL4_+250.4*_IL12p70_-28.6*_TNFa_**			**-10.0+25.1*_IL12p70_-27.0*_TNFa_**		
	ATC^{pred}	**TAC^{pred}**	**ISO^{pred}**	**ATC^{pred}**	**TAC^{pred}**	**ISO^{pred}**
ATC	12	0	1	13	0	0
TAC	0	8	0	0	7	0
ISO	3	0	7	0	0	9
	Accuracy = 87.1% $p = 0.020$			Accuracy = 100% $p = 0.031$		

Best prediction models for skin and muscle and their respective logistic prediction functions and classifier performance including confusion table (assessed by an 8-fold cross validation procedure) are summarized.

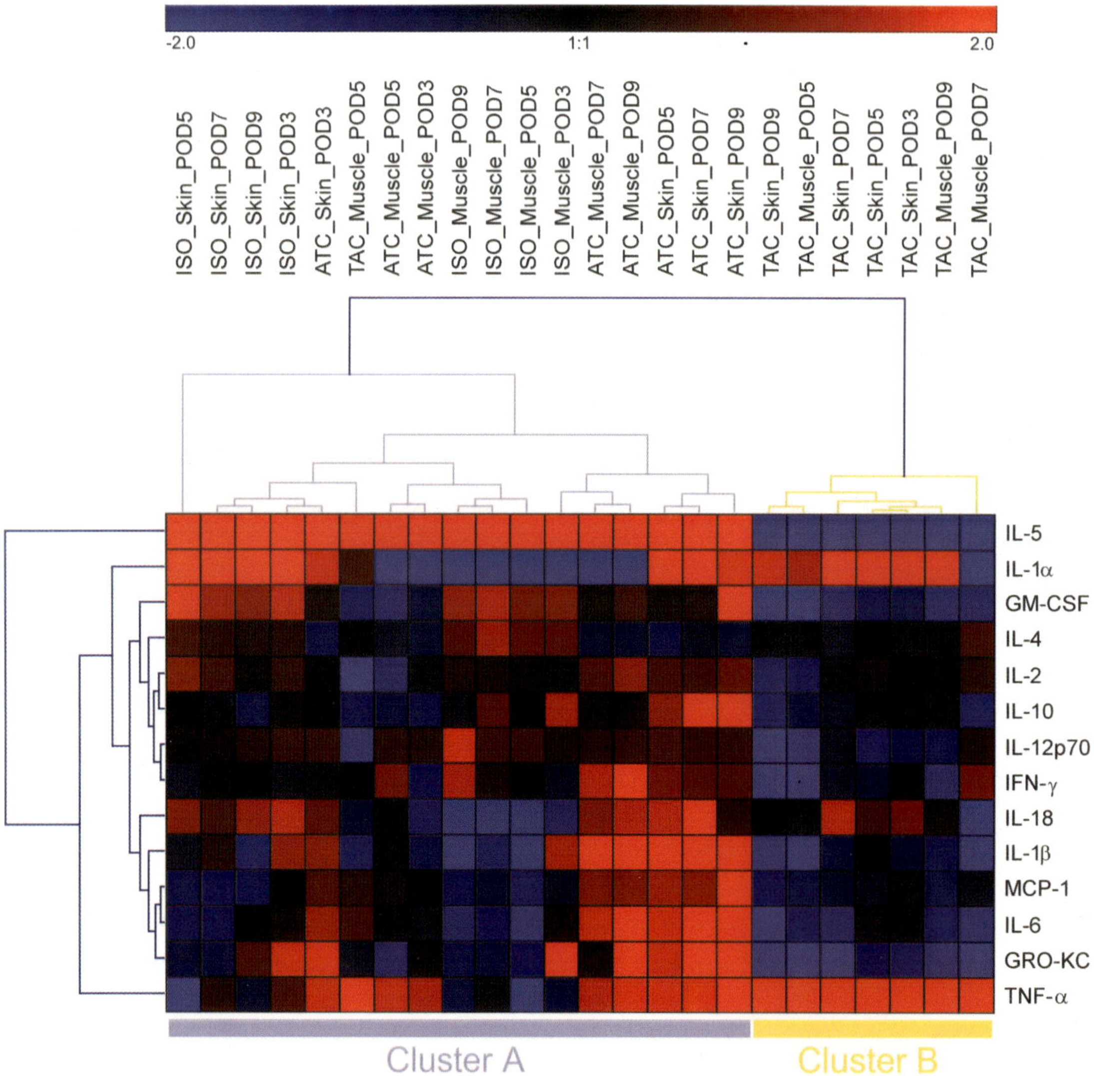

Figure 3. Similarity of sample groups and association between inflammatory mediators in rat limb transplantation models based on their profiles of mean levels in each condition. Heatmap as a result of complete linkage hierarchical clustering on log2-transformed and mean centered data. Log2-fold differences against the respective mean levels of each inflammatory mediator are color coded (red means higher inflammatory mediator levels and blue means lower inflammatory mediator levels than the mean levels of the respective inflammatory mediator according to the color scheme at the top). Dendrograms (trees) show similarity between different conditions and different inflammatory mediator profiles, respectively.

overlap in the expression pattern of the isografts and the rejecting animals for IL-5, IL-1α, IL-18, and GRO-KC.

Mediators relevant for classifications and progression of rejection

Random forest (RF) classification was performed for skin and muscle samples in all three cohorts at POD 3–9. The overall out-of-bag error rate was 6.7% for skin and 7.0% for muscle. The classification tables are shown in Figure 4. The importance of a variable in discriminating among study groups was demonstrated by ranked mean decrease accuracy as depicted in Figure 4. The mediator best capable of differentiating among experimental groups samples was MCP-1 in skin and TNF-α in muscle. Discriminant analysis suggested that the mediators best capable of discriminating among experimental groups in the early postoperative time points were GM-CSF, IL-4, IL-12p70, IL-5, and TNF-α; these mediators also appear within the seven top-ranked mediators in the RF analysis.

To identify inflammatory cytokines with high dynamic variability, we performed principal component analysis (PCA) on the combined mean-centered dataset including the whole postoperative time series over all study groups and tissues. The PCA scores of the first four principle components (explaining >70% of the variance) of all 14 cytokines were ranked based on the sum of the absolute PCA scores (loadings) of all 4 PCs (Figure 5). The top prioritized cytokines IL-1α, IL-18, IL-1β, and IL-4 might be promising candidates for new therapeutic regimens.

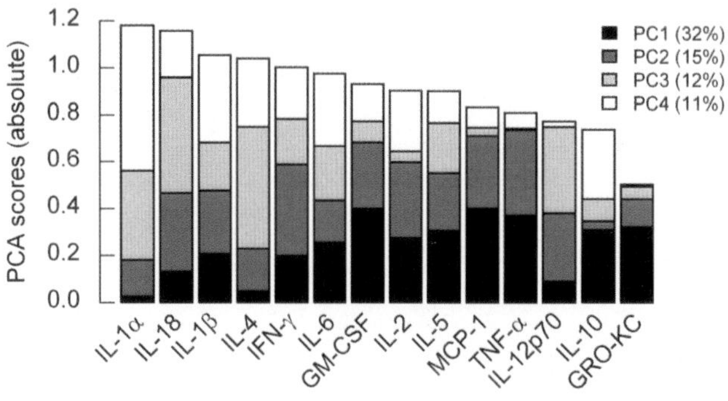

Figure 5. Most variable mediators identified by principal component analysis (PCA) suggesting new potential targets for therapeutic interventions to suppress limb transplant rejection. PCA scores (loadings) for the first four principal components (PCs), which represent more than 70% of information within the data, are displayed in a stacked bar plot for all inflammatory mediators (ranked by the overall PCA score of the 4 PCs).

Discussion

Experimental transplant rejection can be detected reliably in advance of the current clinical gold standard of histologic evaluation, using computational modeling that involves 14 inflammatory mediators in this model. These findings support the hypothesis that the immune signaling associated with rejection follows specific patterns of expression and is driven by different principal components than those associated with inflammation following syngeneic transplantation.

Detailed cellular and molecular assessment provides valuable insights into the role of the immune/inflammatory response in post-transplant pathophysiology [14,15]. Translation of these findings into biomarkers applied clinically, however, has been very limited. It remains a major challenge to reduce the complexity of dynamic biological systems to elements with diagnostic or therapeutic clinical value [16,17]. Data-driven investigations of genomic and proteomic studies in combination with mechanistic computational modeling based on measurements of circulating inflammatory mediators have given insight into the

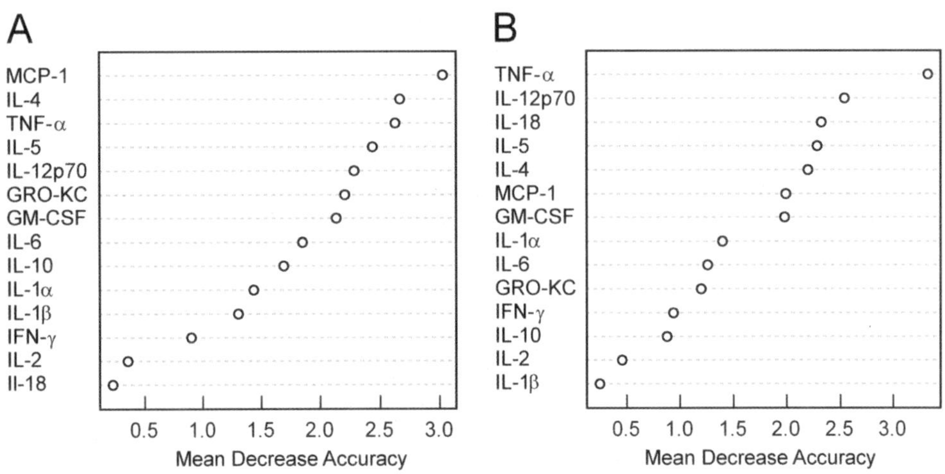

Skin	ATC^{pred}	TAC^{pred}	ISO^{pred}	class error
ATC	22	0	2	8.3 %
TAC	0	16	0	0.0 %
ISO	2	0	18	10.0 %
error rate (OOB)				6.67 %

Muscle	ATC^{pred}	TAC^{pred}	ISO^{pred}	class error
ATC	23	0	1	4.2 %
TAC	1	14	0	6.7 %
ISO	2	0	16	11.1 %
error rate (OOB)				7.02 %

Figure 4. Results from Random Forest classification of the different rejection groups (ISO, TAC, ATC) using over the whole time course (POD 3, POD 5, POD 7, POD 9) measured inflammatory mediators in skin (A) and muscle (B) samples of rat limb transplantation models. Most important mediators for the decision trees based classification approach are evident by ranked mean decrease accuracy. Performances of the classifiers are indicated by the confusion table and the out-of-bag (OOB) error rate.

pathophysiology of trauma, shock as well as organ transplantation [18–22].

Herein, we demonstrate that data-driven and expression pattern-oriented analyses of a high-content dataset can help to decipher the complexity of acute inflammation in VCA. In the present study, these advanced computational algorithms allowed to diagnose rejection in advance of gross histological damage. We suggest that measuring inflammatory mediators expressed in skin and muscle is clinically feasible in the setting of VCA since skin and muscle are more accessible as compared to solid organs. Isografts were compared to allografts and tacrolimus treated allografts in order to delineate between surgery/trauma/ischemia induced inflammation and allograft rejection. Tacrolimus treatment was sufficient to diminish rejection (but not completely eliminate the immune response).

In the samples analyzed in the present study, skin rejection was detected in advance of histological alterations based on the inflammatory mediators IL-4, IL-12p70 and TNF-α, with a prediction accuracy of >87%. In muscle rejection, IL-12p70 and TNF-α were identified as best and accurate classifiers. TNF-α, a canonical inflammatory mediator, is mainly produced by activated monocytes, macrophages, and T-cells, and exerts a direct effect on the proliferation, apoptosis, necrosis, differentiation, and function of virtually every cell type [23]. In the skin, mast cells appear to be the predominant source of preformed TNF-α, which can be released upon inflammatory stimuli [24]. TNF-α activates T-cells; increases the release of other inflammatory mediators; and induces neutrophil adherence, infiltration and the production of enzymes and reactive oxygen. These mechanisms are harmful to the allograft, and subsequently cause tissue injury as well as organ dysfunction [23]. Several studies have demonstrated increased TNF-α levels in the serum during episodes of rejection in liver, kidney and pancreas transplant recipients [25–27]. Interestingly, the increase in TNF-α levels occurred two days before clinical manifestation of rejection.

The production of IL-12 strongly promotes the development of IFN-γ producing helper T (TH)-cells. IL-12 may not only be essential for macrophage-mediated allograft rejection via induction of TH1 responses, but IL-12 may be involved in delaying rejection via induction of inducible nitric oxide synthase (iNOS) and indolamine 2,3 dioxygenase (IDO) [28]. This positive effect was shown in several skin or heart allograft models, as well as in the course of graft-versus-host disease (GVHD) [29–31].

Good performance of the multinomial logistic regression model, which models linear decision boundaries effectively, indicates that the patterns of inflammatory mediator expression in skin are fundamentally different in isograft and allograft skin tissue, and that this difference can be captured with reasonable performance by computationally efficient algorithms. Multinomial logistic regression performance for discrimination of rejection is even stronger and the consistency with which this distinction is made across a rather complex set of features implies a high level of biological significance. In other words, not only is the specific inflammatory mediator, but also the particular combination of mediators in the local inflammatory milieu seems to play a determinative role in the nature and progression of inflammation expressed.

The RF classification approach including more time points (POD 3-POD 9) achieves high levels of accuracy and continues to improve with the addition of variables. This finding implies that there are specific inflammatory mediator interactions that are relevant only under certain contexts [32], and that these interactions can be leveraged to identify potential targets for therapeutic intervention.

We hypothesized that mediators with time-dependent changes might be important in the different dynamic processes and describe principal drivers (principal components, PC), which could turn out as therapeutic targets. We were focusing on the first four PCs since they comprise more than 70% of the total variance. The four top-ranked mediators were IL-1α, IL-18, IL-1β, and IL-4 (Figure 5).

To discern the effect of the inflammatory mediators within each group, we performed the same PCA procedure for each group individually (Figure S1). The impact of IL12p70 already shown as potential early diagnostic marker for rejection was not as pronounced in the tacrolimus-treated animals as in the isograft and allograft study group. Interferon-γ and IL-4 had a high ranking in all groups (ISO, TAC, ATC) indicating a more unspecific effect in inflammation; In contrast, IL-1α and IL-18 exhibited an expression profile which indicates a possible key role in VCA rejection and makes these cytokines interesting candidates for therapeutic interventions.

Our studies identified IL-1α and IL-18 as possible candidates for the treatment of skin rejection. These inflammatory mediators share similarities regarding structure, receptor family, signal transduction pathways, and biological effects. Both inflammatory mediators are produced by monocytes/macrophages but also constitutively expressed by keratinocytes [33]. IL-1α plays an important role in sterile inflammation. During necrotic cell death, the IL-1α precursor is released [34] and binds to its receptor expressed on adjacent macrophages and epithelial cells, which in turn triggers a pro-inflammatory response characterized by an influx of neutrophils followed by macrophages [35,36]. IL-18, together with IL-2, IL-12, and IL-15, is a dominant IFN-γ inducing factor. Several human diseases, such as systemic lupus erythematosus, rheumatoid arthritis, Crohn's disease, psoriasis and graft-versus-host-disease are thought to be mediated in part by IL-18 [37]. Moreover, IL-18 stimulates ICAM-1 expression on monocytic cell lines, which is important for the recruitment of T-cells and other immune cells to the skin. Lymphocyte recruitment is known as a key mechanism in inflammatory skin disorders and [38,39]. Hautz et al. showed, that expression of ICAM-1 correlated closely with severity of skin rejection [8].

Based on our findings, IL-1α and IL-18 appear as interesting potential targets for intervention. Yuan J et al. already showed the efficacy of IL-1 receptor antagonist (IL-1ra) gene transfer treatment for acute corneal graft rejection in a rat model [40] The group demonstrated during acute rejection, that TGF-β1, RANTES and IL-1 levels were lower in the IL-1ra treatment group. Thus antagonizing the biological activitiy of IL-1 could effectively prolong graft survival. IL-ra, a specific inhibitor of both IL-1α and IL-β generically known as anakinra is clinically applied for the treatment of rheumatoid arthritis. IL-18-binding protein (IL-18BP), a specific inhibitor or IL-18 which neutralizes IL-18 bioactivity, was discovered during the search for soluble IL-18 receptors in humane urine [41]. A clinical preparation of human IL-18BP has been shown to be safe and effective in patients with RA or plaque psoriasis [42]. A soluble form of the IL-18 receptor accessory protein (sIL-18Rβ) has recently been identified as novel IL-18 inhibitor in collagen-induced arthritis in mice [43].

In summary, we herein provide information, which could help identifying a diagnostic profile and novel targets for treatment of skin rejection in VCA. The present study demonstrates that the application of advanced computational methods can be successfully applied in molecular assessment of skin rejection and provides novel insights into the inflammatory mediator communication patterns. The study remains observational in its nature and investigational trials are warranted in order to address the true functional value of the postulated treatment targets.

Supporting Information

Figure S1 Most variable (influential) mediators identified by principal component analysis (PCA) for each of the three study groups (ISO/TAC/ATC). PCA scores (loadings) for the first four principal components (PCs), which represent more than 75% of information, are displayed in a stacked bar plot for all inflammatory mediators (ranked by the overall PCA score of the 4 PCs) and a scatter plot of the first two PCs.

Figure S2 Distribution of inflammatory mediator levels (boxplots) at postoperative day 5 in rat limb transplantation models for selected inflammatory mediators. Adjusted p-values from Wilcoxon rank-sum test between the rejection group (ATC) versus Tacrolimus treated group (TAC) are provided.

Acknowledgments

We gratefully acknowledge the effort of Dr. Mario Cherubino and Dr. Yong Wang for performing a major part of hindlimb transplants. The help of Prof. Bernhard Zelger in preparing and evaluating histological sections and the editorial work by Mary Margreiter are also gratefully acknowledged.

Author Contributions

Conceived and designed the experiments: DW SS GB RS WAL YV. Performed the experiments: DW DB TH NE HH. Analyzed the data: DW HH RS TH NE BZ. Contributed reagents/materials/analysis tools: YV JP GP. Wrote the paper: DW HH SS.

References

1. Cendales LC, Kanitakis J, Schneeberger S, Burns C, Ruiz P, et al. (2008) The Banff 2007 working classification of skin-containing composite tissue allograft pathology. Am J Transplant 8: 1396–1400.
2. Kanitakis J, Jullien D, Nicolas JF, Frances C, Claudy A, et al. (2000) Sequential histological and immunohistochemical study of the skin of the first human hand allograft. Transplantation 69: 1380–1385.
3. Kanitakis J (2008) The challenge of dermatopathological diagnosis of composite tissue allograft rejection: a review. J Cutan Pathol 35: 738–744.
4. Schneeberger S, Gorantla VS, van Riet RP, Lanzetta M, Vereecken P, et al. (2008) Atypical acute rejection after hand transplantation. Am J Transplant 8: 688–696.
5. Hautz T, Wolfram D, Grahammer J, Starzl R, Krapf C, et al. (2012) Mechanisms and mediators of inflammation: potential models for skin rejection and targeted therapy in vascularized composite allotransplantation. Clin Dev Immunol: 1–9.
6. Tarca AL, Carey VJ, Chen XW, Romero R, Draghici S (2007) Machine learning and its applications to biology. PLoS Comput Biol 3: e116.
7. Coin L, Bateman A, Durbin R (2003) Enhanced protein domain discovery by using language modeling techniques from speech recognition. Proc Natl Acad Sci U S A 100: 4516–4520.
8. Hautz T, Zelger B, Grahammer J, Krapf C, Amberger A, et al. (2010) Molecular markers and targeted therapy of skin rejection in composite tissue allotransplantation. Am J Transplant 10: 1200–1209.
9. Benjamini Y, Hochberg Y (1995) Controlling the false discovery rate: A practical and powerful approach to multiple testing. J R Statist Soc B 57: 289–300.
10. Sturn A, Quackenbush J, Trajanoski Z (2002) Genesis: cluster analysis of microarray data. Bioinformatics 18: 207–208.
11. Breiman L (2001) Random Forests. Machine Learning 45: 5–32.
12. Mi Q, Constantine G, Ziraldo C, Solovyev A, Torres A, et al. (2011) A dynamic view of trauma/hemorrhage-induced inflammation in mice: principal drivers and networks. PLoS One 6: e19424.
13. Namas RA, Namas R, Lagoa C, Barclay D, Mi Q, et al. (2012) Hemoadsorption reprograms inflammation in experimental gram-negative septic peritonitis: insights from in vivo and in silico studies. Mol Med 18: 1366–1374.
14. Page EK, Dar WA, Knechtle SJ (2012) Biologics in organ transplantation. Transpl Int 25: 707–719.
15. Sarwal MM (2006) Chipping into the human genome: novel insights for transplantation. Immunol Rev 210: 138–155.
16. Vodovotz Y (2006) Deciphering the complexity of acute inflammation using mathematical models. Immunol Res 36: 237–245.
17. Mesarovic MD, Sreenath SN, Keene JD (2004) Search for organising principles: understanding in systems biology. Syst Biol (Stevenage) 1: 19–27.
18. Calvano SE, Xiao W, Richards DR, Felciano RM, Baker HV, et al. (2005) A network-based analysis of systemic inflammation in humans. Nature 437: 1032–1037.
19. Warren HS, Elson CM, Hayden DL, Schoenfeld DA, Cobb JP, et al. (2009) A genomic score prognostic of outcome in trauma patients. Mol Med 15: 220–227.
20. Chow CC, Clermont G, Kumar R, Lagoa C, Tawadrous Z, et al. (2005) The acute inflammatory response in diverse shock states. Shock 24: 74–84.
21. Bohra R, Klepacki J, Klawitter J, Thurman JM, Christians U (2013) Proteomics and metabolomics in renal transplantation-quo vadis? Transpl Int 26: 225–241.
22. Azhar N (2013) Analysis of serum inflammatory mediators identifies unique dynamic networks associated with death and spontaneous survival in pediatric acute liver failure.
23. Grenz A, Schenk M, Zipfel A, Viebahn R (2000) TNF-alpha and its receptors mediate graft rejection and loss after liver transplantation. Clin Chem Lab Med 38: 1183–1185.
24. Walsh LJ, Trinchieri G, Waldorf HA, Whitaker D, Murphy GF (1991) Human dermal mast cells contain and release tumor necrosis factor alpha, which induces endothelial leukocyte adhesion molecule 1. Proc Natl Acad Sci U S A 88: 4220–4224.
25. Imagawa DK, Millis JM, Olthoff KM, Derus LJ, Chia D, et al. (1990) The role of tumor necrosis factor in allograft rejection. I. Evidence that elevated levels of tumor necrosis factor-alpha predict rejection following orthotopic liver transplantation. Transplantation 50: 219–225.
26. Bubnova LN, Kabakov A, Serebrianaya N, Ketlinky S (1992) Interleukin-1 beta and tumor necrosis factor-alpha serum levels in renal allograft recipients. Transplant Proc 24: 2545.
27. Grewal HP, Kotb M, Salem A, el Din AB, Novak K, et al. (1993) Elevated tumor necrosis factor levels are predictive for pancreas allograft transplant rejection. Transplant Proc 25: 132–135.
28. Goriely S, Goldman M (2008) Interleukin-12 family members and the balance between rejection and tolerance. Curr Opin Organ Transplant 13: 4–9.
29. Piccotti JR, Chan SY, Goodman RE, Magram J, Eichwald EJ, et al. (1996) IL-12 antagonism induces T helper 2 responses, yet exacerbates cardiac allograft rejection. Evidence against a dominant protective role for T helper 2 cytokines in alloimmunity. J Immunol 157: 1951–1957.
30. Verma ND, Boyd R, Robinson C, Plain KM, Tran GT, et al. (2006) Interleukin-12p70 prolongs allograft survival by induction of interferon gamma and nitric oxide production. Transplantation 82: 1324–1333.
31. Dey BR, Yang YG, Szot GL, Pearson DA, Sykes M (1998) Interleukin-12 inhibits graft-versus-host disease through an Fas-mediated mechanism associated with alterations in donor T-cell activation and expansion. Blood 91: 3315–3322.
32. Nathan C, Sporn M (1991) Cytokines in context. J Cell Biol 113: 981–986.
33. Dinarello CA (1999) IL-18: A TH1-inducing, proinflammatory cytokine and new member of the IL-1 family. J Allergy Clin Immunol 103: 11–24.
34. Carmi Y, Voronov E, Dotan S, Lahat N, Rahat MA, et al. (2009) The role of macrophage-derived IL-1 in induction and maintenance of angiogenesis. J Immunol 183: 4705–4714.
35. Rider P, Carmi Y, Guttman O, Braiman A, Cohen I, et al. (2011) IL-1alpha and IL-1beta recruit different myeloid cells and promote different stages of sterile inflammation. J Immunol 187: 4835–4843.
36. van de Veerdonk FL, Netea MG (2013) New Insights in the Immunobiology of IL-1 Family Members. Front Immunol 4: 167.
37. Dinarello CA (2009) Immunological and inflammatory functions of the interleukin-1 family. Annu Rev Immunol 27: 519–550.
38. Robert C, Kupper TS (1999) Inflammatory skin diseases, T cells, and immune surveillance. N Engl J Med 341: 1817–1828.
39. Schon MP, Ludwig RJ (2005) Lymphocyte trafficking to inflamed skin—molecular mechanisms and implications for therapeutic target molecules. Expert Opin Ther Targets 9: 225–243.
40. Yuan J, Liu Y, Huang W, Zhou S, Ling S, et al. (2013) The experimental treatment of corneal graft rejection with the interleukin-1 receptor antagonist (IL-1ra) gene. PLoS One 8: e60714.
41. Novick D, Kim SH, Fantuzzi G, Reznikov LL, Dinarello CA, et al. (1999) Interleukin-18 binding protein: a novel modulator of the Th1 cytokine response. Immunity 10: 127–136.
42. Tak PP, Bacchi M, Bertolino M (2006) Pharmacokinetics of IL-18 binding protein in healthy volunteers and subjects with rheumatoid arthritis or plaque psoriasis. Eur J Drug Metab Pharmacokinet 31: 109–116.
43. Veenbergen S, Smeets R, Bennink M, Arntz O, Joosten L, et al. (2010) The natural soluble form of IL-18 receptor beta exacerbates collagen-induced arthritis via modulation of T-cell immune responses. Ann Rheum Dis 69: 276–283.

22

Intramuscular Connective Tissue Differences in Spastic and Control Muscle: A Mechanical and Histological Study

Marije de Bruin[1], Mark J. Smeulders[1], Michiel Kreulen[1,2], Peter A. Huijing[3], Richard T Jaspers[3]*

1 Department of Plastic, Reconstructive and Hand Surgery, Academic Medical Center, Amsterdam, The Netherlands, **2** Department of Plastic, Reconstructive and Hand Surgery, Red Cross Hospital, Beverwijk, The Netherlands, **3** Laboratory for Myology, MOVE Research Institute Amsterdam, Faculty of Human Movement Sciences, VU University Amsterdam, Amsterdam, The Netherlands

Abstract

Cerebral palsy (CP) of the spastic type is a neurological disorder characterized by a velocity-dependent increase in tonic stretch reflexes with exaggerated tendon jerks. Secondary to the spasticity, muscle adaptation is presumed to contribute to limitations in the passive range of joint motion. However, the mechanisms underlying these limitations are unknown. Using biopsies, we compared mechanical as well as histological properties of flexor carpi ulnaris muscle (FCU) from CP patients ($n=29$) and healthy controls ($n=10$). The sarcomere slack length (mean 2.5 μm, SEM 0.05) and slope of the normalized sarcomere length-tension characteristics of spastic fascicle segments and single myofibre segments were not different from those of control muscle. Fibre type distribution also showed no significant differences. Fibre size was significantly smaller (1933 μm^2, SEM 190) in spastic muscle than in controls (2572 μm^2, SEM 322). However, our statistical analyses indicate that the latter difference is likely to be explained by age, rather than by the affliction. Quantities of endomysial and perimysial networks within biopsies of control and spastic muscle were unchanged with one exception: a significant thickening of the tertiary perimysium (3-fold), i.e. the connective tissue reinforcement of neurovascular tissues penetrating the muscle. Note that this thickening in tertiary perimysium was shown in the majority of CP patients, however a small number of patients ($n=4$ out of 23) did not have this feature. These results are taken as indications that enhanced myofascial loads on FCU is one among several factors contributing in a major way to the aetiology of limitation of movement at the wrist in CP and the characteristic wrist position of such patients.

Editor: Maurilio Sampaolesi, Stem Cell Research Institute, Belgium

Funding: This study was supported by the Phelps Stichting voor Spastici (Grant No. 2006009). The funders had no role in study design, data collection and analysis, decision to publish, or preparation of the manuscript.

* Email: r.t.jaspers@vu.nl

Introduction

Spasticity in the forearm due to cerebral palsy (CP) is associated with a limited range of active and passive movement around the wrist and elbow. The flexor carpi ulnaris muscle (FCU) is held largely responsible for the limited range of motion and the contracture around the wrist. Presumed muscle adaptation induced by longstanding spasticity is regarded as the major contributor to the passive movement limitation. Therefore, this muscle is frequently subject of surgical treatment of the spastic arm [1]. In patients with CP, development of lower extremity muscles (triceps surae and hamstrings) has been reported to be compromised, causing shortness [2,3] and/or an increased passive muscle stiffness [4,5,6].

The mechanisms by which spasticity of the FCU results in a limited passive movement around the wrist and elbow are unknown. Several pathophysiological mechanisms may underlie the altered spastic FCU development. Due to the spasticity and the related reduced ability of CP patients to extend the wrist, FCU is largely maintained in a shortened position. Based on effects found for immobilization of experimental animal muscle in a shortened position [7,8], both impeded growth of myofibre diameter and diminished addition of serial sarcomeres within myofibres have been presumed in spastic muscle [9]. However, to our knowledge, quantitative data regarding spasticity related differences in serial sarcomere number are insufficient and hard to obtain, as this requires isolation of myofibres along their full length.

For pennate muscle, such as FCU, myofibre diameter is also a major determinant of both muscle slack and optimum length [10,11]. As such, changes in myofibre cross-sectional size could result in a shift in the muscle operating length range *in vivo*, and affect the wrist range of motion. Regarding the cross-sectional size of spastic myofibres, both atrophy and hypertrophy of slow, as well as fast myofibre types, have been reported in muscles from different limbs without a clear relation to the degree of limitation of joint movement [12,13,14,15,16,17]. In addition, some studies reported similar cross-sectional areas of spastic and control myofibres comparing several muscles from different limbs [18,19]. From the above we can conclude that alleged muscle stiffness is not unequivocally related to myofibre cross-sectional size and muscle shortness in CP.

Other factors that may affect muscle stiffness are (1) a change in the intrinsic, mechanical properties of the myofibres (i.e. myofibre stiffness [20]), (2) the intramuscular connective tissue [13,21], or (3) altered myofascial loads of the epimuscular myofascial connections of the spastic muscle with extramuscular connective tissues, synergists and/or antagonist muscles [22].

Single myofibre segments obtained from different spastic muscles of the forearm have been reported to be stiffer than those of control muscle [20]. However, fascicle segments of spastic muscles have been reported to be more compliant than similar segments in control muscle, suggesting spasticity related deterioration of intramuscular connective tissue [23]. Furthermore, the analysis of the amount of connective tissue in human muscle tissue obtained from muscles in the leg and arm has shown diverse results (cf. [6,13,16,18,21,23]). Above-mentioned variability in results may exist because comparisons were made between biopsies obtained from different muscles within one limb, muscles of different limbs or from biopsies taken from different locations within a muscle. The purpose of this study was to test the hypothesis that the limited range of wrist motion is caused by enhanced stiffness of spastic muscle as affected by intrinsic characteristics of myofibres and fascicles. To test this, we investigated mechanical and histological characteristics of spastic and healthy muscle biopsies taken from the same part of FCU muscle.

Methods

Ethics

All subjects older than 18 years of age gave written informed consent for the study. Subjects younger than 18 years of age participated in this study with written informed consent from their parents (as well as from the children themselves, if aged 12 years or over). The study and informed consent procedure were approved by the local Medical Ethics Committee of the Academic Medical Centre of Amsterdam. The study adhered to the ethical guidelines of the 1975 Declaration of Helsinki

Subjects

Undergoing upper extremity surgery between 2006 and 2009, 29 patients (mean age 19 years, range 5–40, 15 male) with CP and a Zancolli type IIa or IIb grasp and release pattern [24] took part in the study. Patients that have a type Zancolli IIa or IIb grasp and release pattern, have active finger extension that is accompanied by a wrist flexion angle greater than 20°. Furthermore, in type Zancolli IIa pattern the wrist can be actively extended with flexed fingers whereas in type Zancolli IIb pattern there is no active wrist extension [24].

Healthy control subjects (n = 10; mean age 45 years; range 21–62; 3 male), who required upper extremity surgery due to cut or ruptured tendons (n = 5), bone deformities (n = 3), or traumas (n = 2) were also studied. Because of technical failure causing loss of the frozen parts of the biopsies, one of the control subjects and three to six of the patients were excluded from the histological measurements (depending on the type of staining).

Collection and storage of muscle biopsies

During surgery, muscle biopsies (size ~10×0.5×5 mm) were collected from the most distal part of FCU. Each biopsy was divided in two parts. The long axis of both samples was taken parallel to the longitudinal direction of the myofibres. One part to be used for mechanical measurements was put in a 50% muscle relaxing, 50% glycerol solution and stored at −20°C until further use. The relaxing solution consisted of: EGTA, 7.5 mM; potassium proprionate, 170 mM; magnesium acetate, 2 mM; imidazole, 5 mM; creatine phosphate, 10 mM; adenosine triphosphate (ATP), 4 mM; leupeptin, 17 µg/ml; and protease inhibitor E64, 4 µg/ml. Storage time did not affect sarcomere length-tension strain characteristics. All chemicals were obtained from Sigma Aldrich (the Netherlands) unless stated otherwise. The other part, to be used for histological and histochemical analysis, was frozen and stored in liquid nitrogen for maximally one week. Using a cryomicrotome, serial cross-sections (10 µm thick) were cut at −25°C, and then stored at −80°C until further use.

Mechanical measurements

Segments of a fascicle (containing 15–30 myofibres, mean length 6.0 mm ±1.2), as well as single myofibre segments (mean length 5.6 mm ±1.7) were microscopically dissected in 12 of the 29 patient samples and all control samples. Force transducer limitations (maximal load 0.12 N) limited the size of fascicle segments that could be measured. Small platinum hooks (50 µm thick) were tied to both ends of the segments using 20 µm diameter polyamide thread (Ethicon).

At a mean sarcomere length of 2.7 µm, the largest (a) and smallest (b) segment diameters were measured at three locations along the length of the segment (in the middle and 1 mm from each endpoint) by rotating the segment and using an ocular scale. The cross-sectional area at each of the three positions along the segment was calculated assuming an ellipsoidal cross-section (1/4*π times the product of the largest and smallest segment diameters). The mean of these three values was taken as the cross-sectional area of the segment.

One end of the segment was connected to a force transducer (AE801, SensoNor, Horten, Norway) and the other end was connected to a micromanipulator. To measure passive elastic properties, the myofibre and fascicle segments were elongated in steps of 250 µm, starting at passive slack length. Measurements were performed in 100% muscle-relaxing solution described in paragraph "Collection and storage of muscle biopsies" (20°C). In a pilot study, tensions and sarcomere lengths were measured immediately following lengthening and after 2, 4 and 6 minutes, to take the effects of stress-relaxation into account (Fig. 1). Such effects were present up to 4 minutes. Therefore, all further analyses were carried out on tensions measured 4 minutes after imposing each strain increment. The segments were elongated until sarcomere lengths were beyond the physiological range (≥ 4.1 µm) [25,26] or until mechanical failure occurred.

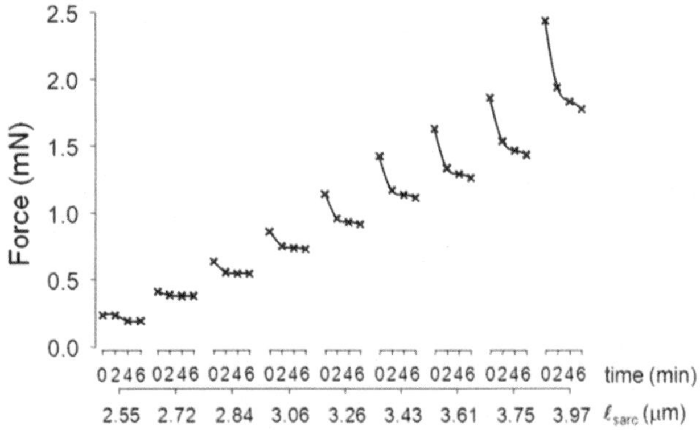

Figure 1. Stress relaxation of myofibres and fascicles at different sarcomere lengths. Representative passive forces of a spastic single myofibre segment from a spastic FCU as a function of sarcomere length (ℓsarc). Forces were measured immediately (time = 0 min), and 2, 4, and 6 minutes after imposing each sarcomere strain increment. Note that effects of stress relaxation are small after at least 4 minutes, therefore sarcomere length-tension curves of myofibre and fascicle segments were assessed based on the forces measured after 4 minutes.

To compare mechanical properties of the myofibre and fascicle segments, tensions were normalized to the cross-sectional area. Data for tension as a function of sarcomere length were least square fitted by a polynomial function. The polynomial order that best described the experimental data was selected with one-way analysis of variance (ANOVA). Third order polynomial curves turned out to provide the best description for all curves (mean $R^2_{myofibre} = 0.993 \pm 0.005$; mean $R^2_{fascicle} = 0.990 \pm 0.01$). These polynomials were used for averaging of data and calculation of standard errors at set sarcomere lengths. The slope of the fitted curve (i.e. stiffness) was calculated within the physiological range by differentiation and considered an estimate of static passive stiffness of the myofibres and fascicles.

Histology

Hematoxilin and eosine (HE) staining. To compare global morphology and spatial distribution of myonuclei, sections were fixed for 10 min in 4% formaldehyde in 0.1 M sodium phosphate buffer, pH 7.4, and stained with hematoxylin and eosin [27].

Myofibrillar ATPase staining. Myofibre typing was performed according to Brook and Kaiser [28]. Optimal myofibre type differentiation was attained at pH 4.5, at which type I myofibres stained black, type IIA myofibres white and fibres that express type IIX or co-express type A and X stained (dark) grey (referred to as IIAX) [29] .

Sirius red staining. Connective tissue was visualized using a modification of the Sirius red staining protocol by Junquiera et al. [30]. To minimize cytoplasmic staining, sections were first fixed in acetone at 0°C for 30 minutes and subsequently in Bouin's solution (75 ml Picric acid, 25 ml 10% formalin, and 5 ml glacial acetic acid) at 20°C for 30 minutes. Following this, sections were stained using a picrosirius red F3BA 0.1% (C.I. 35782; Direct red 80; Sigma Aldrich, the Netherlands) for 30 minutes in a dark environment. After staining, sections were washed in 10 mM HCl and then rinsed two times in absolute ethanol. Subsequently, the sections were submerged in Xylene for 10 seconds and again in Xylene for 2 minutes. Finally, slides were covered with Entallan mounting medium (Merck, Darmstadt, Germany) and a glass cover slip.

Image analyses. Images were obtained using a Zeiss microscope (Axioskop 50) coupled to a AxioCam (Zeiss, Germany) and were analysed with ImageJ (v. 1.41o,; USA National Institute of Health, http://rsbweb.nih.gov/ij/). Within each ATPase-stained sample cross-section, the cross-sectional area of the myofibres (A_{MF}) and fibre perimeter were measured in at least 30 randomly selected cells per myofibre type by manually tracking the fibres. Sections with myofibres at the edge of sections and obliquely cut fibres (circularity <0.30) were excluded from analysis. To measure connective tissue parameters in Sirius red stained sections, contrast between yellow cytoplasm and red connective tissue was enhanced by image-filtering (green-filter [31]) using ImageJ. Subsequently, a binary threshold was applied such that a black overlay covered only the gray values above threshold (i.e. the connective tissue (red stained) areas). For all measurements, we used the Maximum Entropy threshold method by Jarek Sasha (http://ij-plugins.sf.net) prepared for ImageJ. This method minimizes erroneous detection of collagen in the cytoplasm.

Within the fascicle, the endomysium is defined as the connective tissue surrounding single myofibres. In the images, we selected areas containing only myofibres and endomysium. The black areas within the selection represented the absolute endomysium cross-sectional area (A_E). To normalize for myofibre cross-sectional area (A_{MF}), the absolute surface area of endomysium per myofibre (A_E/MF) was determined as: A_E divided by the number of myofibres in the selected regions containing only endomysia and myofibres. The number of myofibres in this region was estimated by dividing the total surface area of the myofibres by the mean A_{MF} of the myofibres (measured on the myofibres of which the entire cross-section was contained within the selected region). Mean endomysium thickness per myofibre (ℓ_E) was calculated by dividing A_E/MF by the measured mean perimeter of the myofibres fulfilling the above criterion.

Traditionally, two domains are distinguished for the perimysium: primary perimysium embedding smallest fascicles of myofibres and secondary perimysium embedding larger fascicles, containing several primary fascicles [32]. We propose distinction of a specialized third level of perimysium. This tertiary perimysium borders parts of the secondary fascicles, but is thickened compared to secondary perimysium and traverses the muscle. The thickness of primary and secondary perimysium in cross-sections ($\ell_{P1\&P2}$) was measured every 25 μm along the perimeter of the fascicle of at least 5 fascicles within the cross-section. The tertiary perimysium thickness (ℓ_{P3}) was measured every 25 μm along its length over a length of at least 1 mm.

Assessment of functional implication of extramuscular connections

To visualize effects extramuscular myofascial connections on length changes of FCU *in vivo*, we collected video data of a boy (14 years old) undergoing tendon transfer surgery. The first step before transfer of the FCU tendon was tenotomy performed just proximal to the pisiform bone causing complete release from its insertion but leaving extramuscular connections of the fascial surroundings to the muscle belly intact. After FCU distal tenotomy the wrist was moved towards maximal flexion and extension by the surgeon. The distal tendon of the FCU and its surroundings was filmed while moving the wrist dynamically. In a subsequent step, FCU muscle belly was dissected partially free from its surrounded connection tissue and photographs were taken.

Statistics

A mixed design repeated measures analysis of covariance (ANCOVA) with one between subjects factor (SPSS Statistics 17.0) and age as covariate was performed to determine if there was a difference between the control and spastic passive sarcomere length-tension curves and the slopes of these curves of myofibre segments and fascicle segments. Slack lengths, muscle morphology and histochemical results of control and spastic groups were compared using *t*-tests. A non-parametric test of independent samples was used to compare myofibre type distributions and perimysial tissue variables, as these were not normally distributed. Non-parametric Spearman's correlations were used to test for age effects (A_{MF}, fibre type proportions, and several connective tissue variables). As the CP group consisted of both children and adults, and literature shows that myofibre size in typically developing children generally increases up to the age of 20 years (cf. [33,34,35,36,37]), additional *t*-tests were performed to test for differences in A_{MF} between CP and control subjects both aged ≥ 20 years (CP n = 7; controls n = 10). For the CP group, effects of sex were tested using *t*-tests. Differences were considered significant at $p < 0.05$. All data are presented as mean±standard error of the mean (SEM).

Results

Subject characteristics

As a result of an age restriction for control subjects due to medical ethical considerations, control subjects ($n = 10$, mean age

44.8±4.3 years) were significantly older than spastic patients ($n = 29$, mean age 18.9±1.6 years).

Mechanical characteristics

All myofibre segments could be strained up to a sarcomere length of at least 4.0 µm. However, for six out of 22 fascicle segments, force transducer limitations prevented us from determining stress-strain characteristics up to this length (two were strained up to 3.5 and 3.6 respectively, and four others were strained up to 3.8 µm). Mean sarcomere slack length was neither significantly different between CP (2.52±0.08 µm) and control myofibre segments (2.44±0.06 µm) nor between CP (2.51±0.07 µm) and control fascicle segments (2.49±0.05 µm) (Fig. 2A). Over the whole range of sarcomere lengths, passive tensions of spastic and control myofibre segments and fascicle segments did not differ significantly (Fig. 2A). No significant differences were found between the passive length-tension curves of control and spastic myofibre segments or between control and spastic fascicle segments. No interaction was present with main factors sarcomere length and CP and type of segment (myofibre or fascicle).

Similarly, sarcomere length-slope of tension curves of spastic myofibre segments and fascicle segments did not differ from sarcomere length-slope of tension curves of control myofibre segments and fascicle segments (Fig. 2B). Again, no interactions were found between sarcomere length, spasticity and type of muscle segment (fibre or fascicle). Thus, increasing sarcomere length had the same result on slope of both control and spastic myofibre segments and fascicle segments.

For both myofibres and fascicle segments, mechanical characteristics were not related to age nor was there a difference between male and female CP patients.

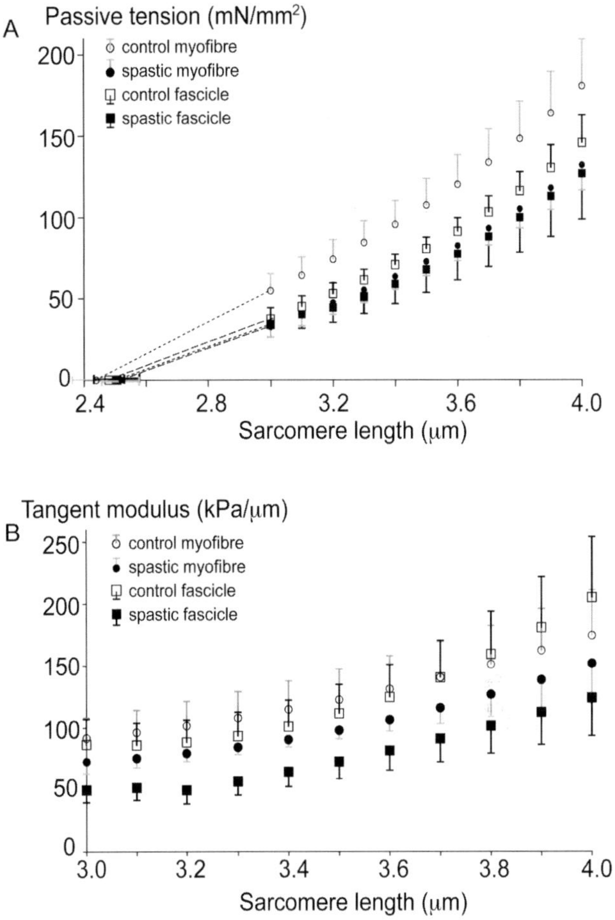

Figure 2. Passive length-tension characteristics of single myofibre segments and fascicle segments in spastic and control FCU. (**A**) passive tension as function of sarcomere length. Sarcomere length-passive tension curves were neither significantly different comparing spastic and control (n = 10) single myofibre segments (both n = 10), nor comparing spastic and control fascicle segments (both n = 10). The same was found for comparing single myofibre segments to fascicle segments within each group. (**B**) slopes of passive length-tension as function of sarcomere length. The curves describing the slopes were neither significantly different comparing spastic and control (n = 10) single myofibre segments (both n = 10), nor comparing spastic and control fascicle segments (both n = 10). The same was found for comparing single myofibre segments with fascicle segments within each group. Means and SEM are plotted.

Myofibre histology

HE staining. Normal localization of myonuclei was found for control subjects as well as patients (Fig. 3A and B), except for one patient. In that particular biopsy, central localization of nuclei was shown in a majority of myofibres (Fig. 3C). These results indicate that, in general, the spastic myofibres do not exhibit this sign of muscle damage.

Myofibre type distributions. Figure 4 shows examples of ATPase stained cross-sections of control and spastic fascicles. Counting of myofibres shows that in control subjects, the biopsies consisted on average for 38% of type I myofibres, 39% of type IIA and for 23% of type IIAX myofibres. The myofibre type distribution in spastic muscle (all CP children) did not differ significantly from that in control muscle (Fig. 4C). However, within the spastic group, the percentage type I fibres correlated negatively with age (Spearman's $\rho = 0.46$, $p<0.016$). In contrast, the percentages type IIA and IIAX did not correlate with age. In addition, fibre type distributions of spastic muscles, did not differ significantly between male and female CP patients.

Myofibre size. Regardless myofibe type, A_{MF} of spastic muscle (testing data for all CP subjects) was significantly smaller than that of control muscle (Fig. 4D, $p<0.01$). However, comparing A_{MF} exclusively for adult CP and control subjects (age ≥20 years), no significant difference was found (t-test). In addition, for spastic muscles, A_{MF} did not differ between adult male and female CP patients.

For spastic muscle of all ages taken together, Spearman's coefficient of correlation for A_{MF} and age was moderately high ($\rho = 0.57$, $p<0.001$). In combination with the lack of difference for A_{MF} between adult spastic and control muscles, this indicates that the correlation found for age and A_{MF}, should be ascribed to age effects in young spastic myofibre size.

Intramuscular connective tissue. Figure 5 shows typical examples of Sirius Red stained cross-sections of control and spastic muscle biopsies. In general, we found no differences between spastic and control muscles for variables describing the endomysial or primary and secondary perimysial parts of intramuscular stroma: No significant differences were found for (1) A_E (Fig. 5C), (2) A_E/MF (data not shown), (3) ℓ_E and (4) $\ell_{P1\&P2}$ (Figs. 5 D-E). However, there was one exception: for the tertiary level of perimysium, a difference was found between control and spastic muscle (Fig. 6). The mean thickness of tertiary perimysium (ℓ_{p3}) in spastic muscle (95.1±11.7 µm) was threefold that of control muscle (31.6±7.1 µm, $p<0.01$; Fig. 6C). However, note also that for some individual spastic muscles (n = 4 out of 23) the value of this variable (ℓ_{p3}) was similar to that of controls, possibly indicating

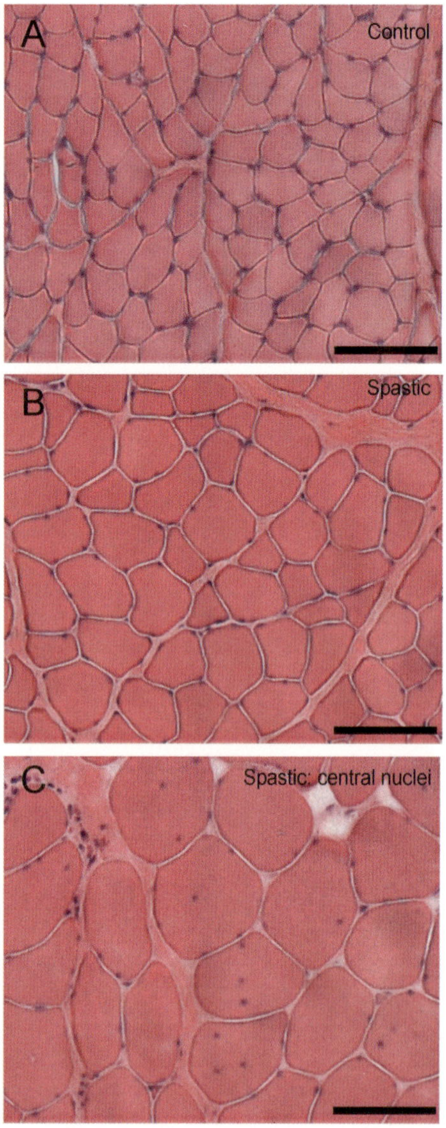

Figure 3. Light micrographic comparison of HE stained cross-sections of fascicles from spastic and control FCU. (**A**) Typical example of a cross-sectional image within control FCU. (**B**) Typical example of a cross-sectional image within spastic FCU. (**C**) example of the pathological sign of central nuclei observed in one CP patient exclusively. Bars represent 100 μm.

diverging properties of individual CP subjects. As the reverse is also true for some control subjects (i.e. fairly high values, n = 3), this indicates that individual variation of ℓ_{p3} may be a confounding factor.

For both groups, no significant rank correlations could be shown for age and any of these variables.

Extramuscular connections and functional implications

In a majority of our CP subjects, thickening of intramuscular neurovascular tracts within spastic FCU may be indicative of adaptation to enhanced loading of these structures. Such loading likely occurs via extramuscular neurovascular tracts. To assess whether myofascial loading of spastic FCU occurs, we imaged effects of distal tenotomy on FCU during surgery (an example is shown, Movie S1). On distal FCU tenotomy the muscle retracts somewhat. Subsequent moving of the wrist joint back and forth between maximal dorsal and palmar flexion causes FCU to be lengthened and shortened repeatedly, despite the fact this muscle no longer crosses the wrist joint. These observations indicate the presence of myofascial loads exerted by neighbouring tissues onto FCU.

Tissues that remain intact after tenotomy consist of fascial extramuscular connective tissue surrounding the muscle belly. Important candidates for mediation of this effect are neurovascular tracts that enter the muscle belly (Fig. 7A) at several locations along its length.

Discussion

The results of this study suggest that movement limitations in the spastic wrist are not explained by differences in FCU myofibre size, myofibre type or in thickness or quantity (absolute or normalized) of intramuscular connective tissues consisting of endomysia and perimysia. A notable exception is the tertiary perimysium being threefold as thick as spastic muscle compared to control muscle, suggesting accumulation of collagen in perimysium reinforcing major blood vessels, nerves and lymphatics,

Limitations of the study

A major limiting factor of this study is the age difference between our patient and control groups. This age difference could not be prevented in our study design. Upper extremity tendon transfer surgery in CP patients often takes place in the second decade of life. But, due to medical ethical considerations, we were not allowed to include control subjects under the age of 18. However, we were able to include some CP patients aged over 20 years and used this subgroup for additional comparisons with the (adult) control group.

Our CP group consisted of similar numbers of males and females, but not our control group (n = 3 vs. n = 7, respectively). For the CP group, none of the variables studied differed between males and females. If this holds also for controls remains to be determined in future work.

Sarcomere length-tension measurements were performed on myofibre and fascicle segments rather than whole myofibres and fascicles. Consequently, we could not compare the series number of sarcomeres within whole myofibres with spastic and control muscle. However, passive and active length-force characteristics of partially dissected FCU in the spastic arm [38] were shown to be similar to those predicted for healthy muscle [39,40]. This suggested that the overstretching of sarcomeres due to a decrease of number of sarcomeres in series may not be the primary cause for the movement limitation in the wirst joint [38].

Our measurements were performed at 20°C. However, sarcomere stiffness increases with temperature, particularly at high length [41]. At 37°C, effects of sarcomere length changes on myofibre and fascicle tension are expected to be higher than shown in our present results.

Comparison of mechanical properties of fascicle and single myofibre segments

For myofibre segments obtained from spastic arm muscles, increased stiffness was reported previously [20,23]. Also, based on previous reports [20,23], the slope of the length-tension curve for spastic fascicle segments may be expected to be lower than for control segments [23]. However, in agreement with previous work from our group [38], neither differences in passive tension nor in slope of the sarcomere length-tension curve could be confirmed by our present results.

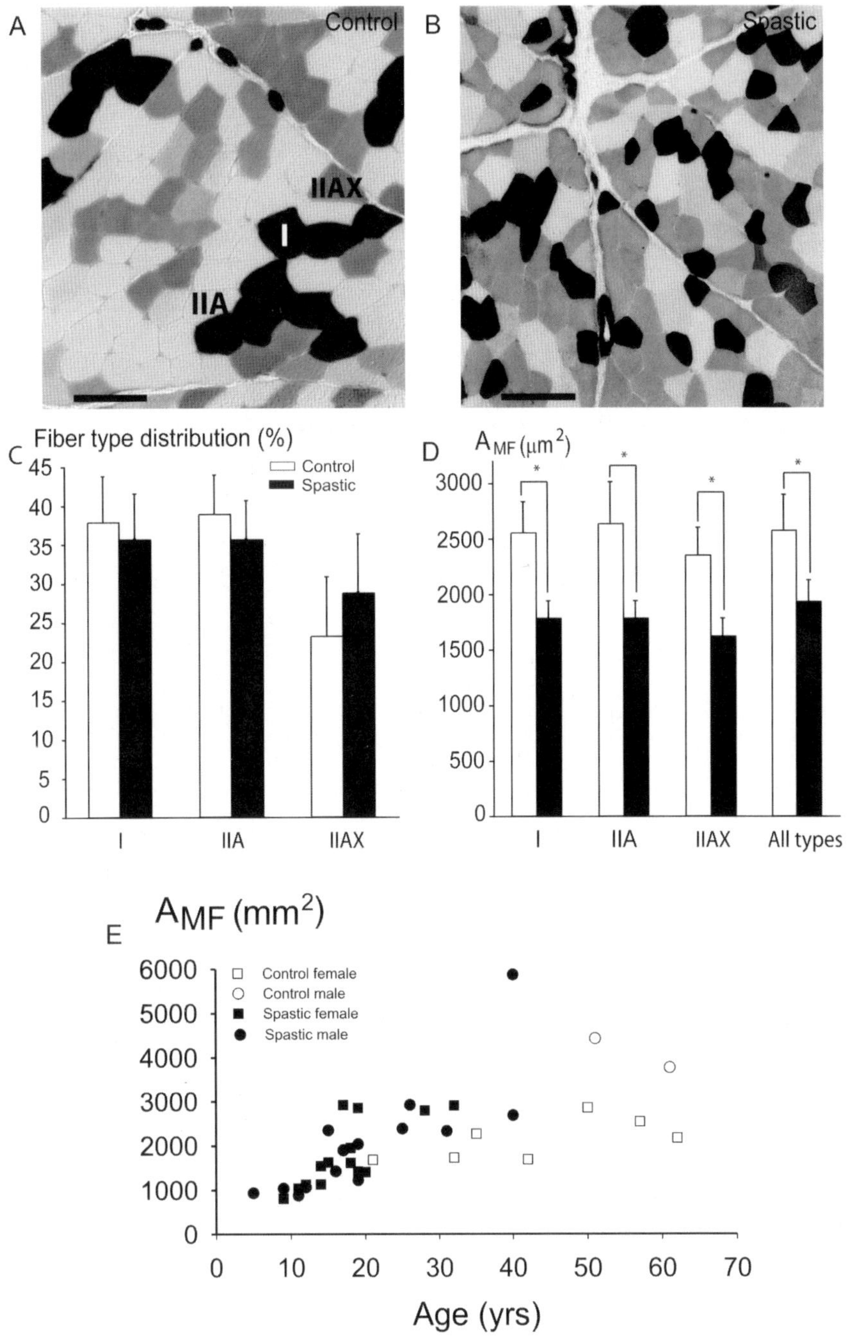

Figure 4. Myofibre typing and myofibre cross-sectional area within fascicles from spastic and control FCU. Typical examples of light micrographs of ATPase stained cross-section of biopsies from: (**A**) Control muscle, (**B**) Spastic muscle. Myofibre types I, IIA and IIAX are assigned; bars represent 100 μm. (**C**) Fibre type distribution within cross-sections from FCU. Fibre type distribution was not significantly different between CP (n = 26) and control (n = 10) samples. (**D**) For all fibre types, myofibre cross-sectional area (A_{MF}) in all spastic samples was significantly smaller than in controls. (**E**). Individual data for A_{MF} plotted as a function of age. For spastic muscle of all ages taken together, Spearman's Rank coefficient of correlation for A_{MF} and age was significant and moderately high. Note that A_{MF} of spastic patients ≥20 years was not significantly different from that of (adult) control muscles. Means and SEM are shown; * indicates significant difference between spastic and control FCU.

Comparison of tension of spastic myofibre segments as function of sarcomere length reported previously [20,23] with our present results indicates that our values of stiffness of spastic myofibre and fascicle segments are higher than those reported previously. An explanation for this difference may be found in age differences: the mean ages of CP patients of the studies cited (7.8 [20] and 9.3 years [23]) were smaller than those of our present CP group (tested for mechanical properties, mean age 20.5 years). Although mechanical variables and age are not correlated (present results), it is conceivable that spastic myofibre and fascicle segments of CP children earlier in their childhood (i.e. age <10 years) may be more compliant than those of adolescents and adults. As muscle myofibre passive stiffness is associated with titin isoform expression [42], we speculate that during childhood a longer (more

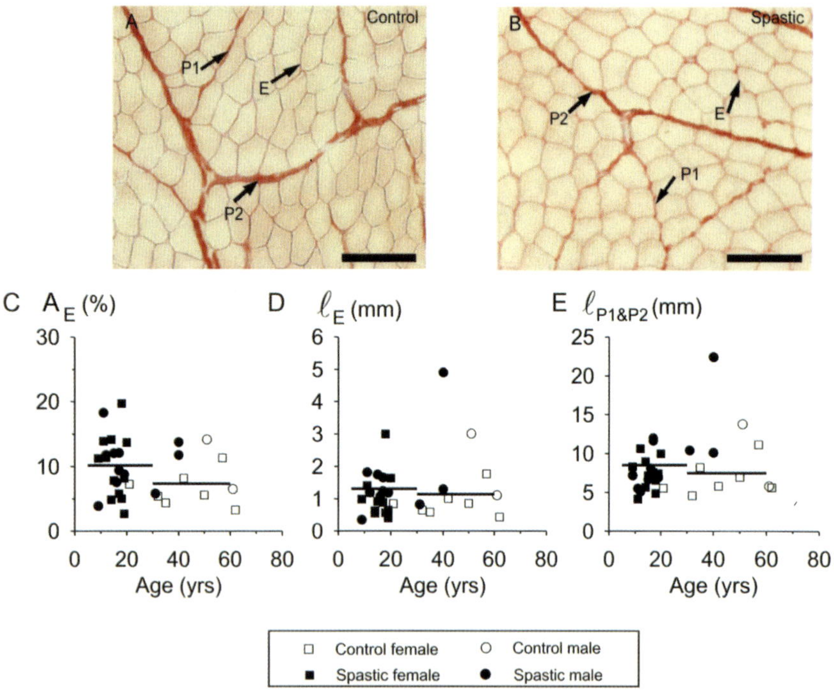

Figure 5. Variables of endomysium, primary and secondary perimysium in cross-sections of spastic muscle. Typical examples of light micrographs of Sirius Red stained cross-sections of FCU biopsies: (**A**) Sample of a 20-year old control subject. (**B**) Sample of an 18-year old CP subject. Bars represent 100 μm. (**C**) Individual data for cross-sectional area of endomysium within FCU plotted as a function of age. The mean (area) proportion taken up by endomysium (i.e. A_E expressed as % of total measured area) was not significantly different between cross-sections of CP (n = 23) and control subjects (n = 9). (**D**) Individual data for endomysium thickness (ℓ_E) within FCU plotted as a function of age. The mean thickness of endomysium per myofibre cross-section was not significantly different in CP and control subjects. (**E**) Individual data for primary and secondary perimysial thickness ($\ell_{P1\&P2}$) within FCU plotted as a function of age. Mean thickness of perimysium within cross-sections of spastic muscle were not different from those in control muscle. Horizontal lines indicate mean values.

compliant) titin isoform may be replaced by a shorter (and stiffer) isoform. However, such young age effects do not explain the low stiffness of single myofibre segments reported for controls as the mean ages of that group were 37.4 [20] and 27.5 years [23]. This suggests that other factors are likely to be involved in explaining the differences results.

Comparison of our methods with those of previous studies shows methodological differences, which may contribute to the contrasting results: (1) some of the studies were conducted on several muscles from different muscle groups in the forearm, upper arm, and shoulder [20,23] compared to only FCU biopsies in the present study. (2) Single myofibre and fascicle cross-sectional area analysis was previously based on the measurement of one diameter on the assumption of a circular shape [20,23], yielding in either an over- or underestimation of cross-sectional area. Assuming a circular myofibre cross-section may lead to a mean deviation of 20% of the actual area, whereas our present assumption of an elliptical cross-section limits this error to a mean deviation of 4% of the actual area [43]. (3) An acknowledged drawback [6] of previous studies concerns tangent calculations of length-tension curves based on two points that were not equidistant at all times [20,23]. In addition, sometimes points for tangent calculations were taken at sarcomere lengths up to 8.0 μm. This is likely to involve damage of the myofibre segment and/or fascicle segment [23]. In the present study we did not exceed 4.0 μm i.e. lengths which is far over the length of minimal thick and thin filament overlap (near 4.0 μm).

Myofibre size

Regarding effects of spasticity on cross-sectional area of spastic myofibres, the literature remains inconsistent. Compared to control myofibres, some studies report growth deficits of spastic myofibres [12,13,15,16,17], whereas others report hypertrophy [13]. Also, similar myofibre sizes in spastic and control muscle have been reported [18,44]. We found mean A_{MF} (data of all CP patients) to be significantly smaller in spastic muscle than in healthy muscle. In children, adolescents and young adults, A_{MF}, mainly of leg muscles, increases with age until approximately 20 years of age (cf. [13,33,34,36,37,45]). However, the fact that adult spastic and control muscles did not differ, indicates that there was no myofibre diameter growth deficit in adult spastic FCU. In any case, if there were a growth deficit within the CP group it disappears on reaching adulthood. Regarding myofibre growth of young CP children, our data does not allow us to exclude unequivocally such a growth deficit.

The coefficient of variance of A_{MF} has been claimed to be significantly higher in spastic muscle [17,19]. Our results do not confirm that conclusion. It has been shown that oxidative capacity of myofibres is inversely related to myofibre cross-sectional area [46,47]. Because no differences in myofibre type composition were found between spastic and control muscle, this variable does not likely affect our results regarding A_{MF}.

For pennate muscle, such as FCU, myofibre diameter is a major co-determinant of the muscle slack and optimum length [10,11] and as such the joint range of motion. Taken together, based on the above elaborations on myofibre size differences, we cannot

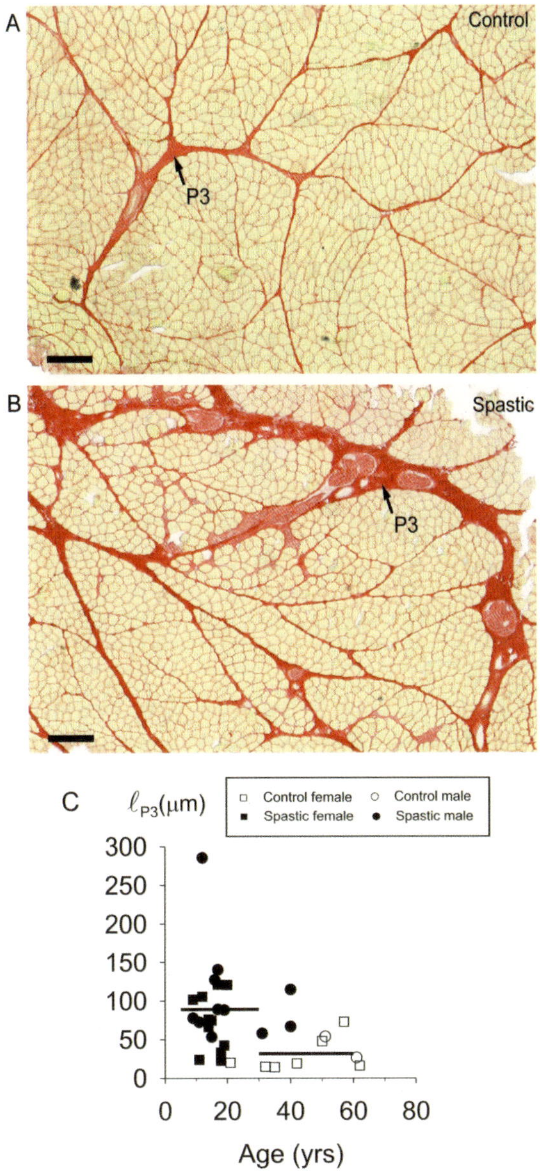

Figure 6. Increased thickness of tertiary perimysium within cross-sections of fascicles within spastic muscle. Typical examples of light micrographs of Sirius Red stained cross-sections of FCU biopsies: (**A**) control muscle. (**B**) Spastic muscle. Bars represent 250 μm. (**C**) Individual data of tertiary perimysium thickness within FCU biopsies plotted as function of age. Mean thickness of tertiary perimysium in FCU (indicated by horizontal lines) of spastic subjects (n = 23) was significantly higher than in FCU of control subjects (n = 9).

attribute the occurrence of postural changes of the wrist in CP to changes in myofibre diameter.

Myofibre typing

Skeletal muscle is well known to adapt to the quantity and type of neural activity [48]). Increase in muscular activity, for instance by means of exercise, may induce fast-to-slow transitions in myofibre types and expression of corresponding myosin isoforms [49]. Slow myofibre predominance has been reported in spastic muscle of the leg and arm [12,13,17,18], however no comparison to a control group was made in those studies. Within the spastic forearm, flexor muscles are reported to have higher proportions of fast myofibres compared to extensor muscles [15,19]. One of these authors later proposed that these results could best be explained by disuse [50]. In agreement with these results, the negative Spearman's Rank correlation found for myofibre type I percentage and age of our spastic FCU group indicates for this group that the fraction of type I fibres decreases with age. Therefore, spasticity may cause a myofibre type shift from slow to fast types, unless for controls similar effects would be present, in which case the effects should be ascribed to growth rather than as effects of spasticity. However, data on fibre type distributions in controls of similar age are required to draw any conclusions on this issue.

Connective tissue

Without actual quantification, it has been suggested, that intramuscular connective tissue may be increased in spastic muscle [6,12,13,21]. In addition, others reported that gene expression profiles of spastic muscle yields evidence for connective tissue remodelling [51] and the concentrations of connective tissue (not distinguishing endomysium, perimysium, and epimysium) in spastic vastus lateralis and semitendinosus muscles were reported to be increased [6,21]. However, these studies made no distinction with regard to connective tissue structures within muscle. As the perimysium constitutes a relatively big fraction of intramuscular connective tissues [52] it is also considered a major contributor to extracellular sources of passive resistance to stretching of muscle [53,54]. Hence, if contractures of spastic muscle would be caused by a change in intramuscular connective tissue content, the perimysium is likely an important factor in this. We distinguish the endomysium and three levels of perimysium.

In our biopsies, variables related to intramuscular connective tissue content (endomysium, as well as primary and secondary perimysium) did not differ between CP and control subjects, nor were they a function of age. Intramuscular connective tissue content in muscle of rodents much further along their life span than our subjects has been shown to be increased compared to that in young muscle [55,56]. However, effects of age on intramuscular connective tissue content within human muscle is not unequivocal [57,58,59]). These studies indicate that fibrosis occurs within very old human muscle and even may be physiological.

The lack of increase in endomysium, as well as primary and secondary perimysium within spastic muscle is in accordance with our finding that the slopes of the length-tension curves of control and spastic single myofibre segments, as well as of control and spastic fascicles segments were not different. Therefore, our results for FCU are different from those for spastic vastus lateralis and semitendinosus muscles, in which collagen content, as assessed by hydroxyproline content, was increased [6]. This suggests that secondary effects of spasticity may differ between muscles in the upper and lower extremities.

Tertiary perimysial structures constitute a connection between collagen fibre reinforcements of intra- and extramuscular elements of neural, venous, arterial and lymphatic tissues. In fact the tertiary perimysia are continuations of (extramuscular) branches of the main neurovascular tracts. Note that the tertiary perimysia, that arethickened in spastic FCU, do not envelop fascicles or groups of fascicles from their origin to insertion, but rather enter and cross the muscle transversely at certain levels. By selection, tertiary perimysia were absent in the fascicle segments used for mechanical measurements. Enhanced thickness and presumably stiffness of such tertiary perimysium will more likely affect muscle function via its extramuscular connections by myofascial force transmission, rather than affect the stiffness of an isolated FCU. In other words its connections are crucial for enhanced stiffness.

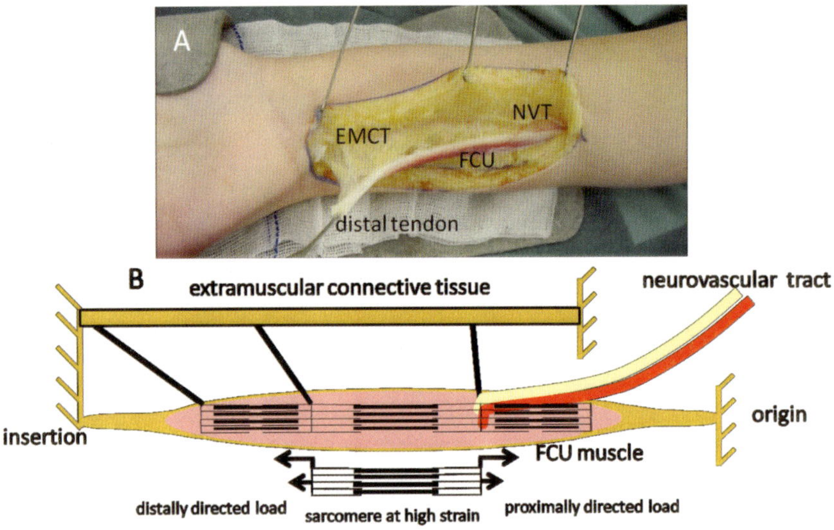

Figure 7. Neurovascular tract and simple schematics of connections. (**A**) Photograph of the tenotomised FCU and its myofascial connections to extramuscular connective tissue (EMCT) consisting of general fascia and neurovascular tracts (NVT). Note that, although not visible in the image, there are also connections to the epimysia of surrounding muscles (i.e. m. extensor carpi ulnaris and flexor digitorum superficialis/profundus). Via these connections, force can be transmitted between the stroma of FCU and extramuscular connective tissue such as general fascia, septa or NVT (i.e. epimuscular force transmission) and other muscles. This will cause loading in proximal as well as distal directions on a fraction of FCU. Distal loading of spastic FCU via myofascial connections has been shown after FCU tenotomy suggesting enhanced epimuscular loading (Movie S1) [64]. As branches of the NVTs generally enter the muscle from proximal directions, loading of the NVTs may chiefly yield proximally directed epimuscular loading of FCU. (**B**) Schematic diagram illustrating how concurrent proximal and distal epimuscular loads may cause high local sarcomere strains. Myofibres are represented by three sarcomeres in series, with myofascial connections to extramuscular connective tissues.

Thickening and presumed stiffening of the tertiary perimysium as apparent in a majority of our CP subjects, suggests that, in spastic muscle, these structures are loaded relatively more than in controls. Such increased loading occurs by enhanced force transmission (further referred to as epimuscular force transmission) from the muscular stroma to structures other than the muscle's origin or insertion tendons [11]. Epimuscular force transmission may occur from the intramuscular stroma onto the epimysium of synergistic muscles or extramuscular neurovascular tracts, as well as onto other structures such as septa, general fascia, interosseal membrane and periost. Epimuscular loads exerted on a muscle can have distal or proximal directions [60,61,62]. In CP patients, the presence of enhanced distal loads on FCU seems evident from the observations that after distal FCU tenotomy the muscle is kept at length and that subsequently extending the wrist stretches both passive (Movie S1) and active FCU muscle [63,64]. These distal loads applied to FCU are exerted via extramuscular connective tissue structures (Fig. 7). Branches of the neurovascular tracts that are embedded in these structures generally enter the muscle from proximal directions. If neurovascular tracts are thicker, such loading will chiefly yield in proximal epimuscular loads on FCU. Myofascial force transmission via such tracts has also been shown to be effective in rodents [61]. If the extramuscular connective tissue is stiffer in spastic patients, extending the wrist will cause simultaneous proximally and distally directed epimuscular loads to be exerted on FCU.

A very special effect of oppositely directed myofascial loads on FCU is that force can be transmitted locally through the muscle without being exerted at its origin and insertion [22]. Because of this condition, it is feasible that a very small fraction of the sarcomeres arranged in series within FCU myofibres is kept at high length, whereas simultaneously the remainder of the sarcomeres within those fibres are at low lengths (Fig. 7) [22]. Note that in spastic patients, it is conceivable that such specific local conditions have sizable effects on joints involved without being very apparent in muscular morphology.

The following conclusions are drawn. No significant differences between control and spastic muscle were found regarding slope of the passive length-tension curves of myofibre segments, cross-section or myofibre type proportions. The altered connective tissue composition of FCU, secondary to spasticity, is manifest exclusively by thickening of its tertiary perimysium in a majority of our CP subjects. This is in contrast to assumptions that spasticity may cause thickening of all of the muscular connective tissue stroma. There are indications that tertiary perimysial tracts in mechanical interaction with extramuscular connective tissues surrounding FCU may play a role in the aetiology of the typical CP wrist joint postures. The substantial individual variation, however, also indicates that this may not be the exclusive mechanism contributing to these wrist postures.

Supporting Information

Movie S1 Passive excursion of the FCU of a child with cerebral palsy after tenotomy of the distal tendon. The movie shows a cut distal tendon of FCU in a patient undergoing a tendon transfer surgery. Note that, after distal tenotomy, the muscle is prevented from shortening. As the wrist is moved alternately into full extension and flexion, FCU lengthens and shortens, respectively. The distally directed loads exerted on FCU have to be transmitted via extramuscular connective tissue (i.e. shared epimysia of neighbouring muscles, and/or general fascia and septa), whereas the proximally oriented loads are likely to be exerted onto FCU via neurovascular tracts.

Acknowledgments

We acknowledge Guus Baan for his contributions to developing the experimental set-up.

Author Contributions

Conceived and designed the experiments: MdB MJS MK PAH RTJ. Performed the experiments: MdB MJS RTJ. Analyzed the data: MdB MJS PAH RTJ. Contributed reagents/materials/analysis tools: MdB PAH RTJ. Wrote the paper: MdB MJS MK PAH RTJ.

References

1. Hoffer MM (1993) The use of the pathokinesiology laboratory to select muscles for tendon transfers in the cerebral palsy hand. Clin Orthop Relat Res 288: 135–138.
2. Fry NR, Childs CR, Eve LC, Gough M, Robinson RO, et al. (2003) Accurate measurement of muscle belly length in the motion analysis laboratory: potential for the assessment of contracture. Gait Posture 17: 119–124.
3. Barber L, Hastings-Ison T, Baker R, Barrett R, Lichtwark G (2011) Medial gastrocnemius muscle volume and fascicle length in children aged 2 to 5 years with cerebral palsy. Dev Med Child Neurol 53: 543–548.
4. Benard MR, Jaspers RT, Huijing PA, Becher JG, Harlaar J (2010) Reproducibility of hand-held ankle dynamometry to measure altered ankle moment-angle characteristics in children with spastic cerebral palsy. Clin Biomech (Bristol, Avon) 25: 802–808.
5. Sinkjaer T, Magnussen I (1994) Passive, intrinsic and reflex-mediated stiffness in the ankle extensors of hemiparetic patients. Brain 117: 355–363.
6. Smith LR, Lee KS, Ward SR, Chambers HG, Lieber RL (2011) Hamstring contractures in children with spastic cerebral palsy result from a stiffer extracellular matrix and increased in vivo sarcomere length. J Physiol 589: 2625–2639.
7. Tardieu C, Tabary JC, Gagnard L, Lombard M, Tabary C, et al. (1974) Change in the number of sarcomeres and in isometric tetanic tension after immobilization of the cat anterior tibialis muscle at different lengths. J Physiol (Paris) 68: 205–218.
8. Williams PE, Goldspink G (1978) Changes in sarcomere length and physiological properties in immobilized muscle. J Anat 127: 459–468.
9. Tardieu C, Tardieu G, Colbeau-Justin P, Huet de la Tour E, Lespargot A (1979) Trophic muscle regulation in children with congenital cerebral lesions. J Neurol Sci 42: 357–364.
10. Heslinga JW, te Kronnie G, Huijing PA (1995) Growth and immobilization effects on sarcomeres: a comparison between gastrocnemius and soleus muscles of the adult rat. Eur J Appl Physiol Occup Physiol 70: 49–57.
11. Huijing PA, Jaspers RT (2005) Adaptation of muscle size and myofascial force transmission: a review and some new experimental results. Scand J Med Sci Sports 15: 349–380.
12. Ito J, Araki A, Tanaka H, Tasaki T, Cho K, et al. (1996) Muscle histopathology in spastic cerebral palsy. Brain Dev 18: 299–303.
13. Castle ME, Reyman TA, Schneider M (1979) Pathology of spastic muscle in cerebral palsy. Clin Orthop Relat Res 142: 223–232.
14. Lieber RL, Steinman S, Barash IA, Chambers H (2004) Structural and functional changes in spastic skeletal muscle. Muscle Nerve 29: 615–627.
15. Ponten E, Friden J, Thornell LE, Lieber RL (2005) Spastic wrist flexors are more severely affected than wrist extensors in children with cerebral palsy. Dev Med Child Neurol 47: 384–389.
16. Romanini L, Villani C, Meloni C, Calvisi V (1989) Histological and morphological aspects of muscle in infantile cerebral palsy. Ital J Orthop Traumatol 15: 87–93.
17. Rose J, Haskell WL, Gamble JG, Hamilton RL, Brown DA, et al. (1994) Muscle pathology and clinical measures of disability in children with cerebral palsy. J Orthop Res 12: 758–768.
18. Marbini A, Ferrari A, Cioni G, Bellanova MF, Fusco C, et al. (2002) Immunohistochemical study of muscle biopsy in children with cerebral palsy. Brain Dev 24: 63–66.
19. Ponten E, Gantelius S, Lieber RL (2007) Intraoperative muscle measurements reveal a relationship between contracture formation and muscle remodeling. Muscle Nerve 36: 47–54.
20. Friden J, Lieber RL (2003) Spastic muscle cells are shorter and stiffer than normal cells. Muscle Nerve 27: 157–164.
21. Booth CM, Cortina-Borja MJ, Theologis TN (2001) Collagen accumulation in muscles of children with cerebral palsy and correlation with severity of spasticity. Dev Med Child Neurol 43: 314–320.
22. Huijing PA (2007) Epimuscular myofascial force transmission between antagonistic and synergistic muscles can explain movement limitation in spastic paresis. J Electromyogr Kinesiol 17: 708–724.
23. Lieber RL, Runesson E, Einarsson F, Friden J (2003) Inferior mechanical properties of spastic muscle bundles due to hypertrophic but compromised extracellular matrix material. Muscle Nerve 28: 464–471.
24. Zancolli EA, Ziadenberg C, Zancolli E Jr. (1987) Biomechanics of the trapeziometacarpal joint. Clin Orthop Relat Res 220: 14–26.
25. Gollapudi SK, Lin DC (2009) Experimental determination of sarcomere force-length relationship in type-I human skeletal muscle fibers. J Biomech 42: 2011–2016.
26. Lieber RL, Ljung BO, Friden J (1997) Intraoperative sarcomere length measurements reveal differential design of human wrist extensor muscles. J Exp Biol 200: 19–25.
27. Jaspers RT, Feenstra HM, van Beek-Harmsen BJ, Huijing PA, van der Laarse WJ (2006) Differential effects of muscle fibre length and insulin on muscle-specific mRNA content in isolated mature muscle fibres during long-term culture. Cell Tissue Res 326: 795–808.
28. Brooke MH, Kaiser KK (1970) Muscle fiber types: how many and what kind? Arch Neurol 23: 369–379.
29. Schiaffino S (2010) Fibre types in skeletal muscle: a personal account. Acta Physiol (Oxf) 199: 451–463.
30. Junqueira LC, Junqueira LC, Brentani RR (1979) A simple and sensitive method for the quantitative estimation of collagen. Anal Biochem 94: 96–99.
31. Marshall PA, Williams PE, Goldspink G (1989) Accumulation of collagen and altered fiber-type ratios as indicators of abnormal muscle gene expression in the mdx dystrophic mouse. Muscle Nerve 12: 528–537.
32. Nishimura T, Fang S, Wakamatsu J, Takahashi K (2009) Relationships between physical and structural properties of intramuscular connective tissue and toughness of raw pork. Anim Sci J 80: 85–90.
33. Lexell J, Taylor CC (1991) Variability in muscle fibre areas in whole human quadriceps muscle: effects of increasing age. J Anat 174: 239–249.
34. Oertel G (1988) Morphometric analysis of normal skeletal muscles in infancy, childhood and adolescence. An autopsy study. J Neurol Sci 88: 303–313.
35. Aherne W, Ayyar DR, Clarke PA, Walton JN (1971) Muscle fibre size in normal infants, children and adolescents. An autopsy study. J Neurol Sci 14: 171–182.
36. Lexell J, Taylor CC, Sjostrom M (1988) What is the cause of the ageing atrophy? Total number, size and proportion of different fiber types studied in whole vastus lateralis muscle from 15- to 83-year-old men. J Neurol Sci 84: 275–294.
37. Vogler C, Bove KE (1985) Morphology of skeletal muscle in children. Arch Pathol Lab Med 109: 238–242.
38. Smeulders MJ, Kreulen M, Hage JJ, Huijing PA, van der Horst CM (2004) Overstretching of sarcomeres may not cause cerebral palsy muscle contracture. J Orthop Res 22: 1331–1335.
39. Lieber RL, Friden J (1997) Intraoperative measurement and biomechanical modeling of the flexor carpi ulnaris-to-extensor carpi radialis longus tendon transfer. J Biomech Eng 119: 386–391.
40. Burkholder TJ (2001) Age does not influence muscle fiber length adaptation to increased excursion. J Appl Physiol 91: 2466–2470.
41. Ranatunga KW (1996) Endothermic force generation in fast and slow mammalian (rabbit) muscle fibers. Biophys J 71: 1905–1913.
42. Prado LG, Makarenko I, Andresen C, Krüge rM, Opitz CA, et al. (2005) Isoform diversity of giant proteins in relation to passive and active contractile properties of rabbit skeletal muscles. J Gen Physiol 126: 461–480.
43. Blinks JR (1965) Influence of osmotic strenght on cross-section and volume of isolated single muscle fibres. J Physiol (Lond) 177: 42–57.
44. Ponten EM, Stal PS (2007) Decreased capillarization and a shift to fast myosin heavy chain IIx in the biceps brachii muscle from young adults with spastic paresis. J Neurol Sci 253: 25–33.
45. Aherne W, Ayyar DR, Clarke PA, Walton JN (1971) Muscle fibre size in normal infants, children and adolescents. An autopsy study. J Neurol Sci 14: 171–182.
46. van Wessel T, de Haan A, van der Laarse WJ, Jaspers RT (2010) The muscle fiber type-fiber size paradox: hypertrophy or oxidative metabolism? Eur J Appl Physiol 110: 665–694.
47. Rivero JL, Talmadge RJ, Edgerton VR (1998) Fibre size and metabolic properties of myosin heavy chain-based fibre types in rat skeletal muscle. J Muscle Res Cell Motil 19: 733–742.
48. Pette D, Vrbova G (1999) What does chronic electrical stimulation teach us about muscle plasticity? Muscle Nerve 22: 666–677.
49. Pette D, Staron RS (2001) Transitions of muscle fiber phenotypic profiles. Histochem Cell Biol 115: 359–372.
50. Lieber RL (1986) Skeletal muscle adaptability. III: Muscle properties following chronic electrical stimulation. Dev Med Child Neurol 28: 662–670.
51. Smith LR, Ponten E, Hedstrom Y, Ward SR, Chambers HG, et al. (2009) Novel transcriptional profile in wrist muscles from cerebral palsy patients. BMC Med Genomics 2: 44.
52. Purslow PP (1989) Strain-induced reorientation of an intramuscular connective tissue network: implications for passive muscle elasticity. J Biomech 22: 21–31.
53. Rowe RW (1981) Morphology of perimysial and endomysial connective tissue in skeletal muscle. Tissue Cell 13: 681–690.
54. Borg TK, Caulfield JB (1980) Morphology of connective tissue in skeletal muscle. Tissue Cell 12: 197–207.
55. Ramaswamy KS, Palmer ML, van der Meulen JH, Renoux A, Kostrominova TY, et al. (2011) Lateral transmission of force is impaired in skeletal muscles of dystrophic mice and very old rats. J Physiol 589: 1195–1208.
56. Alnaqeeb MA, Al Zaid NS, Goldspink G (1984) Connective tissue changes and physical properties of developing and ageing skeletal muscle. J Anat 139: 677–689.

57. Overend TJ, Cunningham DA, Paterson DH, Lefcoe MS (1992) Thigh composition in young and elderly men determined by computed tomograpy. Clin Physiol 12: 629–640.
58. Rice C, L, Cunningham DA, Paterson DH, Lefcoe MS (1989) Arm and leg composition determined by computed tomography in young and elderly men. Clin Physiol 9: 207–220.
59. Haus JM, Carrithers JA, Trappe SW, Trappe TA (2007) Collagen, cross-linking, and advanced glycation end products in aging human skeletal muscle. J Appl Physiol 103: 2068–2076.
60. Huijing PA, Maas H, Baan GC (2003) Compartmental fasciotomy and isolating a muscle from neighboring muscles interfere with myofascial force transmission within the rat anterior crural compartment. J Morphol 256: 306–321.
61. Maas H, Meijer HJ, Huijing PA (2005) Intermuscular interaction between synergists in rat originates from both intermuscular and extramuscular myofascial force transmission. Cells Tissues Organs 181: 38–50.
62. Meijer HJ, Rijkelijkhuizen JM, Huijing PA (2007) Myofascial force transmission between antagonistic rat lower limb muscles: effects of single muscle or muscle group lengthening. J Electromyogr Kinesiol 17: 698–707.
63. de Bruin M, Smeulders MJ, Kreulen M (2011) Flexor carpi ulnaris tenotomy alone does not eliminate its contribution to wrist torque. Clin Biomech (Bristol, Avon) 26: 725–728.
64. Smeulders MJ, Kreulen M, Hage JJ, Huijing PA, van der Horst CM (2005) Spastic muscle properties are affected by length changes of adjacent structures. Muscle Nerve 32: 208–215.

23

Unaccustomed Eccentric Contractions Impair Plasma K^+ Regulation in the Absence of Changes in Muscle Na^+,K^+-ATPase Content

Craig A. Goodman[1,2], Jason A. Bennie[1], Murray J. Leikis[1,3], Michael J. McKenna[1]*

1 Institute of Sport, Exercise and Active Living (ISEAL), Muscle, Ions and Exercise Group, Victoria University, Melbourne, Victoria, Australia, **2** Department of Comparative Biosciences, School of Veterinary Medicine, University of Wisconsin-Madison, Madison, Wisconsin, United States of America, **3** Department of Nephrology, Royal Melbourne Hospital, Department of Medicine, University of Melbourne, Melbourne, Victoria, Australia

Abstract

The Na^+,K^+-ATPase (NKA) plays a fundamental role in the regulation of skeletal muscle membrane Na^+ and K^+ gradients, excitability and fatigue during repeated intense contractions. Many studies have investigated the effects of acute concentric exercise on K^+ regulation and skeletal muscle NKA, but almost nothing is known about the effects of repeated eccentric contractions. We therefore investigated the effects of unaccustomed maximal eccentric knee extensor contractions on K^+ regulation during exercise, peak knee extensor muscle torque, and vastus lateralis muscle NKA content and 3-O-MFPase activity. Torque measurements, muscle biopsies, and venous blood samples were taken before, during and up to 7 days following the contractions in six healthy adults. Eccentric contractions reduced peak isometric muscle torque immediately post-exercise by 26±11% and serum creatine kinase concentration peaked 24 h post-exercise at 339±90 IU/L. During eccentric contractions, plasma [K^+] rose during Set 1 and remained elevated at ~4.9 mM during sets 4–10; this was despite a decline in work output by Set 4, which fell by 18.9% at set 10. The rise in plasma [K^+].work^{-1} ratio was elevated over Set 2 from Set 4– Set 10. Eccentric contractions had no effect on muscle NKA content or maximal in-vitro 3-O-MFPase activity immediately post- or up to 7 d post-exercise. The sustained elevation in plasma [K^+] despite a decrease in work performed by the knee extensor muscles suggests an impairment in K^+ regulation during maximal eccentric contractions, possibly due to increased plasma membrane permeability or to excitation-contraction uncoupling.

Editor: Luis Eduardo M. Quintas, Universidade Federal do Rio de Janeiro, Brazil

Funding: The authors have no support or funding to report.

* Email: michael.mckenna@vu.edu.au

Introduction

The Na^+,K^+-ATPase (NKA) plays a fundamental role in skeletal muscle contractility via the regulation of skeletal muscle membrane excitability (for review see [1,2]). The NKA actively counteracts the action potential-induced passive influx of Na^+ into, and efflux of K^+ from, the muscle fiber [1,3]. An inability to maintain the steep Na^+ and K^+ concentration gradients across the sarcolemmal and transverse tubular membranes during repeated intense contractions may lead to membrane depolarization and the loss of muscle force generation, referred to as fatigue [2,4,5]. The NKA thus acts in concert with other mechanisms that include a decline in membrane Cl^- conductance and intracellular acidosis, to preserve muscle membrane excitability during intense contractions [2,5,6].

To date, the majority of studies that have investigated the effects of acute exercise on K^+ regulation have utilized experimental models that involve predominantly concentric muscle contractions, such as sprint or endurance cycling, and isolated knee extension exercise [7–11]. These studies have consistently shown a net release of K^+ from contracting skeletal muscle, indicating an inability of the NKA to fully counteract the excitation-induced loss of K^+ from the muscle *in-vivo* [5]. For example, during sub-maximal cycling exercise, venous and arterial plasma [K^+] have been reported to be between 5.5–7.0 mM [12], and can exceed 8 mM during brief, high intensity treadmill exercise [13]. Micro-dialysis studies have reported muscle interstitial [K^+] of 11–13 mM during intense concentric knee extension contractions [9,10,14–16]. In sharp contrast to these studies utilising repeated concentric contractions, almost nothing is known about K^+ regulation during or after repeated intense eccentric muscle contractions.

During intense concentric exercise, a relationship exists between work output and plasma [K^+], as seen during intermittent cycling exercise, where a reduction in work output was associated with a concomitant reduction in plasma [K^+] [17,18]. Unaccustomed eccentric, or lengthening, contractions, which are associated with increased sarcolemma and/or t-tubular membrane permeability [19,20] have the potential to alter this relationship such that during intermittent eccentric exercise, plasma [K^+] may increase or remain elevated despite a reduction in work output. Furthermore, acute eccentric exercise has previously been shown to reduce the abundance of important membrane transport proteins such as GLUT-4 [21,22] and the lactate/H^+ transporter [23]. The NKA is located in the sarcolemmal and T-tubular membranes, in association with the cytoskeleton proteins β-spectrin and ankyrin 3

[24]. Thus, there is the possibility that intense eccentric contractions may also adversely affect the abundance and/or activity of the NKA, which, in combination with increased membrane permeability, could adversely affect K^+ regulation during exercise. To date, however, no studies have examined the effect of unaccustomed intense eccentric contractions on plasma $[K^+]$ regulation during exercise and on NKA content.

Therefore, this study investigated the effects of repeated sets of unaccustomed maximal eccentric contractions on K^+ regulation during exercise, muscle force production and the content of the membrane ion transporter NKA in skeletal muscle of untrained individuals for up to 7 days after exercise. We utilised a bout of unaccustomed maximal eccentric contractions that would induce muscle damage, as indicated by a post-exercise increase in plasma creatine kinase (CK) activity, and cause a prolonged reduction in peak muscle torque production that would each recover by 7 d post-contractions. We tested two hypotheses. Firstly that there would be a progressive increase in plasma $[K^+]$ during repeated eccentric contractions which, together with a fall in work output, would lead to an increase in the rise in plasma $[K^+]$/total work ratio ($\Delta[K^+].work^{-1}$). Secondly, we hypothesized that repeated damaging eccentric contractions would induce a reduction in the NKA content after the eccentric contractions.

Materials and Methods

Ethics Statement

Six healthy, recreationally active subjects (3 M and 3 F; age, 26.3±8.1 yr; body mass, 76.3±14.9 kg; height 173.7±17 cm; Means ± SD) volunteered for the study after being informed of all risks and giving written informed consent. Ethical approval was obtained from the Victoria University Human Research Ethics Committee (application HREC 04/44; HRETH 021/04). All subjects were physically active, however, none were currently, nor had in the last 6 months, participated in resistance training.

Overview of Exercise Trials

Subjects attended the laboratory for a total of six testing sessions. These comprised a familiarization trial; two trials to determine variability of muscle strength; the eccentric exercise trial and follow up tests at 1 d and 7 d post-eccentric exercise. All quadriceps muscle function tests were performed using an isokinetic dynamometer (Cybex Norm 770, Henley Health Care,

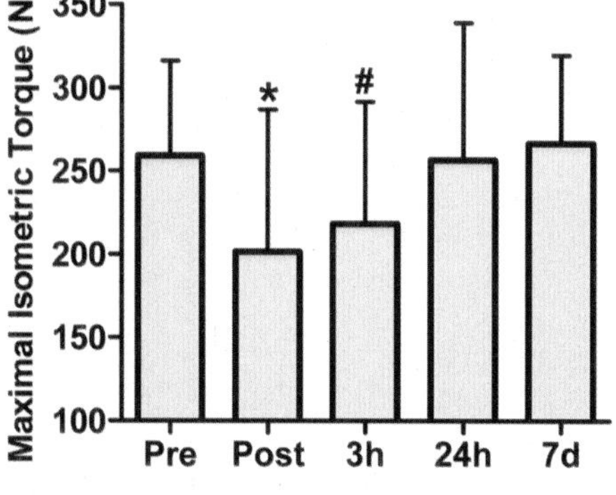

Figure 1. The effect of maximal eccentric knee extensor contractions on maximal knee extensor isometric torque. Measurements were taken before (Pre), immediately after (Post), and 3 h, 24 h, and 7 days following the eccentric contractions. Values are means ± SD; $n = 6$. *$P<0.05$– significantly different from Pre.

Massachusetts, U.S.A). During the course of this study subjects were instructed to avoid involvement in any strenuous exercise activities.

Familiarization and Variability Trials for Maximal Isometric Torque

During the first testing session, subjects were familiarized with the isokinetic dynamometer for testing maximal knee extensor isometric torque and for performing repeated maximal isokinetic contractions. During the next two testing sessions, subjects performed a test of maximal isometric peak torque of the knee extensors. These repeated tests were used to determine the subject's variability in isometric peak torque.

Experimental Trials

At least 2 days after the last maximal isometric torque variability trial, subjects returned to the laboratory to perform repeated sets of maximal eccentric knee extensor exercise, designed to induce localised muscle fatigue and muscle damage. Quadriceps muscle function was assessed by performing maximal isometric knee extensor contractions before and immediately after the eccentric exercise bout. Venous blood samples were taken to determine exercise-induced changes in plasma $[K^+]$ and creatine kinase (CK), while muscle biopsies were also obtained pre- and immediately-post exercise to determine exercise-induced changes in muscle NKA content and 3-O-MFPase activity as a marker of NKA activity in resting muscle. Subjects returned to the laboratory at 24 h and at 7 d after the eccentric exercise bout for an additional maximal isometric torque test, blood sample and muscle biopsy.

Maximal Isometric Knee Extensor Torque Test

Maximal isometric knee extensor torque was determined using an isokinetic dynamometer. Each test comprised three 5 s maximal isometric contractions at a knee joint angle of 45°, with a 30 s recovery between contractions. A visual real-time display of the isometric torque generated during each contraction was provided to each subject during the test and strong verbal encouragement was also provided to encourage the subject to exert maximal force throughout contractions. To evaluate the eccentric exercise-induced loss of muscle strength, maximal isometric peak torque of knee extensors was assessed pre- and immediately-post eccentric exercise, and at 3 h, 24 h and 7 d post-eccentric exercise.

Maximal Eccentric Contractions

The eccentric exercise bout was also performed on the same isokinetic dynamometer and comprised 300 maximal eccentric contractions (10 sets of 30 repetitions), at a velocity of 30°/s, with a 1 min rest interval between sets. This protocol was chosen because previous studies have shown that this number of eccentric contractions induces a significant post-exercise force deficit and increase in muscle membrane permeability as indicated by an increased plasma [CK] [25–27]. A visual real-time display of the torque and work for each contraction was provided to each subject during the bouts and strong verbal encouragement was also provided to encourage the subject to exert maximal force throughout all eccentric contractions.

Muscle Biopsies

A total of five muscle biopsies were taken from the middle third of the vastus lateralis muscle of each subject, at pre-, immediately-post, 3 h, 24 h and 7 d post- eccentric exercise. After injection of a

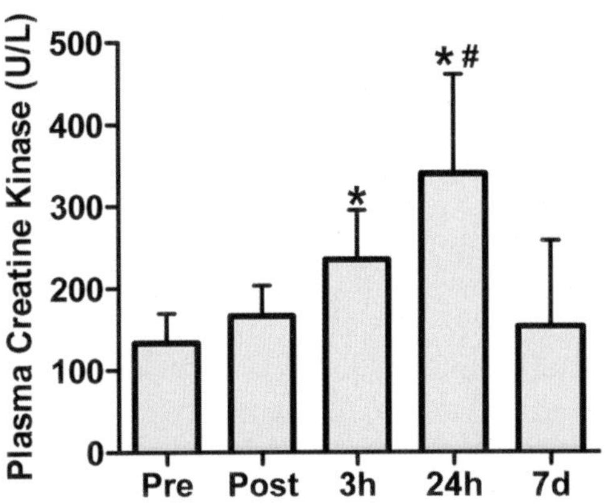

Figure 2. The effect of maximal eccentric knee extensor contractions on plasma creatine kinase (CK) activity. Measurements were taken before (Pre), immediately after (Post), and 3 h, 24 h, and 7 days following the eccentric contractions. Values are means ± SD; $n = 6$. $^{*}P<0.05$– significantly different from Pre, Post and 7 d. # $P<0.05$– significantly different from all other time points.

local anaesthetic into the skin and fascia (1% lidocaine (Xylocaine)), a small incision was made and a muscle sample taken (~120 mg) using a Stille biopsy needle, with suction applied to the needle via a 50 ml syringe. Each biopsy was taken by the same experienced medical practitioner from separate incisions, at a constant depth. Samples were immediately blotted on filter paper and then frozen in liquid N_2 until assayed later for NKA content and 3-O-MFPase activity [28].

Blood Sampling and Processing

Prior to the eccentric knee extension bout, a teflon catheter (20G, Jelco) was inserted into a dorsal hand vein for arterialised venous blood sampling, as previously described [17]. Subjects were seated on the isokinetic dynamometer 15 min before the first pre-exercise arterialized venous blood was taken. Further blood samples were taken whilst seated during the last 5 repetitions of Sets 1, 2, 4, 8 and 10 of eccentric exercise. Blood samples were analysed in triplicate measurements for plasma K^+ concentration ($[K^+]$) using an automated analyser (Ciba Corning 865, Bayer). Serum CK concentration ([CK]) was determined in arterialized venous blood sampled pre- and immediately-post eccentric exercise, and from an antecubital vein at 3 h, 24 h, and 7 d. Each sample was placed into a plain evacuated test tube, and blood allowed to coagulate for 30 min at room temperature and then centrifuged at 1,500 *g* for 10 min. The serum was removed and frozen at −20°C until analyzed in duplicate for [CK] using an Olympus GmbH AU1000 analyzer (Olympus Diagnostics, Clare). The normal reference range of [CK] using this method is 45–130 U/L.

Muscle Na^+, K^+-ATPase content

Approximately 20 mg of frozen muscle was used to determine the NKA content using the vanadate–facilitated [^{3}H]-ouabain method [29,30]. Each sample was cut into small pieces of 2–4 mg wet weight. Samples were washed at 0°C for 20 min (2×10 min) in a vanadate buffer (10 mM Tris-HCl, 250 mM sucrose, 3 mM $MgSO_4$ and 1 mM vanadate, pH 7.3). Muscle samples were then incubated for 2 h at 37°C in vanadate buffer with the addition of [^{3}H]-ouabain (10^{-6} M, 2.0 μCi mL^{-1}; Amersham Pharmacia Biotech, Castle Hill, NSW, Australia). We have previously shown that ^{3}H-ouabain binding reaches saturation after 2 h of incubation in cut sections of both control and stimulated rodent skeletal muscle that are significantly larger than the pieces muscle analysed in this study [31]. Following incubation, the muscle samples were washed for 4×30 min in ice-cold vanadate buffer to remove any unbound [^{3}H]-ouabain, blotted on filter paper and weighed before being soaked overnight in vials containing 500 μL 5% trichloroacetic acid and 0.1 mM ouabain. After approx. 20 h of soaking, 2.5 mL of scintillation cocktail (Opti-Fluor, Packard, Perkin Elmer, Boston, MA, USA) was added prior to liquid scintillation counting of [^{3}H] activity. The content of [^{3}H]-ouabain binding sites was calculated on the basis of the sample wet weight and the specific activity of the incubation medium and samples, and was expressed as pmol.g^{-1} wet wt.

Muscle 3-*O*-MFPase activity assay

The K^+-stimulated 3-*O*-methylfluorescein phosphatase (3-*O*-MFPase) activity assay was determined as a marker of the maximal muscle NKA activity, as previously used in human skeletal muscle in our laboratory [8,32]. This method has recently been criticised as being an inadequate measure of NKA activity during exercise, when intracellular sodium concentration is expected to be elevated and which activates the NKA [33]. Although the method is Na^+-insensitive, it remains valid as a marker of NKA activity in resting muscle, when intracellular Na^+ is not raised. Further, we and others have shown that the assay can be completely inhibited by ouabain, and is therefore selective for the NKA [32], and that the 3-*O*-MFPase activity is highly correlated with the [^{3}H]-ouabain binding site content [28]. Before analysis, muscle homogenates were freeze–thawed 4 times and then diluted 1/5 in cold homogenate buffer. The 3-*O*-MFPase activity was measured in an assay medium containing 5 mM $MgCl_2$, 1.25 mM EDTA, 100 mM Tris and an 80 nM 3-*O*-methyl fluorescein standard at pH 7.40. A 30 *μl* homogenate was incubated in 2.5 ml of assay medium at 37°C for 5 min before addition of 40 *μl* of 10 mM 3-*O*-MFP to initiate the reaction. After 60 s, 10 *μl* of 2.58 M KCl was added to stimulate K^+-dependent phosphatase activity and the reaction was measured for a further 60 s. All assays were performed at 37°C, using continuous stirring, with data sampled at 1 Hz on a spectrofluorimeter (Aminco Bowman AB2 SLM, Thermospectronic, Madison, WI, USA). Excitation wavelength was 475 nm and emission wavelength 515 nm, with 4 nm slit widths. The 3-*O*-MFPase activity was calculated from the slope after addition of 10 *μm* KCl minus the slope prior to KCl addition. Measurements of 3-*O*-MFPase activity data are expressed as nmol per gram wet weight.

Statistical Analysis

Data were analysed with a one-way repeated measures ANOVA, and the Newman-Keul's Multiple Comparison post-hoc test. The agreement between the two variability trials was assessed using an intra-class correlation coefficient (ICC). Significance was accepted at $p<0.05$. All data was reported as mean ± SD.

Results

Maximal Isometric Torque

The maximal knee extensor isometric torque did not differ between variability trials 1 and 2 being 262±68 and 267±60 Nm, respectively. An intraclass correlation co-efficient (ICC) of 0.96 was found for peak torque for the two variability trials. The eccentric exercise bout depressed maximal isometric torque by 26±11% immediately post-exercise ($P<0.05$, Figure 1) and, although not statistically significant, remain depressed (19±17%)

at 3 h post-exercise before returning to pre-exercise values by 24 h and at 7 d.

Plasma [CK]

By 3 h post-exercise, plasma [CK] was higher than Pre, Post, and 7 d post-exercise time points (P<0.05; Figure 2), and by 24 h, plasma [CK] was higher than all other time points (P<0.05). Plasma [CK] had returned to resting levels by 7 d.

Eccentric Work and Plasma [K$^+$]

The work completed during the 10 sets of 30 repetitions of maximal eccentric exercise totalled 32,738±267 J. There were no differences in the cumulative work performed during Sets 1 to 5; however, the cumulative work performed during each of Sets 6, 7, 8, 9 and 10 was depressed by 14.6, 18.0, 16.1, 20.8 and 18.9% compared to Set 1, respectively (P<0.05, Figure 3A). Plasma [K$^+$] was elevated above rest during the final contractions of Set 1 of eccentric exercise to ~4.8 mM (P<0.05), and remained elevated during the final contractions of Sets 2, 4, 6, 8 and 10 at ~4.9 mM (P<0.05, Figure 3B). The calculated rise in plasma [K$^+$]/work ratio (Δ[K$^+$].work^{-1}) during eccentric exercise was elevated at Set 4 above Set 2 (P<0.05) and despite declining work output, remained elevated at this level during Sets 6, 8 and 10 (P<0.05) (Figure 3C).

Muscle [^{3}H]ouabain binding site content and maximal *in vitro* 3-*O*-MFPase activity

There was no significant effect of eccentric exercise on [^{3}H]ouabain binding site content (P = 0.314, Figure 4A) or maximal *in vitro* K$^+$-stimulated 3-*O*-MFPase activity (P = 0.414, Figure 4B).

Discussion

This is the first study to investigate the effects of unaccustomed intense eccentric contractions on K$^+$ regulation during exercise and on skeletal muscle NKA content and 3-*O*-MFPase. The findings of this study supported our hypothesis that the eccentric contraction-induced increase in plasma [K$^+$] would remain elevated despite a decrease in work output, resulting in an elevated Δ[K$^+$]/work ratio. These data suggest that eccentric contractions, which lead to skeletal muscle damage, may impair plasma [K$^+$] regulation during contractions and have an impact on intramuscular K$^+$ handling. However, in contrast to our hypothesis, we found no eccentric contraction-induced decrease in muscle NKA content or the 3-*O*-MFPase as a marker of NKA activity in resting muscle.

Evidence of muscle damage

A reduction in isometric muscle torque and an increase in plasma [CK] were used in this study as evidence for the presence of eccentric exercise-induced muscle damage [34,35]. Whilst maximal isometric torque was depressed by 26% immediately

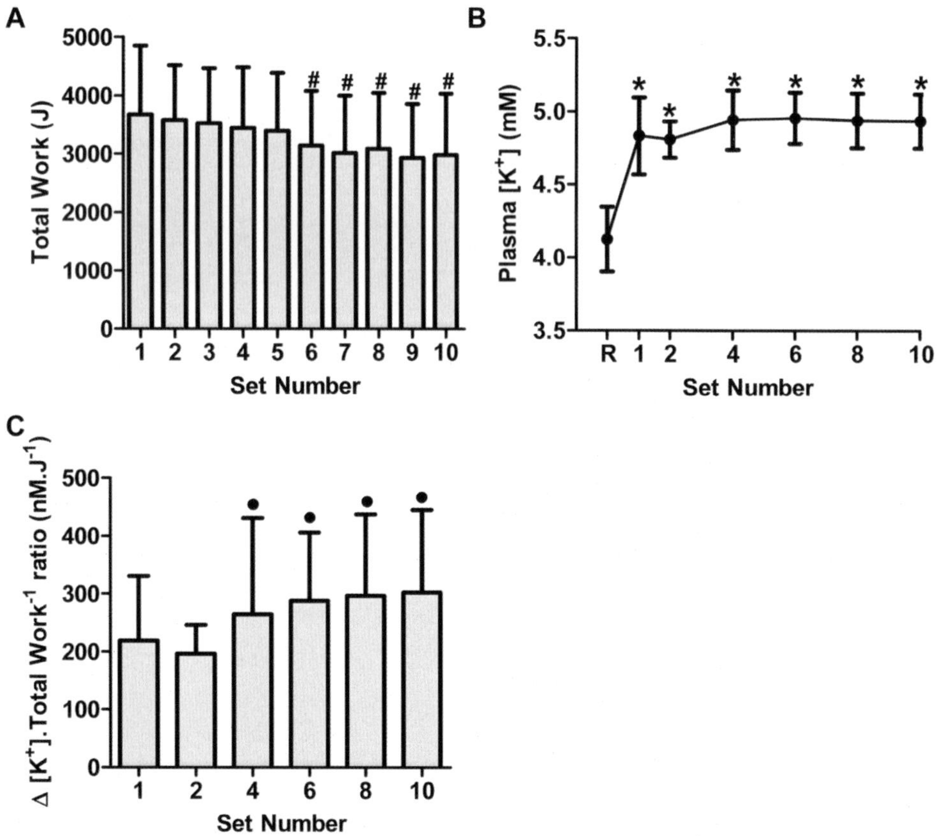

Figure 3. Total work performed (A), Plasma [K$^+$] (B), and the rise in plasma [K$^+$] relative to work performed (ΔK$^+$].work^{-1} ratio) (C) during 10 sets of 30 maximal eccentric knee extensor contractions. Values are means ± SD; *n* = 6. # *P*<0.05– significantly different from Set 1. **P*<0.05– significantly different from Rest. • *P*<0.05– significantly different from Set 2.

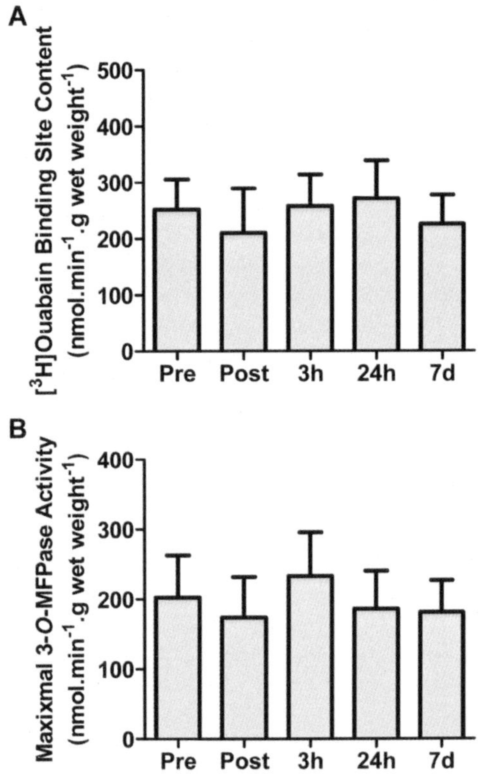

Figure 4. The effects of maximal eccentric knee extensor contractions on [^{3}H]ouabain binding site content (a) and maximal *in vitro* K^+-stimulated 3-*O*-methylfluorescein phosphatase (3-*O*-MFPase) activity (b). Measurements were made on muscle biopsy samples taken from the vastus lateralis muscle before (Pre), immediately after (Post), and 3 h, 24 h, and 7 days following the eccentric contractions. Values are means ± SD; $n = 6$.

post-exercise, this reduction in the force generating capacity post-eccentric exercise could include an element of muscle damage combined with muscle fatigue. However, the tendency for torque to remain depressed at 3 h post-exercise (19%), and the expected elevation in plasma [CK], confirms that our protocol did induce skeletal muscle damage and suggests that the integrity of the sarcolemma had been altered. The doubling of plasma [CK] at 24 h post-eccentric exercise (339±90 IU/L) in this study is similar to a previous study that also performed 300 eccentric contractions (327±156 IU/L at 24 h post-exercise) and which also demonstrated a loss of cytoskeletal protein desmin and the disruption of normal sarcomeric structure [27]. Thus, these measures confirmed that our exercise protocol was sufficient to induce a moderate level of muscle damage.

Impaired plasma [K^+] regulation during eccentric contractions

During concentric exercise, such as intense intermittent cycling exercise, a relationship exists between work output and plasma [K^+] where a reduction in work output is associated with a concomitant reduction in plasma [K^+] [17,18]. In contrast, in the present study, plasma [K^+] was increased above rest by the first set of eccentric contractions and, despite work output decreasing from set 6 to 10, plasma [K^+] remained elevated for the duration of the exercise bout. As a result, the plasma [K^+]/work ratio also remained elevated. This dissociation between plasma [K^+] and work output suggests a possible disturbance in K^+ regulation during the eccentric contractions, which may indicate an increased leakage of K^+ from the muscle and/or decreased clearance of K^+ from the plasma. This disturbance in K^+ regulation could have contributed to a depolarizing effect on the sarcolemmal and T-tubular membranes and thus may have contributed to a fatiguing effect which, along with muscle damage, are likely responsible for the reduction in total work. Possible reasons for this disturbance in K^+ regulation include the eccentric contraction-induced damage to the active muscle, and thus presumably also the sarcolemmal and T-tubular membranes, leading to an excess K^+ release from the damaged muscle (and increased Na^+ influx), or that there may have been a decrease in NKA content or activity. However, there are likely to be multiple factors contributing to muscle fatigue during eccentric contractions including an impairment in SR Ca^{2+} release [36]. In regard to the NKA content, however, we found no significant depressive effect of acute eccentric contractions immediately after exercise on NKA content as measured by [^{3}H]ouabain site content. We also found no effect on the maximal NKA activity as measured by the *in vitro* 3-*O*-MFPase activity assay. Although this assay has recently been criticised as an invalid marker of NKA activity during exercise due its Na+-insensitivity, this method would appear valid for activity measures in resting muscle, as it is inhibited by ouabain and strongly correlated with [^{3}H]ouabain binding measures [8,28]. Another possible explanation for the elevated plasma [K^+], despite a fall in work output, is eccentric contraction-induced excitation-contraction (E–C) uncoupling. In this case, eccentric contractions may have disrupted the normal communication between the dihydropyridine receptor/voltage sensor located in the T-tubular membranes and the ryanodine receptor/calcium release channels located in the sarcoplasmic reticulum membrane [37,38]. Such a scenario would result in a fall in muscle force output due to reduced calcium release despite normal action potential propagation and associated K^+ release [39]. Indeed, E–C coupling in mouse muscles has previously been shown to be impaired immediately post-eccentric contractions in the absence of significant changes in action potential conduction [38–40]. More studies are required to further explore the extent of this phenomenon in human subjects and the underlying intracellular mechanisms.

The peak plasma [K^+] of 4.96 mmol.l^{-1} observed at the end of the 6th set of eccentric contractions was similar to values previously reported during concentric contractions of knee extensor muscles on the same isokinetic dynamometer in our laboratory [8,30]. For example, Fraser *et al.*, [8] found a peak plasma [K^+] of 4.69 mmol.l^{-1} after 50 repetitions of maximal concentric knee extension, while Petersen *et al.*, [30] found a peak plasma [K^+] of 4.89 mmol.l^{-1} after ~ 3 min of fatiguing submaximal knee extensor contractions. The similarity in peak plasma [K^+] between this study and Fraser *et al.*, [8] and Petersen *et al.*, [30], is somewhat surprising, as a unique characteristic of eccentric contractions is that they are considered not to be as metabolically demanding as purely concentric contractions [41,42]. This decrease in metabolic demand during eccentric contractions compared to concentric is ascribed to mechanical detachment of cross-bridges during eccentric (lengthening) contractions while, in contrast, concentric contractions are dependant upon ATP-dependant cross-bridge detachment to develop force [43]. Thus, given the lower ATP utilization during eccentric exercise, it is reasonable to assume that the ionic disturbances associated with eccentric muscle contractions would also be less than during concentric contractions. Another possible reason for similar peak plasma [K^+] during concentric and eccentric contractions may involve the enzyme AMP-activated protein kinase (AMPK). Indeed, activated AMPK has been shown to increase muscle

NKA activity and lower plasma [K^+] [44–46]. Therefore, the lower metabolic demand during fatiguing eccentric contractions may lead to a lower level of activation of AMPK which, in turn, may lead to a plasma [K^+] that is similar to that found with fatiguing concentric contractions during which AMPK is substantially activated [47].

NKA content after eccentric exercise

Previous studies have shown that an acute bout of eccentric exercise reduces the expression of the membrane-bound proteins, GLUT-4 [21,22] and the lactate/H^+ transporter [23]. Moreover, eccentric contractions induce the loss or disruption of cytoskeletal proteins such as dystrophin [20] and desmin [27]. Dystrophin and desmin are components of structures known as costameres which play a key role in the proper alignment of the sarcolemma and sarcomeres, and thus in lateral force transmission [48]. Importantly, the NKA is also a component of costameres and is associated with the cytoskeleton proteins, β-spectrin and ankyrin 3 [24,48]. Thus, we hypothesized that unaccustomed eccentric exercise would lead to a decrease in NKA protein abundance as indicated by the number of [^{3}H]ouabain binding sites. However, we found no significant change in [^{3}H]ouabain binding sites immediately after exercise nor at 3 and 24 h post-exercise when our marker of muscle damage, plasma [CK], was elevated. Likewise, there was no sign of a compensatory upregulation of [^{3}H]ouabain binding sites 7 d after eccentric exercise. These data were also supported by our finding of no significant change in NKA activity, as indicated by the maximal *in vitro* K^+-stimulated 3-*O*-MFPase activity which, in resting muscle, has been shown to be proportional to the number of [^{3}H]ouabain binding sites [8,28]. These findings suggest that NKA protein expression may be regulated differently to other cytoskeletal/costameric proteins in response to eccentric contractions and/or that a greater level of muscle damage is required to induce a significant change in NKA expression and function. Further work is warranted to examine if a threshold of muscle damage exists, beyond which, NKA expression is changed and whether this would further alter K^+ regulation during exercise.

One potential limitation of this study is the inclusion of both male and female subjects with a moderate range of ages. For example, sex and age related variability in NKA content or activity could potentially mask changes to these parameters in response to eccentric exercise. To date, however, there is no evidence that resting NKA content (^{3}H-ouabain binding) or activity (3-*O*-MFPase activity) is different between males and females within the age range and physical activity level of the subjects in this study [see [49–51]). Furthermore, to the best of our knowledge there is currently no evidence that estrogens play a role in the regulation of NKA content and/or activity in skeletal muscle. Thus, based on current evidence, it is unlikely that the inclusion of both male and female subjects would have impacted NKA content or activity values found in the current study. Nevertheless, future studies should specifically investigate the existence of potential sex-based differences in potassium regulation and NKA content and activity in response to exercise, including eccentric exercise.

Conclusion

In conclusion, eccentric contractions that led to moderate levels of muscle damage induced a dissociation between plasma [K^+] and work output, leading to an elevated ratio of the rise in plasma [K^+] relative to work during eccentric contractions. This most likely indicates an impairment in K^+ regulation; however, we found no evidence of a significant change in muscle NKA content after unaccustomed eccentric exercise of the leg extensor muscles. These results may indicate the presence of excitation-contraction uncoupling during eccentric exercise. These findings highlight the need to conduct further research into K^+ dynamics and the regulation of NKA abundance and function during eccentric exercise.

Acknowledgments

The current address for M. J. Leikis is the Capital & Coast District Health Board Renal Service, Wellington, New Zealand.

Author Contributions

Conceived and designed the experiments: CAG JAB MJM. Performed the experiments: CAG JAB MJL MJM. Analyzed the data: CAG JAB MJM. Contributed reagents/materials/analysis tools: CAG MJM. Wrote the paper: CAG JAB MJL MJM.

References

1. Clausen T (2003) Na+-K+ pump regulation and skeletal muscle contractility. Physiol Rev 83: 1269–1324.
2. McKenna MJ, Bangsbo J, Renaud J-M (2008) Muscle K+, Na+, and Cl disturbances and Na+-K+ pump inactivation: implications for fatigue. J Appl Physiol 104: 288–295.
3. Clausen T (2008) Role of Na+,K+-pumps and transmembrane Na+,K+-distribution in muscle function. Acta Physiol 192: 339–349.
4. Sejersted OM, Sjogaard G (2000) Dynamics and Consequences of Potassium Shifts in Skeletal Muscle and Heart During Exercise. Physiol Rev 80: 1411–1481.
5. Cairns SP, Lindinger MI (2008) Do multiple ionic interactions contribute to skeletal muscle fatigue? J Physiol 586: 4039–4054.
6. Pedersen TH, Nielsen OB, Lamb GD, Stephenson DG (2004) Intracellular acidosis enhances the excitability of working muscle. Science 305: 1144–1147.
7. McKenna MJ, Medved I, Goodman CA, Brown MJ, Bjorksten AR, et al. (2006) N-acetylcysteine attenuates the decline in muscle Na+,K+-pump activity and delays fatigue during prolonged exercise in humans. J Physiol 576: 279–288.
8. Fraser SF, Li JL, Carey MF, Wang XN, Sangkabutra T, et al. (2002) Fatigue depresses maximal in vitro skeletal muscle Na(+)-K(+)-ATPase activity in untrained and trained individuals. J Appl Physiol 93: 1650–1659.
9. Juel C, Pilegaard H, Nielsen JJ, Bangsbo J (2000) Interstitial K+ in human skeletal muscle during and after dynamic graded exercise determined by microdialysis. Am J Physiol – Regul Integr Comp Physiol 278: R400–R406.
10. Nielsen JJ, Mohr M, Klarskov C, Kristensen M, Krustrup P, et al. (2004) Effects of high-intensity intermittent training on potassium kinetics and performance in human skeletal muscle. J Physiol 554: 857–870.
11. McKenna MJ, Heigenhauser GJ, McKelvie RS, MacDougall JD, Jones NL (1997) Sprint training enhances ionic regulation during intense exercise in men. J Physiol 501 (Pt 3): 687–702.
12. Vollestad NK, Hallen J, Sejersted OM (1994) Effect of exercise intensity on potassium balance in muscle and blood of man. J Physiol 475: 359–368.
13. Medbo JI, Sejersted OM (1990) Plasma potassium changes with high intensity exercise. J Physiol 421: 105–122.
14. Nordsborg N, Mohr M, Pedersen LD, Nielsen JJ, Langberg H, et al. (2003) Muscle interstitial potassium kinetics during intense exhaustive exercise: effect of previous arm exercise. Am J Physiol Regul Integr Comp Physiol 285: R143–148.
15. Mohr M, Nordsborg N, Nielsen JJ, Pedersen LD, Fischer C, et al. (2004) Potassium kinetics in human muscle interstitium during repeated intense exercise in relation to fatigue. Pflugers Arch 448: 452–456.
16. Street D, Nielsen JJ, Bangsbo J, Juel C (2005) Metabolic alkalosis reduces exercise-induced acidosis and potassium accumulation in human skeletal muscle interstitium. J Physiol 566: 481–489.
17. McKenna MJ, Schmidt TA, Hargreaves M, Cameron L, Skinner SL, et al. (1993) Sprint training increases human skeletal muscle Na(+)-K(+)-ATPase concentration and improves K+ regulation. J Appl Physiol 75: 173–180.
18. Hargreaves M, McKenna MJ, Jenkins DG, Warmington SA, Li JL, et al. (1998) Muscle metabolites and performance during high-intensity, intermittent exercise. J Appl Physiol 84: 1687–1691.
19. Yeung EW, Balnave CD, Ballard HJ, Bourreau JP, Allen DG (2002) Development of T-tubular vacuoles in eccentrically damaged mouse muscle fibres. J Physiol 540: 581–592.

20. Lovering RM, De Deyne PG (2004) Contractile function, sarcolemma integrity, and the loss of dystrophin after skeletal muscle eccentric contraction-induced injury. Am J Physiol Cell Physiol 286: C230–238.
21. Asp S, Kristiansen S, Richter EA (1995) Eccentric muscle damage transiently decreases rat skeletal muscle GLUT-4 protein. J Appl Physiol 79: 1338–1345.
22. Asp S, Daugaard JR, Richter EA (1995) Eccentric exercise decreases glucose transporter GLUT4 protein in human skeletal muscle. J Physiol 482: 705–712.
23. Pilegaard H, Asp S (1998) Effect of prior eccentric contractions on lactate/H+ transport in rat skeletal muscle. Am J Physiol 274: E554–559.
24. Williams MW, Resneck WG, Kaysser T, Ursitti JA, Birkenmeier CS, et al. (2001) Na,K-ATPase in skeletal muscle: two populations of beta-spectrin control localization in the sarcolemma but not partitioning between the sarcolemma and the transverse tubules. J Cell Sci 114: 751–762.
25. MacIntyre DL, Sorichter S, Mair J, Berg A, McKenzie DC (2001) Markers of inflammation and myofibrillar proteins following eccentric exercise in humans. Eur J Appl Physiol 84: 180–186.
26. Murphy RM, Goodman CA, McKenna MJ, Bennie J, Leikis M, et al. (2007) Calpain-3 is autolyzed and hence activated in human skeletal muscle 24 h following a single bout of eccentric exercise. J Appl Physiol 103: 926–931.
27. Beaton LJ, Tarnopolsky MA, Phillips SM (2002) Contraction-induced muscle damage in humans following calcium channel blocker administration. J Physiol 544: 849–859.
28. Nordsborg N, Goodman C, McKenna MJ, Bangsbo J (2005) Dexamethasone up-regulates skeletal muscle maximal Na+,K+ pump activity by muscle group specific mechanisms in humans. J Physiol 567: 583–589.
29. Norgaard A, Kjeldsen K, Clausen T (1984) A method for the determination of the total number of 3H-ouabain binding sites in biopsies of human skeletal muscle. Scand J Clin Lab Invest 44: 509–518.
30. Petersen AC, Murphy KT, Snow RJ, Leppik JA, Aughey RJ, et al. (2005) Depressed Na+-K+-ATPase activity in skeletal muscle at fatigue is correlated with increased Na+-K+-ATPase mRNA expression following intense exercise. Am J Physiol Regul Integr Comp Physiol 289: R266–274.
31. McKenna MJ, Gissel H, Clausen T (2003) Effects of electrical stimulation and insulin on Na+-K+-ATPase ([3H]ouabain binding) in rat skeletal muscle. J Physiol 547: 567–580.
32. Fraser SF, McKenna MJ (1998) Measurement of Na+, K+-ATPase activity in human skeletal muscle. Anal Biochem 258: 63–67.
33. Juel C, Nordsborg NB, Bangsbo J (2013) Exercise-induced increase in maximal in vitro Na,K-ATPase activity in human skeletal muscle. Am J Physiol – Regul Integr Comp Physiol 304: R1161–R1165.
34. Clarkson PM, Sayers SP (1999) Etiology of exercise-induced muscle damage. Can J Appl Physiol 24: 234–248.
35. Clarkson PM, Hubal MJ (2002) Exercise-induced muscle damage in humans. Am J Phys Med Rehabil 81: S52–69.
36. Nielsen JS, Sahlin K, Ortenblad N (2007) Reduced sarcoplasmic reticulum content of releasable Ca2+ in rat soleus muscle fibres after eccentric contractions. Acta Physiol 191: 217–228.
37. Takekura H, Fujinami N, Nishizawa T, Ogasawara H, Kasuga N (2001) Eccentric exercise-induced morphological changes in the membrane systems involved in excitation-contraction coupling in rat skeletal muscle. J Physiol 533: 571–583.
38. Ingalls CP, Warren GL, Williams JH, Ward CW, Armstrong RB (1998) E-C coupling failure in mouse EDL muscle after in vivo eccentric contractions. J Appl Physiol 85: 58–67.
39. Warren GL, Ingalls CP, Shah SJ, Armstrong RB (1999) Uncoupling of in vivo torque production from EMG in mouse muscles injured by eccentric contractions. J Physiol 515: 609–619.
40. Warren GL, Ingalls CP, Lowe DA, Armstrong RB (2001) Excitation-contraction uncoupling: major role in contraction-induced muscle injury. Exerc Sport Sci Rev 29: 82–87.
41. Bonde-Petersen F, Knuttgen HG, Henriksson J (1972) Muscle metabolism during exercise with concentric and eccentric contractions. J Appl Physiol 33: 792–795.
42. Ryschon TW, Fowler MD, Wysong RE, Anthony A, Balaban RS (1997) Efficiency of human skeletal muscle in vivo: comparison of isometric, concentric, and eccentric muscle action. J Appl Physiol 83: 867–874.
43. Enoka RM (1996) Eccentric contractions require unique activation strategies by the nervous system. J Appl Physiol 81: 2339–2346.
44. Ingwersen M, Kristensen M, Pilegaard H, Wojtaszewski JP, Richter E, et al. (2011) Na,K-ATPase Activity in Mouse Muscle is Regulated by AMPK and PGC-1α. J Membr Biol 242: 1–10.
45. Zheng D, Perianayagam A, Lee DH, Brannan MD, Yang LE, et al. (2008) AMPK activation with AICAR provokes an acute fall in plasma [K+]. American Journal of Physiology – Cell Physiology 294: C126–C135.
46. Benziane B, Björnholm M, Pirkmajer S, Austin RL, Kotova O, et al. (2012) Activation of AMP-activated Protein Kinase Stimulates Na+,K+-ATPase Activity in Skeletal Muscle Cells. J Biol Chem 287: 23451–23463.
47. Chen Z-P, Stephens TJ, Murthy S, Canny BJ, Hargreaves M, et al. (2003) Effect of Exercise Intensity on Skeletal Muscle AMPK Signaling in Humans. Diabetes 52: 2205–2212.
48. Bloch RJ, Capetanaki Y, O'Neill A, Reed P, Williams MW, et al. (2002) Costameres: repeating structures at the sarcolemma of skeletal muscle. Clin Orthop: S203–210.
49. Murphy KT, Aughey RJ, Petersen AC, Clark SA, Goodman C, et al. (2007) Effects of endurance training status and sex differences on Na+,K+-pump mRNA expression, content and maximal activity in human skeletal muscle Acta Physiologica 189: 259–269.
50. Green HJ, Duscha BD, Sullivan MJ, Keteyian SJ, Kraus WE (2001) Normal skeletal muscle Na+-K+ pump concentration in patients with chronic heart failure. Muscle & Nerve 24: 69–76.
51. Norgaard A (1986) Quantification of the Na,K-pumps in mammalian skeletal muscle. Acta Pharmacol Toxicol (Copenh) 58 Suppl 1: 1–34.

24

An Examination of Resveratrol's Mechanisms of Action in Human Tissue: Impact of a Single Dose *In Vivo* and Dose Responses in Skeletal Muscle *Ex Vivo*

Cameron B. Williams[1], Meghan C. Hughes[3], Brittany A. Edgett[1], Trisha D. Scribbans[1], Craig A. Simpson[2], Christopher G. R. Perry[3], Brendon J. Gurd[1]*

1 School of Kinesiology and Health Studies, Queen's University, Kingston, Ontario, Canada, **2** Department of Emergency Medicine, Queen's University, Kingston, Ontario, Canada, **3** School of Kinesiology and Health Science, York University, Toronto, Ontario, Canada

Abstract

The current study tested the hypothesis that a single, moderate dose of RSV would activate the AMPK/SIRT1 axis in human skeletal muscle and adipose tissue. Additionally, the effects of RSV on mitochondrial respiration in PmFBs were examined. Eight sedentary men (23.8±2.4 yrs; BMI: 32.7±7.1) reported to the lab on two occasions where they were provided a meal supplemented with 300 mg of RSV or a placebo. Blood samples, and a muscle biopsy were obtained in the fasted state and again, with the addition of an adipose tissue biopsy, two hours post-prandial. The effect of RSV on mitochondrial respiration was examined in PmFBs taken from muscle biopsies from an additional eight men (23.4±5.4 yrs; BMI: 24.4±2.8). No effect of RSV was observed on nuclear SIRT1 activity, acetylation of p53, or phosphorylation of AMPK, ACC or PKA in either skeletal muscle or adipose tissue. A decrease in post absorptive insulin levels was accompanied by elevated skeletal muscle phosphorylation of p38 MAPK, but no change in either skeletal muscle or adipose tissue insulin signalling. Mitochondrial respiration in PmFBs was rapidly inhibited by RSV at 100–300 uM depending on the substrate examined. These results question the efficacy of a single dose of RSV at altering skeletal muscle and adipose tissue AMPK/SIRT1 activity in humans and suggest that RSV mechanisms of action in humans may be associated with altered cellular energetics resulting from impaired mitochondrial ATP production.

Editor: Cedric Moro, INSERM/UMR 1048, France

Funding: Funding was provided by NSERC (CGRP and BJG) and the Canaian Foundation for Innovation (CFI) (BJG). The funders had no role in study design, data collection and analysis, decision to publish, or preparation of the manuscript.

* Email: gurdb@queensu.ca

Introduction

Resveratrol (RSV), a plant derived polyphenol, has recently garnered significant interest due to its purported beneficial effects on glucose homeostasis and metabolic health [1]. In animal models, in addition to the prevention of diet induced obesity and improved metabolic health [2–5], chronic RSV treatment improves insulin sensitivity [4,6–9], and increases mitochondrial content in both adipose tissue and skeletal muscle [2]. While it is widely accepted that RSV acts through the AMPK/SIRT1/PGC-1αpathway [2,10], an energy sensing network linking cellular metabolic state to mitochondrial adaptation [11], the mechanisms by which RSV activates this pathway remain controversial.

In animal and cell line models, while there are reports that RSV interacts with and directly activates SIRT1 [12,13], the direct link between SIRT1 and RSV has been questioned [14,15]. The specific actions of RSV are further complicated by evidence that RSV activates AMPK in muscle [16,17] and adipose tissue [17] and findings that the activation of AMPK is required for the beneficial effects of RSV to manifest [17]. These findings have led to the speculation that RSV activates both SIRT1 and AMPK with direct activation of SIRT1 stimulating AMPK activity via LKB1 [18] or indirect activation of SIRT occurring via AMPK subsequent to an effect of RSV on PDE/cAMP signalling [19]. Alternatively, there is evidence that RSV is capable of inhibiting ATP synthase [20] and reducing ATP concentrations in a variety of cell lines [21–23]. While there is evidence that this effect may be dose dependent [18], and impaired ATP production has yet to be demonstrated *in vivo*, the idea that RSV mediated activation of AMPK results from a disturbance in energy status is compelling.

In contrast to animal studies, chronic RSV supplementation in humans has yielded conflicting results for metabolic outcomes. Specifically, several studies have reported improved insulin sensitivity following chronic RSV supplementation [24–26], while others have not [27,28]. Interestingly, positive effects of RSV have been primarily observed in obese or insulin insensitive/resistant individuals suggesting that an overweight/obese population may be more sensitive to the effects of RSV than lean healthy individuals. The activation of the AMPK/SIRT1 pathway implicated in the mechanism of RSV action in animals has been observed in skeletal muscle and adipose tissue following some [24], but not all [27,28] RSV trials in humans. Thus whether RSV is able to activate AMPK and/or SIRT1 in humans is currently controversial. Further complicating the interpretation of these chronic supplementation studies is the sampling of AMPK/SIRT1 after the intervention, when chronic adaptations induced by RSV may be altering the impact of RSV on signalling pathways. While it is clear that adaptation results from an accumulation of repeated stimuli following repeated daily RSV supplementation, examining the acute effects of RSV may provide new insight into the mechanisms by which chronic adaptations occur. At present much of the information regarding RSVs mechanism(s) of action have been gleaned from chronic feeding studies, however, there is evidence from various cell lines that a single exposure to RSV can activate the AMPK/SIRT1 signalling pathway [17–19,21]. Should similar acute activation occur in human tissue, this would provide an opportunity to observe the mechanisms of RSV action without the confounding influence of chronic adaptations inherent in prolonged feeding studies. Thus, the controversial results from human trials, and the timing of AMPK/SIRT1 measures made in humans to date, make it difficult to discern whether the mechanisms of RSV action proposed from cellular and animal models are conserved in human tissue.

In an attempt to address the mechanisms of RSV action in human tissue we conducted 2 studies with the following purposes: 1) to determine if the mechanisms of RSV action previously described in cellular and animal models [18,19], specifically the AMPK/SIRT1 pathway, are activated in human skeletal muscle and adipose tissue following a single dose of RSV, and 2) to examine the effects of a wide range of RSV concentrations on skeletal muscle mitochondrial oxidative metabolism *ex vivo* utilizing permeabilized muscle fibre bundles (PmFBs). We hypothesize that an acute dose of RSV would activate AMPK and SIRT1 signalling in both skeletal muscle and adipose tissue *in vivo*, and, consistent with observations in rat brain, liver [20] and muscle cells [21], RSV would inhibit mitochondrial oxidative metabolism in human PmFBs, but only at supra-physiological concentrations.

Methods

All experimental procedures performed on human participants were approved by the Health Sciences Human Research Ethics Board at Queen's University and conformed to the Declaration of Helsinki. Verbal and written explanation of the experimental protocol and associated risks was provided to all participants prior to obtaining written informed consent.

Experimental Design

The current study involved the completion of two distinct experiments. The first experiment examined the effects of RSV on skeletal muscle and adipose tissue intracellular signaling and whole body fatty acid oxidation in overweight/obese males. This experiment consisted of the administration of a single dose of RSV (300 mg) or placebo supplement on two separate occasions using a randomized cross over, double-blind design. A 300 mg dose was chosen for the current study as it represents a moderate dose, falling between the lowest (10 mg/day; [25]) and highest (1–2 g/day; [26]) doses reported in the human literature. Each condition was separated by a seven day wash out period. For the second experiment, PmFBs were isolated from muscle biopsies obtained from lean males and the effects of RSV on ADP stimulated respiration were examined.

Participants

In total, 16 men volunteered to participate in this study (participant characteristics are presented in Table 1). Participants in experiment one reported less than one hour per week of structured exercise at enrollment (aerobic training, resistance training, etc.) and were overweight (waist circumference of greater than 94 cm) [29]. Participants were instructed to maintain exercise and nutritional habits, and to avoid the use of nutritional supplements and foods high in naturally occurring resveratrol (grapes, some teas, and peanuts) for the duration of the study. Participants in experiment two were recreationally active and were not involved in a specific training program at the time of recruitment. All participants were instructed to avoid exercise, caffeine, drugs, and alcohol for a minimum of 24 hours prior to each visit.

Experiment 1

Baseline Testing. Participants ($n = 8$; see Table 1 for detailed characteristics) reported for the first laboratory visit a minimum of 72 hours prior to any intervention day. During this visit anthropometric measures were obtained and VO_2peak was assessed on a friction-braked cycle ergometer (Monark, Ergomedic 874E, Vansbro, Sweden) using an incremental ramp protocol. The VO_2peak ramp protocol consisted of a five minute loadless warm-up followed by a step increase to 80 W for one minute and subsequent increases in work rate of 24 $W \cdot min^{-1}$ to volitional exhaustion (determined by the inability of the participant to maintain a cadence of 60 RPM). Gas exchange was measured continuously using a metabolic cart (Moxus AEI Technologies, Pittsburgh, PA). Relative VO_2peak, absolute VO_2peak, and peak hear rate were calculated as the average of their respective values measured in the final 30 seconds of the protocol.

Supplement Intervention Protocol. Participants reported to the laboratory on two subsequent occasions to participate in a placebo and a RSV supplement intervention in random order. On the evening prior to each experimental visit, participants were provided a standardized dinner which included a Stouffer's Sauté Sensations Country Beef Pot Roast (540 kcal; 56 g carbohydrate (CHO), 20 g fat, 14 g protein), 500 mL of 2% milk (260 kcal; 12 g CHO, 5 g fat, 9 g protein) and a Dole Apple Cinnamon Fruit Crisp (160 kcal; 30 g CHO, 3.5 g fat, 2 g protein) before reporting to the lab having fasted overnight (≥12 hours). Participants were asked to drive or walk slowly to the lab, and take the elevator in order to limit their physical activity. Participants then rested for 10 minutes before gas exchange measures were collected for 15 minutes (Moxus AEI Technologies, Pittsburgh, PA) while participants rested in a seated position. Immediately following gas exchange collection, a blood sample and muscle biopsy were obtained while participants rested in a supine position (for details please see *Physiological Measurements*). Subsequently, participants were fed a standardized breakfast consisting of a plain bagel (190 kcal; 36 g CHO, 1 g fat, 7 g protein), 15 g of cream cheese (45 kcal; 1 g CHO, 4 g fat, 1 g protein), and 200 mL of orange juice (100 kcal; 23 g CHO, 0 g fat, 1 g protein), which they were given 10 minutes to eat. This meal was similar to that typically ingested by the participants and reflects a traditional North American diet. Ingestion of breakfast was immediately followed by the ingestion of unlabeled identical capsules containing either 300 mg of RSV supplement (resVida, DSM, Heerlen, Netherlands) or microcrystalline cellulose placebo supplement (PCCA Canada, London, ON) with 200 mL of water. Following ingestion of the supplement, participants rested in bed for 105 minutes and were provided water *ad libitum*, after which post-prandial gas exchange values were recorded for 15 minutes. A post-prandial blood sample, muscle biopsy, and adipose tissue biopsy were then obtained (120 minutes following supplement ingestion) in the same order as the fasted samples described above. The supplement order was randomized and given in a double-blind fashion on consecutive visits, a minimum of seven days apart.

Table 1. Subject characteristic summary.

	Experiment 1 (n = 8)	Experiment 2 (n = 8)
Age (yrs)	23.8±2.4	23.4±5.4
Height (cm)	182.5±10.2	183.6±6.1
Weight (kg)	111.3±37.5	83.2±12.7*
BMI	32.7±7.1	24.4±2.8*
Waist Circumference (cm)	106.4±21.2	84.1±6.3*
VO_2 peak (ml min^{-1} kg^{-1})	34.0±7.3	50.0±8.7*

Values are mean ± SD. yrs, years; cm, centimeters; kg, kilograms; BMI, body mass index.
*Significantly different ($p<0.05$) than participants from experiment 1.

Physiological Measurements. Resting blood samples were collected by venipuncture from an antecubital vein in sterile tubes (BD Vaccutainer, Franklin Lakes, NJ) coated with ethylenediaminetetra acetic acid (EDTA) as an anticoagulant. Plasma was separated by centrifugation at 1300 rcf for 10 minutes at 4°C. Samples were stored at −80°C until analysis. Muscle biopsy samples were obtained using the Bergstrom needle biopsy technique [30] with the addition of manual suction from the vastus lateralis following local anaesthetization (2% lidocaine). For each experimental visit both muscle biopsies (fasted and post-prandial) were obtained from the same leg from separate incisions approximately 2–3 cm apart. Repeated biopsies from separate incisions have been shown to be unaffected by previous biopsies to the same leg [31,32]. Adipose tissue biopsies were also obtained using a Bergstrom needle with the addition of manual suction following local anaesthetization (2% lidocaine). Adipose tissue biopsies were obtained from the abdomen with the incision made approximately 5 cm lateral to the umbilicus and the needle being directed laterally once through this incision. Both muscle and adipose tissue were immediately blotted, snap-frozen in liquid nitrogen, and stored at −80°C until analysis.

Plasma Glucose, Insulin, Glycerol, and Respiratory Exchange Ratio. Plasma glucose was analyzed via a hexokinase reaction assay performed at Kingston General Hospital (Kingston, Ontario). Plasma insulin was determined with a commercially available enzyme-linked immunoabsorbent assay (ELISA) kit (Alpco Diagnositics, Salem, NH). Plasma glycerol was analyzed using the commercially available Free Glycerol Reagent (Sigma, Oakville, ON). All samples were run in duplicate with the coefficient of variation being <10% for all values. Respiratory exchange ratio (RER) was determined from recorded gas exchange values at fasted and post-prandial time points. A 10 minute average was taken from 3–13 minutes of recorded gas exchange values to minimize the impact of any adjustment period following putting on the mask and/or participant anticipation of the mask being removed. RER was used to estimate relative substrate contribution to total substrate oxidation assuming a linear relationship between an RER of 0.7 (100% fat, 0% CHO), and 1.0 (0% fat, 100% CHO) at rest. Specifically, the fat derived component for energy expenditure at each time point was calculated according to the following formula [33]: fat (g·min-1) = 1.695 · O_2 production (l·min-1) −1.701 · CO_2 production (l·min-1). To convert fatty acid oxidation rates to kcal·min-1 resulting values were multiplied by 9 kcal·g-1.

Nuclear SIRT1 Activity. Nuclei were isolated from muscle (~50 mg frozen tissue) using a commercially available kit (Pierce Biotechnology, Rockford, IL) as we, and others have done previously [34–37]. Nuclear extract purity was confirmed via the absence of cytosolic contamination (lactate dehydrogenase) by western blotting as we have done previously [34,35]. A representative blot demonstrating the purity of our nuclear samples is presented in Figure 1A. Nuclear SIRT1 activity was measured with a commercially available SIRT1 fluorometric assay kit (BIOMOL, Plymouth Meetings, PA), as described previously [34]. Briefly, 25 μL of nuclear extract was incubated with 15 μL of Fluor de Lys-SIRT1 substrate (100 μM) and NAD^+ (100 μM) for 30 minutes at 37°C. The reaction was stopped with the addition of 50 μL of developer and nicotinamide (2 mM). The change in fluorescence (Arbitrary Fluorescence Units (AFU)) per minute was normalized to the amount of total muscle (mg wet weight) used for the nuclear extraction procedure.

Western Blot Analysis. Frozen skeletal muscle samples (30–50 mg) were homogenized in 2 mL of lysis buffer (210 mM sucrose, 2 mM EGTA, 40 mM NaCl, 30 mM Hepes, 20 mM EDTA) supplemented with both protease inhibitor (cOmplete ULTRA tables, Roche, Mannheim, Germany) and phosphatase inhibitor (PhosSTOP, Roche, Mannheim, Germany) cocktails. 40–50 mg of frozen adipose tissue were homogenized in 275 μL of lysis buffer also supplemented with inhibitor cocktails. Both types of tissue were added to tubes filled with the appropriate amount of pre-chilled (4°C) lysis buffer. Samples were subsequently homogenized for three seconds at 20 000 RPM (muscle) or 15 000 RPM (adipose) (Polytron PT10/35 GT Benchtop Homogenizer, Kinematic, Luzern, Switzerland). Protein concentrations were determined for all homogenates using a commercially available protein assay kit (Pierce, Rockford, IL). Samples were diluted to equivalent concentrations with a mixture of 4× Laemmli sample buffer and H_2O and then denatured by heating to 95°C for five minutes. Proteins were separated by SDS-PAGE using 8% (phospho-ACC, ACC), 10% (phospho-AMPK, AMPKα, phospho-Akt Ser473 and Thr308, pan-Akt, phospho-AS160 Thr642, phospho-(Ser/Thr) PKA Substrate, acetyl-p53 Lys379, GAPDH), and 15% (phospho-p38 MAPK, p38 MAPK) polyacrylamide gels and were subsequently transferred to a polyvinylidene difluride membrane. For the detection of proteins, commercially available antibodies were used for GAPDH (Millipore, Billerica, MA) and phospho-p38 MAPK Thr180/Tyr182, p-38 MAPK, phospho-AMPKα Thr172, AMPKα, phospho-ACC Ser79, ACC, acetyl-p53 Lys379, phospho-Akt Ser473, phospho-Akt Thr308, pan-Akt, phospho-AS160 Thr642, and phospho-(Ser/Thr) PKA Substrate (Cell Signaling Technologies, Danvers, MA). Membranes were blocked with 5% BSA in TBS-T (0.1%) and immunoblotted with primary antibody. Proteins were visualized by chemiluminescence detection according to the manufacturer's instructions (Millipore, Billerica, MA). Blots were imaged using the FluorChem Cell Biosciences imaging system (ProteinSimple, Santa Clara, CA) and quantified using

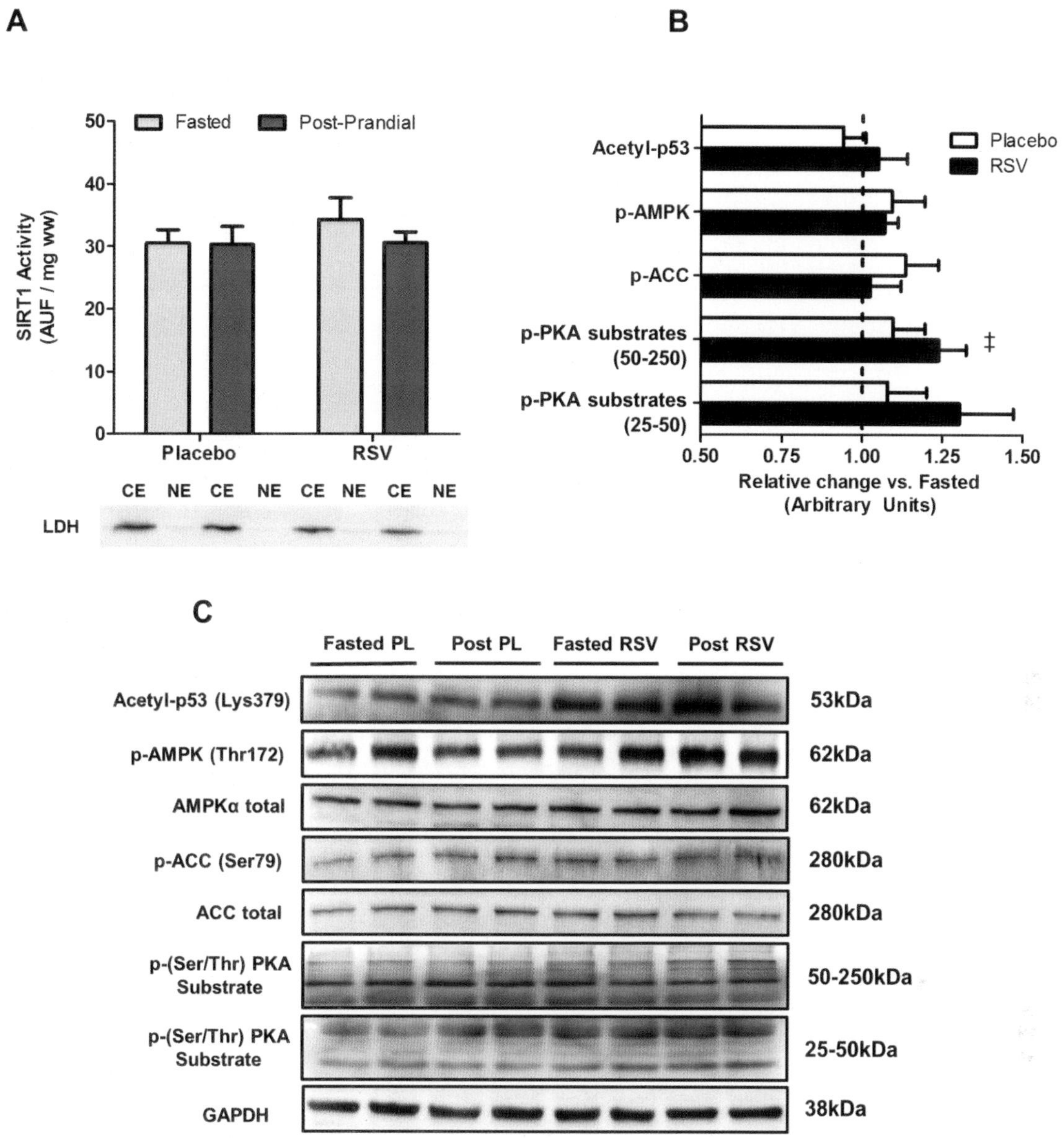

Figure 1. Both the activation of proteins implicated in SIRT1 activation and nuclear SIRT1 activity are unaltered following an acute dose of resveratrol in human skeletal muscle. Skeletal muscle nuclear SIRT1 activity (A) in the fasted (light bars) and post-prandial state (dark bars) in both conditions; and cytosolic contamination (LDH protein content) of nuclear extracts is also shown. The change in phosphorylated and acetylated protein content (B) in the post-prandial (post) state (expressed relative to fasting) in the placebo (PL; open bars) and resveratrol (RSV; shaded bars) conditions. Representative blots for all proteins are shown (C). ‡ Significant effect ($P<0.05$) of time on phosphorylated protein content.

AlphaView technology (ProteinSimple, Santa Clara, CA). Equal protein loading for all western blots was confirmed using ponceau staining for total protein. Equal protein loading for all skeletal muscle western blots was additionally confirmed using GAPDH as a loading control. Due to the limited size of the adipose tissue samples and low protein yield, western blot analysis of adipose tissue protein was limited to the proteins reported in the results section below.

Experiment 2

Participants ($n=8$; see Table 1 for detailed characteristics) reported for the first laboratory visit a minimum of 72 hours prior to any intervention day. During this visit anthropometric measures were obtained and VO_2peak was assessed on a friction-braked cycle ergometer as described above. Subsequently, participants reported to the laboratory at 9am having already consumed breakfast (participants were instructed to consume a breakfast that was high in CHO and low in fat similar to what they would eat on a normal morning). Upon arrival at the lab, participants rested for 10 minutes after which a muscle biopsy was obtained from the vastus lateralis while participants rested in the supine position (for details please see *Physiological Measurements* above). A portion of this biopsy was immediately placed into ice-cold BIOPS (described below) and used to prepare permeabilized fibre bundles (PmFBs).

Preparation of PmFBs. This technique is partially adapted from previous methods [38,39] and has been described in detail by us previously [40,41]. Briefly, small portions (~25 mg) of muscle were dissected from each biopsy and placed in ice-cold BIOPS.

The muscle was trimmed of connective tissue and fat and divided into several small muscle bundles (~2–7 mm, 1.0–2.5 mg wet weight). Each bundle was gently separated along their longitudinal axis with a pair of anti-magnetic needle-tipped forceps under magnification (Zeiss Stemi). Bundles were then treated with 30 μg·ml^{-1} saponin [42] in BIOPS and incubated on a rotor for 30 minutes at 4°C. Following permeabilization, PmFBs were washed at 4°C (<30 min) in MiR05 (see below) until respiratory measurements were initiated.

Mitochondrial Respiration and RSV Titration Experiments. High-resolution respirometry were conducted in 2 ml of respiration medium (MiR05) using the Oroboros Oxygraph-2k (Oroboros Instruments, Corp., Innsbruck, Austria) with stirring at 750 rpm. The composition of MiRO5 has been described previously [43]. All experiments were conducted in the Oxygraph chamber with an initial [O_2] of 300 μM and completed before the oxygraph chamber [O_2] reached 150 μM. 25 μM Blebbistatin (BLEB), dissolved in DMSO (5 mM stock), was used to prevent PmFB spontaneous contraction and ensure respiratory kinetics were assessed in a relaxed state [40]. We determined the effect of resveratrol on mitochondrial respiratory responses to a variety of substrates that generate NADH for complex I-supported respiration (A, 10 mM glutamate; C, 10 mM pyruvate), $FADH_2$ for complex II-supported respiration (B, 10 mM succinate) or both (D, 40 μM palmitoyl carnitine) in the presence of 5 mM malate as required for the above reactions. Each protocol began with the induction of state 3 respiration (5 mM ADP) supported by one of the above substrates in the presence of 5 mM malate as required for the reactions to proceed. The respiratory responses to resveratrol were monitored beginning with an initial dose of 1 μM up to 1500 μM, a titration protocol that began at or below plasma concentrations of RSV reported in humans following RSV supplementation [44]. Polarographic oxygen measurements were acquired in two second intervals, with the rate of respiration derived from 40 data points. Cytochrome *c* was added to test for mitochondrial membrane integrity, with all experiments demonstrating <10% increase in respiration.

Statistical Analysis

For experiment one, a two-way, repeated measures analysis of variance (ANOVA) was used to compare the effect of condition (RSV and placebo) and time (fasted and post-prandial) for blood measures, gas exchange analysis, and all muscle biopsy derived data. A Bonferonni correction was used for post-hoc pairwise comparison of means for main effects and significant interactions. As adipose tissue biopsies were obtained at a single time point, paired t-tests were used to compare the effect of placebo or RSV on protein content and phosphorylation or acetylation status. For experiment two, due to missing data, complete data sets were not available for several participants for either the RSV or vehicle conditions (please see results for details). As a result, a two-way ANOVA with repeated measures for concentration only was utilized to compare the effects of condition (RSV and vehicle) with concentration. A bonferonni correction for post-hoc comparisons of main effects and interactions. Data analysis was completed with GraphPad Prism v 5.01 (GraphPad Software Inc., La Jolla, CA). Statistical significance was accepted at $p<0.05$.

Results

RSV and Skeletal Muscle Signalling

No effect of time (fasted vs. post-prandial) or RSV was observed for nuclear SIRT1 activity (Fig. 1A). Further, while there was a significant effect of time ($P<0.05$) observed for p-PKA substrates between 50 and 250 kDa (but not 25–50 kDa), no effects of time or RSV were observed for the acetylation status of p53 (SIRT1 substrate), p-AMPK or p-ACC (Fig. 1B). No effects of time or RSV were observed for total AMPK, total ACC or GAPDH. Representative blots for all protein measured are presented in Fig. 1C.

RSV and Adipose Tissue Signaling

There was no effect of RSV on the acetylation status of p53 or the phosphorylation status of p38 MAPK, AMPK, ACC, Akt (Ser473 and Thr308) (Fig. 2A). Representative blots for all protein measure in adipose tissue are presented in Fig. 2B.

Whole Body VO_2 and Fatty Acid Oxidation

VO_2 increased in both conditions (Table 2) with no effect of RSV observed. Respiratory exchange ratio (RER) was unchanged post-prandial in both placebo and RSV (Table 2) with no effect of RSV observed. Estimated rates of fatty acid oxidation increased in a time-dependent fashion approaching significance (main effect of time, $P=0.08$; Table 2). No effect of group and no interaction effects were observed for fatty acid oxidation rates. Plasma glycerol, a marker of systemic lipolysis, demonstrated a significant effect of time ($P<0.05$; Table 2) with no effect of RSV observed.

Blood insulin and Intracellular Insulin Signalling

A significant interaction effect ($P<0.05$) and main effect of time ($P<0.05$) were observed for plasma insulin concentration with a lower plasma insulin concentration observed in the post-prandial state in RSV compared to placebo (Table 2; Fig. 3A). There was no effect of time (fasted vs. post-prandial) or condition (placebo vs. RSV) on plasma glucose concentrations (Table 2; Fig. 3B). A significant interaction effect ($P<0.05$) was observed for p38 MAPK with a reduction in phosphorylation observed following placebo (−27±11%), and an increase following RSV (+36±19%). p-AKT (Ser473) increased in a time dependent fashion ($P<0.05$) following both RSV (+73±21%) and placebo (+82±22%), with no interaction or group effect. Similarly, p-AS160 increased in a time dependent fashion ($P<0.05$) with no independent effect of RSV observed. There were no significant changes with time (fasted vs. post-prandial) or condition (placebo vs. RSV) on p-Akt (Thr308) (Fig. 3C). Representative blots for all protein measured are presented in Fig. 3D.

RSV and Mitochondrial Respiration

As a result of tissue limitations full data sets were not available for all participants (i.e. some participants were missing either a vehicle or a RSV sample). When a participant was missing a sample for a given substrate, their data for that substrate were excluded from the analysis resulting in an final n of 7, 5, 6, and 6 for glutamate, succinate, pyruvate and palmitoyl CoA respectively. RSV resulted in a significant reduction in mitochondrial respiration with significant ($P<0.05$) effects of time, group and group by time interactions observed for glutamate (Fig. 4A), succinate (Fig. 4B), pyruvate (Fig. 4C), and palmitoyl carnitine (Fig. 4D). Post-hoc analysis revealed that the RSV concentration required to impair respiration was 300 μM, 100 μM, 200 μM, and 300 μM for glutamate, succinate, pyruvate and palmitoyl carnitine, respectively.

Discussion

The present study examined both the effect of a single dose of RSV (300 mg) on skeletal muscle and adipose tissue intracellular signalling, and whole body fatty acid oxidation *in vivo* in

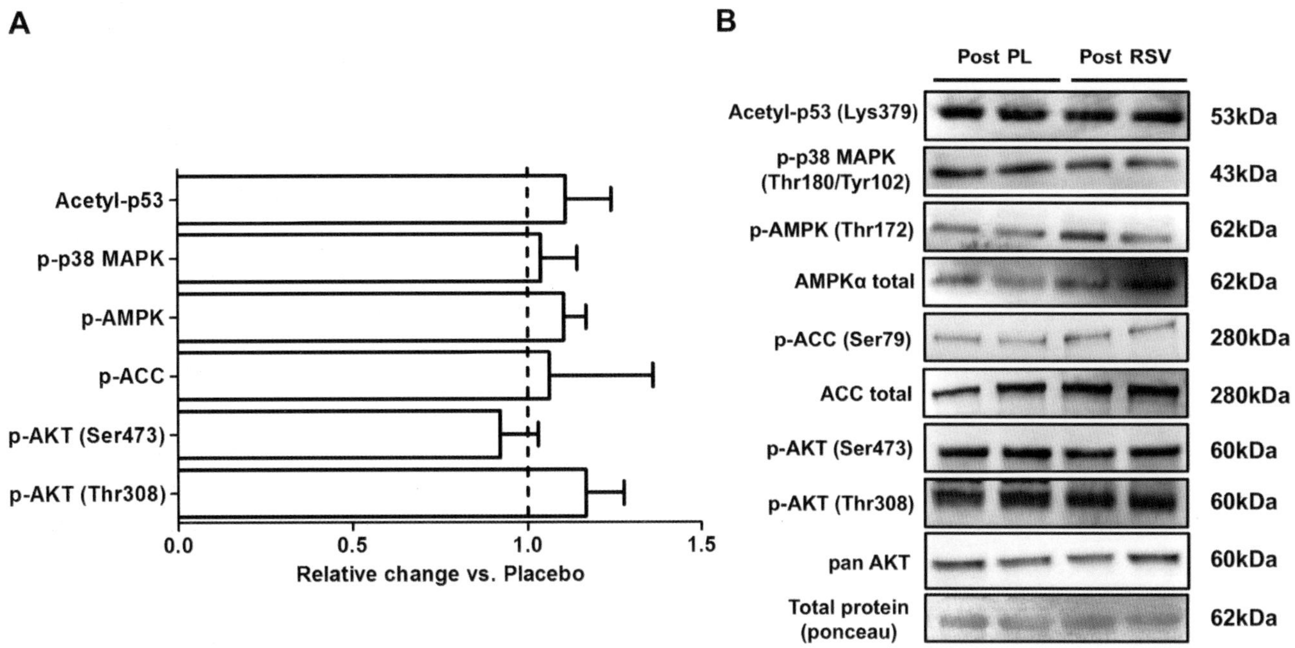

Figure 2. Adipose tissue signaling is unaltered by resveratrol. Phosphorylated protein content (A) in the post-prandial (post) state following resveratrol (RSV) expressed relative to placebo (PL). Representative blots for all proteins are also shown (B).

overweight young men, as well as the effects of RSV on mitochondrial respiration in skeletal muscle mitochondria obtained from lean adult men *ex vivo*. Our *in vivo* results indicate that a single oral dose of RSV appears to have no effect on the activation of the intracellular signalling pathways (specifically AMPK and SIRT1) through which RSV is proposed to alter cellular function in either skeletal muscle (Fig. 1) or adipose tissue (Fig. 2). Interestingly, RSV reduced post-prandial blood insulin concentrations; however, this response was not explained by altered insulin signalling in either skeletal muscle or adipose tissue. Finally, we present novel data demonstrating that higher concentrations of RSV inhibit mitochondrial respiration in PmFBs from human skeletal muscle obtained from lean adults. These results suggest that either a single dose of resveratrol is not adequate to activate intracellular signalling pathways, or that relatively low orally administered doses of RSV are unable to acutely impact skeletal muscle and adipose tissue function in overweight humans *in vivo*. Further, the inhibition of mitochondrial respiration by RSV suggests that caution is warranted should future studies attempt to increase the bioavailability of RSV in humans *in vivo*.

RSV Mechanism of Action in Skeletal Muscle and Adipose Tissue In Vivo

In both muscle cells, and in rodent skeletal muscle, RSV exposure induces the activation of SIRT1 which translates into positive effects on mitochondrial biogenesis through the deacetylation of PGC-1α [2,4,10,18,19]. Based on these results several models have been proposed regarding RSV's mechanism of action in skeletal muscle including both indirect activation of SIRT1 through cAMP dependent activation of AMPK and increased availability of SIRT1 substrate [10,19], and direct activation of SIRT1 by RSV and the subsequent activation of AMPK via

Table 2. Changes in metabolic and plasma measures from fasting to the post-prandial state in both the Placebo and RSV conditions.

	Placebo		RSV	
	Fasted	**Post-prandial**	**Fasted**	**Post-prandial**
VO_2 (ml/min) ‡	307±108	340±97	373±111	387±124
RER	0.82±0.05	0.81±0.05	0.81±0.06	0.82±0.07
Fatty Acid Oxidation (kcal/min)	0.87±0.15	1.04±0.22	0.97±0.19	1.11±0.18
Plasma Glycerol (mmol/L) ‡	0.08±0.02	0.07±0.03	0.10±0.03	0.08±0.04
Plasma Insulin (μIU/L) †‡	7.2±3.5	27.6±5.7	7.8±3.3	19.0±2.5
Plasma Glucose (mmol/L)	5.1±0.2	5.2±0.2	5.3±0.3	5.0±0.3

Values are means ± SD. VO_2, Oxygen uptake; RER, Respiratory Exchange Ratio; ml, millimeters; kcal, kilocalories; mmol, millimole; mIU, micro international units.
‡Significant effect ($P<0.05$) of time.
†Significant interaction ($P<0.05$).

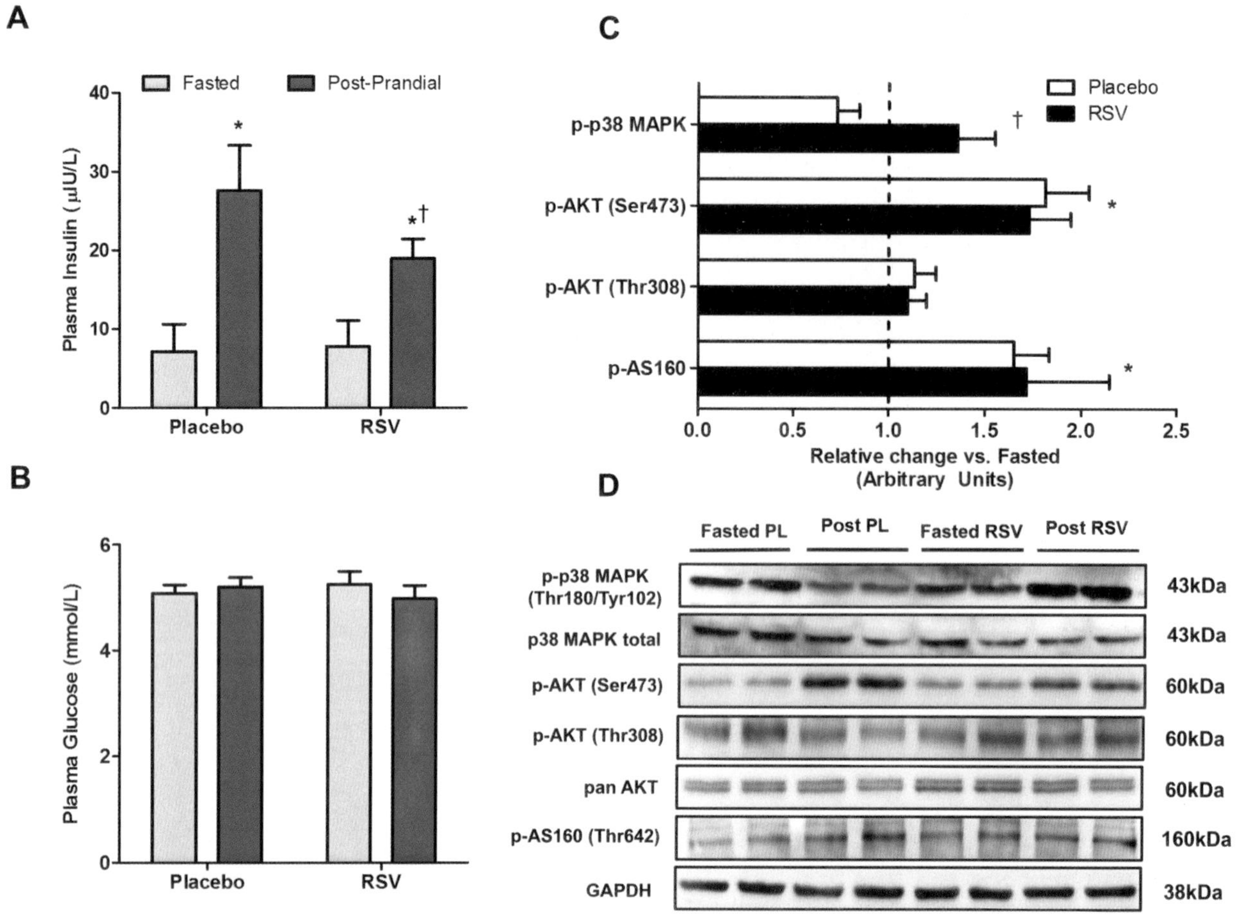

Figure 3. Impact of an acute dose of resveratrol on 2 hour blood insulin and glucose concentrations and insulin signaling in muscle. Plasma insulin (A) and plasma glucose (B) concentrations in the fasted (light bars) and post-prandial (dark bars) state. The change in phosphorylated protein content (C) in the post-prandial (post) state (expressed relative to fasting) in the placebo (PL; open bars) and resveratrol (RSV; shaded bars) conditions. Representative blots for all proteins are shown (D). * Significantly different ($P<0.05$) from fasted within same condition. † Significant interaction ($P<0.05$) between RSV and placebo.

LKB1 [13,18]. In these models, while the position of AMPK, either upstream [19] or downstream [18] of SIRT1 is controversial, its activation remains an essential component of both proposed RSV-SIRT1 pathways [17]. In the current study, a single dose of RSV in overweight adults had no effect on markers of either AMPK (p-AMPK and p-ACC) or SIRT1 (nuclear SIRT1 [muscle only] and acetyl-p53) activity in either skeletal muscle (Fig. 1) or adipose tissue (Fig. 3). Further, there was no effect of RSV on p-PKA substrates in skeletal muscle (Fig. 1), a result that is consistent with unaltered cAMP and PDE activity, a proposed target of RSV in animal tissue [18]. In contrast to evidence from cellular models where a single dose of RSV can activate AMPK and SIRT1 [17–19,21], these results suggest that a single 300 mg dose of RSV administered to overweight adults does not activate SIRT1 in human skeletal muscle or adipose tissue *in vivo*.

The lack of an acute effect of RSV on intracellular signalling in either skeletal muscle or adipose tissue in the current study likely reflects poor bioavailability of RSV following a single intraoral dose [45]. This potential bioavailability limitation of RSV in humans may help explain several recent reports that chronic administration of RSV has no effect on skeletal muscle or adipose tissue [27,28]. Alternatively, the lack of an effect of RSV observed in the current study, and in previous reports [27,28] may be attributed to the healthy populations studied (current study, overweight men; [27], non-obese women; [28], obese men). However, this is difficult to reconcile with the positive effects observed by Timmers et al. [24] in otherwise healthy obese men. The results from Timmers et al. [24] are also in contrast to the potential bioavailability limitation to RSV action in humans as they reported elevated AMPK phosphorylation, increased protein content of both SIRT1 and its downstream targets following chronic RSV administration. These results raise the possibility that an additive effect of repeated RSV ingestion may increase bioavailability within skeletal muscle and other peripheral tissues, although accumulation of RSV in plasma samples have not been observed following repeated RSV dosages at a similar dose to that used by Timmers et al. [24] or in the current study [46]. It remains difficult to reconcile the positive effects of RSV observed by Timmers et al. [24] with recent studies demonstrating no effects [27,28] of chronic RSV and the current data demonstrating no effect of an acute dose of RSV. It should be mentioned that several RSV metabolites have also been shown to have biological effects [47], however, if these metabolites were elevated following a single RSV dose in the current study, they appear not to have impacted skeletal muscle or adipose tissue. This suggests that either 1) a single 300 mg dose does not produce enough active metabolites to activate musculoskeletal pathways, and/or 2) that these metabo-

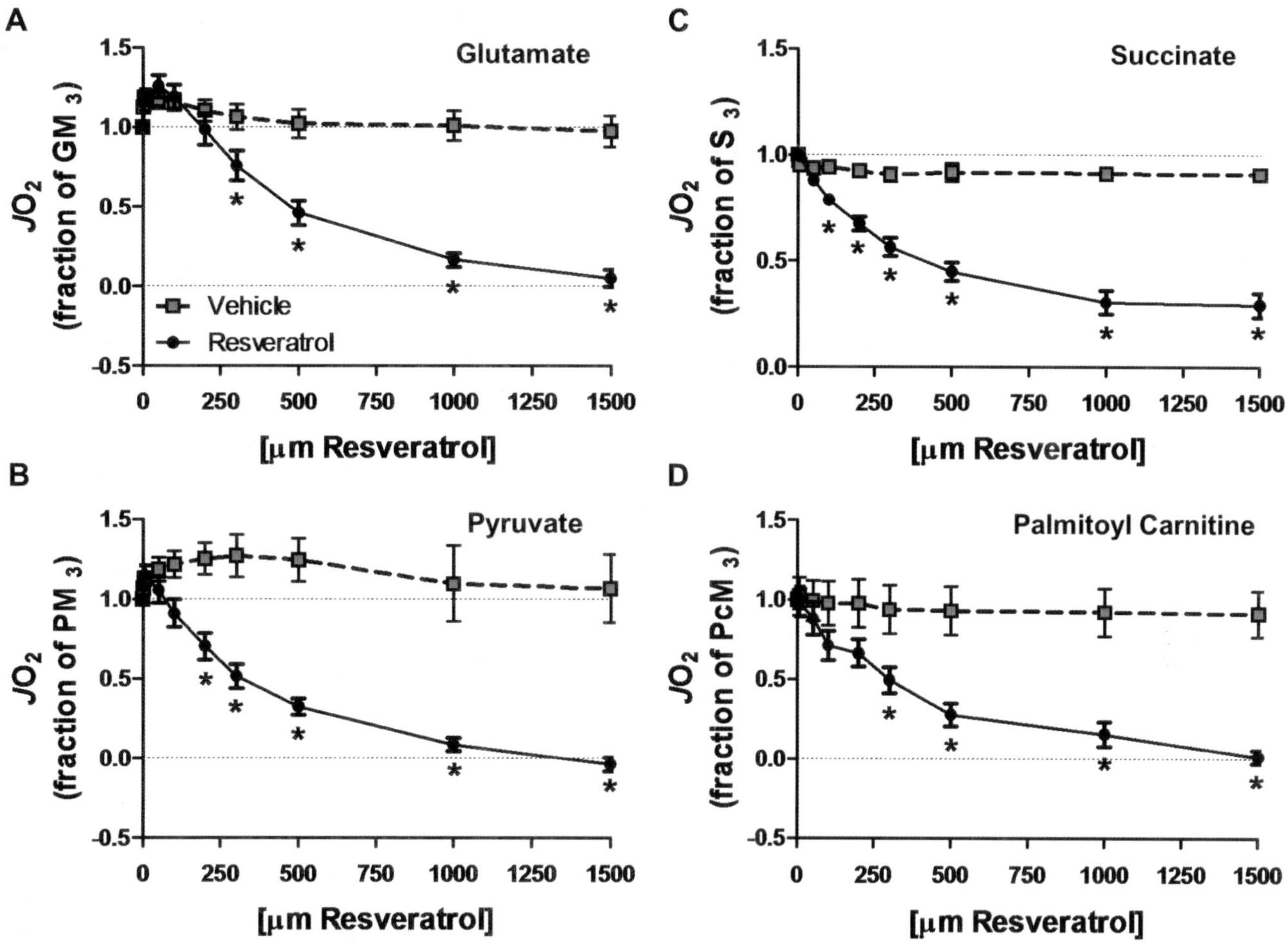

Figure 4. Resveratrol inhibits mitochondrial respiration in permeabilized muscle fibre bundles. The effect of resveratrol or vehicle (DMSO) on substrate-specific respiration was determined by titrating resveratrol following the induction of state 3 respiration with either 10 mM glutamate (A), 10 mM succinate (B), 10 mM pyruvate (C) or 40 µM palmitoyl carnitine (D) with 5 mM malate in all protocols. Changes in mitochondrial respiration are expressed relative to maximal state 3 respiration determined immediately prior to the resveratrol titration. * Significantly different ($P < 0.05$) from vehicle treatment.

lites are not responsible for the proposed effects on skeletal muscle energetic pathways.

An Alternative Mechanism Explaining the Activation of AMPK and SIRT1 in Skeletal Muscle

While there is evidence that RSV can interact directly with signalling molecules such as SIRT1 in skeletal muscle [13,18,19,48] it is also possible that RSV mediated activation of pathways associated with AMPK may result from an acute impairment in the ability of mitochondria to produce ATP [18,21–23]. Consistent with the latter mechanism, we have demonstrated, for the first time in intact human skeletal muscle fibres (obtained from lean adult men), that RSV impairs mitochondrial oxidation of multiple substrates, including fatty acids and pyruvate (Fig. 4). While the mechanism underlying the observed inhibition is unclear, two potential mechanisms exist. First, RSV-meditated inhibition of ATP synthase [20] would directly inhibit mitochondrial respiration regardless of which substrate is oxidized. Conceivably, this may impair energy homeostasis leading to activation of AMPK. Second, SIRT3 inhibition by RSV [49] may indirectly inhibit respiration via acetylation-based regulation of substrate catabolism though altered substrate provision to the electron transport chain [50]. Regardless of the mechanism(s), our results support the possibility that activation of AMPK/SIRT1 *in vivo* may result from RSV-mediated inhibition of ATP production/mitochondrial respiration.

This possibility positions RSV as a potential hormetic agent, a topic that has received recent attention in several other fields [51], but to date has been generally dismissed in skeletal muscle and metabolic health research [1]. While toxic effects of RSV have been demonstrated in muscle cells [21], this effect was observed at concentrations (20–50 µM) above those generally observed in human plasma *in vivo* (<5 µM) [45]. Our results also demonstrated impaired mitochondrial respiration at seemingly supraphysiological levels (~100–300 µM depending on the substrate examined) a result that is consistent with the lack of an effect of RSV on whole body VO_2 observed in experiment #1. While this logic has been used in the past to dismiss a possible toxic effect of RSV *in vivo* [1], our results suggest that attempts to increase RSV bioavailability using high oral dosages [28] or alternative methods of delivery [52] be approached with caution such that [RSV] be controlled within a hormetic zone far below toxic levels.

The current results contribute to a rapidly growing number of chronic RSV supplementation trials and the significant controversy regarding RSVs mechanism(s) of action in animals. The findings of acute inhibition of mitochondrial respiration in intact skeletal muscle from lean adult men provide a potential alternative mechanisms of RSV action and underscore the dearth of information regarding how and/or if RSV alters cellular function in humans, highlighting the need for future work to reconcile the divergent acute and chronic effects of RSV.

RSV and Control of Blood Insulin

Interestingly, we observed that an acute dose of RSV decreased blood insulin (compared to placebo) 2 hours post meal challenge in overweight men (Fig. 3). The similar post-prandial phosphorylation of Akt and AS160, two of the critical intermediates in the insulin-signaling pathway, observed in skeletal muscle (Fig. 2C) and adipose tissue (Akt only; Fig. 2A), despite a lower plasma insulin concentration with RSV, suggests that RSV may improve insulin sensitivity and glucose clearance in peripheral tissue. While this effect may have been related to the elevated p38 MAPK phosphorylation observed in the RSV condition (Fig. 3), p38 MAPK is implicated as both a contributor to insulin sensitivity [53,54] and an activator of GLUT4 mediated glucose transport [55], this is speculative at this juncture and it is difficult to draw any solid conclusions regarding the mechanisms underlying the lower post-prandial insulin levels from the current data set. Further, it is unclear whether lower insulin 2 hours post meal would have been reflected in different glucose/insulin kinetics during the immediate post meal period (i.e. <2 hours) and this represents an interesting question worthy of future study. Alternatively, RSV-mediated decreases in plasma insulin may have resulted from other tissues not examined in the current study. For example, RSV is known to impact liver function [4] and can inhibit pancreatic insulin production in isolated pancreatic islets [56].

Regardless of mechanism, the observed change in blood insulin 2 hours post meal with RSV contributes to previous data demonstrating an insulin sensitizing effect of chronic RSV supplementation [24–26]. While not all studies in humans have observed improved insulin sensitivity [27,28], our findings suggest a potentially novel clinical outcome. Specifically, that RSV may acutely boost endogenous insulin action, possibly in addition to the therapeutic/preventative benefit associated with the chronic adaptations. However, given the poor time resolution of the current study, the acute effects of RSV on glucose kinetics, uptake by peripheral tissue along with changes in insulin secretion by the pancreas represent important areas for future study.

Conclusions

The current study examined both the effect of a single dose of RSV (300 mg) on several metabolic outcomes and intracellular signaling pathways hypothesized to be affected by RSV in overweight humans *in vivo*, as well as the impact of RSV on human skeletal muscle mitochondrial respiration in PmFBs obtained from lean men *ex vivo*. Our *in vivo* results demonstrate that a single dose of RSV appears to have no impact on skeletal muscle and adipocyte intracellular signalling in overweight men, likely resulting from limited bioavailability. Interestingly, the lower blood insulin observed following RSV may reflect acute effects of RSV on either hepatic or pancreatic function. Finally, we have demonstrated that RSV impairs mitochondrial oxidation of multiple substrates including fatty acids and pyruvate in human PmFBs obtained from lean adult men. The latter result suggests a mito-toxic nature of resveratrol that has not previously been considered in human muscle and may stimulate hormetic improvements in metabolic capacities; however, this effect would appear to only occur at supra-physiological concentrations of RSV. Future studies should continue to examine the mechanisms by which RSV alters physiological function in humans with the important caveat that caution is warranted should higher doses, or alternative means of administration aimed at increased RSV bioavailability be pursued.

Author Contributions

Performed the experiments: CBW MCH BAE TDS CAS CGRP BJG. Analyzed the data: CBW MCH BAE TDS CAS CGRP BJG. Contributed reagents/materials/analysis tools: CGRP BJG. Contributed to collection, interpretation and analysis of data: CBW CAS CGRP BJG CBW MCH BAE TDS CAS CGRP BJG. Primary writers of the manuscript while all authors contributed to critical interpretation and manuscript preparation: CBW BJG. Approved the final manuscript: CBW MCH BAE TDS CAS CGRP BJG.

References

1. Chung JH, Manganiello V, Dyck JR (2012) Resveratrol as a calorie restriction mimetic: therapeutic implications. Trends Cell Biol 22: 546–554. S0962-8924(12)00114-6 [pii];10.1016/j.tcb.2012.07.004 [doi].
2. Lagouge M, Argmann C, Gerhart-Hines Z, Meziane H, Lerin C, et al. (2006) Resveratrol improves mitochondrial function and protects against metabolic disease by activating SIRT1 and PGC-1alpha. Cell 127: 1109–1122. S0092-8674(06)01428-0 [pii];10.1016/j.cell.2006.11.013 [doi].
3. Dal-Pan A, Blanc S, Aujard F (2010) Resveratrol suppresses body mass gain in a seasonal non-human primate model of obesity. BMC Physiol 10: 11. 1472-6793-10-11 [pii];10.1186/1472-6793-10-11 [doi].
4. Baur JA, Pearson KJ, Price NL, Jamieson HA, Lerin C, et al. (2006) Resveratrol improves health and survival of mice on a high-calorie diet. Nature 444: 337–342. nature05354 [pii];10.1038/nature05354 [doi].
5. Pearson KJ, Baur JA, Lewis KN, Peshkin L, Price NL, et al. (2008) Resveratrol delays age-related deterioration and mimics transcriptional aspects of dietary restriction without extending life span. Cell Metab 8: 157–168. S1550-4131(08)00182-4 [pii];10.1016/j.cmet.2008.06.011 [doi].
6. Su HC, Hung LM, Chen JK (2006) Resveratrol, a red wine antioxidant, possesses an insulin-like effect in streptozotocin-induced diabetic rats. Am J Physiol Endocrinol Metab 290: E1339–E1346. 00487.2005 [pii];10.1152/ajpendo.00487.2005 [doi].
7. Kang W, Hong HJ, Guan J, Kim DG, Yang EJ, et al. (2012) Resveratrol improves insulin signaling in a tissue-specific manner under insulin-resistant conditions only: in vitro and in vivo experiments in rodents. Metabolism 61: 424–433. S0026-0495(11)00269-1 [pii];10.1016/j.metabol.2011.08.003 [doi].
8. Andersen G, Burkon A, Sulzmaier FJ, Walker JM, Leckband G, et al. (2011) High dose of dietary resveratrol enhances insulin sensitivity in healthy rats but does not lead to metabolite concentrations effective for SIRT1 expression. Mol Nutr Food Res 55: 1197–1206. 10.1002/mnfr.201100292 [doi].
9. Marchal J, Blanc S, Epelbaum J, Aujard F, Pifferi F (2012) Effects of chronic calorie restriction or dietary resveratrol supplementation on insulin sensitivity markers in a primate, Microcebus murinus. PLoS ONE 7: e34289. 10.1371/journal.pone.0034289 [doi];PONE-D-11-25547 [pii].
10. Canto C, Gerhart-Hines Z, Feige JN, Lagouge M, Noriega L, et al. (2009) AMPK regulates energy expenditure by modulating NAD+ metabolism and SIRT1 activity. Nature 458: 1056–1060. nature07813 [pii];10.1038/nature07813 [doi].
11. Canto C, Auwerx J (2009) PGC-1alpha, SIRT1 and AMPK, an energy sensing network that controls energy expenditure. Curr Opin Lipidol 20: 98–105. 10.1097/MOL.0b013e328328d0a4 [doi];00041433-200904000-00004 [pii].
12. Howitz KT, Bitterman KJ, Cohen HY, Lamming DW, Lavu S, et al. (2003) Small molecule activators of sirtuins extend Saccharomyces cerevisiae lifespan. Nature 425: 191–196. 10.1038/nature01960 [doi];nature01960 [pii].
13. Hubbard BP, Gomes AP, Dai H, Li J, Case AW, et al. (2013) Evidence for a common mechanism of SIRT1 regulation by allosteric activators. Science 339: 1216–1219. 339/6124/1216 [pii];10.1126/science.1231097 [doi].
14. Kaeberlein M, McDonagh T, Heltweg B, Hixon J, Westman EA, et al. (2005) Substrate-specific activation of sirtuins by resveratrol. J Biol Chem 280: 17038–17045. M500655200 [pii];10.1074/jbc.M500655200 [doi].
15. Pacholec M, Bleasdale JE, Chrunyk B, Cunningham D, Flynn D, et al. (2010) SRT1720, SRT2183, SRT1460, and resveratrol are not direct activators of SIRT1. J Biol Chem 285: 8340–8351. M109.088682 [pii];10.1074/jbc.M109.088682 [doi].
16. Park CE, Kim MJ, Lee JH, Min BI, Bae H, et al. (2007) Resveratrol stimulates glucose transport in C2C12 myotubes by activating AMP-activated protein

kinase. Exp Mol Med 39: 222–229. 2007043011 [pii];10.1038/emm.2007.25 [doi].
17. Um JH, Park SJ, Kang H, Yang S, Foretz M, et al. (2010) AMP-activated protein kinase-deficient mice are resistant to the metabolic effects of resveratrol. Diabetes 59: 554–563. db09-0482 [pii];10.2337/db09-0482 [doi].
18. Price NL, Gomes AP, Ling AJ, Duarte FV, Martin-Montalvo A, et al. (2012) SIRT1 is required for AMPK activation and the beneficial effects of resveratrol on mitochondrial function. Cell Metab 15: 675–690. S1550-4131(12)00143-X [pii];10.1016/j.cmet.2012.04.003 [doi].
19. Park SJ, Ahmad F, Philp A, Baar K, Williams T, et al. (2012) Resveratrol ameliorates aging-related metabolic phenotypes by inhibiting cAMP phosphodiesterases. Cell 148: 421–433. S0092-8674(12)00030-X [pii];10.1016/j.cell.2012.01.017 [doi].
20. Zheng J, Ramirez VD (2000) Inhibition of mitochondrial proton F0F1-ATPase/ATP synthase by polyphenolic phytochemicals. Br J Pharmacol 130: 1115–1123. 10.1038/sj.bjp.0703397 [doi].
21. Higashida K, Kim SH, Jung SR, Asaka M, Holloszy JO, et al. (2013) Effects of Resveratrol and SIRT1 on PGC-1alpha Activity and Mitochondrial Biogenesis: A Reevaluation. PLoS Biol 11: e1001603. 10.1371/journal.pbio.1001603 [doi];PBIOLOGY-D-13-00038 [pii].
22. Zang M, Xu S, Maitland-Toolan KA, Zuccollo A, Hou X, et al. (2006) Polyphenols stimulate AMP-activated protein kinase, lower lipids, and inhibit accelerated atherosclerosis in diabetic LDL receptor-deficient mice. Diabetes 55: 2180–2191. 55/8/2180 [pii];10.2337/db05-1188 [doi].
23. Hawley SA, Ross FA, Chevtzoff C, Green KA, Evans A, et al. (2010) Use of cells expressing gamma subunit variants to identify diverse mechanisms of AMPK activation. Cell Metab 11: 554–565. S1550-4131(10)00112-9 [pii];10.1016/j.cmet.2010.04.001 [doi].
24. Timmers S, Konings E, Bilet L, Houtkooper RH, van de Weijer T, et al. (2011) Calorie restriction-like effects of 30 days of resveratrol supplementation on energy metabolism and metabolic profile in obese humans. Cell Metab 14: 612–622. S1550-4131(11)00386-X [pii];10.1016/j.cmet.2011.10.002 [doi].
25. Brasnyo P, Molnar GA, Mohas M, Marko L, Laczy B, et al. (2011) Resveratrol improves insulin sensitivity, reduces oxidative stress and activates the Akt pathway in type 2 diabetic patients. Br J Nutr 106: 383–389. S0007114511000316 [pii];10.1017/S0007114511000316 [doi].
26. Crandall JP, Oram V, Trandafirescu G, Reid M, Kishore P, et al. (2012) Pilot study of resveratrol in older adults with impaired glucose tolerance. J Gerontol A Biol Sci Med Sci 67: 1307–1312. glr235 [pii];10.1093/gerona/glr235 [doi].
27. Yoshino J, Conte C, Fontana L, Mittendorfer B, Imai S, et al. (2012) Resveratrol supplementation does not improve metabolic function in nonobese women with normal glucose tolerance. Cell Metab 16: 658–664. S1550-4131(12)00399-3 [pii];10.1016/j.cmet.2012.09.015 [doi].
28. Poulsen MM, Vestergaard PF, Clasen BF, Radko Y, Christensen LP, et al. (2013) High-dose resveratrol supplementation in obese men: an investigator-initiated, randomized, placebo-controlled clinical trial of substrate metabolism, insulin sensitivity, and body composition. Diabetes 62: 1186–1195. db12-0975 [pii];10.2337/db12-0975 [doi].
29. Lean ME, Han TS, Morrison CE (1995) Waist circumference as a measure for indicating need for weight management. BMJ 311: 158–161.
30. Bergstrom J (1975) Percutaneous needle biopsy of skeletal muscle in physiological and clinical research. Scand J Clin Lab Invest 35: 609–616.
31. Vissing K, Andersen JL, Schjerling P (2005) Are exercise-induced genes induced by exercise? FASEB J 19: 94–96. 04-2084fje [pii];10.1096/fj.04-2084fje [doi].
32. Guerra B, Gomez-Cabrera MC, Ponce-Gonzalez JG, Martinez-Bello VE, Guadalupe-Grau A, et al. (2011) Repeated muscle biopsies through a single skin incision do not elicit muscle signaling, but IL-6 mRNA and STAT3 phosphorylation increase in injured muscle. J Appl Physiol (1985) 110: 1708–1715. japplphysiol.00091.2011 [pii];10.1152/japplphysiol.00091.2011 [doi].
33. Holloway GP, Bezaire V, Heigenhauser GJ, Tandon NN, Glatz JF, et al. (2006) Mitochondrial long chain fatty acid oxidation, fatty acid translocase/CD36 content and carnitine palmitoyltransferase I activity in human skeletal muscle during aerobic exercise. J Physiol 571: 201–210. jphysiol.2005.102178 [pii];10.1113/jphysiol.2005.102178 [doi].
34. Gurd BJ, Yoshida Y, McFarlan JT, Holloway GP, Moyes CD, et al. (2011) Nuclear SIRT1 activity, but not protein content, regulates mitochondrial biogenesis in rat and human skeletal muscle. Am J Physiol Regul Integr Comp Physiol 301: R67–R75. ajpregu.00417.2010 [pii];10.1152/ajpregu.00417.2010 [doi].
35. Holloway GP, Gurd BJ, Snook LA, Lally J, Bonen A (2010) Compensatory increases in nuclear PGC1{alpha} protein are primarily associated with subsarcolemmal mitochondrial adaptations in ZDF rats. Diabetes. db09–1519 [pii];10.2337/db09-1519 [doi].
36. Little JP, Safdar A, Bishop D, Tarnopolsky MA, Gibala MJ (2011) An acute bout of high-intensity interval training increases the nuclear abundance of PGC-1alpha and activates mitochondrial biogenesis in human skeletal muscle. Am J Physiol Regul Integr Comp Physiol 300: R1303–R1310. ajpregu.00538.2010 [pii];10.1152/ajpregu.00538.2010 [doi].
37. Little JP, Safdar A, Cermak N, Tarnopolsky MA, Gibala MJ (2010) Acute endurance exercise increases the nuclear abundance of PGC-1alpha in trained human skeletal muscle. Am J Physiol Regul Integr Comp Physiol 298: R912–R917. 00409.2009 [pii];10.1152/ajpregu.00409.2009 [doi].
38. Kuznetsov AV, Tiivel T, Sikk P, Kaambre T, Kay L, et al. (1996) Striking differences between the kinetics of regulation of respiration by ADP in slow-twitch and fast-twitch muscles in vivo. Eur J Biochem 241: 909–915.
39. Tonkonogi M, Fernstrom M, Walsh B, Ji LL, Rooyackers O, et al. (2003) Reduced oxidative power but unchanged antioxidative capacity in skeletal muscle from aged humans. Pflugers Arch 446: 261–269. 10.1007/s00424-003-1044-9 [doi].
40. Perry CG, Kane DA, Lin CT, Kozy R, Cathey BL, et al. (2011) Inhibiting myosin-ATPase reveals a dynamic range of mitochondrial respiratory control in skeletal muscle. Biochem J 437: 215–222. BJ20110366 [pii];10.1042/BJ20110366 [doi].
41. Perry CG, Kane DA, Lanza IR, Neufer PD (2013) Methods for assessing mitochondrial function in diabetes. Diabetes 62: 1041–1053. 62/4/1041 [pii];10.2337/db12-1219 [doi].
42. Kane DA, Lin CT, Anderson EJ, Kwak HB, Cox JH, et al. (2011) Progesterone increases skeletal muscle mitochondrial H2O2 emission in nonmenopausal women. Am J Physiol Endocrinol Metab 300: E528–E535. ajpendo.00389.2010 [pii];10.1152/ajpendo.00389.2010 [doi].
43. Pesta Gnaiger (2012) Mitochondrial Bioenergetics. Methods in Molecular Biology 810: 25–58.
44. Boocock DJ, Faust GE, Patel KR, Schinas AM, Brown VA, et al. (2007) Phase I dose escalation pharmacokinetic study in healthy volunteers of resveratrol, a potential cancer chemopreventive agent. Cancer Epidemiol Biomarkers Prev 16: 1246–1252. 16/6/1246 [pii];10.1158/1055-9965.EPI-07-0022 [doi].
45. Patel KR, Scott E, Brown VA, Gescher AJ, Steward WP, et al. (2011) Clinical trials of resveratrol. Ann N Y Acad Sci 1215: 161–169. 10.1111/j.1749-6632.2010.05853.x [doi].
46. Brown VA, Patel KR, Viskaduraki M, Crowell JA, Perloff M, et al. (2010) Repeat dose study of the cancer chemopreventive agent resveratrol in healthy volunteers: safety, pharmacokinetics, and effect on the insulin-like growth factor axis. Cancer Res 70: 9003–9011. 0008-5472.CAN-10-2364 [pii];10.1158/0008-5472.CAN-10-2364 [doi].
47. Lasa A, Churruca I, Eseberri I, Andres-Lacueva C, Portillo MP (2012) Delipidating effect of resveratrol metabolites in 3T3-L1 adipocytes. Mol Nutr Food Res 56: 1559–1568. 10.1002/mnfr.201100772 [doi].
48. Horowitz JF (2003) Fatty acid mobilization from adipose tissue during exercise. Trends Endocrinol Metab 14: 386–392. S1043276003001437 [pii].
49. Gertz M, Nguyen GT, Fischer F, Suenkel B, Schlicker C, et al. (2012) A molecular mechanism for direct sirtuin activation by resveratrol. PLoS ONE 7: e49761. 10.1371/journal.pone.0049761 [doi];PONE-D-12-24873 [pii].
50. White AT, Schenk S (2012) NAD(+)/NADH and skeletal muscle mitochondrial adaptations to exercise. Am J Physiol Endocrinol Metab 303: E308–E321. ajpendo.00054.2012 [pii];10.1152/ajpendo.00054.2012 [doi].
51. Calabrese EJ, Mattson MP, Calabrese V (2010) Resveratrol commonly displays hormesis: occurrence and biomedical significance. Hum Exp Toxicol 29: 980–1015. 29/12/980 [pii];10.1177/0960327110383625 [doi].
52. Walle T, Hsieh F, DeLegge MH, Oatis JE, Jr., Walle UK (2004) High absorption but very low bioavailability of oral resveratrol in humans. Drug Metab Dispos 32: 1377–1382. 10.1124/dmd.104.000885 [doi];dmd.104.000885 [pii].
53. Somwar R, Perreault M, Kapur S, Taha C, Sweeney G, et al. (2000) Activation of p38 mitogen-activated protein kinase alpha and beta by insulin and contraction in rat skeletal muscle: potential role in the stimulation of glucose transport. Diabetes 49: 1794–1800.
54. Thong FS, Derave W, Urso B, Kiens B, Richter EA (2003) Prior exercise increases basal and insulin-induced p38 mitogen-activated protein kinase phosphorylation in human skeletal muscle. J Appl Physiol 94: 2337–2341. 10.1152/japplphysiol.00036.2003 [doi];00036.2003 [pii].
55. Furtado LM, Somwar R, Sweeney G, Niu W, Klip A (2002) Activation of the glucose transporter GLUT4 by insulin. Biochem Cell Biol 80: 569–578.
56. Szkudelski T (2007) Resveratrol-induced inhibition of insulin secretion from rat pancreatic islets: evidence for pivotal role of metabolic disturbances. Am J Physiol Endocrinol Metab 293: E901–E907. 00564.2006 [pii];10.1152/ajpendo.00564.2006 [doi].

Permissions

All chapters in this book were first published in PLOS ONE, by The Public Library of Science; hereby published with permission under the Creative Commons Attribution License or equivalent. Every chapter published in this book has been scrutinized by our experts. Their significance has been extensively debated. The topics covered herein carry significant findings which will fuel the growth of the discipline. They may even be implemented as practical applications or may be referred to as a beginning point for another development.

The contributors of this book come from diverse backgrounds, making this book a truly international effort. This book will bring forth new frontiers with its revolutionizing research information and detailed analysis of the nascent developments around the world.

We would like to thank all the contributing authors for lending their expertise to make the book truly unique. They have played a crucial role in the development of this book. Without their invaluable contributions this book wouldn't have been possible. They have made vital efforts to compile up to date information on the varied aspects of this subject to make this book a valuable addition to the collection of many professionals and students.

This book was conceptualized with the vision of imparting up-to-date information and advanced data in this field. To ensure the same, a matchless editorial board was set up. Every individual on the board went through rigorous rounds of assessment to prove their worth. After which they invested a large part of their time researching and compiling the most relevant data for our readers.

The editorial board has been involved in producing this book since its inception. They have spent rigorous hours researching and exploring the diverse topics which have resulted in the successful publishing of this book. They have passed on their knowledge of decades through this book. To expedite this challenging task, the publisher supported the team at every step. A small team of assistant editors was also appointed to further simplify the editing procedure and attain best results for the readers.

Apart from the editorial board, the designing team has also invested a significant amount of their time in understanding the subject and creating the most relevant covers. They scrutinized every image to scout for the most suitable representation of the subject and create an appropriate cover for the book.

The publishing team has been an ardent support to the editorial, designing and production team. Their endless efforts to recruit the best for this project, has resulted in the accomplishment of this book. They are a veteran in the field of academics and their pool of knowledge is as vast as their experience in printing. Their expertise and guidance has proved useful at every step. Their uncompromising quality standards have made this book an exceptional effort. Their encouragement from time to time has been an inspiration for everyone.

The publisher and the editorial board hope that this book will prove to be a valuable piece of knowledge for researchers, students, practitioners and scholars across the globe.

List of Contributors

Trisha D. Scribbans, Brittany A. Edgett, Jennifer B. L. Matusiak and Brendon J. Gurd
School of Kinesiology and Health Studies, Queen's University, Kingston, Ontario, Canada

Kira Vorobej, Andrew S. Mitchell and Joe Quadrilatero
Department of Kinesiology, University of Waterloo, Waterloo, Ontario, Canada

Sophie D. Joanisse and Gianni Parise
Department of Kinesiology, McMaster University, Hamilton, Ontario, Canada

Ji-Guo Yu
Department of Surgical and Perioperative Sciences, Sports Medicine Unit, Umeå University, Umeå, Sweden

Jing-Xia Liu, Lena Carlsson, Lars-Eric Thornell and Per S. Stål
Department of Integrative Medical Biology, Section for Anatomy, Umeå University, Umeå, Sweden

Bethannie Golden, Marybeth Camboni, Kumaran Chandrasekharan and Rui Xu
Center for Gene Therapy, The Research Institute at Nationwide Children's Hospital, Columbus, Ohio, United States of America

Paul T. Martin
Center for Gene Therapy, The Research Institute at Nationwide Children's Hospital, Columbus, Ohio, United States of America
Department of Pediatrics, The Ohio State University College of Medicine, Columbus, Ohio, United States of America
Department of Physiology and Cell Biology, The Ohio State University College of Medicine, Columbus, Ohio, United States of America

Kevin M. Flanigan
Center for Gene Therapy, The Research Institute at Nationwide Children's Hospital, Columbus, Ohio, United States of America
Department of Pediatrics, The Ohio State University College of Medicine, Columbus, Ohio, United States of America

Jonathan Okerblom and Ajit Varki
Departments of Medicine and Cellular and Molecular Medicine, University of California, San Diego, La Jolla, California, United States of America

Joe N. Kornegay
Department of Veterinary Integrative Biosciences, Texas A and M University, College Station, Texas, United States of America

Håvard Hatle, Per Kristian Støbakk, Harald Edvard Mølmen, Arnt Erik Tjønna, Ulrik Wisløff, Charlotte Björk Ingul and Øivind Rognmo
K.G. Jebsen Centre of Exercise in Medicine, Norwegian University of Science and Technology (NTNU), Trondheim, Norway
Department of Circulation and Medical Imaging, NTNU, Trondheim, Norway

Eivind Brønstad and Sigurd Steinshamn
K.G. Jebsen Centre of Exercise in Medicine, Norwegian University of Science and Technology (NTNU), Trondheim, Norway
Department of Circulation and Medical Imaging, NTNU, Trondheim, Norway
Department of Pulmonary Medicine, St Olav University Hospital, Trondheim, Norway

Eirik Skogvoll
Department of Circulation and Medical Imaging, NTNU, Trondheim, Norway
Evelyn B. Parr, Donny M. Camera and José L. Areta
Exercise and Nutrition Research Group, School of Medical Sciences, RMIT University, Bundoora, Victoria, Australia

Louise M. Burke
Department of Sports Nutrition, Australian Institute of Sport, Canberra, ACT, Australia

Stuart M. Phillips
Exercise Metabolism Research Group, Department of Kinesiology, McMaster University, Hamilton, Ontario, Canada

John A. Hawley
Exercise and Nutrition Research Group, School of Exercise Science, Australian Catholic University, Fitzroy, Victoria, Australia
Research Institute for Sport and Exercise Sciences, Liverpool John Moores University, Liverpool, United Kingdom

Vernon G. Coffey
School of Exercise and Nutrition Sciences and Institute of Health and Biomedical Innovation, Queensland University of Technology, Kelvin Grove, Queensland, Australia

Cameron J. Mitchell, Tyler A. Churchward-Venne, Gianni Parise, Leeann Bellamy and Stuart M. Phillips
Exercise Metabolism Research Group, Department of Kinesiology, McMaster University, Hamilton, Ontario, Canada

Steven K. Baker
Department of Neurology, School of Medicine, McMaster University, Hamilton, Ontario, Canada

Kenneth Smith and Philip J. Atherton
Metabolic and Molecular Physiology Research Group, MRC-ARUK Centre of Excellence for Musculoskeletal Ageing Research, School of Graduate Entry Medicine and Health, Derby, United Kingdom

Ilse G. M. Slot, Bram van den Borst, Valéry A. C. V. Hellwig, Annemie M. W. J. Schols and Harry R. Gosker
Department of Respiratory Medicine, NUTRIM School for Nutrition, Toxicology and Metabolism, Maastricht University Medical Center+, Maastricht, The Netherlands

Esther Barreiro
Pulmonology Department-Muscle and Respiratory System Research Unit (URMAR), Research Institute of Hospital del Mar (IMIM), Department of Experimental and Health
Sciences (CEXS), Pompeu Fabra University (UPF), Barcelona Biomedical Research Park (PRBB), Barcelona, Spain
Network of Excellence in Respiratory Research (CIBERES), Institute of Health Carlos III (ISCIII), Bunyola, Majorca, Balearic Islands, Spain

Igor L. Chernyavsky, Huguette Croisier, Jonathan E. Hiorns and Bindi S. Brook
School of Mathematical Sciences, University of Nottingham, Nottingham, United Kingdom

Lloyd A. C. Chapman and Laura S. Kimpton
Mathematical Institute, University of Oxford, Oxford, United Kingdom

Oliver E. Jensen
School of Mathematics, University of Manchester, Manchester, United Kingdom

Charlotte K. Billington, Ian P. Hall and Simon R. Johnson
Department of Therapeutics and Molecular Medicine, University of Nottingham, Nottingham, United Kingdom

Mark Screen, Jeanette Holmlund-Hampf, Per Harald Jonson and Peter Hackman
Folkhälsan Institute of Genetics and Department of Medical Genetics, Haartman Institute, University of Helsinki, Helsinki, Finland

Olayinka Raheem
Neuromuscular Research Unit, Department of Neurology, University Hospital and University of Tampere, Tampere, Finland

Sanna Huovinen
Neuromuscular Research Unit, Department of Neurology, University Hospital and University of Tampere, Tampere, Finland
Department of Pathology, Fimlab Laboratories, Tampere University Hospital and University of Tampere, Tampere, Finland

Bjarne Udd
Folkhälsan Institute of Genetics and Department of Medical Genetics, Haartman Institute, University of Helsinki, Helsinki, Finland
Neuromuscular Research Unit, Department of Neurology, University Hospital and University of Tampere, Tampere, Finland
Department of Pathology, Fimlab Laboratories, Tampere University Hospital and University of Tampere, Tampere, Finland

Claudia Langhans, Franziska Schmidt, Jida Hamati, Melanie Kny, Xiaoxi Zhu, Doerte odka, Simone Spuler and Michael Boschmann
Experimental and Clinical Research Center (ECRC), a Cooperation between Max Delbrück Center and Charité Universitätsmedizin Berlin, Campus Buch, Berlin, Germany

Steffen Weber-Carstens, Tobias Wollersheim, Susanne Koch, Martin Krebs and Claudia Spies
Charité Universitätsmedizin Berlin, Campus Virchow and Campus Mitte, Anesthesiology and Operative Intensive Care Medicine, Berlin, Germany

Herbert Schulz, Kathrin Saar, Norbert Hubner and Gunnar Dittmar
Max Delbrück Center for Molecular Medicine, Berlin, Germany

Siegfried Labeit
Universitätsmedizin Mannheim, Mannheim, Germany

Joachim Spranger
Experimental and Clinical Research Center (ECRC), a Cooperation between Max Delbrück Center and Charité Universitätsmedizin Berlin, Campus Buch, Berlin, Germany

Charité Universitätsmedizin Berlin, NeuroCure Clinical Research Center, Berlin, Germany
Charité Universitätsmedizin Berlin, Department of Endocrinology, Diabetes and Nutrition, Berlin, Germany

Gillian Butler-Browne and Vincent Mouly
Institut de Myologie, Institut national de la santé et de la recherche mé dicale, and L'Université Pierre et Marie Curie Paris, Paris, France

Jens Fielitz
Experimental and Clinical Research Center (ECRC), a Cooperation between Max Delbrück Center and Charité Universitätsmedizin Berlin, Campus Buch, Berlin, Germany
Charité Universitätsmedizin Berlin, Campus Virchow, Cardiology, Berlin, Germany

Amirtharaj Francis, Kandavalli Vinodh, Shiva Krishna Katkam and Kumarasamy Thangaraj
CSIR-Centre for Cellular and Molecular Biology, Hyderabad, India

Balaraju Sunitha and Narayanappa Gayathri
Department of Neuropathology, National Institute of Mental Health and Neurosciences, Bengaluru, India

Kiran Polavarapu Atchayaram Nalini and Sailesh Modi
Department of Neurology, National Institute of Mental Health and Neurosciences, Bengaluru, India

M. M. Srinivas Bharath
Department of Neurochemistry, National Institute of Mental Health and Neurosciences, Bengaluru, India

Michael S. Davis
Department of Physiological Sciences, Oklahoma State University, Stillwater, Oklahoma, United States of America

Arend Bonen, Laelie A. Snook and Swati S. Jain
Department of Human Health and Nutritional Sciences, University of Guelph, Guelph, Ontario, Canada

Kenneth Bartels
Department of Veterinary Clinical Sciences, Oklahoma State University, Stillwater, Oklahoma, United States of America

Raymond Geor
Department of Large Animal Clinical Science, Michigan State University, East Lansing, Michigan, United States of America

Karsten Hueffer
Department of Veterinary Medicine, University of Alaska-Fairbanks, Fairbanks, Alaska, United States of America

Khetam Ghannam, Lorena Martinez-Gamboa, Lydia Spengler, Biljana Smiljanovic, Marc Bonin, Salyan Bhattarai, Gerd-R. Burmester, Thomas Häupl and Eugen Feist
Department of Rheumatology and Clinical Immunology, Charité University Hospital, Berlin, Germany

Sabine Krause
Friedrich Baur Institute, Ludwig Maximilians University, Munich, Germany

Andreas Grützkau
German Arthritis Research Center, Berlin, Germany

Marta Fernandez-Fuente and Richard J. Piercy
Comparative Neuromuscular Diseases Laboratory, Department of Clinical Sciences and Services, Royal Veterinary College, London, United Kingdom

Cesare M. Terracciano
Laboratory of Cell Electrophysiology, Imperial College London, Myocardial Function, National Heart and Lung Institute, Hammersmith Hospital, London, United Kingdom

Pilar Martin-Duque
Universidad Francisco de Vitoria, Facultad de Ciencias Biosanitarias: Pozuelo de Alarcón (Madrid), Madrid, Spain

Susan C. Brown
Comparative Biomedical Sciences, Royal Veterinary College, London, United Kingdom

Georges Vassaux
Laboratoire TIRO, UMRE 4320, iBEB, DSV, Commissariat a' l'Energie Atomique, Nice, France

Chantal Beekman, Jessica A. Sipkens, Janwillem Testerink, Stavros Giannakopoulos, Dyonne Kreuger, Judith C. van Deutekom, Giles V. Campion, Sjef J. de Kimpe and Afrodite Lourbakos
Prosensa Therapeutics BV, Leiden, the Netherlands

Kevin Murach, Ulrika Raue, Brittany Wilkerson, Kiril Minchev, Bozena Jemiolo, James Bagley, Nicholas Luden, Scott Trappe
Human Performance Laboratory, Ball State University, Muncie, Indiana, United States of America

Joakim M. Bischoff, Thomas K. Ringsted, Marian Petersen and Mads U. Werner
Multidisciplinary Pain Center 7612, Neuroscience Center, Rigshospitalet, Copenhagen University, Copenhagen, Denmark

Claudia Sommer and Nurcan Üçeyler
Department of Neurology, University Hospital of Würzburg, Würzburg, Germany

Mats I. Nilsson, Lauren G. Macneil, Yu Kitaoka, Fatimah Alqarni, Rahul Suri, Mahmood Akhtar, Maria E. Haikalis, Pavneet Dhaliwal, Munim Saeed and Mark A. Tarnopolsky
Department of Pediatrics and Medicine, Neuromuscular Clinic, McMaster University Hospital, Hamilton, Ontario, Canada

Vincent Meininger
Département des Maladies du Système Nerveux, Assistance Publique - Hôpitaux de Paris, Centre de Référence Maladies Rares SLA, Groupe Hospitalier Pitié-Salpêtrière
Université Pierre-et-Marie-Curie, Paris, France

Andrea Corse
Neuromuscular Pathology Lab, Johns Hopkins University School of Medicine, Baltimore, Maryland, United States of America

Safa Al-Sarraj
Department of Clinical Neuropathology, Kings College Hospital/Kings College London, London, United Kingdom

Benjamin Rix Brooks
Carolinas Neuromuscular/Amyotrophic Lateral Sclerosis-Muscular Dystrophy Association Center Department of Neurology, Carolinas Medical Center and University of North Carolina School of Medicine-Charlotte Campus, Charlotte, North Carolina, United States of America

James B. Caress
Wake Forest School of Medicine, M Reynolds Tower, Medical Center Boulevard, Winston-Salem, North Carolina, United States of America

Merit Cudkowicz
Department of Neurology, Massachusetts General Hospital, Harvard Medical School, Boston, Massachusetts, United States of America

Stephen J. Kolb
Department of Neurology, The Ohio State University Wexner Medical Center, Columbus, Ohio, United States of America

Dale Lange
Department of Neurology, Weill Cornell School of Medicine, New York, New York, United States of America

P. Nigel Leigh
Trafford Centre for Biomedical Research, Brighton and Sussex Medical School, Falmer, Sussex, United Kingdom

Thomas Meyer
Department of Neurology, Charité - Universitätsmedizin Berlin, Berlin, Germany

Stefano Milleri
Centro Ricerche Cliniche, University Hospital G.B. Rossi, Verona, Italy

Karen E. Morrison
School of Clinical and Experimental Medicine, University of Birmingham and Neurosciences Department, Queen Elizabeth Hospital, Birmingham, United Kingdom

Richard W. Orrell
Department of Clinical Neuroscience, Institute of Neurology, University College London, London, United Kingdom
Department of Neurology, Royal Free London NHS Foundation Trust, London, United Kingdom

Gary Peters
GlaxoSmithKline Clinical Unit Cambridge, Addenbrooke's Hospital, Cambridge, United Kingdom,

Jeffrey D. Rothstein
Brain Science Institute, Johns Hopkins University, Department of Neurology, Baltimore, Maryland, United States of America

Jeremy Shefner
Department of Neurology, SUNY Upstate Medical University, Syracuse, New York, United States of America

Arseniy Lavrov
Neurosciences Therapy Area Unit, Medicines Discovery and Development, GlaxoSmithKline, Stockley Park, Uxbridge, Middlesex, United Kingdom

Nicola Williams and Phil Overend
Clinical Statistics, GlaxoSmithKline, Stevenage, Hertfordshire, United Kingdom

Jeffrey Price
Clinical Pharmacology, Science and Study Operations, BioPharm and Infectious Diseases, GlaxoSmithKline, Stevenage, Hertfordshire, United Kingdom

Stewart Bates and Bams Abila
BioPharm Translational Medicine, GlaxoSmithKline, Stevenage, Hertfordshire, United Kingdom

Jonathan Bullman
Clinical Pharmacology Modelling and Simulation (Neurosciences), GlaxoSmithKline, Stevenage, Hertfordshire, United Kingdom

David Krull
Safety Assessment, GlaxoSmithKline, Research Triangle Park, North Carolina, United States of America

Alienor Berges and Guy Meno-Tetang
Clinical Pharmacology Modelling and Simulation, GlaxoSmithKline, Stockley Park, Uxbridge, Middlesex, United Kingdom

Jens Wurthner
Oncology Translational Medicine, Novartis Basel, Switzerland

Pierre-François Pradat
Département des Maladies du Système Nerveux, Assistance Publique – Hôpitaux de Paris, Centre de Référence Maladies Rares SLA, Groupe Hospitalier Pitié-Salpêtrière, Université Pierre-et-Marie-Curie, Paris, France
Unité Mixte de Recherche-678, Institut National de la Santé et de la Recherche Médicale - Université Pierre-et-Marie-Curie, Groupe Hospitalier Pitié - Salpeêtrière, Paris, France

Grégoire Millet
ISSUL Institute of Sport Sciences University of Lausanne, Lausanne, Switzerland
Department of Physiology, University of Lausanne, Lausanne, Switzerland

David J. Bentley
Faculty of Health Science, University of Adelaide, Adelaide, South Australia, Australia

Belle Roels
ORION, Clinical Services Ltd, London, England

Lars R. Mc Naughton
Department of Sport and Physical Activity, Edge Hill University, Ormskirk, Lancashire, England

Jacques Mercier
Laboratoire de physiologie des Interactions EA 701, Institut de Biologie, Montpellier, France

David Cameron-Smith
School of Nutrition and Exercise Sciences, Deakin University, Melbourne, Victoria, Australia
Liggins Institute, University of Auckland, Auckland, New Zealand

Valeria Beltrame, Paolo Ortolan, Alessandro Coran, Riccardo Zanato, Matteo Gazzola and Roberto Stramare
Department of Medicine, Section of Radiology, University of Padova, Padova, Italy

Annachiara Frigo
Department of Cardiac, Thoracic and Vascular Sciences, University of Padova, Padova, Italy

Luca Bello and Elena Pegoraro
Department of Neurosciences, University of Padova, Padova. Italy

Julia Etich, Vera Bergmeier, Christian Frie, Sandra Kreft and Lena Bengestrate
Center for Biochemistry, Medical Faculty, University of Cologne, Cologne, North Rhine-Westphalia, Germany

Bent Brachvogel
Center for Biochemistry, Medical Faculty, University of Cologne, Cologne, North Rhine-Westphalia, Germany
Center for Molecular Medicine Cologne (CMMC), Medical Faculty, University of Cologne, Cologne, North Rhine-Westphalia, Germany

Sabine Eming
Center for Molecular Medicine Cologne (CMMC), Medical Faculty, University of Cologne, Cologne, North Rhine-Westphalia, Germany
Department of Dermatology, University of Cologne, Cologne, North Rhine-Westphalia, Germany

Cornelia Mauch and Beate Eckes
Department of Dermatology, University of Cologne, Cologne, North Rhine-Westphalia, Germany

Hikmet Ulus
Clinic for Paediatric Surgery, Cologne, North Rhine-Westphalia, Germany

Frances E. Lund
Department of Medicine, University of Rochester Medical Center, Rochester, New York, United States of America

Gunter Rappl and Hinrich Abken
Center for Molecular Medicine Cologne (CMMC), Medical Faculty, University of Cologne, Cologne, North Rhine-Westphalia, Germany
Tumorgenetics, Department I of Internal Medicine, Medical Faculty, University of Cologne, Cologne, North Rhine-Westphalia, Germany

Mats Paulsson
Center for Biochemistry, Medical Faculty, University of Cologne, Cologne, North Rhine-Westphalia, Germany
Center for Molecular Medicine Cologne (CMMC), Medical Faculty, University of Cologne, Cologne, North Rhine-Westphalia, Germany
Cologne Excellence Cluster on Cellular Stress Responses in Aging - Associated Diseases (CECAD), Cologne, North Rhine-Westphalia, Germany

Dolores Wolfram, Nadine Eberhart and Gerhard Pierer
Department of Plastic, Reconstructive and Aesthetic Surgery, Innsbruck Medical University, Innsbruck, Austria

Ravi Starzl
Language Technologies Institute, Carnegie Mellon University, Pittsburgh, Pennsylvania, United States of America

Hubert Hackl
Division of Bioinformatics, Biocenter, Innsbruck Medical University, Innsbruck, Austria

Derek Barclay and Yoram Vodovotz
Department of Immunology, University of Pittsburgh, Pittsburgh, Pennsylvania, United States of America

Theresa Hautz and Johann Pratschke
Department of Visceral, Transplant and Thoracic Surgery, Innsbruck Medical University, Innsbruck, Austria

Bettina Zelger
Department of Pathology, Innsbruck Medical University, Innsbruck, Austria

Gerald Brandacher, W. P. Andrew Lee and Stefan Schneeberger
Department of Plastic and Reconstructive Surgery, Johns Hopkins University School of Medicine, Baltimore, Maryland, United States of America

Marije de Bruin and Mark J. Smeulders
Department of Plastic, Reconstructive and Hand Surgery, Academic Medical Center, Amsterdam, The Netherlands

Michiel Kreulen
Department of Plastic, Reconstructive and Hand Surgery, Academic Medical Center, Amsterdam, The Netherlands
Department of Plastic, Reconstructive and Hand Surgery, Red Cross Hospital, Beverwijk, The Netherlands

Peter A. Huijing and Richard T Jaspers
Laboratory for Myology, MOVE Research Institute Amsterdam, Faculty of Human Movement Sciences, VU University Amsterdam, Amsterdam, The Netherlands

Jason A. Bennie and Michael J. McKenna
Institute of Sport, Exercise and Active Living (ISEAL), Muscle, Ions and Exercise Group, Victoria University, Melbourne, Victoria, Australia

Craig A. Goodman
Institute of Sport, Exercise and Active Living (ISEAL), Muscle, Ions and Exercise Group, Victoria University, Melbourne, Victoria, Australia
Department of Comparative Biosciences, School of Veterinary Medicine, University of Wisconsin-Madison, Madison, Wisconsin, United States of America,

Murray J. Leikis
Institute of Sport, Exercise and Active Living (ISEAL), Muscle, Ions and Exercise Group, Victoria University, Melbourne, Victoria, Australia
Department of Nephrology, Royal Melbourne Hospital, Department of Medicine, University of Melbourne, Melbourne, Victoria, Australia

Cameron B. Williams, Brittany A. Edgett, Trisha D. Scribbans and Brendon J. Gurd
School of Kinesiology and Health Studies, Queen's University, Kingston, Ontario, Canada

Craig A. Simpson
Department of Emergency Medicine, Queen's University, Kingston, Ontario, Canada

Meghan C. Hughes and Christopher G. R. Perry
School of Kinesiology and Health Science, York University, Toronto, Ontario, Canada

Index